Thieme

Textbook and Atlas of Neural Therapy

Diagnosis and Therapy with Local Anesthetics

Hans Barop, MD
Private Practice
Hamburg, Germany

182 illustrations

Thieme
Stuttgart • New York • Delhi • Rio de Janeiro

Library of Congress Cataloging-in-Publication Data is available from the publisher.

This book is an authorized translation of the 2nd German edition published and copyrighted 2015 by Karl F. Haug Verlag in MVS Medizinverlage Stuttgart GmbH & Co. KG, Stuttgart. Title of the German edition: Lehrbuch und Atlas Neuraltherapie

Translator: tolingo translation agency, Hamburg/Germany

Illustrator: Reinhold Henkel, Heidelberg/Germany

Body-Painting: Heike Dimler, MD, Hamburg/Germany

1st Italian edition 2003

Thieme Publishers Stuttgart
Rüdigerstrasse 14, 70469 Stuttgart, Germany
+49 [0]711 8931 421, customerservice@thieme.de

Thieme Publishers New York
333 Seventh Avenue, New York, NY 10001, USA
+1-800-782-3488, customerservice@thieme.com

Thieme Publishers Delhi
A-12, Second Floor, Sector-2, Noida-201301
Uttar Pradesh, India
+91 120 45 566 00, customerservice@thieme.in

Thieme Publishers Rio, Thieme Publicações Ltda.
Edifício Rodolpho de Paoli, 25º andar
Av. Nilo Peçanha, 50 – Sala 2508
Rio de Janeiro 20020-906 Brasil
+55 21 3172 2297 / +55 21 3172 1896

Cover design: Thieme Publishing Group
Typesetting by Ditech, India

Printed in Germany by CPI Books GmbH 5 4 3 2 1
ISBN 978-3-13-241049-7

Also available as an e-book:
eISBN 978-3-13-241050-3

MIX
Papier aus verantwortungsvollen Quellen
FSC® C083411
www.fsc.org

Many thanks to the brothers Ferdinand and Walter Huneke and all subsequent physicians dedicated to the development of neural therapy as a comprehensive new treatment method for the benefit of patients.

Contents

Part 1
History and Theory

Part 2

The Practice of Neural Therapy

Part 3

Injection Technique and Indications

Part 4
Indications and Therapy

Part 5
Appendix

Preface

The first observations of the "side effects" of local anesthetics started at the same time as local anesthesia was developed for surgical purposes. As so often happens in applied medicine, ultimately a new therapy concept with a very broad scope of application emerged as a result of attentive and detailed observation. Thanks to the consistent work of the physicians and brothers Ferdinand and Walter Huneke, this treatment method, initially based on individual observations with local anesthetics, was able to be developed and spread through numerous applications.

In 1963, Peter Dosch published the first comprehensive neural therapy textbook in which he summarized more than 60 years' experience in the therapeutic potential of local anesthetics, thus making this information available for teaching. Other major contributors to the spread of neural therapy are the countless doctors whose observations - to some extent even before Huneke - confirmed the efficacy of the first experiences in the therapeutic use of local anesthesics and thereby helped to stabilize the method and enable its further expansion.

The 1st German edition of my textbook "Lehrbuch und Atlas Neuraltherapie ...." was published 20 years ago. On the one hand, it was based on the enormous variety of therapeutic experience published over decades by neural therapists as reproducible "empirical medicine". On the other hand, the medical knowledge of the neuroanatomical and neurophysiological principles of the autonomic nervous system were used as the scientific basis of neural therapy.

The scientific facts about the neuroanatomy and neurophysiology of the autonomic nervous system have grown significantly in the meantime. Numerous studies and trials have shown substantial involvement of this system in the pathogenesis of various diseases (e.g. inflammation, pain, degeneration). Many anatomical and neurophysiological textbooks and individual works published in the last 20 years increasingly detail the interaction of autonomic dysfunctions in numerous diseases. Here the focus is on the regulation of microcirculation and simultaneous organ and tissue function through the autonomic nervous system. At the same time, an intensive search began for ways to therapeutically implement these findings. The current thinking primarily points in the direction of drug therapy methods.

The epistemological foundations of neural therapy have been strongly integrated with this greatly increased knowledge of the autonomic nervous system. Further experiences in the practice of neural therapy, the gradual acceptance of certain components of the method in different fields of medicine and the introduction of neural therapy as a subject for medical students at some universities indicate an increasing integration of neural therapy as an independent method of treatment.

This book can give students the opportunity to learn the basics of neural therapy and, in particular, it is designed to illustrate the influence of the autonomic nervous system on numerous diseases. Qualified physicians should use this textbook along with practical 2-year training to expand their therapeutic options in practice, independently of their specialist training.

Neural therapy offers the opportunity to answer the still-open question of the therapeutic realization of pathogenetic correlations between different disorders related to dysfunctions of the autonomic nervous system, especially the sympathetic nervous system. To this end, the decades of experience in pragmatic neural therapy are available. Through thoughtful and critical approaches, academic medicine has a proven therapy concept in the form of valuable and reliable practical experience which makes a further search for e.g. medications influencing the autonomic system unnecessary. On the other hand, neural therapy gratefully expands and confirms its theoretical foundations from comprehensive academic findings.

The second German edition of "Lehrbuch und Atlas Neuraltherapie" was expanded to include the growing evidence of neurovegetative anatomy and physiology. The anatomical details of autonomic end formation have become clearer through modern imaging methods such as immunohistochemistry, tracer techniques and electron microscopy. At the same time, the knowledge of the diversity of transmitter substances has increased, resulting in more clarity in the etiology and pathogenesis of diseases with regard to the interdependence of stimulus and stimulus response, the physiological and pathological processes that occur via the autonomic nervous system with simultaneous feedback. This not only confirms the observations by Rickers, which he summarized in relations pathology, but also illustrates the logical therapeutic conclusion which can be conceptionally rediscovered in neural therapy.

The creation of the second German edition was made possible by the cooperation and exchange of ideas between neural therapists and academic institutes of anatomy and neurophysiology, among others. The empirical data resulting from the treatment of patients can be placed on a comprehensive scientific basis in continuous discussion with academic medicine, providing both sides – neural therapists as well as researchers - with clearer ideas about the function of the autonomic nervous system, its influence on the body, and the potential for therapeutic use.

This English edition of *Textbook and Atlas Neural Therapy* grew out of the international dissemination of neural therapy, and the diagnostic and therapeutic use of local anesthetics. Neural therapy originated and developed in the German speaking world and until now, most of the literature was written in German. The growing international interest in this method has necessitated a translation of the new edition into the international medical language. It is our hope that an important gap can be filled.

Acknowledgement

First, I must thank my editor Ms. Angelika-M. Findgott, Thieme Publishers Stuttgart – Germany, for her consistently friendly support. She organized and supervised the various steps of the translation and the overall development of this textbook for which I am very grateful.

I would also like to thank Professor J. Giebel und Professor T. Koppe from the Anatomical Institute at the University of Greifswald for continuous consultation and discussion about the anatomy of the neural autonomic system both in the dissection room and in literary recommendations. For the countless detailed conversations and discussions about observations in the practice of neural therapy in conjunction with the scientific foundations, I would like to thank Professor L. Fischer, professor and chair of neural therapy at the University of Berne, author of the textbook "Neuraltherapie, Neurophysiologie, Injektionstechnik und Therapieempfehlungen" (now in its 4th edition), who continues to publish many papers on the scientific nature, efficacy and cost-effectiveness of neural therapy.

Furthermore, my special thanks go to Dr. S. Resch, neural therapist and senior physician at the Headache Clinic in Königstein, for her detailed assistance in the revision and editing of the textbook.

Last but not least, my thanks go to my patients. Each of them, as individual cases, provided me with the majority of empirical data without which the practice of neural therapy — in balance with the scientific principles — would not have been possible.

Hamburg, Fall 2017
Hans Barop

Part 1
History and Theory

1 History of Local Anesthesia and Neural Therapy

1.1 Introduction

The history of anesthesia,[274] whether used prophylactically before surgery or therapeutically to treat existing pain, occupies a prominent place in medicine, because pain caused by illness or injury is one of the most common symptoms in everyday medical practice. The methods of targeted pain treatment were highly variable until the end of the 19th century. In addition to medicinal forms, various methods of localized pain reduction for surgical procedures were developed, such as tissue compression, and later nerve compression with truss pad, and the application of cold to specific sites.

A completely new form of localized pain treatment was first described in 1839 by **Lundy, Taylor**, and **Washington**. Using precursors of the modern syringe, they tried administering morphine solutions under the skin to achieve a reduction in pain. With the development of the syringe by the French **Pravaz** (1843), and the hollow cannula by the Scottish **Wood** in the same year, it was possible for the first time to achieve pain relief through targeted injections of morphine solutions into painful areas and nerves. However, local anesthesia, i.e., the complete alleviation of pain, could not be achieved with morphine solutions.

Koller, an ophthalmologist at the University of Vienna, came into contact with **Freud** in 1883 during his neurological training.[274,282] Freud had experience with cocaine, which he used to treat heart diseases and nervous exhaustion or depression. In a self-test, Freud determined the analeptic effect of cocaine in addition to its anesthetic effect on the tongue and oral mucosa, and reported this to his colleague. Koller was able to experience this anesthetic effect in his own self-test, especially when suffering from a painful gum inflammation, which he daubed with a cocaine solution on the advice of Freud.

In contrast to Freud, as a surgical ophthalmologist Koller saw the obvious potential for pain-free surgery using cocaine. He applied this property of cocaine therapeutically and, after preliminary trials with animals, performed the first cataract surgery using local anesthesia on September 11, 1884. At a meeting of doctors in Vienna on October 17, 1884, he first reported the successful use of cocaine for local anesthesia of the eye. This was also the starting point for the use of local anesthesia throughout surgery worldwide, which then evolved with breathtaking speed.

Only then was it clear to Freud what a groundbreaking discovery he had been involved in. In a report in Heitler's *Zentralblatt für die gesamte Therapie*, he had already reported on the anesthetic effect of cocaine before Koller, and considered the use of cocaine for localized painful infections. Freud was more interested in the therapeutic use than the possibility of a local anesthetic for surgical procedures. He recommended that the ophthalmologist von Königstein use cocaine on iritis and trachoma. He himself had experimentally (and unsuccessfully) attempted to treat trigeminal neuralgia with a cocaine injection targetedto the trigeminal nerve. Worth mentioning is the 1863 report published in Paris by the Peruvian general physician **Moreno y Maiz** on an animal experiment in which a bullfrog leg was anesthetized by way of cocaine infiltration.

1.2 Anesthesia and the Treatment of Pain

1.2.1 Local Anesthesia

Considering the initial phase of local anesthesia thus far, at this very early stage there were already two different pathways for the newly discovered drug, cocaine:

1. Targeted local anesthesia, i.e., anesthesia for surgical purposes, which was eagerly awaited by the world of surgical treatment.
2. Slightly overshadowed by local anesthesia, the therapeutic use of local anesthesia for existing pain, whether due to neuralgia or tissue inflammation (Freud).

When keeping this two-pronged development in mind and not allowing the concept of pure local anesthesia for surgical purposes to dominate at first sight, local anesthesia and neural therapy can be easily differentiated.

Knowledge about both pathways is still required, since the technique of local anesthesia in the implementation of neural therapy falls into the realm of the technical.

Infiltration, Block, and Spinal Anesthesia

In the rapid development of local anesthesia for surgical purposes, the names **Halstedt, Hall**, and **Hartley** are representative of infiltration anesthesia and block anesthesia, which they used in animal experiments and later in human surgery. The first major drawbacks of the drug cocaine came to light: overdoses and dependence with repeated use. Halstedt had become addicted to cocaine through numerous self-tests but was cured after undergoing detoxification; Hall, who had also become addicted, died.

On the one hand, increased experience with the drug **cocaine** resulted in successful local anesthesia for surgery; on the other hand, an increase in overdose deaths occurred. Thanks to the Parisian surgeon **Reclus**, the cocaine dosage was corrected after the initial euphoria and a number of iatrogenic deaths, and the use of cocaine for local anesthesia could be continued and developed further. The 20 to 30% cocaine solution first used for topical anesthesia resulted in severe intoxication and even death. Reclus was able to prevent both intoxication and deaths by reducing the concentration initially to 2 to 3% and later to 0.5% solutions.

Block anesthesia, the selective suppression of sensitive peripheral nerves, evolved from infiltration anesthesia, i.e., local numbing through local infiltration of cocaine. With more centrally acting local anesthesia, **Bier** developed spinal anesthesia, which he first successfully performed on August 15, 1898. His idea was to use the more centrally implemented anesthesia to create a more comprehensive anesthesia with lesser amounts of cocaine than were used in pure block anesthesia. He achieved this by intrathecal injection in the lumbar region with 3 mL of an 0.5% solution of cocaine. Bier was also able to report on the "postspinal headache" after the self-test with this new neuraxial anesthesia.

The American neurologist **Corning** had successfully performed neuraxial anesthesia before Bier, though not in preparation for surgical treatment, but for treating existing pain. To what extent this involved true spinal anesthesia with intrathecal administration or epidural anesthesia remains unclear.

With regard to the history of local anesthesia, this meant a breakthrough in surgical development in the public eye. With the advancement of local anesthesia, the number of general narcosis procedures previously using chloroform and ether could be reduced and thus many, sometimes fatal, incidents involving general narcosis could be avoided.

Emergence of Segmental Therapy

Less exciting, however, was the development in the therapeutic use of local anesthetics, since it suffered from a lack of attention that still exists even today in the medical landscape of surgery. On closer inspection, however, it turns out that the use of local anesthetics for purely therapeutic use has at least as much potential as local anesthesia for surgery.

In the analysis of the history of neural therapy, it is useful to provide some preliminary guidance for clarifying its fundamental difference from purely local anesthesia. The names representing the beginning of neural therapy are partly the same as those for the development of local anesthesia. These are predominantly the names of surgically qualified doctors who used the injection of local anesthesia in their daily practice. The first observations pointing the way toward neural therapy were made when local anesthetic was not applied to surgical procedures but to preexisting pain.[446,469,470] Now, it was frequently observed that despite the local anesthesia wearing off, the preexisting pain symptoms were reduced or even completely disappeared.

Reconsider the earliest days of local anesthesia when Freud shared with Koller his first observations on mucosa anesthesia after oral ingestion of cocaine. Freud's logical, rather intuitive decision to apply a local anesthetic for therapy and not for anesthesia would prove to be correct in the shadow of the rapid development of local anesthesia in surgery. At the same time that the French surgeon **Reclus** reduced the concentration of cocaine and ultimately prevented its decline in use due to frequent toxic complications, the German **Schleich** developed "refined local anesthesia" also by reducing the cocaine concentration, by targeted infiltration of nerves, and by additional cooling of the tissue with ethyl chloride.

This combination resulted in a radical reduction of the toxic effects of cocaine, so that the local anesthetic in this "defused form" prevailed.

Schleich also used a 0.5 to 1% strength solution of cocaine for purely therapeutic purposes.[446] In 1898, he was the first to observe that not only local infiltration of cocaine alleviated rheumatic symptoms during the anesthetized period, but also the rheumatic symptoms were alleviated for a long time thereafter, or recurred only to a lesser extent. This first documented successful application of local anesthetics for therapeutic purposes can be characterized as the birth of neural therapy. The method was refined over the next few years and developed into the first part of neural therapy, namely segmental therapy.

Independently of Schleich, **Spiess** also observed in clinical use that repeated anesthesia resulted in not only a strikingly pain-free surgical wound beyond the duration of the anesthesia, but at the same time wound healing, in this case in the throat area after a tonsillectomy, that was clearly less prone to irritation than without the repeated local anesthesia.[469,470] In addition, he observed that existing inflammatory wound healing disorders were resolved faster and without irritation. Spiess published these new clinical observations in 1906 in the "*Münchner Medizinische Wochenschrift*" ["Munich Weekly Medical Journal"] under the title "The Healing Effect of Anesthetics."[470]

1.2.2 Neural Therapy

Development

Parallel to the use of local anesthesia and neural therapy, pharmacologists were intensively researching alternative substances to cocaine with the aim of achieving comparable anesthetic quality without the toxic side effects. In 1905, **Einhorn** succeeded in producing a local anesthetic with the same anesthetic quality as cocaine, but without any addictive side effects. The substance was procaine (p. 37), which was used worldwide as a local anesthetic after 1905 and is used today for purely therapeutic purposes because of its short duration of action.

Once cocaine, which was used until 1905, was replaced with procaine, the path was cleared for the use of less dangerous local anesthesia and neural therapy. After the first reports of therapeutic applications from **Schleich** and **Spiess** made little impression, the works of **Leriche** and colleagues garnered attention.[299] Leriche's extensive neurosurgical experience certainly contributed to this, having first used the effect of local anesthesia intraoperatively.[302]

Specifically, the study of the sympathetic nervous system, at first purely surgically and later also using neural therapy, provided **Leriche** with important information on the wide range of possible applications of local anesthetic for therapy. The surgical removal of the stellate ganglion for therapeutic purposes—published in 1920—and the therapeutic "stellate infiltration," also first performed by him, basically gave comparable results; consequently, repeated stellate ganglion block prior to the extirpation was considered by him to be a less traumatic procedure. The term "bloodless knife of the surgeon,"[301,302] as coined by Leriche, stems from the application of this method. His therapeutic recommendations resulted from impressive clinical trials involving the infiltration of local anesthetics into sympathetic nerve structures to affect diseases that could not yet be treated satisfactorily. Stellatum injections in the case of pulmonary embolism, cerebral embolism, and vascular dyskinesias after injury or for various headache disorders are just a few examples. Leriche's other observation, that the consolidation of a fracture occurred in half the time under repeated procaine infiltration, underscores the value of the sympathetic nervous system. No less important are his observations on the intra- and periarterial application of local anesthetics for the treatment of vasomotor disorders. His book *The Surgery of Pain* convincingly presents his decades of experience in neurosurgery and neural therapy.[302]

Without knowledge of the therapeutic use of local anesthetics already practiced by Leriche, **Ferdinand Huneke**, a general practitioner in Dusseldorf, unintentionally became aware of the local anesthetic procaine when he injected his migraine-suffering sister with a mixed preparation recommended by another colleague, whereby the migraine abruptly disappeared.[223] He injected atophanyl, a drug meant for the treatment of rheumatic symptoms, which was available in two versions: for intravenous injection as pure atophanyl and for intramuscular injection with the addition of procaine. He had inadvertently given the intramuscular injection intravenously, which did not lead to the complication of cardiovascular depression as indicated by the manufacturer. When the injection was repeated, the migraine did not abate as expected; this time he had used the drug intended for intravenous injection without the addition of procaine. Thus, Huneke found that the actual active substance responsible for these two different responses was procaine. In fact, on the occasion of his sister's next migraine attack, he injected pure procaine intravenously and was able to curtail the migraines. He and his brother **Walter Huneke,** who was also a general practitioner, began to use the product for a variety of disorders. In addition to traditional drug therapy through intravenous and intramuscular administration, they developed targeted injection into painful tissue structures, nerves and blood vessels, joints, and ganglia.

When the first paravenous injection of a patient with headache showed the same therapeutic effect as intravenous injection, already frequently performed, the idea developed that it was not the general distribution of procaine in the body that provided the crucial therapeutic effect, but rather this "healing process" must obviously proceed over neural structures because of their repeatedly striking rate of occurrence. The Huneke brothers suspected the autonomic system as guiding this process and published their collective therapeutic experience with procaine in the article "Unknown remote effect of local anesthesia"[223] for the first time in 1928. Over time, they characterized their therapy with local anesthetics as "healing anesthesia." They had not yet departed from the idea of anesthesia, which in this case means only the reversible suppression of pain-conducting fibers. The pharmacological basis of membrane research, which would prove the stabilizing effect of general anesthetics on each membrane and not only on nerve cells, was not known at that time. The healing processes which repeatedly proceeded analogously in a variety of diseases caused the brothers to focus on the idea of uniform involvement of the autonomic system.

Lightning Reaction—The Discovery of the Interference Field

In 1940, **Ferdinand Huneke** first observed something entirely new.[236] A female patient, who he had just treated unsuccessfully for a very painful functional disorder of the left shoulder, presented again due to exacerbated chronic recurrent osteomyelitis in the right lower leg. Knowing that inflammation could be successfully treated using procaine, he infiltrated the inflamed lower leg section with **impletol**, a 2% procaine solution with a caffeine additive. Immediately thereafter, the painful left shoulder became completely mobile and symptom-free, to the surprise of the doctor as well as the patient. The reaction in the left shoulder, which had occurred directly after the remote infiltration in the right lower leg, suggested a connection between the two diseases. The Huneke brothers focused on this result, as it was key to many chronic diseases which could not be healed with previous therapeutic procedures.

This first "lightning reaction" meant the revision of the idea formulated much earlier by **Pässler**, which had defined the focal site as bacterially contaminated tissue with metastatic distribution of bacteria and their toxins throughout the body. The speed at which the patient's left shoulder became pain-free was evidence that the nerves involved in the left shoulder disorder were controlled by the inflammation of the right lower leg. It was therefore possible that chronic diseases may be caused or maintained by focal sites and could be cured only through their "suppression" by means of local anesthetic or surgical removal (e.g., teeth), whereby the effect of the suspected focal site is only revealed after injection into the site. It is to the undeniable credit of the brothers **Ferdinand** and **Walter Huneke** that they recognized the fundamental nature of this singular observation and newly coined the term "focal site." They introduced the concept as "nerval interference field" and developed the interference field test as a therapeutic principle. This resulted in three ground rules:

1. Any chronic illness may be due to an interference field.
2. Any illness or injury can leave behind an interference field.
3. Each interference field disorder is curable only by "suppression" of the interference field.

Certainly, similar observations had been made before Huneke. Some dentists no doubt learned from their patients that after removal of a diseased tooth, for example, long-lasting back pain suddenly disappeared. As early as 1936, **Leriche** observed and described the cessation of remote pain after infiltration of a nonirritated scar. However, the therapeutic consequences of this observation were first recognized and implemented by **Ferdinand** and **Walter Huneke**.

Term

The word "neural," previously used in context to distinguish therapeutic use from the local anesthesia practiced only for surgical procedures, was established in 1940 after the discovery of the lightning reaction by Huneke.

In 1938 **von Roques**,[430] who also worked with neural therapy like many other doctors, started the English to German translation of a book of basic principles by **Speransky.**[467] (He was familiar with the extensive neurological and experimental work that had been carried out by Speransky in Russia.) Thus, von Roques coined the term "neural therapy according to Huneke," which is still used today. Before that time, the therapeutic use of local anesthetics was paraphrased with other terms such as "procaine therapy," "impletol treatment," and "healing anesthesia." Since a particular drug is not essential to the therapy, since other local anesthetics can be used, neither is local anesthesia the basis of the therapy, but only a partial property of the local anesthetic, the term neural therapy was certainly more comprehensive.

The suffix "according to Huneke" is not primarily regarded as a tribute to the "inventor," but rather indicates that it consists of the following two parts:

1. Segmental therapy, which was practiced before 1940. It included local treatment with local anesthetics "in the diseased segment."
2. Interference field therapy; this means the ubiquitous possible therapeutic use of local anesthetics, detached from the segment, depending on the location of the suspected interference field.

The term "therapeutic local anesthesia," which is still in use today, was coined by **Gross**[179] after 1940 to characterize neural therapy. But this is confusing in that local anesthesia does not account for the therapy. Painless diseases without the neural therapeutically negligible side effect of a local anesthetic can also be treated, e.g., hyperthyroidism, vertigo, and chronic sinusitis.

2 Theoretical Foundations and Practice-Based Hypotheses

2.1 Introduction

In order to make the basic principles of neural therapy understandable, it is first necessary to describe the anatomical substrate that enables a diagnostic and therapeutic approach to the organism. A prerequisite is the realization that all bodily functions are linked to an information system, which coordinates these functions using control loops and ensures homeostasis. Major significance must be attributed to the autonomic nervous system with regard to causal relationships in physiological or pathophysiological functions.[69,425]

The separate analysis of an anatomical structure serves to identify it more clearly, albeit with partial loss of insight into its functional relationships. The anatomical isolation of the autonomic nervous system illustrates this particularly well, as the central and peripheral connections to other anatomical structures are extremely obvious. Knowledge of the anatomy and physiology of the autonomic nervous system is still not sufficiently disseminated in medicine and therefore does not receive the necessary consideration in diagnosis and therapy.

The basic function of the autonomic nervous system is the rapid antagonistic and coordinated control of individual tissue functions of an organism in order to enable homeostasis—or, better, homeodynamics—and to properly respond to external influences to which the organism is continuously exposed. The aim is to keep individual organ functions in balance. Thus, the autonomic nervous system represents the conductive structure on which all qualitatively uniform but quantitatively variable stimuli proceed as a steadily changing flow of information.

In order to control vital functions such as breathing, digestion, metabolism, secretion, water balance, electrolyte balance, temperature, blood pressure, and reproduction, a distribution of the system up to the terminal vascular bed and a high degree of cross-linking are necessary to enable a feedback-based information exchange between the individual organ and functional areas which are independent from one another. Thus, the autonomic nervous system requires a "nervous circulation", with afferent and efferent branches similar to the vascular system with its arterial and venous branches.

2.2 Autonomic Nervous System

2.2.1 Anatomy and Function

In terms of function, it is useful to understand the anatomy of the **stimulus pathway** in terms of both the efferent and afferent systems. The centers of the sympathetic and the parasympathetic branches can be found in the diencephalon in the hypothalamus region and represent the overriding functional link between the autonomic, somatic, and endocrine systems. Anatomical differentiation in this autonomic organization level between the sympathetic and parasympathetic parts is not possible because there is close anatomical and functional networking of both systems. The experimentally structured stimulus or severing of these diencephalic centers results in overriding antagonistic functions for entire organ areas. **Rohen** has created a table that illustrates the influences of the organ systems (▶Table 2.1).[429]

Here, Rohen develops the terms **ergotropic** (sympathetic adrenergic) and **trophotropic** (parasympathetic, cholinergic) **reaction conditions** to clarify the functional relationships. The region of the hypothalamus with the corresponding autonomic nucleic regions has an afferent and efferent interconnection with the cranial nerves, pituitary, and the cortex, and thus has a promotional or inhibitory effect on perception organs, hormone-forming organs (pituitary, thyroid, parathyroid, kidneys and adrenal glands, gonads), and somatomotor activity and somatic sensitivity. Further peripherally, the anatomy of the autonomic nervous system is far clearer, as the anatomical mapping of the segmental structure of the **sympathetic nervous system** at the level of the spinal cord becomes less complex and therefore differentiable.

Although the **parasympathetic nervous system** has no segmental distribution, its course is defined with the cranial nerves III (oculomotor nerve), VII (facial nerve), and IX (glossopharyngeal nerve) and the parasympathetic cranial ganglia (ciliary ganglion, pterygopalatine ganglion, otic ganglion, submandibular ganglion).

The most extensive parasympathetic portion is represented by the cranial nerve X, the vagus nerve. The sacral portion of the parasympathetic nervous system from segments S2–S4 completes the picture of the parasympathetic nervous system, which becomes anatomically and functionally comprehensible and thus diagnostically and therapeutically accessible by way of the described topography.

Cellular structure is common to the sympathetic as well as the parasympathetic portions. The relatively small nerve cells generally have multiple nerve fibers per cell unit, which efferently ensure the principle of divergence and combine impulses from the periphery using the afferent pathway. This is the basis for the autonomic nervous system's typical divergence, which enables widely divergent information transmission on the efferent branch and thereby has a harmonizing effect on entire organ areas. The conduction rate of the autonomic nervous system is significantly slower than that of the somatic system. Since the nerve fibers are poorly myelinated or unmyelinated and have a very small diameter in the peripheral organ distribution of up to 0.3 µm, the conduction rate is between a maximum of 25 m/s (afferent A-δ fiber) and a maximum of 0.5 m/s (C fiber).

► **Table 2.1** Influence of the organ systems according to Rohen[429]

Organ	Effect of the (ortho-) sympathetic nervous system (adrenergic effects)	Effect of the parasympathetic nervous system (cholinergic effect)
Eye		
• Iris	• Mydriasis	• Miosis
• Ciliary muscle	• Disaccommodation	• Accommodation
Heart		
• Rate	• Accelerating	• Decelerating
• Contraction strength	• Increased	• –
• Rhythm	• Ventricular extrasystoles, tachycardia, fibrillation	• Bradycardia, atrioventricular block, vagal cardiac arrest
• Conduction time	• Shortened	• Prolonged
Vessels		
• Coronary arteries	• Expansion	• Narrowing?
• Muscle vessels	• Narrowing	• –
• Intestinal vessels	• Narrowing	• Expansion
Lung		
• Bronchial musculature	• Slackness	• Contraction
• Bronchial mucosa	• Decreased secretion	• Increased secretion
Gastrointestinal canal		
• Peristalsis	• Inhibited contraction	• Increased
• Sphincters	• ?	• Slackness
• Glandular secretion	• Decreased	• Promoted
Extrahepatic bile ducts and gall bladder	Slackness	Contraction
Spleen (musculature)	Contraction	Slackness
Salivary glands	Secretion (thick secretion)	Secretion (thin secretion)
Pancreatic islets of Langerhans	Decreased insulin secretion	Increased insulin secretion
Liver	Glycogenolysis	Biliary discharge
Adrenal medulla	Discharge of adrenaline and noradrenaline	Reduction in the release of adrenaline and noradrenaline
Bladder		
• Musculature	• Slackness	• Contraction
• Sphincter	• Contraction	• Slackness
Cerebral cortex	General activation, increased awareness	Inhibition, loss of consciousness
General response	Ergotropic "output nerve"	Trophotropic "recovery nerve"

In addition to different cell types, the autonomic ganglia also have strong vascularization. This certainly serves not only the nutritional supply of the nerve cells, but also probably the metabolic functions mediated via neurotransmitters.[429] Switch processes take place in the ganglia, e.g., from the preganglionic to the postganglionic neurons. Not only do cholinergic synapses transmit the information further, but so do dopamine-containing cells (SIS) with dopaminergic synapses that terminate at the perikarya of the postganglionic neurons and affect their conduction through modulation.

2.2.2 Sympathetic Efferent

The nucleic regions of the sympathetic nervous system are in the intermediolateral nucleus of the spinal cord at the level of segments C8–L2 (L3). The preganglionic fibers exiting the spinal canal via the intervertebral foramen together with the anterior root portions initially course for a short distance together with the spinal nerves in order to leave them via the myelinated white ramus communicans for the paravertebral ganglion. Here, they become connected partly synaptically with the nerve cells of the ganglion cells of higher and deeper segments and leave after switching to the second neuron via the gray ramus communicans in order to extend in the direction of the periphery with the spinal nerve bundle.

This results in the **first** efferent **distribution pathway** of the sympathetic nervous system, which is directed toward the periphery all the way to the effector organs. It includes the sympathetic supply to the skin and extremities. As a result, the peripheral, segmentally structured somatomotor and somatosensory nerves always proceed accompanied by sympathetic postganglionic fibers. These sympathetic fibers in turn originate from several paravertebral ganglia of the sympathetic chain, resulting in a wider divergence compared to the somatomotor and somatosensory innervation area. The somatosensory innervation area of skin regions is more precisely delineated, while the sympathetic supply to the skin does not have such strict, segment-bound division.

The **second distribution pathway** of the sympathetic nervous system proceeds from the intermediolateral nucleus of the spinal cord via the ganglia without switching to the prevertebral ganglia (e.g., celiac ganglion, aorticorenal ganglion, superior and inferior mesenteric ganglion). The switch to the second neuron occurs only in these prevertebral ganglia. From here, the sympathetic nervous system reaches the abdominal and pelvic organs, primarily accompanied by the arterial and venous vessels as well as free nerve bundles. The sympathetic supply of the thoracic cavity and the thoracic organs and the entire head and upper extremities proceeds via the three cervical ganglia, in which the switch to the second neuron takes place, and via the first six thoracic sympathetic ganglia; the cervical and thoracic ganglionic section receive their preganglionic fibers from the intermediolateral nuclei of segments C8–T6. The sympathetic supply of the abdominal cavity, the retroperitoneal space, the pelvis, and the lower extremities proceeds with overlap from segments T5–L2 (L3) and the associated lumbar (abdominal, sacral, coccygeal) ganglia.

Thus, the efferent sympathetic nervous system proceeds together with the brain and spinal nerves as well as with the blood vessels up to the capillary end flow path in order to reach the periphery. This anatomically describes its ubiquitous distribution. Therefore, the efferent sympathetic nerve supply to the periphery proceeds together with spinal nerves and blood vessels down to the capillary system. The parasympathetic nervous system does not have this generalized distribution, since—according to current knowledge—it is not involved in the supply of the extremities and the skin.

The **third distribution path** of the sympathetic nervous system can be called interganglionic. Over the beadlike connection of the 23 individual ganglia, there are homolateral connections in cranial and caudal directions, as well as in the contralateral direction via interganglionic nerve branches to the para- and prevertebral sympathetic ganglia. The 23 paravertebral and 5 prevertebral ganglia groups only face 15 sympathetic nucleic origin areas in the spinal cord. Thus, in accordance with the divergence, numerous preganglionic fibers of a spinal segment must be switched to the second neuron in several ganglia. This results in greater "security" of the impulse transfer in the vertical homolateral direction, i.e., the failure of a ganglion does not cause any significant restriction in function of the sympathetic nervous system. However, at the spinal level with unilateral sympathetic stimulation, the co-reaction—albeit limited—of the sympathetic nervous system on the contralateral side is possible through the horizontally extending interganglion branch. This explains why the degeneration of the hip joint, which is linked to reduced blood supply—i.e., increased sympathetic stimulation, among other things—initially occurs on one side and later on the other side; it also explains the clinical observation that CRPS (complex regional pain syndrome) on one side of the body can also occur like a "mirror image" on the contralateral side, or explains the phenomenon of "contralateral pain therapy" in which segmental therapy on the "healthy side" mirrors the therapeutic effect on the "affected side."

Special consideration needs to be given to the sympathetic nervous system in the periphery, i.e., in the **area of the terminal vessels**, in which the conducted impulse at the axon terminal is to be transmitted to the target organ. Around 1925, Stoehr was the first to deal with the anatomy of the autonomic nervous system in the area of the terminal vessels, i.e., with the terminating fiber portion in the periphery. He created the concept of the "**terminal reticulum**" which describes the fact that the finest unmyelinated autonomic nerve endings terminate in the interstitial space as inextricable fiber material without direct contact with other cells.[477,478] Thus, the transmission of information via the autonomic nervous system to the organs to be supplied proceeds via the interstitium.

Pischinger et al managed a further significant step.[399,400] They described the terminal autonomic fiber materials as a component of the interstitium to be defined as a system. As further components, they combined the three capillary structures (arterial, venous, lymphatic), the cellular portion (fibrocyte, macrophage), and the extracellular fluid (ground substance) into the so-called interstitial regulation system (p. 13). Thus, the efferent sympathetic nervous system ends as a free "synapse" in the interstitium where the impulse transmission of nerve fibers proceeds through the release of neurotransmitters into the extracellular fluid and thus influences both the capillary system and the cell system of the interstitium.

In addition to the free termination of the efferent sympathetic nervous system, in numerous animal species Fujita et al reported synapses between the end formation of the sympathetic nervous system and the so-called paraneurons.[154] These are special cells in the epithelial lining of hollow organs, glandular ducts, and blood vessel walls that produce transmitters, whose release is modulated by direct autonomic synapses. Similar conditions are found in the skin and mucosa in the dendritic cells, whose function, among others, is the modulation of immunological processes (monocyte–macrophage system) through the absorption of antigenic material and transfer to the lymphocytes.

The description of the function of the efferent sympathetic nervous system incorporating the interstitial regulation system and the paraneurons emphasizes its ubiquitous distribution in the whole organism. On this neurophysiological basis, the sympathetic nervous system can engage as an information system in regulatory activity of all tissue structures.

2.2.3 Sympathetic Afferent

The classification of nerve fibers into A, B, and C fibers does not allow a complete description of the fiber portions allocated to the afferent sympathetic nervous system. Clearly defined is the **sympathetic efferent**, which proceeds from its nucleic regions in the intermediolateral nucleus of the spinal cord (segments C8–L2), over the anterior root, the white ramus communicans of the sympathetic trunk, and the prevertebral ganglia together with the vessels and spinal or cranial nerves. The preganglionic fibers make their way as myelinated fibers to the para-and prevertebral ganglion, and the postganglionic fibers as slightly myelinated or nonmyelinated fibers to the interstitium of the target organ. The **sympathetic afferent** is identified not only through the fiber characteristics (little or no myelinization), but also primarily from its afferent function. (Remaining questions on the microanatomy of this region can currently only be addressed via the clinical, physiological, and pathophysiological functions.)

This divisive view of the efferent sympathetic nervous system and sole designation of the efferent as the sympathetic nervous system[436] is to be challenged, since the designation of the sympathetic nervous system comes from its function. This can only be inferred from the consideration of efferent **and** afferent, i.e., via the neural conduction arc. By analogy, it is equally useful to construct the term "vascular system" from the efferent arterial branch and the venous and lymphatic afferent branch in order to satisfy the related purpose of the vascular system.

Thus, the sympathetic afferent does not result in a uniform picture when considering only the fiber quality. Rather, a sensible approach considers the direct or indirect informing function of the afferent via the posterior horn to the efferent nucleic region in the spinal cord, the reticular formation in the brain and in the hypothalamus. In this respect, fiber quality of the sympathetic afferent results in a mixed picture:

- A-fibers: for pressure, warmth, and stretching (heart, veins, arteries, and lungs).
- B-fibers: for visceral sensitivity, atria, and lungs.
- C-fibers: for warmth, cold, itching, dull surface pain, deep protopathic pain, and visceral pain.

The afferent impulses are conducted from the periphery toward the center and form the reflex arc with the sympathetic efferent fibers. They are connected with the somatic nervous system through numerous circuits and generally course in the same nerve bundles as the corresponding efferent sympathetic nerve fibers. In this case, the identical, now converging, distribution pathway is defined as in the diverging—efferent—sympathetic system.[69] The fiber course thus proceeds via:

- Sensory fibers of the spinal nerves via spinal ganglion and posterior root to the spinal cord.
- Sensory nerves, but then via the white ramus communicans to the ganglion and the gray ramus communicans; then via the anterior and posterior root to the spinal cord: the corresponding ganglion cells are in the spinal ganglion, but probably also in the sympathetic trunk ganglia and the para- and prevertebral sympathetic ganglia.
- Pure autonomic nervous bundles; visceral branch, splanchnic nerves directly to the sympathetic trunk.
- Sympathetic perivascular plexuses to the sympathetic trunk and further via the rami communicantes to the anterior and posterior root of the spinal nerves to the spinal cord.

The afferent fiber processes and the associated localization of the synaptic connections result in the complex transfer of information within the sympathetic nervous system, and especially between the somatosensory and somatomotor systems in the head and the cranial nerves. This is how the autonomic functional area regulates itself in pure autonomic connectivity. The purely autonomic self-regulation is relativized where there are neural connections to the somatic nervous system. In some cases, these narrow autonomic and somatic connections are already at the receptor organ, e.g., at the lamellar bodies. These proprioception organs discharge both an afferent myelinated and unmyelinated afferent autonomic fiber, so that the autonomic nervous system receives both functional and somatosensory supply from one and the same "information organ."[69] Similar relationships are found, among others, in the muscle spindles, on Dogiel's corpuscles, and at Krause's end bulbs.[69]

The functions of the sympathetic afferents are highly variable. They impart the feeling of discomfort (e.g, distension of the bladder) up to pain (overfilled bladder), or vascular pain with irritation of the sympathetic perivascular plexus (e.g., from an infection). When the sympathetic trunk of the throat or the sympathetic carotid plexus is stimulated, the afferent sympathetic branch responds with head, face, neck, tooth, and ear pain.[69]

Considering the comprehensive supply of the entire organism through the efferent sympathetic nervous system, which reaches both the individual organs and the vascular system, the influence of the sympathetic nervous system becomes clear. The efferent sympathetic nervous system modulates organ function in two ways: on the one hand, it controls organ function directly via the interstitial distribution in the interstitial regulation system; on the other hand, it controls the microcirculation of the same organs via the vasomotor system. The efferent role of the sympathetic nervous system along with the afferent impulse inputs not only ensures the purely sympathetic conduction arc, but it also exists in numerous direct and indirect afferent contacts with the parasympathetic nervous system (e.g., intestinal lining) and the somatosensory and somatomotor systems. These functions illustrate the capacity of sympathetic nervous system throughout the whole body. Quite simply, no other peripheral nervous system has the functional range of the sympathetic nervous system.

2.2.4 Parasympathetic Efferent

In contrast to the sympathetic nervous system, which has preganglionic neurons present in the intermediolateral nucleus of the spinal cord in segments C8–L2/L3, the preganglionic neurons of the parasympathetic nervous system are found in various nucleic regions. Unlike the sympathetic nervous system, with the exception of the vagus nerve, these neurons do not form any independent nerves and use cranial and sacral spinal nerves as conductors. Since there is no parasympathetic trunk in which the switching takes place on the second neuron, the fiber length of the preganglionic neurons is very long in contrast to those of the sympathetic nervous system. The switch to the second neuron takes place either shortly before the target organ in parasympathetic ganglia or in the target organ itself.

There is differing information about the location of the source cells of the parasympathetic branch. Clara differentiates cranial, spinal, and sacral components, which is no longer found in modern anatomy textbooks.[69] These three components are taken into consideration in another form through the definition of the "continuous" postganglionic neurosecretion of acetylcholine. This is a defining feature of the parasympathetic nervous system and signifies its difference from the sympathetic nervous system, which secretes noradrenaline.

Also included in this new definition are the names of "sympathetic adrenergic" and "sympathetic cholinergic" efferent innervation that are based on the immunohistochemical detection of the neurotransmitters of the sympathetic and parasympathetic nervous systems.[420,428]

The cranial parasympathetic portion extends in four cranial nerves: oculomotor, facial, glossopharyngeal, and vagus nerves. The parasympathetic preganglionic fibers, which course with the oculomotor nerve, originate from the Edinger–Westphal nucleus, are switched in the ciliary ganglion, and supply the sphincter pupillae and ciliary muscles.

The preganglionic fibers coursing with the facial nerve originate in the superior salivatory nucleus, are switched in the pterygopalatine ganglion, and supply the tear ducts and the glands of the nose and palate via the zygomatic nerve. In the pterygopalatine ganglion, there are further neurons that modulate cerebral circulation intracranially as vasodilators with the cranial nerves (internal carotid artery).[558]

Further parasympathetic fibers from the facial nerve course via the chorda tympani to the lingual nerve, are switched to the second neuron in the submandibular ganglion, and supply the glands at the base of the oral cavity. Finally, parasympathetic fibers course with the peripheral branches of the facial nerve and supply a part of the facial sweat glands.

The preganglionic parasympathetic fibers, which course with the glossopharyngeal nerve, originate from the inferior salivatory nucleus and extend to the otic ganglion, where they are switched to the second neuron, and supply the parotid gland as well as the lip and cheek glands.

The vagus nerve forms the largest cranial part of the parasympathetic nervous system, whose source lies in the dorsal nucleus of the vagus nerve. The area supplied includes the chest and abdomen, whereby the switching to the second neuron takes place in the ganglion of the vagus nerve itself (superior ganglion and inferior ganglion) or in ganglia directly before or within the target organs. The main task of the vagus nerve is the motor supply of the palate and pharynx muscles as well as the entire larynx muscles; the sensory supply of the posterior fossa, a portion of the tympanic membrane, a portion of the skin of the external auditory meatus, the outer ear, and the larynx; and the sensory, secretory, and motor supply of all thoracic and abdominal organs up to the middle third of the transverse colon (Cannon–Böhm point). The rest of the large intestine and the pelvic viscera is supplied via the sacral parasympathetic nervous system.

The second section of the parasympathetic nervous system is the spinal portion of C1–S1 with its root cells from the midportion of the spinal cord, which send their nerve fibers over both the posterior and the anterior root of the spinal cord.[69] The efferent, thin-caliber myelinated fibers of the posterior root have a skin-vasodilating, perspirant, and pilomotor effect. Immunohistochemical studies of the abundant innervation of the sweat glands, sebaceous glands, hair follicles, and arrector pili muscle confirm the NO secretion, as is typical of the parasympathetic nervous system, but refer to them as "sympathetic-cholinergic." In smaller amounts, "sympathetic-adrenergic" fibers and parasympathetic fibers are found in connection with blood vessels of the skin.[74,428]

The efferent fibers, which extend across the anterior root, cannot be distinguished from the sympathetic fibers in the chest and upper lumbar spinal cord. Their function is partly in segment-related sweat secretion, and they may also be significant with regard to muscle tone.

The third parasympathetic section is the sacral portion and includes the segments S2–S4. From the sacral intermediolateral nucleus, the efferent nerve fibers radiate as pelvic nerves into the pelvic plexus via the anterior root. The question remains whether the parasympathetic efferents in their course with the spinal nerves and the blood vessels penetrate all the way into the skin, analogous to the sympathetic nervous system. Clinically, irritation of the skin over the sacrum (S1–S5) can lead to reactions of the rectum (e.g., diarrhea) as an indication of increased parasympathetically induced colon activity. The switch to the second neuron takes place in the pelvic ganglia and in the intramural ganglia of the target organs. The area supplied by the sacral parasympathetic portion comprises the last third of the transverse colon, descending colon, sigmoid colon, rectum and anus, the bladder with urethra, and internal and external sex organs. Bowel and bladder emptying is supported by muscular contraction and relaxation of the internal sphincter muscles. The pelvic splanchnic nerves relax the blood vessels of the external genitals, resulting in blood filling the corpus cavernosum.

The distribution proceeds partly with the vessels, similar to the sympathetic system, in some cases freely without vascular accompaniment via the mesentery and the hollow organs. On and in the hollow organs, myelinated fibers—which are preganglionic up to that point—are switched to the second neuron in numerous intramural ganglia. They supply both the myenteric plexus (Auerbach), which innervates the smooth muscles of the gastrointestinal tract, and the submucosal plexus (Meissner), which is responsible for the mucosa of the gastrointestinal tract. A stimulation of the efferent cholinergic parasympathetic system therefore results in an increased peristalsis and an increased secretion of mucous, with simultaneous cholinergic-induced vasodilation of the supplying blood vessels. On the one hand, the outgoing parasympathetic fibers terminate blindly in the interstitial space. On the other hand, as already described in the sympathetic system, according to Heine[204] and Fujita et al,[154] there are numerous synaptic connections to the paraneurons that are located in the network of the mucosal lining of the hollow organs. The question remains whether the paraneurons receive impulses from both the sympathetic and the parasympathetic system or only from one of these two branches. Given the large number of neurotransmitters formed by the paraneurons, which are transmitted both to the intestine and in the interstitium underneath the basement membrane, the sympathetic and parasympathetic innervation of paraneurons is quite conceivable. The intramural nervous system ensures a separate autonomy for the gastrointestinal tract. Consequently, an isolated, vessel-supplied intestinal segment continues to maintain directed peristalsis as well as mucous membrane function and thus, inter alia, can be used for bladder reconstruction surgery or intestinal interposition.

2.2.5 Parasympathetic Afferent

Although center-directed, the parasympathetic afferents show the same course as the efferents, i.e., an efferent parasympathetic nerve bundle also guides afferent fibers simultaneously. These converge in the vagus nerve and the pelvic nerves (▶Fig. 2.1). The view expressed in several textbooks that the afferent fibers of the parasympathetic nervous system form only an insignificant proportion of the neural structure is in contrast to the published 1994 studies of Linda Rinaman (University of Pittsburgh, Pennsylvania, United States) and Grundy (University of Sheffield, South Yorkshire, England). The study results indicate that approximately 80% of the fibers of the vagus nerve have an afferent function and only about 20% have an efferent function. This means that there is a very close relationship between the entire gastrointestinal tract, the brain stem, and the hypothalamus. A portion of the afferent fibers of the vagus nerve connects with the spinal nucleic regions of the trigeminal nerve, but especially with the terminal nucleus of the spinal tract and the posterior column of the first and second cervical segments.[69] Therefore, through irritation of the afferent parasympathetic fibers, illness in the area supplied by the vagus nerve can lead to irritation of the spinal nucleic regions of the trigeminal nerve and the posterior column at the first to third cervical segments, with corresponding clinical symptoms (facial pain, cervicocephalgia).

The sensory supply of the intestine is ensured by the afferent sympathetic system, which is to be regarded as an actual pain-conducting structure, while the afferent parasympathetic system rather imparts specific organic sensations. Thus, the pain of cholecystitis or gastritis is transmitted by the sympathetic nervous system, while malaise, nausea, and vomiting proceed via the parasympathetic afferents.

2.2.6 Afferent of the Phrenic Nerve

A peculiarity which involves the phrenic nerve and does not affect the autonomic nervous system should be mentioned here because it has clinical relevance. The main task of the phrenic nerve is motor supply to the diaphragm. In addition, the following course in the phrenic nerve: sensory afferents of the lower pleura, pericardium, and subdiaphragmal peritoneum as well as the peritoneal lining of the liver and the pancreas. Further clinical observations suggest that a more extensive afferent supply through the phrenic nerve seems likely, especially since shoulder pain and sensorimotor disorders in the third to fifth cervical segments, the nucleus of the phrenic nerve, occur not only with inflammation of the thoracic space and the upper abdomen, but also in diseases of the organs in the small pelvis (adnexa, uterus, seminal vesicles, and prostate). Since the nucleic regions of the phrenic nerve are not only constantly formed in the third to fifth cervical segments, but also time and again distributed over the segments C3–C7 or C8, reflex symptoms in these corresponding neck segments can occur with abdominal disorders.[69]

This somewhat detailed description of the topography, in particular that of the peripheral autonomic structures, is designed to convey to the reader the multiplicity of distribution channels of the sympathetic and parasympathetic systems and to clarify that the structures associated with the course of the peripheral autonomic nervous system can be used for diagnostic and therapeutic applications of local anesthetics.

Note

The topography of the autonomic nervous system is one of the foundations of neural therapy and a prerequisite for the entire injection technique.

Knowledge of the macroscopic and microscopic anatomy and neurophysiological relationships helps to clarify pathogenetic and etiologic correlations of diverse symptomatics of "idiopathic diseases." The differentiated use of this system for diagnosis and therapy enables a multidisciplinary application.

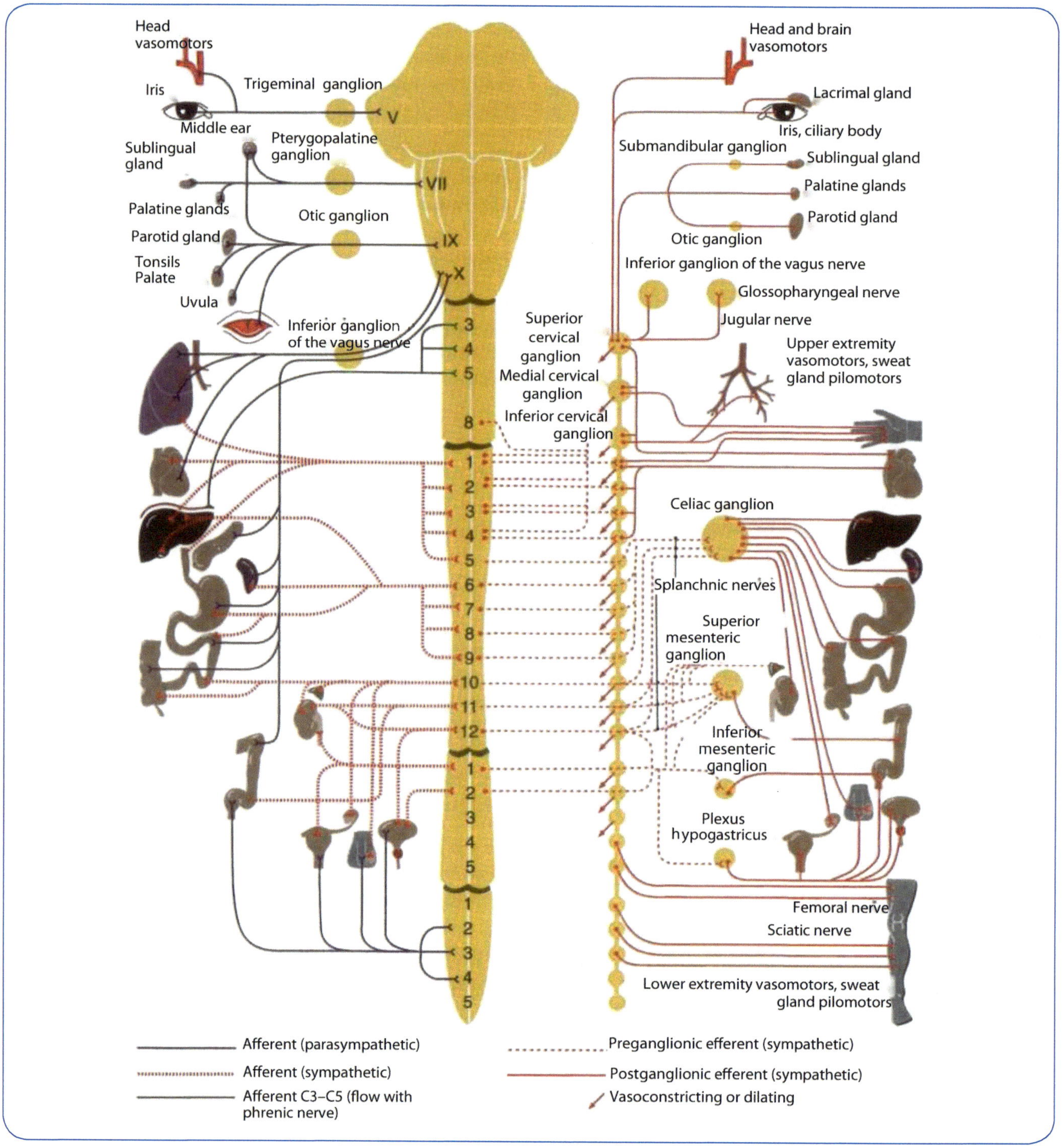

► **Fig. 2.1** Visceral efferent/afferent innervation as the basis of the meso-rhombo-spinal organization of the autonomic reflexes (modified from Fulton).

3 Interstitial Regulation System According to Pischinger and Heine

3.1 Introduction

"The cell concept is, strictly speaking, only a morphological abstraction. Biologically speaking, it cannot be considered without the milieu of the cell."[399,400] This quote by **Pischinger** illustrates the difference between Virchow's cell theory and today's mindset of placing the cell in a functional relationship with the whole organism. **Virchow** believed that each cell of an organism on its own constitutes an elementary organism, which enables the function of the whole through a networked division of labor. According to Pischinger, this view neglects the milieu that is the basis of existence for each cell.

The milieu essentially represents the result of cellular function and therefore, according to Virchow, can be attributed to the cell as the elementary organism. The difference between the mindsets of Virchow and Pischinger is that Virchow considers the cell itself as the source unit of an organism, while Pischinger uses the specific cell efficiency as a starting point. Virchow's mindset created the basis for today's explanation—extending up to the molecular level—regarding the composition of the elementary organism cell, while Pischinger and Heine succeeded in a clarification—extending to molecular sizes—of the function of the nonspecific connective tissue.

Both viewpoints are important for applied medicine. The rather static view of the pathologist Virchow is useful for identification and description of the pathologic structure, while the dynamic mindset of the physiologist and anatomist Pischinger is useful for recognizing disease processes. The consequence of Virchow's cell theory is the linear thinking in diagnosis and therapy which is common today, with the risk that the causal relationships, in particular for chronic illness, are not recognized or incompletely recognized due to lack of consideration of the high level of cross-linking for all organic systems. The result can be found primarily in the symptomatically oriented treatment of chronic diseases by medications (antihypertensives, anti-inflammatory drugs, antipyretics, etc.) that steadily suppress the symptoms of the illness, which also means that the symptoms reoccur when the medication is discontinued. In contrast, harking back to Pischinger, the simultaneous consideration of the interstitial regulation system function in diagnostics and therapy allows for the influence of diseased organs and organ systems through the use of the intrinsic regulation of the organism.

Before Virchow and Pischinger, the pathologists **Bordeu** from Paris (1767) and **Reichert** (1854) from Dorpat indicated the significance of connective tissue, which functions in microcirculation and metabolism between capillaries and the cell system, in addition to its mechanical and supportive function. **Pischinger** recognized that not only the connective tissue played a static filtering role in the cell supply, but also, due to the uniform composition of the extracellular space, a structure had been found that pervades the entire organism and is involved in all cellular functions of the organism as well as the internal and external stimuli affecting it.

The interstitial regulation system is shown in the schematic drawing (▶Fig. 3.1). The cutaway single capillary represents the capillary branch consisting of arterial, venous, and lymphatic capillaries. The inflow and outflow of oxygen and nutrients, messenger molecules, and cell metabolites as well as cells for immunological processes takes place via the vascular system.

The autonomic end formation is represented by two terminal axons whose efferent impulse delivery and neurotransmitters (acetylcholine, adrenaline) enable the afferent impulse uptake, modulated by changes in the basic substance (e.g., metabolites, hormones, neuropeptides). According to **Fujita et al**[154] and **Heine**,[204] there are also synaptic connections of the autonomic end formation with so-called paraneurons, which use the release of transmitters to influence specifically operating cell systems and also have a feedback effect on the interstitium. The free cellular component of the interstitial regulation system is represented by the pluripotent fibrocyte, which communicates via its cell processes with about 30% of all fibrocytes and is responsible for the synthesis of the ground substance and the production of collagen and elastin, as well as the formation of new cells—among others, the immunocompetent cells— represented by the mast cell as an example of a tissue hormone-producing cell and by the defense cell (macrophage), which is responsible for the immunological processing and dissemination of degradation products, viruses, and bacteria. Other cells that have an immunological function and dispose of the ground substance are shown in ▶Fig. 3.1.

The ground substance is represented as a homogeneous extracellular fluid in a network of glycosaminoglycans (hyaluronic acid and heparin) weaving through the entire interstitium as elongated polysaccharide chains studded with brush-shaped, short-chain proteoglycans. Due to their charge and structure, this network is capable of water binding and ion exchange, i.e., for isotonicity, isoiony, and isoosmy. The interstitial regulation system can be found in the entire organism as the interstitium.

3.2 Structure and Function

The **intercellular structure** basically consists of the pluripotent **fibrocytes**, which are responsible for the synthesis of structural components (collagen, elastin) and the intercellular substance of the interstitium, **the macrophages**, whose main function is the phagocytosis of pathological intercellular structures (viruses, bacteria),

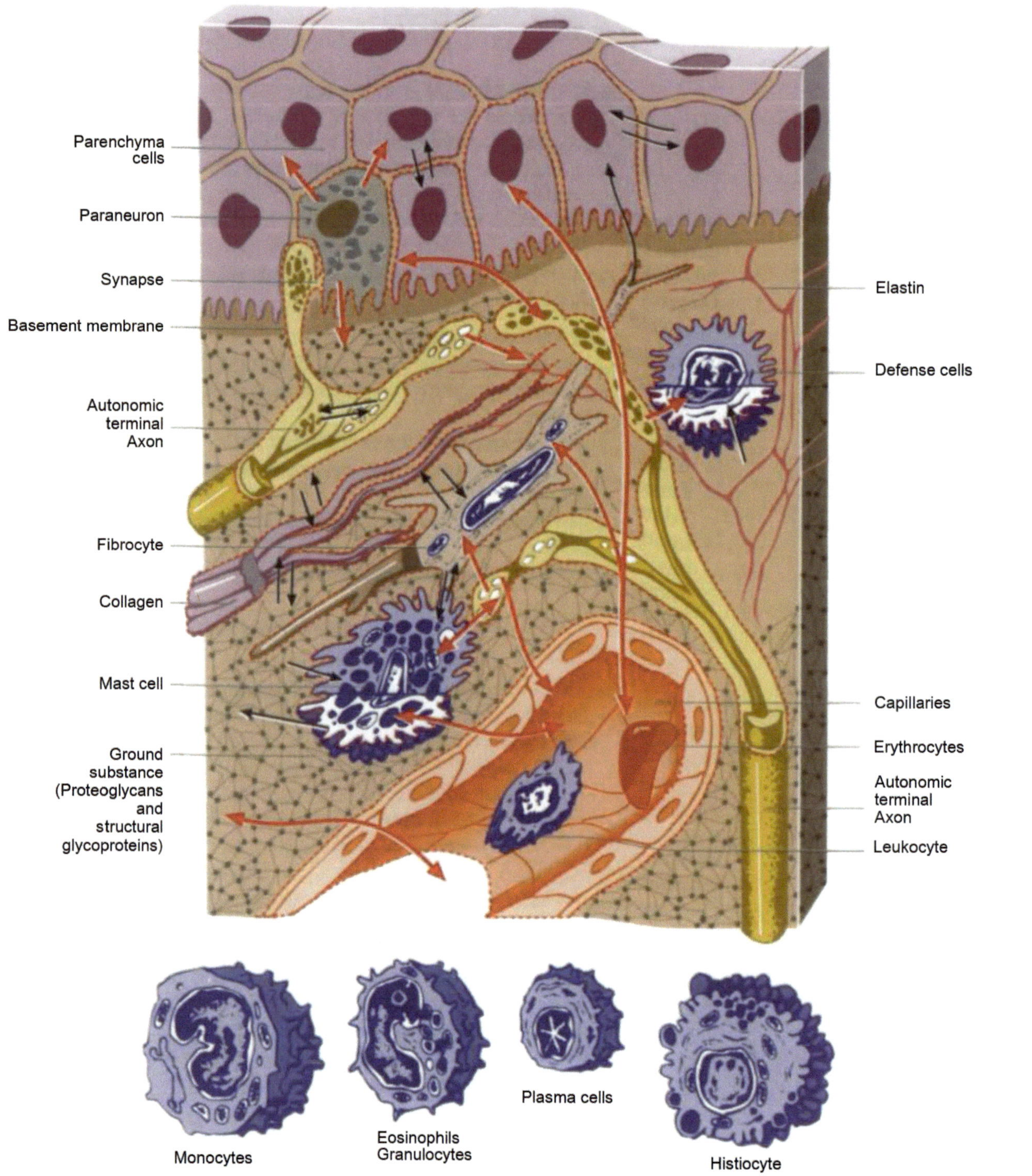

▶ **Fig. 3.1** Schematic diagram of the interstitial regulation system modified according to Pischinger and Heine, based on the functional unit of capillaries, autonomic end formation, free cells, and the ground substance.

the **capillaries** (arterial, venous, lymphatic), the **free autonomic nerve cell endings**, and the structured **intercellular substance** verified by Heine, consisting of proteoglycans and structural glycoproteins.

This system, first formulated by Pischinger as the interstitial regulation system (p. 13), has the following functions:

- Supply of energy to the cells.
- Delivery of building blocks for cells and cell products.
- Removal of cell products (e.g., hormones), cell detritus, and phagocytosis of metabolic products.
- Uptake and transfer of immunological stimuli via macrophages (antigens).
- Initiation of cellular repair or regeneration after injury or disease.
- Information transfer via the capillaries (slow, e.g., by hormones, neuropeptides).

- Information transfer via autonomic nerves (fast, e.g., by neurotransmitters).
- Production of the self-regulated ground substance as needed via fibrocytes.
- Regeneration of the interstitial regulation system.

With the interstitial regulation system, the organism has an available structure through which ultimately every cell of the body is informatively and energetically connected to all other cells. The uniform structure of this system means that a stimulus reaching the organism is answered from the interstitial regulation system in a uniform manner, regardless of its location within the organism; the response is then specified as a second step by the cellular system of the interstitium and the specific tissue (organs). In a feedback process, the interstitial regulation system with all of its parts is influenced by the organ tissue, so that the functional condition of the organs can also be incorporated in the autonomic conduction arc and can be thus modified if necessary. Through this system, the various organs are hemodynamically coordinated.

Note

The normal, undisturbed functioning of the interstitial regulation system provides the basis for the body's health and ability to regenerate. The temporary disruption of this function leads to temporary illness, and chronic disruption leads to chronic illness.

According to present knowledge, factors of this chronic disturbance are all the things that stress the individual components of the interstitial regulation system beyond predetermined tolerance limits. These include chemical, physical, viral, and bacterial noxa as well as endogenous toxicants that are discharged to the interstitium by the interstitial cells and the specific working parenchymal cells.

3.3 Significance of Autonomic End Formation

The part of the interstitial regulation system that is essential to neural therapy is the end formation of the autonomic nervous system in the interstitium. The efferent transfer of information is carried out by the following neurotransmitters in the intercellular space:

- Acetylcholine.
- Vasoactive intestinal peptide (VIP; parasympathetic nervous system).
- Adenosine triphosphate.
- Noradrenaline.
- Neuropeptide γ (sympathetic nervous system).

From the intercellular space via the corresponding cell membrane receptors of the interstitial cells and the parenchymal cells, the corresponding cell function is modulated in an inhibitory or facilitative manner depending on which receptors can take up the stimulus. Ideally, the result of this efferent impulse transmission is the balanced stimulus response of the specific tissues. The physiological state probably results from the continuous equalization of internal and external stimuli, because the body responds permanently to fluctuations in its environment.

This condition, which can be best described by the physical concept of oscillation, only becomes balanced if the change in condition created by the autonomic end formation via the efferent pathway triggers centrally oriented information feedback. This is ensured through the afferent branch of the autonomic end formation.

Although it is not possible to differentiate efferent autonomic neurofibrils from afferent in the interstitium, further centrally the already bundled information flow of the afferent inputs can be interrupted at the ganglionic level, for example, by way of a local anesthetic, with a change in clinical symptoms of the target organs supplied by the autonomic end formation.

The physiological function of the autonomic stimulus conduction system is the electrical stimulus transfer (0.5–2 m/s) and the neurosecretion (norepinephrine/acetylcholine) linked to this. In a physiological functional state, this provides the afferent–efferent coupling that ensures **homeostasis**. If the tolerance range of this system is exceeded over a longer period due to excessive stimulation or increased irritability of the sympathetic nervous system, both the electrical stimulus profile and the neurotransmitter profile change as a result. This causes a change in the microcirculation, which leads to an altered metabolic state of the interstitium and the parenchymal cells/organs:

- Oxygen and nutrient deficiency.
- Change in pH value.
- Release of inflammatory mediators (silent inflammation).
- Activation of nociceptors (e.g., pain).

Interstitial dysregulation with simultaneous disruption of microcirculation leads to a disruption of organ function (e.g., pain based on "silent inflammation") as well as structural changes (e.g., degeneration) in the case of chronicity. In summary, a chronic disease process can thus be explained to be a result of chronic pathological stimulation of the sympathetic nervous system.

3.4 Interstitial Regulation System and Autonomic Nervous System

The balanced physiological impulse emission of the autonomic efferent ensures physical microcirculation, which is essential for the exchange of physiological energy and materials. At the same time, the activity of macrophages is modulated, immunological processes are activated or attenuated. The fibrocytes, which are about 30% connected with each other via their cell processes in the organism, are adaptively regulated with regard to their interstitial function and cell formation, the production of ground substance, collagen and elastin, and the "repair" of specific cell systems. These physiological processes ensure **homeostasis** and thus the balanced, need-based functioning of all systems with one another.

The widespread networking, the high regenerative capacity, and the plasticity of the autonomic nervous system enable the controlled function of an organism in its environment.[428,478,513,514] The inner and outer stimuli are routed through the autonomic nervous system (p. 6) and passed in a facilitative or inhibitory capacity to the specific organ system. The resulting adaptations made accordingly are what determines the fundamental viability of an organism in its environment. Each system however is limited in its capacity for adjustment in response to input from the autonomic nervous system. This limit applies to both ends of the physiological scale and is accompanied by a corresponding range of tolerance in either direction which is individual for each organ.

In an individually differentiated formation of the tolerance ranges, different degrees of stimulation can normally be transmitted from the organism itself and from its environment without causing a disorder in the organism. Simply put, the body would be healthy up to this point. With prolonged stimulation of the autonomic nervous system due to addition of various subliminal afferent stimuli, for example, the autonomic nervous system may become overloaded. Then, from a cybernetic perspective, a persistent shift between actual and target values occurs.

Note

Persistently exceeding the tolerance range leads to disease. This becomes chronic when the irritation beyond the tolerance range cannot be eliminated.

This isolated analysis of the autonomic end formation as an anatomical substrate within the system of stimulus conduction explains the therapeutic aspect of interrupting the conduction of pathological impulses via the infiltration with a local anesthetic during neural therapy. Medicinal interruption of pathological stimulus enables normalization of autonomic stimulus conduction by way of reset, thereby normalizing the function of the interstitial regulation system. This is critical for the therapeutic effect beyond the anesthesia period; otherwise, the pathological stimulus would return after the end of the local anesthetic's medicinal effect.

The transient effect of a local anesthetic, especially that of procaine, not only is important for the peripheral autonomic end formations with all effects on the reflexive, autonomic conduction arc, but also is reflected in additional parts of the interstitial regulation system. **Sealing of the capillaries** and **membrane stabilization** of the cellular portions of the interstitial regulation system (fibrocytes, macrophages, mast cells) occurs, leading to interruption of the pathological delivery of perfusion-disrupting peptides from these cells.

The crucial therapeutic effect is the drug-induced, suddenly improved capillary perfusion and the consequent improvement of microcirculation. The resulting normalization of all portions of the interstitial regulation system including the milieu of the interstitium acts as a relief with the result of normalization of the specific organ cell function controlled by this system. This represents the actual neural therapeutic effect.

3.5 Summary

Neural therapy accesses the organism via the autonomic nervous system, especially the sympathetic nervous system and its end formation in the interstitium. The other parts of the interstitial regulation system are modulated via the autonomic branch of the interstitial regulation system:

- Capillaries.
- Interstitial cell system.
- End formation somatic afferents.

This way, both the local disorder (segment disease) and the interference field disorder are treated. This is only possible through the ubiquitous distribution of the autonomic nervous system, especially the sympathetic nervous system, as well as by its high degree of cross-linking with all other systems (vascular system, immune system, hormonal system) of the organism. Therapeutic access to precise functions of different organ systems takes place via the autoregulation mechanism of specific parts of the interstitial regulation.

4 Ricker's Pathology of Relations

4.1 Introduction

The term "pathology of relations" dates back to Ricker (1870–1948), who was the Head of the Pathology Institute Magdeburg from 1906 to 1933. He managed an essential step in systematizing the etiology of various diseases whose common cause he found to be the pathological irritation of the perivascular sympathetic nervous system. Contesting Virchow's cellular pathology, which held that every disease originates from the cell itself, Ricker realized the logical inadequacy of the static concept of the cell as a basic building block of the organism. He replaced this paradigm with the dynamic concept of cell function, which equates the dependence of the cells to each other with regard to function in both the physiological and the pathological events.

Ricker emphasized that Virchow's theory of cellular pathology with its assumption that the stimulus-impacted cell will function automatically contradicts the functioning of the blood and nervous system. He countered Virchow with the observation that all diverse cell and tissue processes are in casual relationship with the blood and nervous system, whereby the neural systems are chronologically the first (though not predominant) to produce various macro- and micro-anatomical changes according to the cellular and tissue processes involved.[425] Here, we see the difference with Virchow's definition of pathology, the study of the diseases, in particular their origin and the organic–anatomical changes caused by them. While Virchow focuses on the **cellular findings** and derives the etiology of disease from these, Ricker takes the pathological findings into account one step earlier in the **pathological disease process**. Using a microscope, he observed the behavior of the vascular system by pathological stimulation of the perivascular sympathetic nervous system in animal experiments over a long period and recognized the pathological change of the tissue, including the pathological changes in organs.

With experimental proof, Ricker established the relationship of the cellular pathological findings to the blood and vascular system responsible for the supply, which is controlled by the sympathetic nervous system. His view is basically that the descriptive pathology must be inextricably linked to the physiology in order to represent natural science that is distinct, verifiable, and applicable not only in human medicine, but also in the entire field of biology.

Pathology of relations leads to evidence that the pathological stimulus necessary for the emergence of a cellular pathological finding does not primarily attach to the cell itself but to the stimulus conduction system specially designed for this, namely, the sympathetic nervous system. It is noteworthy that Ricker considered the same tissue structure as Pischinger did a few decades later in the description of the interstitial regulation system (p. 13). He divides the nonspecific connective tissue according to its function in the capillary final pathway, the autonomic end formation, interstitial cell system, and the extracellular fluid, which he calls the "**ground substance**." This interstitial regulation system precedes all organs and organ systems in the physiological and pathological processes and has primary involvement with any type of disease. Ricker's investigations were confirmed in detail in studies by Marvar and Harrison and supplemented with further details from neuroimmunology.[428]

4.2 Basics of the Experiments, Stimulus, and Stimulus Effects

Ricker's special contribution lies in microscopic examinations on living animals, which were certainly unique in their wide scope. He and his collaborators demonstrated physiological and pathophysiological processes that were not visible to the naked eye and revealed regularities whose scope and impact on the organism were previously unknown. Experimental measures on living animals developed from the idea that only the **observation of functional sequences** can shed a clear light on the etiology of diseases—unlike the "snapshot" from a histological preparation under the microscope, which can only allow one to make assumptions about a pathological process. They provided reproducible results with respect to the pathological stimulus, its transmission through the perivascular sympathetic nervous system to the arterioles and capillaries, and the changes of the interstitium all the way to the pathological cell reaction.

His textbook *Pathologie als Naturwissenschaft—Relationspathologie* describes pathophysiological processes with remarkable precision and dialectical confrontation with the results of other scientists, along with a critical view of his own results, which he contrasted with the cellular pathology view of Virchow. The difference between **cellular pathology** and **pathology of relations** is demonstrated in the clarity with which the microscopic examinations of stimulus effects of the perivascular sympathetic nervous system demonstrate the pathway from the physiological to the pathophysiological condition of the interstitial regulation system and the sequelae of organ cells and organ systems.

Ricker's experimental design was determined by the need to illustrate the vasal reactions of the capillary vascular system in the interstitium from which the supply and disposal of cell aggregates exercising any specific functions takes place. In the area of this switch point, it was possible to study the reactions of the vascular system on sympathetic nervous system stimulus and the behavior of the capillary blood flow, changes in the interstitium, and the response of the cell aggregate to be supplied. The value of the microscopic imaging was that unique functional relationships could be shown that could not be seen by the naked eye or in a histological preparation under the microscope. With this experimental design, evidence was also provided that the stimulus that leads to cellular pathological findings does not act directly on the cell, but on the corresponding stimulus conduction system, namely, the perivascular sympathetic nervous system.

The following conditions were proven experimentally with regard to stimulus:

- The experimental stimulus which leads to stimulation of the perivascular sympathetic nervous system can be physical (mechanical, thermal, electrical) or generated by chemical substances (neurotransmitters, cytokines, cell metabolites, pH changes in the interstitium, toxins, hormones, viruses and bacteria or their toxins). Any kind of influence that leads to stimulation of the sympathetic nervous system is considered to be stimulus.
- The stimulation consists of increased or decreased impulse emission from the stimulated axons.
- The stimulus quality, consisting of physical or chemical stimulus, or both, only receives a quantitative response from the sympathetic nervous system through variable pulse frequency and pulse strength.
- The stimulus remains transient if it can be reduced or removed from the organism or if the stimulus supply is interrupted. The stimulus remains chronic if it is neither reduced nor removed or interrupted from the outside.

4.2.1 Experiments with the Sympathetic Nervous System

The reaction of the perivascular sympathetic nervous system to a stimulus can only be assessed indirectly under the microscope, since the impulse emission, the increased or decreased impulse conduction, or the excitability are visible only in the reaction of the vascular system supplied. The reaction reveals itself as vessel dilation with the slightest stimulus, as vasoconstriction with strong stimulus, or as excitability with the strongest stimulus. Ricker's microscopic investigation revealed a **"double" sympathetic innervation of the vascular system**: the well-known main portion of the sympathetic nervous system, which produces noradrenaline as a neurotransmitter and leads to vasoconstriction, and a second sympathetic part which, similar to the skin, releases acetylcholine as a neurotransmitter for vasodilation. This enabled Ricker to confirm that vasodilation is not—as is commonly believed—a passive occurrence that comes about by impulse reduction of the vasoconstrictive sympathetic nervous system or its failure, but an active process which is also generated via the sympathetic nervous system. Depending on the stimulus intensity, according to Ricker's observation, there is **active vasoconstriction** (stronger stimulus) and **active vasodilation** (weak stimulus), which exceeds the sympatholytic dilation.

Ricker describes this sympathetic function—which initially seems paradoxical—as a microscopically visible interplay whereby the effect of the constrictive sympathetic system and the dilating sympathetic system is increased or reduced by various stimuli or interrupted by medication. The nucleic regions of the vasodilatory sympathetic nervous system are in the anterior part of the hypothalamus. The skin vessels, particularly those of the face, are modulated via the cervical sympathetic nervous system, the muscle vessels are modulated from the thoracolumbar part of the sympathetic trunk, and the abdominal viscera are modulated via the splanchnic nerves.

The vasodilators are important for organ perfusion. With hyperemia or increased microcirculation, the following affects occur:

- Reduction of inflammation.
- Reduction of pain.
- Decrease in allergic reactions.
- Interruption of degenerative changes.
- Initiation of regeneration.

4.2.2 Particulars of the Sympathetic Nervous System

Ricker described another consequence of stimulus, viz. continuous strong stimulation of the perivascular sympathetic nervous system results in proximally (toward the heart) progressive vasoconstriction until active vascular occlusion occurs, which, along with the observed vasodilation toward the periphery, causes slowing of the blood—up to standstill—especially in the capillary branch. This stimulus sequence is made possible via the reflexive path of the sympathetic afferent by activating the spinal nucleic regions and thus activating the efferent vascular branch, e.g., Sudeck's disease and CRPS (complex regional pain syndrome). It also became clear that the excitability of the perivascular sympathetic nervous system increases from the central region toward the periphery. This means that the same stimulus intensity on the perivascular sympathetic nervous system of the major vessels causes weaker stimulus effects than on the perivascular sympathetic nervous system of the minor vessels.

Another reaction of the perivascular sympathetic nervous system leads to a sustained (engramic) change in excitability of the sympathetic nervous system. The unique, pathological, stronger or longer-lasting stimulation leads to disruption, although it leads to a gradual normalization of vascular, blood, and tissue responses. However, restimulation at the same location or a remote location generates a much stronger stimulus response, regardless of the time interval between the two stimuli. This sensitization of the perivascular sympathetic nervous system after pathological stimulation is to be regarded as a phenomenon, as the cause of this reaction is unexplained. However, the phenomenon has clinical relevance and was described experimentally in another context as "**second-strike**" phenomenon by Speransky.[467]

The microscopic observation of the response patterns of the perivascular sympathetic nervous system after stimulation showed highly differentiated functioning of the antagonistically working vasculature, which is of crucial significance in its effect on the vascular system, the bloodstream, the interstitial space, and the cell system to be supplied, and represents the theoretical basis of segmental disease as well as interference field disease.

4.2.3 Medication-Based Stimulus Disruption

Previously, the reactions of the sympathetic nervous system which take place in experimental (pathological) stimulus were described. Ricker also described the reactions that become visible microscopically through stimulus interruption by medication or by nerve transection:

- Medicinal interruption of stimulus conduction through a local anesthetic at the site of the stimulus certainly prevents the effect of the stimulus when the interruption occurs before the stimulus. If conduction is interrupted after the stimulus at the stimulus site, the stimulus has only an attenuated effect.
- If the vascular sympathetic nervous system proximal to the stimulus location is interrupted prior to the stimulus, the reflexive path that leads to efferent stimulation via the afferents at the spinal level is turned off, so that the stimulus effect on the vascular system and the interstitium is less severe.
- After transection of a peripheral spinal nerve and thus its sympathetic fiber portion, if there is a stimulus in its supply area, the stimulus response is significantly stronger. The nerve transection performed before the stimulus acts as a preforming stimulus of the entire innervated segment, because the sympathetic afferents and efferents that extend beyond the vascular system are preserved. This summation effect explains the enhanced effect of the local stimulus.

4.2.4 Reaction of the Vascular System

As already described, the vascular system reacts via the sympathetic nervous system by active dilation in the case of very weak stimulus and vasoconstriction in the case of stronger stimulus. From observations of the vascular system in living animals, Ricker described a permanent change in the resting phase from mild vasoconstriction and dilation. Depending on the strength and duration of the stimulus, the experimental stimulus results in longer-lasting active vasodilation with a very weak stimulus, while stronger stimulus results in vasoconstriction of the entire vascular section from the site of stimulation to the periphery; further strengthening of the stimulus causes narrowing of the vessel proximal to the stimulus site and dilation distal to the stimulus site. These vascular reactions represent the most significant role in the modulation of blood flow rate through the vascular system, from which the supply to the tissues is directly dependent: the faster the blood flow, the better the microcirculation; the slower the flow rate, the more reduced the interstitial exchange.

Microscopic examination showed that there is also a stimulus-dependent constriction and dilation in the capillary vascular branch that is not supplied with smooth muscle. Here, Ricker observed an active process dependent on the sympathetic nervous system function, which is controlled via capillary nerves that end with button-shaped distension near capillaries. Distinct synapses are not described in this context. This gives rise to the microscopically visible interplay between the constricted and dilated capillaries in vivo and is comparable with the vessels supplied with muscles. In the case of capillary dilation and slowing of the bloodstream, plasma and erythrocytes pass from the capillary lumen into the interstitium.

For this purpose, Ricker described "**stomata**" that open between the individual capillary cells through which the plasma and erythrocyte discharge is observed. The discharge of leukocytes from the vascular lumen occurs not in the capillary branch but from the smallest vein adjoining the capillary system and is the reaction of a slowdown in the bloodstream.

4.2.5 Properties of the Blood and its Components

The detailed observation of the bloodstream in the capillary region yielded the seamless description of the behavior of acellular and cellular blood components in response to vasoconstriction and dilation induced by the sympathetic nervous system. Ricker basically stated that the pathological changes inside and outside of the vascular system are directly dependent on the bloodstream rate. The pathological findings occur in the situation described by Ricker as "**prestasis**," in which the capillary blood flow significantly slows down due to vascular constriction and dilation distal to the stimulus site and progressing from the stimulus site in the proximal direction.

It should be noted beforehand that hyperemia, which macroscopically presents as congestion, is not to be equated with better supply to the tissues. Hyperemia is found both in dilated capillaries with a constricted proximal arterial branch, resulting in a slowdown in the bloodstream, i.e., poorer supply conditions, and in overall dilated vessels with fast blood flow; only in these cases does hyperemia mean improved supply conditions.

Below a certain flow rate, the slowing of the bloodstream results in the discharge of plasma into the interstitium, based on capillary cell leakage (reduced capillary wall tension) in the adhered cell membranes. The result is interstitial edema and, in the case of free cavities, effusion (e.g., joint, chest cavity, abdominal cavity). Plasma discharge from the capillaries with normal blood flow rate was not observed in any case. Furthermore, there can be adhesion of erythrocytes, leukocytes, and platelets, up to standstill (stasis) of the blood column in the capillaries, which Ricker described as "**red stasis**." Even with slow blood flow, erythrocytes do occur in the interstitium due to capillary leakage as described previously. Erythrodiapedesis is more pronounced with a slow progression of prestasis than with a fast progression. Also, a small amount of leukocyte extravasation occurs in the area of the smallest veins adjoining the capillaries. When the blood flow has stopped, no further exit of cells from the vascular system into the interstitium is observed.

When reinitiating the blood flow through termination of the stimulus and thus normalizing the vascular status (poststatic state), there is strong leakage of leukocytes from the smallest veins into the interstitium. The longer the stasis, the more severe the leukocyte extravasation; the shorter the stopped blood flow, the lower the leukocyte discharge.

The most extreme form of the blood's reaction to the sympathetic nervous system–dependent vascular reaction is red and white thrombosis, which occurs with longer blood flow stasis. The fixation of the blood column mainly caused by erythrocytes and fibrin is designated "**red thrombosis**," and the fixation of leukocytes and fibrin in the smallest veins and capillaries after strong erythrodiapedesis is referred to as "**white thrombosis**." In each case, the basis is long cessation of blood flow. In flowing blood, no thrombosis occurs with an intact vascular system and normal coagulation status.

4.2.6 Result of Pathological Sympathetic Nervous System Stimulation

Inflammation, Degeneration, Necrosis, and Hyperplasia

In addition to the already described discharge of plasma, erythrocytes, and leukocytes into the interstitium, there are further reactions of the cellular portion belonging to the interstitium (fibrocytes, macrophages). The reaction of the extracellular fluid is not described by Ricker.

With slowed capillary blood flow and the associated hypoxia, fibrocytes proliferate and new capillaries form. At the same time, there is an increase in the fibrous components of the interstitium, in particular collagen fibers, as an expression of increased fibrocyte activity. Ricker reported that the newly formed capillaries show the same sympathetic nervous system–dependent reaction of constriction and dilation as the old capillaries, i.e., the slowdown of the bloodstream results in increased plasma discharge to the interstitium. Thus he emphasized that the newly formed capillaries are controlled by the sympathetic nervous system.

The previously described reaction of the interstitium is not fully reversible. The cessation of the stimulus with normalization of the sympathetic and vascular function and blood flow causes a drop in the fibrocyte count and capillaries, as well as later-onset degradation of part of the collagen. The final state, in comparison with the normal interstitium, is an interstitium that is richer in fibers and poorer in cell count and capillaries—the scar.

Ricker did not investigate the cell invasion from the capillary vascular system (leukocytes, lymphocytes, plasma cells, mast cells, etc.) also occurring in the interstitium and the new cell formation from the pluripotent fibroblasts. This cellular response is also dependent on stimulus, but it represents a specific immunological, macrophagic cell efficiency that occurs as a secondary result of the stimulation of the perivascular sympathetic nervous system.

The altered capillary perfusion and microcirculation process in the interstitium after pathological stimulation of the sympathetic nervous system corresponds to the clinical inflammatory process. Ricker proved that the inflammation-inducing stimulus primarily attaches to the sympathetic nervous system, regardless of whether it is an inflammatory reaction after trauma or physical, chemical, bacterial, or viral etiology. The four characteristics of inflammation going back to Celsus can be traced to hyperemia (**rubor**) with a slowdown of blood flow, which in turn is the result of strong sympathetic nervous system stimulation. The three additional features **calor**, **dolor**, and **tumor** are only consequences of this first step, and may be partially absent. Therefore, strictly in terms of hard science, Ricker views the term "inflammation" commonly used in applied medicine as untenable.

A value-free, pure description of the inflammatory process is needed to enable a clear scientific assertion. The features of inflammation on the intestinal mucosa during digestion correspond to those of the infectious disease dysentery, and inflammation features on the endometrium before and after menstruation correspond to those of septic endometritis, pneumonia to those of pulmonary infarction, and edema of the subcutaneous fat in nephritis or heart failure to those of phlegmon. The process described can occur locally or generally in the healthy and the diseased state; it always has the same background of a quantitatively variable stimulus at the sympathetic nervous system.

4.2.7 Effect on Specific Tissues

Based on increased and reduced microcirculation, which is primarily dependent on sympathetic function, Ricker described the following as the cornerstone of the tissue response: hyperplasia resulting from sustained increase in microcirculation, and necrosis when circulation is interrupted.[425] In experiments the stimulus result is dependent on the stimulus intensity and the duration of the exposure.

The effect of long-term local stasis is the necrosis of the tissue section, in which the vascular supply area of the affected vascular section is located. Depending on the extent of the arrested metabolism between the vasculature, interstitium, and organ due to stasis, small tissue sections, organ parts, or whole organs can become necrotic. The degree of severity of sequelae depends on the function of the necrotic tissue. Long-term stasis in a small portion of liver tissue has functionally less sequelae than stasis of a large section of tissue. Stasis of part of the brain in the neocortex, brain stem, cerebellum, or spinal cord, for example, or in a portion of heart muscle has more significant clinical effects.

Ricker demonstrated experimentally that the autolytic necrosis of the pancreas is not caused when the primary secretion of the pancreas destroys the pancreatic tissue. Rather, the stimulus of the secretion primarily on the perivascular sympathetic nervous system triggers the stimulus of the same, which results in long-term stasis in the vascular system with subsequent necrosis of the pancreatic tissue; only in this state is the pancreatic tissue vulnerable to the pancreatic secretion.

The same pathophysiological mechanisms occur in the stomach. The primary cause of necrosis of the stomach lining or the stomach wall is not the stomach acid, but local permanent stasis of the vasculature. This is followed by necrosis of the gastric mucosa, whereby the gastric secretions only become active in this tissue state and reach the gastric vessels (bleeding) or the stomach muscles (perforation). The same processes were shown to be present in the kidney, adrenal gland, lung, and brain.

In the **periphery**, the parenchyma disconnected from the bloodstream through stasis can be found both in vivo in animal studies and in the snapshot of a corresponding histological preparation, consistent with the reaction of the vessels, the interstitium, and the parenchyma that occurs due to **peristasis** (alternation of stasis and reduced perfusion). It includes:

- Slowdown of the bloodstream.
- Discharge of erythrocytes and leukocytes.
- Proliferation of collagen fibers initiated by fibrocytes.
- Hypoplasia of the parenchyma cells.

The basis for this is a stimulus-dependent response of the interstitium and parenchyma during the slowdown in capillary blood flow and the resulting reduction in metabolism. Comparing the process that leads to tissue necrosis with the causes of tissue hypoplasia shows the same mechanism, only differing in strength. The clinical result of peristasis **in the transition to necrosis** is degeneration. The clinical result of pure peristasis can be described with the clinical term **involution**.

Other changes in the different tissues that are dependent on peristasis are:

- Formation of granulation tissue (e.g., after an injury).
- Hyperplasia of the nonparenchymal epithelium (e.g., gland ducts of the gastrointestinal tract and urogenital tract).
- Hyperplasia of the epithelium forming on the skin surface (e.g., in chronic inflammation).

Again, the cause can be found in the microcirculation, which fluctuates in peristasis (chronic hypoxia) between weak hyperemia and hyphemia. Permanent hyperemia results in hyperplasia (e.g., adenoma) and hyphemia results in hypoplasia of the tissue (atrophy).

4.3 Ricker's Three Stage Laws

In Ricker's observed responses of the interstitium and the connected tissue, the changes emanating from stimulation of the sympathetic nervous system range from necrosis to hyperplasia, from degeneration to regeneration, and from slight to abscess-forming necrotizing inflammation. In the three stage laws which are outlined below, Ricker described the classification of the reaction of the tissue to be supplied, which starts with pathological stimulation of the perivascular sympathetic nervous system and runs through the vascular system, the blood, and the interstitium.

The three stage laws originated from the microscopic observation of the vascular system before and in the capillary final pathway after stimulus of the perivascular sympathetic nervous system of variable strength and duration. They consist of three stages:

- **First stage:** By exciting the dilators, weak stimuli cause general vascular dilation up to the capillary region with increased blood flow rate and resulting increased microcirculation. The mechanism of active vasodilation while retaining the function of the vasoconstrictors is unknown. With slight stimulation of vasodilators, the vascular process, which consists of interplay between dilation and constriction in a physiological resting state, is unilaterally changed in favor of dilation. Ricker called the result of this vascular reaction "**pathic fluxion**" (hyperfusion).
- **Second stage:** With excitation of the vasoconstrictors, moderate stimulation causes narrowing of the arteries and capillaries from the stimulus site toward the periphery. This results in a **slowdown of blood flow** in the arterial, capillary, and venous branch; stronger stimulus results in occlusion of the arteries and capillaries with **stasis of the arteriovenous blood flow**. Hypoperfusion to ischemia of the tissue to be supplied can occur. The circulation normalizes completely upon termination of the stimulus. Increased cell or plasma discharge is not observed.
- **Third stage:** At the stimulus site, strong stimulus of the perivascular sympathetic nervous system directs the activity of the vasoconstrictors **toward the periphery**; they cannot be stimulated by adrenaline.

Vasodilators that remain excitable for longer periods cause initial vascular dilation until these are also unable to be reached through strong stimul. The continued strong stimulation eventually leads to further progressive vasoconstriction from the site of stimulation proximally by stimulation of the vasoconstrictors (reflexive stimulation flow through the afferent branch). After initial blood flow acceleration, there is a continued slowdown of the blood column up to stasis in the dilated capillaries. The condition before cessation of the bloodstream is called "**prestasis**" and the cessation of the bloodstream is known as "**stasis**"; the condition that comes about after the removal or reduction of the stimulus and enables the blood to flow again is "**poststasis.**" The condition of the bloodstream in pre- and poststasis was named "peristasis" by Ricker (see above).

Weak leukodiapedesis occurs during prestasis, followed by plasma discharge from the capillaries and erythrodiapedesis. In principle, the poststatic state is similar to prestasis; however, the leukodiapedesis is more pronounced in poststasis. The longer the stasis between pre- and poststasis, the more pronounced the leukodiapedesis, which corresponds to the clinical findings of "pus." The result of permanent stasis is tissue necrosis. The first and the second stage are also found in poststasis, i.e., ischemia and fluctuation, partly fleeting or even more pronounced depending on the regression of the strong stimulus leading to stasis. A strong stimulus which triggers the third stage as a result of the stimulus causes a change in the stimulus threshold in terms of sensitization in the sympathetic nervous system.

Note

After a very strong stimulus, the excitability of the sympathetic nervous system does not completely normalize despite the cessation of the stimulus.

This permanently increased excitability (low stimulus threshold, "engrammation," neuroplasticity) of the perivascular sympathetic nervous system leads to a **pathological reaction** with all subsequent consequences to the vasculature, interstitium, and the tissue to be supplied, even with physiological impulse strength.

4.4 Pathology of Relations and Neural Therapy

The experimentally verified evidence that the autonomic nervous system (p. 6), specifically the sympathetic nervous system, is involved first chronologically in every pathophysiological process as a stimulus-conducting, regulative nervous system is the basis of pathology of relations. Ricker thus achieved a clinically applicable scientific statement which resulted in the three stage laws (p. 21). Precise microscopic studies of living animals provided a clear description of the dynamic process after stimulation of the sympathetic nervous system, with all sequelae of the subordinate structures up to the organ or tissue section whose pathological changes lead to the diverse symptoms of disease. At the same time, the function of the sympathetic nervous system as well as its special response to different stimuli could be defined on the basis of in vivo studies. Thus, in many cases the causal relationships of an illness were understandable by way of a unique pathophysiological sequence.

In theory, when summing up Ricker's scientifically derived results while seeking a logical therapeutic concept for applied medicine, this would result in the usage of local anesthetics for therapeutic purposes. This can be found in Huneke's neural therapy concept whose basic principle involves the interruption of pathological stimulus of the sympathetic nervous system, resulting in normalization of its function. The pathological sequelae from the stimulus are removed and the stimulus that initiated the pathophysiological sequence is broken down.

Impressive, but not unique in medicine, is the fact that neural therapy is a purely empirical method that gradually developed from pure observation in working with local anesthetics in clinical experiments, initially without any scientific basis. This, in turn, was concluded by Ricker independently of the development of neural therapy in the form of his pathology of relations. The experience gained through the therapeutic use of local anesthetics corresponds with the experimental findings down to the last detail. Thus, both pathology of relations and the therapeutic concept of neural therapy are clinically confirmed with a scientific basis.

5 Functional Aspects of the Autonomic Nervous System

5.1 Introduction

Two observations, which must be fundamentally distinguished from one another, paved the way for local anesthesia and neural therapy. First, reversible local pain relief was achieved by infiltration of a local anesthetic that was used for surgical procedures. Furthermore, local infiltration of a local anesthetic in an already-painful area of tissue often—but not always—relieved pain lasting far beyond the anesthesia time, the duration of which could be increased with repeated injections until full pain relief was obtained. Thus, from these obervations developed the present form of local anesthesia on the one hand and neural therapy on the other.

In the following, the fundamentals of neural therapy are presented through primary consideration of the autonomic nervous system and based on clinical and experimental studies. In attempting to categorize the first neural therapeutic observations, definite parallels to older forms of treatment can be found. The first neural therapeutic observations of "segmental therapy" were quite similar to the results of locally applied physiotherapy, e.g., massage, application of heat or cold, osteopathic treatment, or other stimulus treatment. For example, painful locally strained back muscles are often successfully treated with repeated use of physiotherapy techniques as well as with neural therapy. The muscles regain a normal state of tension, functional limitations disappear, and pain subsides. Clearly, the body responds uniformly despite the use of different methods. It is worth analyzing this situation in order to identify similarities and functional relationships that lead to normalization. At the same time, this may explain how it is possible that an abundance of very different diseases can be treated with neural therapy. The different diseases are clearly based on a fundamental, identical pathological mechanism.

In the complexity of the connections between the somatic and autonomic nervous systems, the afferent–efferent feedback forms the theoretical basis for the generation of **pain** (particularly chronic), the progression of **inflammation**, the emergence of **degenerative diseases**, and the occurrence of "**allergies**." Depending on which tissue is involved, different diseases with different subjective symptoms (e.g., pain) and objective symptoms (muscle spasms, inflammation, degeneration, metaplasia, hyperplasia) may occur. The common feature of these diseases is secondary disruption of the microcirculation after pathological stimulation of the autonomic nervous system.

Jänig showed the complex effect of pathological stimulation of the sympathetic nervous system, especially in pain physiology.[243] The memory of pain, neuroplasticity with a change in the stimulus conduction and pathways, as well as the functional storage of repetitive stimuli through flexible synapse formation and altered neurotransmitter profiles of different neurons, are an extension of Ricker's local observations, which are also reflected in the pathogenesis of inflammatory or degenerative diseases.[425]

Immunohistochemical studies and tracer-based representations of the autonomic end formation show the modulatory activity of the autonomic nervous system not only in neuronal tissue with the clinical outcome of "pain," but also in **fibrocytes**, in the **monocyte–macrophage system**, and in **mast cells** for the modulation of the immune system (**neuroimmunology**).[428] The pathological stimulus of the sympathetic nervous system initiates a change in the expression of immune-modulating substances of immunocompetent cells. These relationships can be found in the skin and the mucous membranes (Langerhans cells, dendritic cells), the Kupffer stellate cells of the liver, the alveolar macrophages, the surface cells of the synovial membrane, the osteoclasts, and the microglial cells of the brain. This clarifies the neural therapeutic access to the immune system via the modulation of the sympathetic and parasympathetic nervous system with simultaneous improvement of microcirculation in each.

With these innervation relationships, it is possible to present the etiology of various diseases with major involvement of the autonomic nervous system. The existing knowledge of the complex function of the autonomic nervous system is sufficient to classify clinical experiences in neural therapy, obtained empirically, as realistic to provide a scientific theoretical basis and at the same time answer the question of how it is possible to treat different disorders with neural therapy.

The concept of neural therapy, which arose and arises from the detailed observation of patients is continuously validated through clinical experience in various medical specialties. Its neurophysiological basis, logical mechanism of action, and over 80 years of medical practice should be made available to students through academic teaching at university.

5.2 Reaction and Function of the Sympathetic Nervous System

Ricker's microscopic studies in vivo discovered a number of pathological changes in the capillary final pathway, i.e., the interstitial regulation system, that were already known to static pathology, but not as causative components. Edema, leukodiapedesis, and erythrodiapedesis, i.e., the "inflammation" caused by ischemia and stasis, microscopic findings of high clinical relevance, could only be generated individually and repeatably through the gradual stimulation of the perivascular sympathetic nervous system. With the different responses of the vasculature through narrowing and expansion and the resulting change in capillary perfusion, these pathological reactions in the terminal vessels eventually lead to the pathological findings in the organ and the resulting clinically emergent diseases. Ricker emphasized the value of the sympathetic nervous system in the general pathological process, in particular, inflammation and degeneration, and thereby also in the occurrence of pain and allergies.[425]

Note

In its sole function of stimulus conduction and transmitter secretion, the sympathetic nervous system in a pathological state is capable—depending on the strength of the stimulus—of initiating and maintaining different "diseases" through the modulation of capillary perfusion.

In this case, the stimuli may be intrinsic or may come from the environment. The strength of the sympathetic stimulation is dependent on the strength of the stimulus, the sensitivity which is individually variable in humans, and the site of the stimulation. The same stimulus intensity leads to increasingly severe stimulus going from central to peripheral direction.

The sequence of stimulus and stimulus sequelae are as follows:

1. A stimulus occurs.
2. The sympathetic nervous system is stimulated and the stimulus is transmitted directionally along the efferent and afferent pathways.
3. The result of stimulus at the capillary end formation is increased or decreased interstitial perfusion and microcirculation.
4. Finally, with persistent pathological stimulus via the interstitium, there is a pathological response in the connected tissue and, at the same time, a change in the afferent feedback.

These four general steps are the basis of Ricker's three stage laws. Depending on the involved tissue, the following may occur: pain disorders (e.g., headache, joint pain, lower back pain), chronic inflammation with gradual tissue degeneration (e.g., chronic hepatitis with cirrhosis), and chronic mucosal inflammation (arthritis). The pathophysiological changes in the terminal vessels observed by Ricker enable a better understanding of the etiology of "healthy" and "sick."

With "pathology of relations" (p. 17), Ricker created the basis for the pathophysiology of the interstitium and thus the scientific basis of neural therapy. The multidisciplinary, relational diagnostic and therapeutic use of local anesthetics, which is based on the therapeutic use of the properties and functions of the autonomic nervous system, has a clear background in pathology of relations. It is an experimentally verified knowledge base of interstitial pathophysiology, which was clarified about 30 years later by Pischinger's elucidation of the interstitial regulation system (p. 13).

5.3 Therapeutic Use of the Sympathetic Nervous System

The comprehensive view of Ricker's pathology of relations (p. 17) and Pischinger's interstitial regulation system (p. 13) enables the recognition of new, diagnostically and therapeutically relevant functional aspects of the autonomic nervous system.

Limited by its **ubiquitous distribution**, the sympathetic nervous system is the only information system pervading the whole body. It regulates organ function via physiological feedback loops, thus ensuring appropriate adjustment for maximal efficiency. The parasympathetic nervous system is the antagonist in the head region, the neck, and the torso organs, and ensures ACh (acetylcholine)- and VIP (vasoactive intestinal peptide)-induced vasodilation in the case of stimulus, thus increasing the microcirculation.[428] This enables consistent diagnostic and therapeutic access through local application of a local anesthetic by access at any point on the body.

Note

The application of a local anesthetic has a dampening effect in the case of pathologically increased sympathetic activity and thus promotes the mechanisms of autoregulation.

The sympathetic nervous system essentially has two tasks: the control of circulation and the indirect influence on the organ systems via the interstitium. The therapeutic use of a local anesthetic is performed accordingly for:

- Normalization of circulation.
- Normalization of the interstitial regulation system functions.
- Normalization (indirect) of organ function.

The resting state of the terminal vessels consists of ongoing, slightly changing, vascular narrowing and expansion. Microcirculation oscillates between a slight increase and decrease and changes in favor of hyperemia under conditions of stress.

The many changes and processes in the terminal vessels are also a result of stimulation of the perivascular sympathetic nervous system. The result of the stimulus is not dependent on the type of stimulus (physical stimulus or chemical stimulus), but on the amount of stimulus and duration of its effect. The local application of a local anesthetic at the site of stimulation reliably interrupts stimulation of the sympathetic nervous system temporarily, regardless of the type of stimulus and the duration of its effect, resulting in an improvement in the microcirculation of the affected tissue (reset, therapeutic effect) beyond the local anesthetic's period of activity. The application of a local anesthetic before positing of the stimulus also prevents the occurrence of a stimulus, regardless of the stimulus quality and intensity (prophylactic effect).

Thus, the clinical outcome is the disruption of stimulation effects in the interstitium and the organ tissue, or the prevention of stimulus propagation. These effects include inflammation, pain, degeneration to necrosis, hyperplasia, and hypoplasia.

Depending on the clinical findings, examples of the local anesthetic effect are:

- Antiphlogistic.
- Analgesic.
- Anti-inflammatory.
- Antiallergic.
- Antihistaminic.
- Antipyretic.
- Antiarrhythmic.
- Spasmolytic.
- Regenerative.

Also important is the possibility of permanent stimulation of the perivascular sympathetic nervous system by temporally limited stimulation. After removal of the stimulus, the effects of the stimulus gradually normalize up to a return to original condition. However, one-time stimulus can certainly lead to a "sensitization" of the perivascular sympathetic nervous system with a lowering of the threshold and a stronger stimulus response with a new stimulus.[425] Very strong stimulus as well as the multiple repetition of a strong pathological stimulus can lead to an engrammatic lowering of the threshold of the perivascular sympathetic nervous system, which prevents restoration to original condition via autoregulation. The clinical corollary is chronic disease.

In turn, this stimulus sequence can be interrupted by the repeated local application of a local anesthetic at the site of stimulation. Similar to the way that repeated stimulus leads to engrammatic change in the stimulus capacity or sensitization of the sympathetic nervous system, repeated application of the local anesthetic can reverse this engrammatic change and remove the sensitization. The same stimulus intensity generates a qualitatively equal stimulus response in the supply area of the corresponding sympathetic section, whereby peripheral stimulus induces a stronger stimulus response than centrally located stimulus, which is weaker and broader in its stimulus effect.

Practical Advice

The localization of the application of the local anesthetic is crucial for therapeutic success. Whenever possible, it should take place at the primary site of stimulus in order to achieve therapeutic efficacy (note: segmental or interference field disease). If the application does not take place there, transient sympatholysis occurs only for the duration of the local anesthetic's effect, with little or no therapeutic success.

In interference field diseases (primary stimulus not in the disease area), after the drug effect subsides the application acts as an additional stimulus, which triggers intensification of the stimulus sequence through summation. The clinical result is the transitory exacerbation of pain symptoms that regress only back to baseline after removal of the additional "iatrogenic" stimulus from the injection. More details on this can be found in the section "Reaction Phenomenon according to Hopfer" (p. 98). Lastly, it can be established that stimulus of the perivascular sympathetic nervous system is transmitted from the site of stimulation on efferent pathways to the periphery and on afferent pathways toward the center. Through the sympathetic conduction arc, the afferent conduction path also leads to excitation of the efferent sympathetic nervous system proximal to the site of stimulus. Especially with prolonged stimulation, this leads to similar reactions of the vascular system, the interstitium, and the organ cells also proximal to the stimulation site, all structures involved such as CRPS (p. 8), chronic pain maintained solely by the sympathetic nervous system, and the quadrant syndrome.

The stimulus conducted via the sympathetic afferent pathway reaches the nucleic regions of the sympathetic nervous system, where it excites autonomic efferents and can lead to homolateral autonomic "exposure."[34,36,400,473,475] Additional or already existing stimuli in the area of this homolateral stimulated region can trigger a disproportionately strong reaction at any location in the sympathetic nervous system, the interstitium, and the organs, as seen clinically in a focal disease. This form of chronic illness is known as "**focal disease**" or "**interference field disease**," a chronic pathologically stimulated condition caused by local stimulation of the afferent sympathetic nervous system (interference field: e.g., teeth, tonsils) ipsilateral to the efferent sympathetic nervous system. The targeted and generally repeated application of a local anesthetic into this site of first stimulation (interference field) reliably interrupts the chronic disease process and leads to the normalization of the "half-side exposure."

The sympathetic nervous system function is the common basis of empirically based therapies such as massage, osteopathy, acupuncture, hydrotherapy, and neural therapy, which can cause the same medical conditions to subside. The methods differ only in the fact that, in the physiotherapeutic method, a low stimulus enables the first stage of Ricker's three stage laws (p. 21) to be reached, which he described as "pathic fluctuation," and corresponds to improved microcirculation according to the current viewpoint, while neural therapy also triggers the elimination of pathologic afferent/efferent feedback with the help of a local anesthetic in addition to the stimulus from the needlestick.

The pathological sympathetic function becomes particularly evident when the local sympathetic stimulation is interrupted in the case of interference field diseases. Here, the neural therapeutic infiltration of the interference field causes local medicinal interruption of the afferent pathological impulse emission of the sympathetic nervous system and thus the efferent pathological effect on other organs or organ systems. Furthermore, local efferent-oriented sympathicolysis leads to improved microcirculation in the area of the interference field and thus often to sustained relief of the stimulus. Re-infiltration of the interference field can often sustainably remove the effect of the interference field over the entire body.

Taking into consideration the sympathetic nervous system activity, neural therapy makes it possible to pursue multidisciplinary or—even better, converging—diagnostics and treatment, which counteracts the divergent trend of highly specialized medicine and its increasing difficulty of interdisciplinary communication. At the same time, the basic research of Ricker[425] and Jänig[243] provides an understanding of the concept of "regulatory medicine." If it were common knowledge, pathology of relations could help to ensure that knowledge of diseases in human medicine, which is always becoming more detailed, would have a common base and logical synthesis in the analytical pursuit.

Conclusion

In summary, neural therapy is a method that can be used in almost all fields of medicine. The range of indications for neural therapy is oriented not only toward specialist diagnoses, but also more extensively to higher-level general neurophysiological mechanisms of the particular disease and therefore covers diseases from the areas of inflammation, degeneration, allergies, pain disorders, and functional disorders. The mechanism of action is causal, in any case, which means that the disease is terminated by the organism itself via autonomic autoregulation. Neural therapy only induces the "healing process."

6 Concept of the Segment in Neural Therapy

6.1 Definition

What constitutes a segment is oriented by the somatic nervous system. For example, the assignment of defined areas of the skin for segmental division of the spinal cord is used clinically to identify the corresponding somatosensory segmental portion of the spinal cord through the skin in the case of interrupted somatic sensitivity. However, only a portion of the segment is detected in this way. If one imagines cutting a segment slice from the spinal cord and looks at the incoming and outgoing peripheral nervous system structures according to their system affiliation, this comes close to the actual definition of segment. Viewed functionally, the segment includes not only the sensory-motor system, which is also summarized as an oikotropic nervous system, but also an autonomic component system component at the spinal level, which is also referred to as an idiotropic nervous system and is represented by the sympathetic nervous system in segments C8–L2 and to a smaller extent by the parasympathetic nervous system in segments S2–S4.

Particularly under consideration of the peripherally ubiquitous distribution of the sympathetic nervous system, which is more extensive than that of the entire oikotropic nervous system, and incorporating the efferent and afferent pathways, the definition of the segment completely changes, in part via a supply system covering several spinal segments. The actual segmental association is lost and is augmented by organ areas that are not sharply defined in the region of the head, trunk, and extremities. This divergent distribution of the sympathetic nervous system through the afferent pathway on the spinal level has a segment-oriented structure, to the extent that the sympathetic nervous system is closely linked synaptically with the conduction arc of the oikotropic nervous system and thus can be functionally fenced in again segmentally.

Clinically relevant examples in the segmental neural connection of the sympathetic nervous system with the somatic nervous system can be found in the systemized observations of the English neurologist **Head**, who identified **hyperesthetic** or **hyperalgesic skin zones** associated with diseases of internal organs. These skin zones correspond to the segment-associated dermatomes that result from stimulation of the afferent sympathetic nervous system in the case of an "internal disorder," which leads to a simultaneous stimulation of the somatosensory system at the segment level that is responsible for the sympathetic supply of the corresponding internal organ. With this viscerocutaneous reflex, the spinal-segmental supply of the organs by the sympathetic nervous system can be more precisely defined.

The observation of the Scottish surgeon **Mackenzie** of **segment-related muscle guarding** in organ diseases has the same neurological background, whereby in this case the connection between the sympathetic and somatomotor system is clinically demonstrated. Since conduction arcs principally consist of supplying (afferent) and discharging (efferent) neurons that are synaptically connected with one another, stimulation of one neuron leads to simultaneous stimulation of the other. Both facilitative and inhibitory influences on the stimulated neurons are possible in the feedback loop, whereby the principle of the conduction arc is not interrupted. From a cybernetic perspective, this lays the foundation for a **feedback loop**. The stimulus is received via specific receptors, routed via the afferent neuron to the efferent neuron, and then moves from here to the target organ. In turn, the change in the capacity of the target organ is "reported" to the efferent neuron by the afferent neuron via specific receptors in a feedback process. This circular communication of information is necessary in order to maintain the specified target values in their tolerance ranges, in balance with the permanently changing actual values.

6.2 Therapeutic Implications

The systematized observations by Head and Mackenzie are understandable through direct or indirect synaptic connections of different afferent neurons of the somatic and autonomic nervous systems with the efferent neurons of the same systems under the condition of the neural conduction arc. The observations which represent the response of the somatosensory nervous system after stimulation of the autonomic nervous system not only have diagnostic value, but also may—in the reverse order—be used for treatment via the direct or indirect reflex pathway.

Note

A therapeutic effect on internal organs is also possible via targeted, dosed stimulus in the same way that treatment of the organs via the autonomic system can eliminate a pathological finding in the somatosensory system.

Physical therapy methods that perform mechanical, thermal, or electrical stimulation successfully use these mixed conduction arcs for therapeutic purposes. The use of these methods is older than our knowledge of the peripheral nervous system, and much older than the discovery of the autonomic nervous system. In this way, for example, the concept of the cutivisceral reflex originated. The expansion of the therapeutically utilizable reflex pathways gave rise to the terms osteovisceral or myovisceral reflex or explained the treatment path of osteopathy on the fascia accompanying the autonomic nerves, depending on which anatomical structure has a therapeutic effect on internal organs via the segmental-reflexive pathway. Neural therapeutic injection includes both the somatic and the autonomic reflex arc.

However, according to current knowledge, the therapeutically relevant portion is the autonomic reflex arc, since the skin, periosteum, fascia, and muscles are innervated via the afferent and efferent pathways of the sympathetic nervous system like the internal organs.

The segment formulated for neural therapeutic purposes is based primarily on the distribution modalities of the sympathetic nervous system. Spinal-segmental association is possible through the synaptic connections to the somatosensory and somatomotor systems. In the case of spinal root stimulation in the L5 segment, the entire neural segment including the sympathetic nervous system is stimulated, with the possible consequence of a perfusion change in the tissue parts belonging to this segment, including the somatosensory and somatomotor nerves. Segmental identification of irritation is possible by way of the clinical symptoms of somatic nerve irritation. If a local anesthetic is infiltrated at the level of the spinal ganglion, there is immediate improvement or normalization of perfusion of the ganglion as well as the segmental efferents in addition to the interruption of somatic afferents (dorsal root ganglion) and motor efferents (anterior root) via sympatholysis. Clinically, this normalization expresses itself in the cessation of pain beyond the effect of the local anesthetic due to sympatholysis and normalization of perfusion. This neurophysiological process takes place when the sympathetic stimulation is primarily in the corresponding spinal segment, e.g., in the form of a degenerative disk disease. If the stimulus is not primarily at the level of the spinal segment, but outside of this segment, the stimulation of the sympathetic nervous system is elsewhere (interference field), e.g., in the teeth, and the infiltration of the local anesthetic at the level of the spinal segment results in only short-term normalization of symptoms for the length of the anesthesia time. In this case, sympatholysis in the teeth is necessary to resolve the sympathetic nervous system–induced pain in the segment (interference field therapy).

Evidence of the interference primarily carried out via the sympathetic stimulation is provided by the fact that a local anesthetic is used (e.g., procaine 1%), which has little influence on the somatic nervous system because of its weak effect, but which can interrupt the less isolated and therefore more sensitive sympathetic nervous system in its stimulation. Clinically, after infiltration, there is no anesthesia or motor paralysis in segment L5, but only a feeling of warmth due to hyperemia.

Neural diagnostics uses both the comprehensible systematics of somatosensitivity and the well-known subdivision of the sympathetic nervous system to the spinal level in order to locate the suspected organ-related interference in sympathetic nervous system function. All of the structures that are supplied by the sympathetic nervous system are used in applying the therapy. These include:

- Skin.
- Subcutaneous tissue.
- Musculature.
- Tendons.
- Ligaments.
- Capsular tissue.
- Periosteum.
- Pleura.
- Peritoneum.
- Peridural space.
- Peripheral nerves.
- Vascular system.
- Sympathetic and parasympathetic ganglia.

Via these structures, the organs can be reached directly or indirectly on the reflex pathways.

In addition to the classical component, the **segment concept** employed in neural therapy includes the autonomic component which is responsible for regulating the supply of all tissues, including the peripheral nerves (vasa nervorum), the ganglia (vasa ganglionares), and spinal cord.

The connections of different cranial nerve nuclei with each other and at the spinal level in the upper cervical spinal cord with the spinal nucleic regions of the trigeminal nerve and accessory nerve sensorimotor systems must be repeatedly mentioned. This results in segmental disease relationships that are rediscovered clinically through a "mixed" segment-reflexive function and can result in very diverse symptoms that explain "interference field disease" along with the function of the sympathetic nervous system. These include connections of the trigeminal nerve spinal nucleic regions with those of the facial nerve, glossopharyngeal nerve, accessory nerve, and phrenic nerve, and the afferent connections of the vagus nerve to the spinal nucleic regions of the trigeminal nerve, which in turn connect to the upper three sensorimotor cervical segments. This explains the variety of possible segmental reflex symptoms which take place due to a solitary disease in the supplied area of one of the aforementioned nerves. The simultaneous supply of all aforementioned structures by the sympathetic nervous system clarifies the concept of the interference field as a superordinate segmental-reflexive occurrence.

7 Theory and Basic Principles of the Interference Field

7.1 Introduction

The historical concept of the interference field comes from its effect on the organism and is confirmed by the reproducible phenomenon taking place in which a remotely located disease completely subsides—at first temporarily—after infiltration of the interference field with a local anesthetic.[14,102,107,173,236,238,272,383,458,461,509] Upon recurrence of the disease symptoms, the symptom-free period increases with each repetition of the interference field infiltration until the patient is ultimately free of symptoms. The following shows the neuroanatomical and neurophysiological foundations that present the existence of the interference field in an understandable manner.

7.1.1 Stimulus and the Sympathetic Nervous System

After the speed with which this "lightning reaction" (p. 3) takes place, the sympathetic nervous system immediately comes to mind as the transmitter of the disease, since it is the only nervous system that has a ubiquitous distribution and its function is the afferent and efferent supply to each tissue. In physiological and pathophysiological terms, this enables informative connection in the entire organism.

Definition

Interference Field

The interference field is any tissue section with sympathetic innervation, whereby the afferent of this tissue section is in a pathological, chronic state of stimulus and initiates or maintains a generally chronic illness at another site via the distribution system of the sympathetic nervous system.

The regional pathological stimulation of the sympathetic **afferents** in the interference field reaches the sympathetic and somatic efferents continuously with the vessels, partially with the spinal nerves and dorsal root ganglia and eventually via the switch in the posterior horn. Via the sympathetic **efferents**, a sustained pathological tissue reaction is triggered that reverts into the periphery through perfusion failure (segment reflex). Through the converging afferent and divergent efferent distribution of the sympathetic nervous system, "cross-segmental" diseases can be induced. An involvement of the reticular formation of the hindbrain and midbrain, which is superordinate to the spinal system, is quite possible with their effects on organs and organ systems and their function.[429] Last but not least, pathological effects on a diencephalic level, i.e., in the region of the hypothalamus, are conceivable in terms of interlocking systems that control the water balance or regulate the hormonal balance, for example, pathological effects on the brain stem, hypothalamus, thalamus, and cerebrum are also possible.

The pathological stimulation of the sympathetic afferent of the interference field can be caused by a persistent irritation after a previous injury or illness (accident, surgery, infection, etc.) with subsequent local "silent inflammation" (with and without a foreign body) or by continuing increased stimulus of the afferent without persistent irritation through the above-described engrammation, a special feature of the sympathetic nervous system after strong stimulus. Thus, each inherently physiological efferent stimulus leads to a pathological afferent feedback reaction.

Note

The interference field is often clinically asymptomatic, suggesting a subliminal stimulation of the sympathetic nervous system. This means that the chronicity of the stimulus, and not the strength, is the more important criterion of the interference field.

Thus, an otherwise symptom-free scar can be painful, itchy, or become red or swollen when the weather changes, in stressful situations, or by selective stimulation. An infected tooth which normally does not cause symptoms can become painful during a common cold, sudden mechanical stress, or after treatment of another tooth. In these cases, the sum of the additional stimuli leads to above-threshold stimulation of the interference field with the corresponding symptomatology. This process applies to both potential and manifested interference fields. Due to increasingly better understanding of the complex neuroanatomical cross-segmental connections of the sympathetic nervous system to the somatic nervous system and the detailed knowledge of the neurophysiology of the autonomic nervous system, the interference field can become more "demystified" and explained scientifically.

Clinical observations have shown that a significant proportion of interference fields can be found in the innervation area of the trigeminal nerve and vagus nerve (teeth, tonsils, nasal sinuses, gastrointestinal tract, internal genitalia) and that it is crucial to consider the full innervation of an interference field.

The nucleic regions of the trigeminal nerve reach to the spinal segments C3 in the cervical spinal cord, so that with chronic afferent stimulation of the sympathetic trigeminally supplied tissue (e.g., in periodontitis, impacted teeth, chronic sinusitis) a reflex response in the sensorimotor section C1–C3 is also expected. Muscular tension of the upper cervical spine with consequences such as headaches and neck pain is possible, as well as improper strain of the whole spine over muscle chains with corresponding clinical symptoms at remote areas (e.g., lumbar spine, sacroiliac joint).

Disorders of the masticatory muscles (myoarthropathy of the masticatory system) are quite explainable due to sinus or tooth infections (periodontitis, chronic sinusitis), since the afferent trigeminal nerve in the pathological state of irritation leads to a change in potential of the trigeminal-innervated masticatory muscles. Bite correction by occlusal splints is understandable from an orthodontic point of view, but is not a causal therapy.

The connections of the trigeminal nucleic region with the facial nerve (the trigeminal nerve is afferent of the facial nerve), glossopharyngeal nerve, and accessory nerve (C1–C5/C6) significantly extend the clinically emergent interference field disorders via the "segmental reflex system" and paint a diverse picture of most chronic diseases in the area of the mutually corresponding cranial nerves.

Chronic irritation of the intestines, e.g., arising from food allergies, dysbiosis, or after gastrointestinal infections, is likewise responsible for the afferent stimulation of the trigeminal nucleic regions in the cervical cord via the afferents of the vagus nerve and then with corresponding clinically relevant chronic symptoms of the supply region of the trigeminal nerve (e.g., tooth/jaw discomfort, nasal sinus problems, atypical facial pain, headache), the glossopharyngeal nerve (e.g., chronic symptoms of Waldeyer's tonsillar ring, the pharyngeal muscles, neuralgia of the glossopharyngeal nerve), and the accessory nerve (trapezius and sternocleidomastoid muscle tension).

The sympathetic innervation in the supply region of the above-described nerves is involved in each case and represents the afferent "input" that affects the above-described change in the microcirculation of the corresponding tissue components via the sympathetic conduction arc including the somatic nervous tissue (e.g., ganglia, spinal cord). The reflexive symptoms emanating from the sympathetic nervous system and somatic nervous system represent the **interference field disorder**. The interference field disorder, depending on the position of the interference field, in many cases is shown to be a segmental-reflexive occurrence upon closer examination of the innervation relationship, always with the involvement of the "cross-segmental" sympathetic nervous system arising from the segmental concept.

The theory of the interference field derived from clinical experience finds its experimental basis in the extensive animal testing by Ricker, which showed that a one-time stimulation of the sympathetic nervous system can lead to a permanent increase in the excitability of the efferents (vasomotor) (e.g., chronic sinusitis, irritable colon). Each physiological stimulus leads to a pathological stimulus response. This experimentally observed phenomenon corresponds perfectly with the clinical observation of the properties of an interference field.

7.1.2 Causes of Chronic Irritation, Neuroplasticity

Irritation caused by the chronic regional stimulation of the sympathetic afferents of an interference field is nonspecific and can consist of many different factors. Clinically, it has been shown that an interference field effect can emanate from any disease, any kind of injury, or generally from any chronic irritation of the afferent sympathetic nervous system beyond the physiological strength of the irritation. Kellner microscopically examined scar tissue which was excised after it had been identified as an interference field for another disease through the neural therapeutic infiltration of a local anesthetic.[268] In addition to the altered content of collagen fibers, he found nonspecific inflammation foci at organic or inorganic inclusions and some foreign bodies, e.g., talc crystals. This indicated the possible substrate of a chronic irritation.

Also taking into account the possibility of ephapse formation, i.e., the traumatically induced pathological stimulus transmission of different axons among themselves, as occurs in injuries involving the peripheral nervous system, makes pathological stimulus even more tangible. Similar conditions can also occur after severe inflammatory, bacterial, or viral diseases or diseases caused by other toxicants associated with partial tissue destruction, reactive inflammation, and thus scar formation.

In any case, there is a permanent change in the interstitial regulation system and thus the terminal vessels in the sympathetic end formation. The slight irritability of the sympathetic nervous system, which consists of nonmyelinated, poorly insulated C-fibers in its end formation, certainly plays a fundamental role.

7.1.3 Stimulus Interruption—Turning Off the Interference Field

With lightning reactions (p. 3), an interruption of the afferent sympathetic stimulation primarily takes place with clinical, repeatedly significant cessation of various remotely located symptoms. At the same time, however, a change in the substrate of the interference field itself must take place, which causes progressive reduction of the stimulus. Otherwise, increasingly longer cessation of the disorder induced by the interference field could not proceed.

Note

If the irritation cannot be abated, as in the case of a foreign body or a chronic bacterial infection of a tooth, even repeated neural therapeutic infiltration cannot lead to sustained cessation of the disorder induced by the interference field.

With repeated infiltration of procaine in an interference field, a "**hyperperfusion**" (mediated by diethyl aminoethanol), takes place in addition to the cell membrane stabilization (mediated by para-aminobenzoic acid). This process leads to the "**interference field elimination**" effect extending beyond the duration of the anesthesia. The production of inflammatory mediators is interrupted, the regeneration process is initiated (via fibroblasts, etc.), and the increased microcirculation improves the overall trophism and function of the interference field tissue. Thus, the afferent sympathetic input arising from the interference field is interrupted.

The fact that changes in the interference field actually take place is shown by keloid scars, for example, with a clinically proven interference field function, which change into nonirritated scars after repeated infiltration with a local anesthetic. Increased skin resistance of scars normalizes to standard values.[268,474] Elevated transaminases, caused by the liver acting as an interference field in the case of chronic hepatitis, normalize after repeated injection in the celiac ganglion. The same processes can be found in pathological tissue changes that have no interference field function. Normalization of inflamed tissue was also one of the first observations on the therapeutic use of local anesthetics, at a time when the existence of the interference field was still unknown.[470] Cases in which a remotely located chronic disorder was sustainably eliminated only after surgical removal of the interference field (scar, tooth, tonsils, appendix, etc.), after prior neural therapeutic infiltration resulted in only short-term success, prove the neurophysiological value of interference field tissue.

7.2 Pathogenesis of the Interference Field

In considering the origin of the interference field, further clinical observations can be detailed in addition to those previously mentioned, as follows.

7.2.1 Temporal Relationships

Note

The temporal relationships between the emergence of the interference field and the resulting disorder are highly variable.

The medical history of a patient showed that discomfort in the shoulder joint occurred immediately after dental treatment; however, the history of another patient with the same symptomatology showed no temporal link with another injury or illness. With this patient, the tonsillectomy scars, for example, were revealed to be the interference field by way of the lightning reaction (p. 3), whereby the tonsillectomy took place 40 years before the start of the shoulder joint pain.

The origin of the interference field can be easily explained in the first case: the irritation resulting from the dental treatment leads via the afferent sympathetic nervous system to a segmental pathological stimulation of the efferent sympathetic nervous system, resulting in a disturbance of the trophism of the shoulder joint, which appears clinically as a painful shoulder joint disorder. In the second case, the interference field effect probably existed for a long time, but was tolerated by the body.

The pathological impulse emission of the afferent sympathetic nerve system from the area of the tonsillectomy scar could therefore be compensable over a long period. It is quite conceivable that with increasing age, the compensability of pathological impulse emissions of the sympathetic nervous system gradually decreases and thus interference fields start to have a pathological effect, in the same way that all organ systems develop performance limitations with increasing age.

Note

"Stresses" to the body (heavy metal pollution, dietary chemical exposure, deficiency diseases, mental stress) are quite capable of promoting an interference field.[134]

In this case as well, an individually variable, age-dependent regressive development is likely.

7.2.2 Emergence of an Interference Field

The emergence of an interference field after injury or disease is never obligatory. The majority of injuries or illnesses heal without consequences to the sympathetic nervous system. From clinical observation, however, it is clear that some characteristics of the progression of an illness contribute to the development of an interference field.

Note

As opposed to nonirritated clinical progression, a particularly lengthy or severe disease progression with complications more frequently leaves behind an interference field.

Complicated wound healing processes, particularly bacterial **infections of wounds**, **abscesses**, **boils**, **carbuncles**, and **phlegmons**, often leave behind a pathological afferent regional sympathetic stimulation, i.e., a potential interference field. It should never be assumed, however, that a "subclinical disease progression" or "minor injury" cannot also leave behind an interference field. According to current knowledge of the sympathetic nervous system, it can be assumed that this repeatedly clinically confirmed circumstance is dependent on the variably persistent stimulation of the sympathetic nervous system, whereby it appears that stimulation intensity and duration of the extent of the past injury or disease as well as the "healing ability" of the body are relevant.

Furthermore, only taking into account the autonomic nervous system, there are direct connections between the superior cervical ganglion responsible for the head and the parasympathetic inferior ganglion of the vagus nerve and the extracranial ganglion of the glossopharyngeal nerve over the jugular nerve. An interganglionic synaptic connection between the sympathetic nervous system and the vagus nerve or glossopharyngeal nerve is likely but not yet proven. With the sympathetic nucleic regions of the superior cervical ganglion—essentially responsible for the head—from spinal segments C8–T6/T7, there are synaptic connections to the corresponding sympathetic plexus of the chest and abdominal area, as well as to the strictly segmentally arranged sensorimotor nervous system.[69] Independent of the sympathetic supply, there are additional opportunities for an interference field through the cranial nerve supply to the indicated organ areas as well as through connections to the immune system, e.g., via the tonsils. The evidence of the interference field and the disease dependent on it is always linked to the "lightning reaction" (p. 3), i.e., to the reproducible clinical evidence of the abatement of a medical condition.

The interference field can still only be defined based on a few facts, for example, by the experiments of Ricker,[425] which illustrated the functional operation of the sympathetic nervous system and its properties (engrammation ability) and enable theoretical proof of the interference field through experiments or on the basis of investigations by Pischinger, Kellner, Stacher, Siegen, and Bergmann et al,[34,267,399,461,473] who provided histological, physiological, and clinically objectifiable findings with regard to the interference field and its effect. It should be noted that Ricker's investigations were conducted without knowledge of neural therapy and were not influenced by it. Direct evidence of the interference field, which demonstrates the theoretically required pathological impulse emission of the sympathetic nervous system from the interference field to the target organ, is still pending. However, this does not change the clinical relevance of the interference field. Currently, evidence of the interference field is only clinically possible by interrupting the pathological impulse emission by means of a local anesthetic and the reproducible reduction of the disease induced by the interference field.

7.3 Clinical Evidence of the Interference Field

Huneke emphasized the principle that any chronic disease **can** be induced by an interference field. Thus, the diagnosis of an interference field in chronic disease usually occurs after unsuccessful segmental treatment, which must not necessarily consist only of neural therapeutic measures (p. 81).

Due to the case history data, clinical examinations, and experience accumulated over more than 70 years, an individualized interference field test is performed on each patient. For this purpose, the suspected interference field is infiltrated with a local anesthetic. The cause of the disease is then clear if a fully fledged lightning reaction (p. 3) is triggered that can be reproduced with the same infiltration and if the symptom-free period is prolonged. The lightning reaction can be triggered solely by this one interference field. The infiltration of other suspected interference fields causes no lightning reaction, just as other forms of treatment which do not account for the responsible interference field are not successful. The measurement of the theoretically required, pathological sympathetic impulse emission in the interference field and at the "target organ," as well as their permanent normalization after infiltration of the interference field, would be the neurophysiological evidence of the interference field and its effect on the body. However, this is not yet possible with the currently available techniques.

The clinical evidence which is important for the therapy consists of controlling the elimination of a medical condition. The following are clinical parameters which can demonstrate the normalization of a previously interference field–induced disease:

- Sustained pain relief.
- Reduction and normalization of inflammatory tissue reactions macroscopically and via laboratory chemistry.
- Sustained normalization of tissue-specific enzyme levels in serum.
- Lack of allergic reactions to tested allergens.
- Cessation of radiologically controllable, progressive degenerative joint diseases and improvement in their function.
- Sustained normalization of hormone levels previously outside the norm.

7.4 Interference Field and Segmental Disease

7.4.1 Fluid Transition

As shown previously in this chapter (p. 29), without knowledge of the topography of the sympathetic nervous system and its function, acceptance of the interference field and its induced illness is difficult. This is demonstrated by numerous criticisms demanding the scientific evidence and rejecting the interference field phenomenon despite abundant evidence that is clinically reproducible. The farther the interference field is located from the secondary disease site, the less its existence is accepted. Initially confusing is the fact that, on the one hand, chronic illnesses can arise from completely different interference fields and, on the other hand, the same interference fields can initiate and maintain different illnesses in different patients. This lack of systematics, as well as the general possibility that a wide variety of chronic diseases from all fields of medicine can be induced by an interference field, seems implausible.

With special consideration of the sympathetic nervous system, an attempt will now be made to demonstrate the almost seamless transition from the generally accepted, segmental-reflexive disease to the interference field disease. The segment-based relationship between a dental disease and trigeminal neuralgia, neuralgia of the occipital nerve, or a functional disorder of the first three cervical neck segments is clear.[69] When considering the tooth-supplying trigeminal nerve, with its spinal nuclei reaching up to cervical segment C3, the disease correlation between the tooth and the trigeminal nerve or occipital nerve from spinal segments C1–C3 is understandable at first glance (segmental-reflexive system).

However, if the described medical condition originates from a surgically devitalized tooth (root canal treatment, root end surgery), which no longer has a connection to the trigeminal nerve, the sympathetic nervous system is the only remaining possible nerve connection. This supplies the tooth and periodontium, and proceeds along with the trigeminal nerve, the occipital nerves, the vessels accompanying these nerves, and the vasa nervorum, which are responsible for supplying the neurons. The afferent conduction pathway of the sympathetic nervous system responsible for the tooth now opens up completely new aspects of possible disease relationships. The sympathetic supply pathway of the **teeth** is afferent as well as efferent via the cervical sympathetic trunk as well as the corresponding sympathetic ganglia (superior cervical ganglion, stellate ganglion) whose nucleic regions are in segments C8–T7. The same nucleic regions are also the origin of the sympathetic fiber portions which course with the trigeminal nerve, occipital nerves, and the vessels supplying these structures.

Via the sympathetic conduction arc, with stimulus of the afferent branch by the focal tooth, there is possible efferent sympathetic stimulation of the upper cervical spinal cord with corresponding perfusion and therefore the participation of the nucleic regions of the trigeminal nerve, accessory nerve, glossopharyngeal nerve, and thus also the facial nerve and, last but not least, the vagus and occipital nerves.

If we include the vascular supply of the skull, the neck, and the thoracic space as well as the interganglionic connections of the sympathetic trunk when tracing the efferent pathological sympathetic activity, the initially described segmental-reflexive disease relationship is clearer and effectively shows the potential impact of a regional afferent sympathetic stimulation of the tooth/jaw region.

The parasympathetic supply to the brain vessels and arterial vessels of the facial bones for vasodilation with passage from the pterygopalatine ganglion should not be taken into account here.[74,490,491] The innervation relationships between the sympathetic and parasympathetic nervous systems may well play a role, e.g., in trigeminal autonomic head pain or circulation disorders of the brain, with preexisting chronic sinus disorder.

Looking at the wide supply area of the upper sympathetic nucleic regions between C8 and T7, there is a possible influence of the efferent sympathetic nervous system, starting from an infected tooth, the head, the neck, the upper extremities, the chest and abdominal cavity, and the lower extremities. The nucleic regions of the major splanchnic nerve supplying the abdomen start at T5 and, on the way to the celiac ganglion, generate numerous branches to the aortic plexus, which also supplies the vessels of the lower extremities.[69] In this regard, the infected tooth can become an interference field, even if the segmental-reflexive pathway between the trigeminal nerve and the second cervical segment is interrupted.

In summary, the trigeminal or occipital irritation initially perceived as segment related, starting from a tooth with a dead nerve, also involves an interference field disease, since the causal therapy needed to remedy the neuralgia is repeated neural therapeutic infiltration of the diseased tooth or surgical tooth extraction if the infiltration does not result in sustained elimination of the neuralgia. In this case, infiltration in the area of the trigeminal nerve or occipital nerves brings about no lasting change in the medical condition.

Another generally well-known clinical example will illustrate these innervation relationships as a purely segmental-reflexive process. Acute myocardial ischemia in the area of the left ventricle often shows not only precordial pain at the level of T1–T4/T5 on the left, but also a referred pain over the left shoulder extending to the left lower jaw in the C8 segment with pain all the way into the left little finger, often associated with a feeling of heaviness and weakness in the left arm. In this case, the efferent nervous system of segments C8–T4/T5 is stimulated through the stimulus of the afferent sympathetic nervous system starting from the zone of the ischemic heart muscle and progressing over the sympathetic conduction arc. The efferent path then passes through the blood vessels whose sympathetic supply originates, among others, from the sympathetic stellate ganglion and the superior cervical ganglion. The nucleic regions of the efferent sympathetic nervous system, which supplies the heart, among others, start in segment C8, i.e., in the same segment that partially provides sensorimotor as well as sympathetic supply to the upper extremities. Pain in segment C7 or C6, both of which also supply the upper extremities, does not occur as a rule since the sympathetic nucleic regions in the intermediolateral part of the spinal cord do not start until C8.

The segmental nature of this disease process is confirmed by the results of an injection at the stellate ganglion. The suppression of the sympathetic conduction arc, which causes clinical symptoms between segments C8 and T4/T5, hereby achieves clinical effects beyond the duration of the local anesthetic used. Suppression of the stellate ganglion via sympatholysis disrupts the pain-causing viscero-sensory cardiac fibers and also improves perfusion of the heart muscle which leads to the resolution of ischemic pain.

The strict separation of interference field disease and segmental disease is therefore only a didactic necessity, which satisfies the spinal-segmental system of the spinal nervous system. Since there is topographically no isolated "somatic" innervation, but there is afferent and efferent involvement of the sympathetic distribution system in every case of a segmental disease, the step from the segmental disease to the interference field disease is much smaller and easier to understand. The theoretical disease relationships primarily derived from clinical observation and the symptoms seem to indicate a causal, precedent-setting involvement of the sympathetic nervous system in interference field diseases.

Conclusion

In summary, when evaluating segmental and interference field disease, it is necessary to consider the full innervation relationships of an interference field anatomically as well as clinically in order to understand the sympathetic nervous system–dependent neuromodulatory properties of the interference field in their complex clinical picture and consequently carry out any necessary neural therapeutic interventions.

7.5 Case Histories and Interpretation

On the basis of clinical and animal experimental observations, the following cases will show how interference field diseases manifest and why the same interference field can trigger different diseases in different patients.

Two patients suffered whiplash injury (cervical whiplash) with generally known symptoms:

- In the first patient, normalization of the pain could be achieved by local treatment of the cervical spine. The treatment was successfully completed after about 6 weeks.
- In the second patient, with the same trauma and comparable clinical symptoms, the same conservative therapy was performed in the form of physical measures. The treatment was eventually discontinued because of persistent pain despite various therapeutic measures under which there occurred a temporary worsening of symptoms. Owing to the existing recurrent pain in the upper jaw before the whiplash occurred, an impacted wisdom tooth was extracted 1 year after the whiplash. Shortly afterward, the whiplash symptoms subsided without further therapy.

In the first case, conservative treatment was carried out, which supported the elimination of trauma sequelae by utilizing segment-reflexive relationships. In the second case, an interference field in the form of an impacted wisdom tooth already existed before the accident. Whether this involved a manifest or potential interference field can no longer be determined. According to the medical history data of the second patient, there were at least no cervical spine symptoms before the cervical spine injury. It is safe to assume that prior to the accident there must have been a subclinical pathological condition in the cervical spine by way of the tooth acting as an interference field, causing the trauma sequelae to persist. Therefore, in terms of sympathetic nervous system function, before the accident there was already a pathological stimulus in the area, which was subjected to additional stimulus by the accident. With the existing initial stimulus, no normalization of the sympathetic nervous system function could be achieved despite segmental therapy measures. In accordance with Speransky, this is a classic case of so-called **second strike**.[467]

Definition

Second strike

This is a summation of stimulus that the body cannot completely eliminate or compensate for because of the persistence of the initial stimulus.

This second strike phenomenon is often found in everyday clinical practice. Examples are:

- Postcholecystectomy syndrome with the symptoms of gallstone disease but without detectable gallstones.
- "Activated" arthritis that causes persistent pain after minor injury, even though there were no arthritis symptoms before the accident.
- Headache after any form of stress or after consuming particular foods or beverages.
- Herpes simplex infection which always appears at the same site during a common cold or during stress (e.g., short-term nausea).
- Migraine that occurs with the onset of menarche, after the first birth, after menopause, or after a gynecological procedure.

This second strike phenomenon is based on the so-called **first strike** in the form of a preexisting, self-compensating sympathetic stimulation which does not appear clinically, i.e., it progresses asymptomatically, or a preexisting exposure without sympathetic stimulation, consisting of congenital "organ weakness," microorganism exposure, or toxic exposure.

An additional, "second strike", whether caused by a general or regional stimulus leads to a pathological response in the form of chronic disease, as the body fails to compensate. This second stimulus may be completely non-specific, e.g. trauma to any part of the body, or a change in the weather.

Note

If the primary or the secondary stimulus is successfully eliminated by means of a local anesthetic, the pathological stimulus is reduced to the extent that the sympathetic nervous system function is brought back into the physiological performance range and therefore back into the physiological range of autoregulation.

The stimulus is reduced by the infiltration of the interference field with a local anesthetic, whereby the lasting effect is achieved either by repeated infiltration with the above-described "medicinal stimulus removal" or by surgical removal of the interference field.

7.6 Neurophysiological Criteria of the Interference Field

Taking into account the topography of the sympathetic nervous system, this interference field theory arising from observations of animal experiments and clinical observations in patients can be further established. The sympathetic nervous system function operates at different levels, i.e., the sympathetic conduction arc is divided into three areas according to Rohen[429]:

- The spinosegmental area represents the lowest functional level.
- The next level is the reticular formation of the hindbrain and midbrain.
- The highest level is represented by the diencephalon-associated hypothalamus.

The interactions of different organ systems originate in this area; the connections to the central nervous system (CNS) enable the awareness of autonomic functions.

All three levels are interdependent, although certainly not every impulse input reaches all three levels. Starting with the knowledge that not the quality but the quantity of the stimulus determines the function of the autonomic nervous system, it can be assumed that function and responsiveness of the three autonomic levels are subject to this same criterion. In simple terms, this means that primarily the spinosegmental conduction arc is used up to a certain stimulus intensity. With increasing stimulus intensity, the next level up is used until the hypothalmic functional range is achieved with the ability to propagate to the CNS and thus consciousness. This gives the second-strike phenomenon a neurophysiological basis. In general terms, the sum of the stimulus causes the pathological impulses to eventually trigger an illness via all three autonomic functional levels. This theory may also help clarify the question as to why the same interference fields initiate or maintain individually different diseases at different locations of the body and why the same diseases can be caused by various interference fields.

The localization of the disease induced by the interference field depends on the level from which the quantitatively largest pathological impulse output is transmitted in the periphery to the corresponding organ region or body area. Terms originating from clinical experience, such as **inherited or acquired organ weakness, locus minoris resistentiae, or disposition**, can hereby be explained as a first strike in accordance with the concept of neuropathology.

This theoretical foundation also allows us to understand the very different length of time between the emergence of the interference field and the disease induced by it. Also conceivable is that the afferent stimulus arising from the interference field affects the reaching of the higher-level autonomic nucleic regions in the hindbrain and the midbrain or hypothalamus as a second strike, in accordance with Speransky[467]: the irritated afferent causes stimulation of the efferent—which is then no longer only segmentally attached—and can lead at the spinal level to an interference field disease at a completely different location. Furthermore, the efferent response of the sympathetic nervous system, starting from the centers supraordinate to the spinal level, can also determine the localization of the interference field disease. With more diffuse stimulus, one organ area or tissue section may react as a site of illness, whose responsiveness and compensation capacity—congenital or acquired—is limited.

7.7 Summary

The **interference field** is a regional sympathetically-supplied tissue section or organ whose afferent branch chronic pathological stimulus beginning in the interstitium. Due to a persistent, non-specific ("second-strike") stimulus, which cannot be decreased by the body's own mechanisms or by engrammatically increased irritability of the sympathetic nervous system after trauma or disease (Ricker), a lasting pathological reponse will remain in spite of a decrease of the original stimulus. Any type of elapsed or persistent illness or injury may be a cause of chronic nonspecific stimulus. Starting from the interference field, the pathological impulse output is transmitted on the afferent pathway to the nucleic regions of the sympathetic nervous system at the spinal level as well as in the area of the hindbrain and the hypothalamus. From these three functional levels, there is efferent transmission of the pathological impulse output to the periphery, which causes the interference field–induced disease in another portion of tissue or organ. The dysregulation up to the organ change is made possible by the disturbance of microcirculation and organ and tissue capacity, which are controlled by the sympathetic nervous system and also influence the interstitial regulation system.

The diagnostics and causal therapy of the interference field disease is possible via direct neural therapeutic infiltration of the interference field or, if direct infiltration is not possible, indirectly through "segmental therapy" (p. 53) of the interference field, including the responsible autonomic ganglia (e.g., celiac ganglion in diseases of the abdominal organs) or by surgical removal of the interference field (e.g., teeth, appendix, gall bladder).

8 Local Anesthesia in Neural Therapy

8.1 Introduction

The choice of medication used for neural therapy must be based primarily on the fundamental mode of action of this treatment method. Although a drug is needed, it is not drug therapy in the traditional sense, where a general drug level must be reached in order to achieve a therapeutic effect. The effect of neural therapy is achieved through a targeted, short interruption of pathological sympathetic stimulation. This acts as a reset, resulting in a return to physiological impulse output from the sympathetic nervous system.

Practical Advice

The longer the period of interruption by way of the drug, the longer the interruption of the desired autoregulative state. Therefore, a local anesthetic with the shortest possible duration of action and the lowest toxicity is optimal.

8.2 Local Anesthesia as a Neural Therapeutic Agent

Even without medication, the needlestick in the skin provides an initial nonspecific stimulus, which elicits a response through the afferent and efferent pathways by both the rapidly conducting sensitive nervous system and the sympathetic nervous system supplying the skin. A drug can be used to intensify the stimulus, whereby it was observed that the stronger stimulus also shows a stronger effect, which does not necessarily mean that the stimulus response in all cases is therapeutically positive.

The use of distilled water, saline, or other drugs, and even the injection of air are taken as evidence that the choice of a drug in neural therapy is secondary. This is true insofar as the additional or oft-repeated regional stimulus from a needlestick with and without infiltration or the extensive stimulus of a massage, or the application of heat or cold, leads to a segmental-reflexive response in each case. Thus, both the sensorimotor and autonomic nervous systems respond.

However, the neural therapy treatment method comes not just from stimulus of the tissue, but also from the elimination of a stimulus by the infiltration of a local anesthetic. Since a needlestick stimulates nerve tissue through mechanical injury and injures tissue with no conducting function, a protracted response of the stimulus conduction system, starting from the site of tissue injury, is to be expected along with the immediate segmental-reflexive response. Both effects are amplified by an additional drug stimulus unless a membrane-stabilizing drug is used in the form of a local anesthetic, which prevents both the conduction and tissue stimulus.

The neural therapeutic injection to be performed is thus determined by two factors:

- The stimulus from the needlestick.
- The elimination of the stimulus through a local anesthetic.

On the one hand, therapeutic responses are triggered by the stimulus alone indirectly through the segmental-reflexive function of the sympathetic nervous system (perfusion, among others). On the other hand, through infiltration of a local anesthetic, the sympathetic nervous system is brought to a physiological state of irritation as a reset by way of disrupting the sympathetic conduction arc. This second part of the neural therapy injection process is the essential difference to the simple stimulation process and, in particular, is an indispensable prerequisite for the elimination of an interference field.

A drug used in neural therapy must be able, among other things, to disrupt an existing pathological stimulation of the sympathetic nervous system. (Here, we recall the experimental investigations of Ricker, who proved the disease-transmitting pathological stimulation of the sympathetic nervous system). Starting from the principle that every disease progresses with the involvement of the autonomic nervous system, especially the sympathetic nervous system, the selection of a local anesthetic in association with neural therapy is meaningful. It involves targeted stimuli interruption with subsequent therapeutic effect due to the normalization of sympathetic nervous system function, which lasts longer than the drug-induced stimulus interruption. Targeted therapeutic stimulation by a simple needlestick (e.g., acupuncture) or by additional local administration of a nociceptive drug uses inhibitory neurons, for example, on a segmental-reflexive pathway to exert indirect therapeutic influence on the disturbed sympathetic nervous system function.

Note

Only the segment-bound disease is influenced with stimulation therapy, not the interference field–induced disease wherein the actual disruption of the sympathetic nervous system function is outside of the diseased spinal segment.

Strictly speaking, the concept of local anesthesia associated with the local anesthetic is misleading in connection with neural therapy, since this by no means targets local anesthesia. As well, the attempt by Gross to replace the term "neural therapy" with the name "**therapeutic local anesthesia**" does not contribute to clarifying the effect of a local anesthetic in neural therapy.[179] This is only possible by viewing **local anesthetics as lytic substances** and their action, which Fleckenstein described as the general stabilization of membranes.[142] How this process is achieved is still not completely understood, but it has been shown experimentally and clinically.

Membrane stabilization does not mean interruption of conduction in the membrane of a nerve cell or a nerve process. Each local anesthetic interrupts stimulus conduction through blockade of the sodium channel. This applies to the afferent conductive sensory nerve fiber and to any other nerve fiber or nerve cell. If sympathetic nerve fiber stimulus conduction is interrupted, which is important for neural therapy, the sympathetic conduction arc is interrupted. Furthermore, through the cleavage product para-aminobenzoic acid, there is membrane stabilization of all tissue structures reached by procaine.

The crucial neural therapeutic process is **increased microcirculation** of the diseased tissue over the period of the local anesthetic's effect, with normalization of the interstitial milieu (pH, capillary permeability, fibrocytes, macrophages, mast cells, etc.) and subsequent normalization of conduction of the autonomic conduction arc (reset). Since the sympathetic nervous system has an efferent and afferent branch, the reaction of this nervous system can be observed in both directions after interruption of conduction. The interruption of the **efferent** branch means **sympatholysis** in the classical sense, while interruption of the **afferent** branch reduces the stimulus conduction centrally within the sympathetic conduction arc. At the same time, the mixed reflex pathway is influenced, including the sensorimotor system. Here, it is worth recalling the phenomenon—typical of the sympathetic nervous system—that the pathological irritation lasts longer than the stimulus. Furthermore, the interruption of a pathological irritation by a local anesthetic leads to normalization of the sympathetic function lasting well beyond the drug's time of action, and this can last indefinitely when repeating the interruption. The clinical findings present as remission of the symptoms.

Info

The principal difference in the effect of local anesthetics with respect to local anesthesia and neural therapy is that the local anesthetic for prophylactic analgesia primarily applies to the somatosensory system, while neural therapy applies diagnostically and therapeutically to the already disturbed sympathetic nervous system function.
The suppression of the autonomic nervous system during local anesthesia through the topography of the somatic and autonomic nervous systems should be viewed as a side effect and is not critical for the local anesthesia. Conversely, the suppression of the somatosensory and somatomotor activity during neural therapy is therapeutically irrelevant.

8.2.1 Procaine for Neural Therapy

When reviewing local anesthetics for **local anesthesia**, it is logical to seek a drug with the longest possible duration of action available. For this reason, in recent decades local anesthetics with activity duration of up to 3 hours or more were synthesized. This development was initiated by Löfgren, who produced the first amide-structured local anesthetic, "lidocaine," in 1945, 40 years after the synthesis of procaine.

Considering, however, the reaction of the autonomic nervous system relevant to **neural therapy** in both pathological stimulation and stimulus interruption by a local anesthetic, a short-acting local anesthetic is desirable, since the therapeutically achievable normalization of autonomic conduction is only dependent on the interruption of pathological stimulus conduction and not on its duration.

Note

The very short-acting ester-structured procaine is the first choice for neural therapy. Long-acting local anesthetics may also be used, but they offer no improvement of the therapeutic effect.

From the perspective of neural therapy, long-acting anesthetics have an undesirably lengthy effect on the autonomic nervous system (p. 6) and extend the interruption of autoregulation sought by neural therapy.

Comparing the activity profiles of different local anesthetics and evaluating them according to the important criteria either for local anesthesia or for neural therapy, the resulting optimal local anesthetic for neural therapy is procaine in a 1% solution without any additives, in particular without vasoconstrictors and preservatives. As evidence of this, the ester-structured procaine will be contrasted with the representative amide-structured drug, lidocaine.

8.2.2 Comparison of Procaine and Lidocaine

Duration of Action

Depending on the application site, the interruption of stimulus conduction as the primary, clinically important criterion is:

- For procaine: approximately 20 minutes.
- For lidocaine: 60 minutes.

Procaine's duration of action is more favorable for neural therapy than that of lidocaine, as the shorter duration means better controllability of the drug. Furthermore, all side effects (p. 101) that affect the somatic nervous system are significantly shorter under procaine. In practice, this means shorter sensorimotor dysfunction, so that the patient's return to normal function is reached more quickly with procaine.

Pharmacokinetics

In terms of **diffusion capability**, the distribution in tissue and penetration ability of lidocaine is generally superior to procaine. However, since the nerve structure relevant to neural therapy is mainly made of thin C fibers with little or no myelinization and the "insulation" is poor, the lower diffusion and penetration properties of procaine is sufficient for neural therapy. Furthermore, there is relative selection for the **interruption of the stimulus conduction** in favor of the autonomic nervous system and to the disadvantage of the somatic nervous system. The weaker properties of procaine compared with lidocaine are thus assessed as positive. However, procaine's poorer diffusion ability has an adverse effect in that its injection must be more precise than that of lidocaine in order for it to reach the impaired autonomic nerve structure.

Degradation

Procaine is essentially cleaved into para-aminobenzoic acid and diethylaminoethanol "on site" through the nonspecific pseudocholinesterase present in the entire tissue, while lidocaine is transported essentially unchanged from the injection site and cleaved in the liver by oxidation into acetaldehyde and ethylamine acetone 2,6-xylidine.

The **cleavage products** of procaine are responsible for the vasodilatory effect at the injection site (diethylaminoethanol) and for capillary stabilization (para-aminobenzoic acid). Lidocaine lacks these properties. The cleavage products of both local anesthetics are excreted primarily through the kidneys. The additional therapeutically important feature of procaine cleavage products is the exclusion of the liver "organ exposure" of lidocaine. Thus, procaine is more effective than lidocaine for neural therapy in terms of tissue compatibility.

Toxicity

The toxicity of procaine is half that of lidocaine. This difference is particularly clinically relevant when liver impairment is present, as the degradation of lidocaine occurs primarily in the liver. Analogous to this is pseudocholinesterase deficiency at an assumed incidence rate of 1:2,500 in the general population, which must be taken into consideration when administering procaine, since delayed degradation of procaine is to be expected. However, this becomes clinically relevant only if cholinesterase is lacking to the greatest possible extent, which is extremely rare and is assumed to be of the magnitude 1:250,000 in the general population. Because of this toxicity difference, the unit quantity needed for neural therapeutic treatment with procaine is two times higher than with lidocaine. At the same concentration, this amounts to 500 mg for procaine and 250 mg for lidocaine, assuming an average body weight of 70 kg, normal liver function, and the same cholinesterase concentration in the body.

When considering **tissue toxicity**, procaine is once again superior to lidocaine. In any case, the injected quantity and concentration of a particular local anesthetic is locally "toxic" to the tissue in the area of application. The **neurotoxicity** of procaine is lower than that of lidocaine, as evidenced by the amount and strength of the "nerve injury" and the perineural edema formation. This specific toxicity of amide-structured local anesthetics is based on the absence of the capillary obstruction and vasodilatory effects at the injection site and the varied neurotoxicity, myocardial toxicity, and cardiotoxicity. At a macroscopic level, lidocaine's lack of vasodilatory effect compared to procaine is shown by the placement of a wheal. The procaine wheal shows a clear, bright red "hyperemia" in the injection area, while the lidocaine wheal shows a white, anemic color (▶Fig. 8.1).

Special attention must be given to the possibility of toxic and genetic damage (**teratogenicity**). After extensive literature searches, Hahn-Godeffroy established that for procaine and lidocaine there is no increased malformation risk for newborns whose mothers were treated with procaine or lidocaine in the first trimester.[192,193] Both procaine and lidocaine definitely cross the placenta. This means that both substances must also be eliminated from the child's body in the treatment of pregnant women—procaine by pseudocholinesterase and lidocaine in the child's liver. When solely considering the doubly high toxicity of lidocaine compared with procaine, the latter is certainly the more favorable drug to use during pregnancy as well as in obstetrics. Mink,[346] Funk,[155,156] and Goecke,[170] physicians long active in pregnancy care and obstetrics, published identical results on the use of procaine and lidocaine in pregnant women.

General symptoms that might occur under the application of procaine as part of neural therapeutic treatment vary in severity. However, these result in no therapeutic consequences. The most common symptom is a slight dizziness that lasts only a few minutes, without causing measurable changes in blood pressure. A general feeling of warmth, slight sweating, and a metallic taste also occur fairly frequently. Occasionally, patients describe an inner "shaky" feeling, without visible tremor. Short-term lack of concentration, and speech, vision, or hearing disorders lasting a few seconds are reported rarely by patients and resolve spontaneously. It is notable that all of these drug-induced reactions are different from patient to patient. Evidently, they are dependent on the initial autonomic condition. After treatment with procaine, some patients describe a sense of wellbeing and sympatheticotonic people describe a quieter mood while parasympatheticotonic patients are more likely to report the opposite. This rather analeptic action of procaine is an additional positive effect. Using the correct injection technique and strictly taking the procaine dosage into account, all reactions can be observed.

The effects of overdose are divided into an excitation phase and a paralysis phase (▶Table 8.1).[274,565,566] All local anesthetics have the same clinical appearance for **intoxication phases**. However, both phases do not have to occur. The toxic appearance depends on the level of intoxication and the speed with which the local anesthetic reaches the brain. With slow intoxication through absorption of the extravascularly administered toxic dose, there is a 15- to 20-minute progression of intoxication with a first phase and a subsequent second phase.

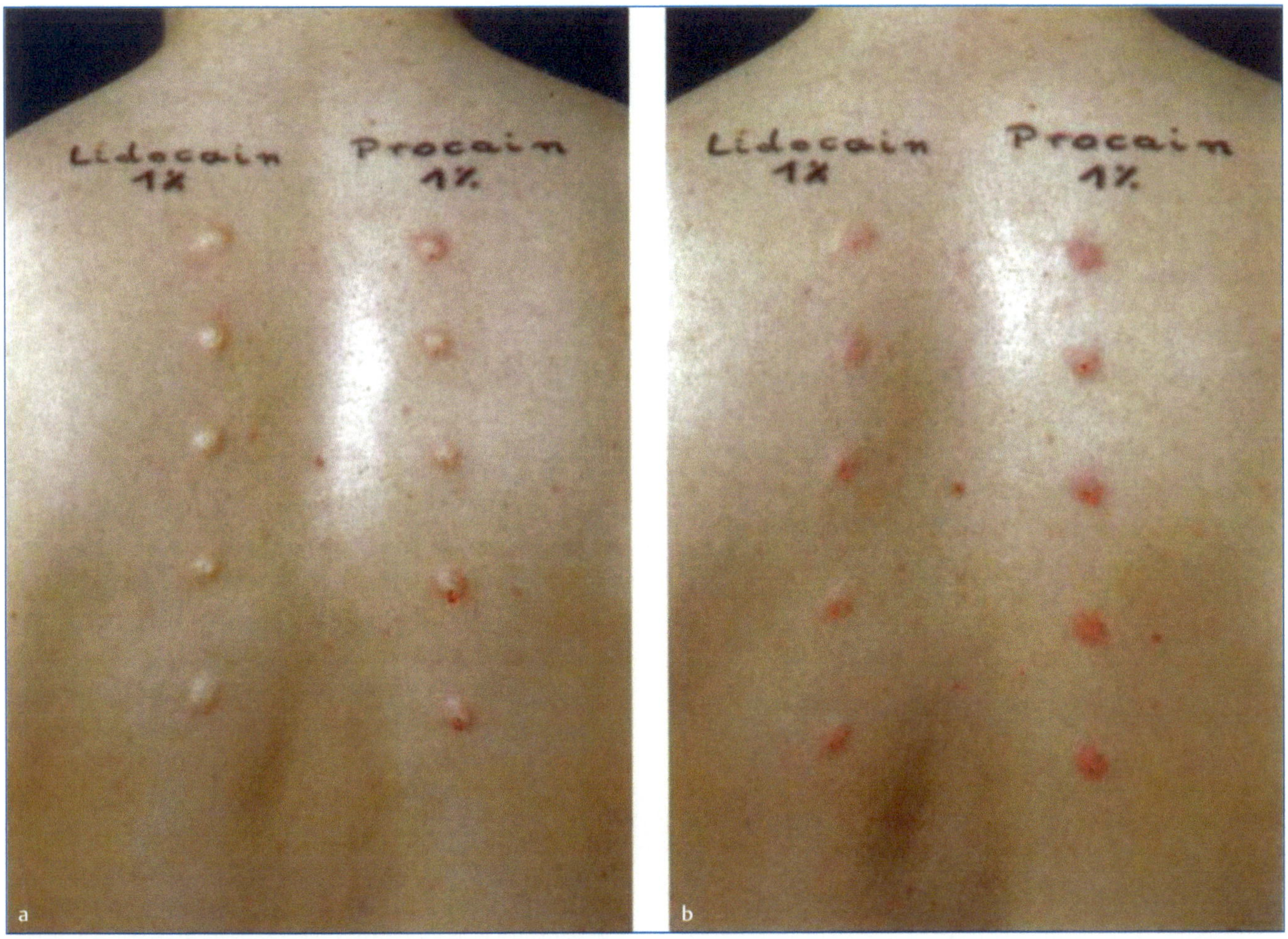

▶ **Fig. 8.1** Example of a wheal series paravertebral to the thoracic spine: left with 1% lidocaine, right with 1% procaine. Left image: 0.5 minutes after injection; right image: 3 minutes, after injection. The reddening from the procaine wheal (dimethylaminoethanol) at the injection site as a sign of vasodilation is lacking in the lidocaine wheal.

Cave

Toxic reactions affecting the whole body are to be expected when the maximum dose of a local anesthetic is exceeded or if an inherently nontoxic effective amount is administered intravenously, or especially intra-arterially, in a vessel leading toward the brain, with consequent suppression of vital parts of the brain.

With rapid intoxication, for example, by inadvertent intra-arterial administration of the local anesthetic in a vessel leading toward the brain (common carotid artery, vertebral artery), a skipping of the first phase of intoxication and thus onset of cardiac/respiratory arrest within seconds is to be expected.[274]

The normally occurring generalized seizures, which serve as a criterion for clinical differentiation of intoxication sequelae and seizure-free anaphylaxis, can also be lacking. Especially when applying amide-structured local anesthetics with their higher local anesthetic potency, the "prodromal" of phase 1 can be skipped so that a narcotic-like state is reached immediately.

8.2.3 The Effects of Procaine Reaction of the Blood Vessels

All local anesthetics have **sympathicolytic** function. However, the reaction of the blood vessels directly at the application site is quite variable and depends on the specific local anesthetic. Thus, the intradermal administration of procaine leads to visible increased circulation to the skin at the injection site; the intradermal administration of lidocaine results in vasoconstriction after initial vasodilatation.[96] The reaction of the capillaries to the injection of procaine is due to the cleavage product of procaine, diethylaminoethanol, as a stimulant of the vasodilators, and the visible local reduced circulation after lidocaine is due to the "toxic" stimulus of the sympathetic nervous system at the injection site with subsequent vasoconstriction. These different properties have therapeutic relevance.

Note

The use of lidocaine for local injection treatment of bacterial infections is contraindicated, while the injection of procaine is ideally suited.

▶ Table 8.1 Symptomatology of intoxication by procaine

First phase: excitation	Second phase: paralysis
• Facial flushing or paleness	• Hearing loss, deafness
• Cold sweat	• Loss of speech
• Talkativeness, internal unrest	• Unconsciousness
• Anxiety, impaired speech	• Vasomotor paralysis (pallor, weakness, symptoms of collapse)
• Pupil dilation, possibly nystagmus	• Complete sensory and motor paralysis
• Confusion, contentiousness	• Dyspnea, increasing cyanosis, possibly apnea
• Slight lightheadedness	• Bradycardia (sometimes tachycardia)
• Disorientation	• Blood pressure drop
• Difficulty breathing; hyperpnea	• Conduction disorders of the heart, arrhythmia
• Tachycardia, palpitation	• Paralysis of all sphincters
• Increase in pulse and blood pressure	• Coma
• Nausea, vomiting	• Cardiac/respiratory arrest
• Tremors, spasms (e.g., facial nerve)	
• Choreiform movements	
• Convulsions	
• Tonic–clonic seizures	
• Increased temperature	

The first experiences of Spiess showing that infected wounds heal faster under procaine already demonstrated this therapeutically useful property of procaine and led to the inclusion of local treatment of bacterially infected wounds in the catalog of indications for neural therapy with procaine.[469,470] Through the **improved microcirculation** at the injection site, the inflammation-associated hypoxia and the pH-value deterioration are eliminated, so that regeneration and the immunological response (fibroblasts, macrophages) is initiated more quickly. This is particularly noteworthy because, from a surgical point of view, local anesthesia of infected tissue sections is generally prohibited and classified as negligence, not only from the aspect of cross-contamination, but also in view of the deterioration of the local tissue trophism by amide-structured lidocaine, which is more commonly used in local anesthesia today.

The cause of procaine's lower **neurotoxicity** compared to the amide-structured local anesthetics is probably the improved trophism by "hyperperfusion" with the result that the infection can be "degraded" faster via the body's immune system, and the generally tissue-friendlier property of procaine in comparison to lidocaine.[104]

In animal experiments, Kilian showed a **capillary stabilizing effect** of procaine after subcutaneous administration, which is lacking in lidocaine.[274] The cleavage product of procaine, para-aminobenzoic acid, is the active factor because the same effect occurred even after direct administration of para-aminobenzoic acid, but not with the second cleavage product, diethylaminoethanol. Of importance here is the fast cleavage of procaine and the associated high influx of para-aminobenzoic acid. Stable ester-structured local anesthetics, e.g., tutocaine, that are cleaved more slowly, showed no capillary stabilizing effect.

The clinical relevance of this capillary-obstructing effect, which is present in procaine and lacking in lidocaine, can be found in the possibility for local use of procaine for inflammatory diseases, regardless of the agent or the specificity of inflammation. Thus, procaine has an excellent "anti-inflammatory" effect.

Influence of the Membrane Potential

"Local anesthetics are nonspecific lytics that exert their effect by displacement of cations of anionic charge carriers or through interactions with hydrophobic groups of proteins or lipids of the membrane. Membrane stabilization can be achieved through these two major possible binding modes, not only in the nerve cell, also but in all cells of the organism."[274]

The sensation of pain (cortical, thalamic) requires stimulation of the afferent neurons responsible for this effect. In addition to exogenous physical and chemical stimuli, endogenous stimuli via substances are produced by the body itself. These include:

- Histamine.
- Serotonin.
- Bradykinin.
- Kallikrein.
- Kallidin.
- Oligo- and polypeptides such as substance P.
- Angiotensin.
- Oxytocin.
- Vasopressin.

According to the experimental studies by Fleckenstein, the mechanism of action for the different causes of pain is sensitization of the nerve through destabilization of the membrane,[141,142] whereby the resting potential is reduced and the nerve is depolarized from stimuli that normally remain below the threshold. Local anesthetics can prevent this reduction of the membrane potential by blocking sodium channels, if they were administered before the application of the pain trigger; if they are given after the application of pain triggers, they normalize the lowered membrane potential so that the stimulus threshold is lowered.

The membrane-stabilizing effect is more or less pronounced in different local anesthetics and depends not only on the purely local anesthetic potency of the drug. Generally, the diverse effects that can be used therapeutically emerge from this property. Therefore, pure local anesthesia as a clinically useful property represents only one of these numerous effects. Membrane stabilization and the resulting effect can be seen in clinical findings on cell or organ efficiency, depending on which cell membrane was stabilized by the local anesthetic.

This property applies to both procaine and lidocaine in various forms. It can be assumed that the membrane-sta-bilizing action of the ester-structured procaine progresses differently than the amide-structured lidocaine, as the effects of procaine and lidocaine vary in their clinical appearance.

In nerve cells, the stabilization of cell membranes means the interruption of stimulus conduction as well as the release of neurotransmitters. Considering other cells, e.g., the mast cell, from which the release of histamine takes place, the local anesthetic becomes an antihistamine by stabilizing the mast cell membrane. In animal studies, bronchospasm produced by intravenous administration of acetylcholine, histamine, or serotonin can be mitigated or eliminated by additional intravenous administration of procaine. Intravenous administration of lidocaine shows no spasmolytic effect on the drug-induced bronchospasm.

Suppression of the Sanarelli–Shwartzman Phenomenon

The versatility of the therapeutic benefits of procaine in more complex tissue processes was demonstrated by Siegen[460,461] and Hirsch.[210] Siegen wrote the following on the Sanarelli–Shwartzman phenomenon: "If a rabbit is injected with 0.5 mL of a particular E. coli infiltrate intradermally in the breast skin (wheal), outwardly nothing more is observed initially than would be observed with an indifferent saline infiltration. However, if a second strike is made after 24 hours with the same infiltrate, this time in the ear vein, this leads to a rapidly progressing necrotic process, sharply delineated to the site of the intradermal first injection. Whole shreds of skin and subcutaneous tissue are shed within a few hours with considerable deterioration of the general condition. For over 30 years, pharmacologists have used this classic allergy model for testing their antiallergenics, central analgesic sedatives, antihistamines, etc., which are usually structured according to humoral aspects. But with a procaine injection targeted to the primarily intracutaneous interference field, another team I am involved with succeeded—as early as the preliminary test—in totally suppressing the recurring process that is otherwise triggered by the intravenous second injection, entirely in accordance with my expectations. The animals literally did not have a hair out of place."[461]

This is how the Sanarelli–Shwartzman phenomenon can be suppressed by procaine. In vital tissue that was sensitized by injecting foreign protein, no "allergic" or necrotizing response occurred when procaine was infiltrated there, before the second injection. The same observation was found experimentally after temporally staggered intravenous administration of foreign proteins when procaine was given intravenously prior to the second protein application. In clinical applications, for example, after an insect sting or bite, no significant local inflammatory response or allergic reaction occurs when procaine is infiltrated immediately after the insect sting. Another medicinal factor of procaine is the suppression of "silent inflammation," which interrupts or prevents the inflammation cycle through the blockade of inflammation-inducing membrane receptors. Siegen's experiments impressively showed the involvement of the sympathetic nervous system in allergic events as well as the involvement in "immunological" sensitization, the "engrammatic ability" of the sympathetic nervous system, and not least the impact of an interference field on the whole body.

Improved Oxygen Supply

Under procaine, hypoxic effects in the tissue are significantly lower or do not occur, thanks to the membrane-stabilizing effect. It could be shown[274] that under procaine perfusion the otherwise irreversible damage to the optic nerve after 1-hour anoxia did not occur. The so-called Eppendorf cardioplegic solution, in which procaine is used, utilizes the vasoconstrictive effects of procaine to "preserve" the heart of a sedated patient during surgery.

The oxygen-conserving effect of procaine can otherwise be generally utilized in all inflammatory or degenerative tissue diseases where a deterioration of the oxygen supply is expected. Procaine therapy can improve the oxygen perfusion in these inflammatory and degenerative disorders and interrupt or weaken cell hypoxia. This it does by the combined action of vasodilation through the "local anesthetic" sympathicolysis and diethylaminoethanol, and the stabilization of the capillaries by the drug itself as well as its cleavage product para-aminobenzoic acid, and "membrane sealing" of any body cell, which maintains and stabilizes the physiological electrolyte balance of the cell interior and cell outer milieu. Lidocaine lacks this combined effect.

Endoanesthesia with Procaine

The membrane stabilization ability is ultimately reflected in the influence on endoreceptors that make the therapeutic and prophylactic use of local anesthetics outside of local anesthesia and neural therapy possible. The concept of endoanesthesia, characterized by Zipf, describes these effects of local anesthetics. With intravenous administration, procaine affects pulmonary tension receptors, which serve proprioceptive reflex-vagal respiratory control and whose elimination leads to improved respiration. The vascular receptors reached by procaine in endoanesthesia are also desensitized like mechanoreceptors and chemoreceptors of the carotid sinus. The effect of procaine is particularly evident in the heart muscle and its stimulus conduction system, which is modulated by sympathetic and parasympathetic nervous systems. Overactivity of the sympathetic or parasympathetic nervous system is offset by intravenous procaine, so that an economization of cardiac function results depending on the initial autonomic condition.[274]

Hahn-Godeffroy has studied the different "effects" of procaine for years and compared them to lidocaine.[192,194,195] Generally, procaine has a local anesthetic, psychoanaleptic, and blood circulation–promoting effect after intravenous administration. The effects in the brain stem and the central nervous system (CNS) are explained by reuptake inhibition of dopamine, serotonin, and norepinephrine, as well as inhibition of monoamine oxidase (MAO).[1] These CNS effects cannot be achieved with lidocaine.

For the purposes of drug therapy, procaine has a balancing effect since cellular functions can be normalized through the membrane stabilization of all cell structures, and procaine can be used for both "overactive" and "underfunctioning" organs and organ systems. The procaine infusion therapy increasingly used in recent years successfully utilizes the pharmacological properties of the drug to exert a nonspecific effect on inflammation, pain, and degenerative as well as mental illnesses (e.g., depression). The results thus far indicate a time/dose-dependent (e.g., 300 mg procaine in 250 mL NaCl/30 min infusion therapy) positive effect.

Like neural therapy, this **general** "reset method" uses the effects of procaine and its cleavage products for the therapy via the autonomic nervous system as well as the CNS. However, success comparable to neural therapy cannot be achieved.

Local Anesthetics and Allergies

There is probably no medication to which an organism cannot respond with an allergy—up to anaphylaxis—after administration. Of course, this also applies to local anesthetics. Therefore, in addition to the appearance of the allergy, the frequency of allergic reactions is crucial for the selection of the local anesthetic. Hahn-Godeffroy researched the topic of procaine allergy and the para group allergy described repeatedly in this context, which theoretically specifies a high risk of allergies for procaine.[7,194,195] Taking into account the international literature and after interviewing physicians who had used procaine for decades, Hahn-Godeffroy found that the total allergy rate for procaine in relation to other local anesthetics or drugs is conspicuously low, i.e., well below the allergy rate of different antibiotics, sulfonamides, nonsteroidal anti-inflammatory drugs, and antihypertensives. With regard to the allergy rate of procaine and lidocaine, there is no difference which could justify the preference of one or the other product.

8.3 Summary

Procaine is preferable to lidocaine as a neural therapeutic agent, since it has more clinically relevant positive properties than lidocaine. Of particular value is the fact that the cleavage products of procaine—para-aminobenzoic acid and diethylaminoethanol—are **therapeutically active substances** that hold a special position in neural therapy. The degradation products of lidocaine, however, are therapeutically worthless.

The efficacy spectrum of procaine and the reactions of different tissue structures to the application of procaine illustrate the therapeutic value of this drug. The term "local anesthetic" represents only one aspect, whereby the purely local anesthetic effect of procaine is more poorly pronounced than that of lidocaine.

When comparing the ester-structured procaine and the amide-structured lidocaine, only manifest procaine allergy indicates the use of lidocaine for neural therapy.

Other ester-structured or amide-structured local anesthetics are certainly possible as drugs for neural therapy. However, amide-structured local anesthetics, in particular, worsen microcirculation at the site of application, thus preventing a part of the neural therapeutic effect and unnecessarily prolonging the interruption of autoregulation via the autonomic nervous system. Preservatives which are intended to prevent contamination with microorganisms certainly degrade the efficacy spectrum of procaine, e.g., by increased tissue toxicity, and increase the risk of allergies.

Note

Additives such as vasoconstrictors, which should lengthen the duration of the local anesthetic action of procaine, are contraindicated for neural therapy.

For the reasons illustrated above, procaine remains the optimal neural therapeutic agent.

Part 2
The Practice of Neural Therapy

9 Clinical Examination

9.1 Neural Therapeutic Medical History

The medical history determines the approach to the diagnosis and treatment of any disease. This is true in particular for neural therapy, because the data gathered are more useful for a clinical picture than with the usual medical history, as will become clear below.

The neural therapeutic history begins with the description of the symptoms to be treated. Focused listening and, above all, allowing the patient to finish speaking are often crucial to the aim of successful causal treatment. The patient should describe every notable detail of his or her symptoms, since what initially seems like a trivial statement quite often results in the essential therapeutic approach. The patient's subjective etiological concepts as well as the highly individually variable perceptions of the symptomology are very valuable. These include the patient's recollections that the symptoms started shortly after an operation, a pregnancy, an accident, or another illness, as well as the observations of simultaneously occurring symptoms at a completely different bodily location, e.g., the ever-recurring feeling of pressure at a certain point in the jaw and chronic recurring lumbago. If the patient does not provide such information spontaneously, these possible connections should be explored through targeted questioning. Sometimes, the patient does not notice these correlations until they are pointed out. The start date of an illness should be defined as precisely as possible; this is easier in the case of acute symptoms versus chronic illnesses.

When taking the current medical history, the patient should also be asked about previous treatments undergone for this symptomology. Therapeutic measures performed for chronic illnesses and the result obtained are especially valuable aspects in the context of neural therapy. The evidence that chronic lumbago shows no sustained improvement, or even possibly worsens temporarily, with repeated physiotherapeutic measures gives rise to suspicion of an interference field–induced disease even while the medical history is being recorded. If other medicinal, surgical, or physiotherapeutic treatments were performed before the neural therapy, this should be documented in the history along with the result.

If the neural therapeutic history is viewed as a verbal diagnostic tool with regard to the possible presence of an interference field–induced illness, the further medical history—outside of the current symptomology requiring treatment—becomes more significant than the traditional medical history. With the traditional medical history, it is irrelevant whether an appendectomy was performed in childhood if the current symptomology shows coxarthrosis or chronic sinusitis. Under the traditional concept of the medical history, hepatitis occurring at age 20 years also has no relationship to a headache disorder that started after age 40 years and is now being treated at age 50 years

Practical Advice

The neural therapeutic history outside of the current symptomology to be treated must include all of the patient's illnesses and injuries to the fullest extent possible, since the concept of neural therapy indicates that every chronic illness can be interference field induced and every illness and injury can leave behind an interference field. Therefore, the information provided in the medical history on previous illnesses or injuries that are far removed from the current symptomology to be treated is of particular importance, especially since these can be viewed in the context of interference field diagnostics.

Clinically, the importance of the medical history is impressively confirmed when, according to the example described above, the painful symptoms of coxarthrosis or chronic sinusitis permanently disappear after infiltration of the appendectomy scar with a local anesthetic, or when the headache disorder ceases after injection to the right celiac ganglion as a neural therapeutic response to the hepatitis experienced.

Overall, the further medical history is more important for neural therapy than for therapeutic methods that do not take into account the potential interference field disease. When the medical history is first prepared, numerous patients do not fully remember their own previous medical history, with the result that some medical history data are provided later on in the course of the neural therapeutic treatment. It is worthwhile repeatedly using targeted questions to evoke memories about minor illnesses and injuries.

During the examination, skin changes or scars are often detected which remind the patient of a long-forgotten childhood injury.

The broader medical history starts with typical **childhood diseases** such as measles (possible interference field after otitis or encephalitis), mumps (possible interference field after orchitis or pancreatitis), chickenpox (possible interference fields: skin scars), and whooping cough (possible interference field: lungs). Scarlet fever, diphtheria and recurrent infections of the middle ear, sinuses, and tonsils often leave an interference field, as can the navel, which may take on interference field characteristics as the first scar.

During further questioning of the patient, it has proven effective not to ask about illnesses in general, but to ask about the **individual body sections** and **organs** from "head to toe" with regard to possible illnesses. This very often results in an unexpected number of diseases that are not spontaneously recalled by the patient. The diseases of individual organs should be listed in as much detail as possible, whereby it is shown again and again that clarity is only achieved by asking about the individual symptoms of a medical condition which are perceived by the patient as normal, as these symptoms have persisted for a long time and are part of the patient's day-to-day life. Often, the question of a paranasal sinus disorder is denied, but the patient is then reminded of symptoms such as varying pain in nasal breathing, morning expectoration from the nasopharyngeal space, the occasional feeling of pressure on the maxillary sinus, or recurrent frontal headache as well as chronic bronchitis as an indication of a sinubronchial syndrome with primary discharge from the paranasal sinuses.

Questions about **operations** are generally answered in full, apparently because the trauma of an operation remains more deeply embedded in the patient's memory. However, it is worthwhile to also specifically ask about small surgical procedures such as the excision of a wart, a nevus, or the incision of a furuncle in childhood. The course of wound healing is also important in connection with an operation because secondary healing or more generally pronounced infected wounds often leave an interference field. Persistent pains in scars, which may itch with a change in the weather or trigger dysesthesia at the slightest touch, are strongly suspected to be associated with an interference field. Symptoms that were not completely resolved despite surgery or that occurred after an operation should also be documented as an indication of the presence of an interference field–induced disease or an interference field caused by the operation. Evidence of this is in the pain symptomology after abdominal procedures paraphrased with the term "adhesion pain" in neural therapy practice, since these symptoms can be resolved for the most part with local treatment or an interference field. Operations should be documented chronologically, if possible indicating the year, since the patient often does not realize these correlations because the start of a chronic illness usually occurs shortly after an operation.

The same is true for all types of **injuries**, which must be queried as the next item in the medical history. In doing so, the same level of detail should be applied in the process of questioning. The simple question: "Have you ever sustained an injury?" results in an incomplete history of injuries. Tear, puncture and cutting wounds, contusions, and fractures should be asked about along with distortions, bruises with hematoma development, tooth injuries in childhood (e.g., incisors), and burns. The listing of various types of injury according to the body region or body part is much more likely to yield a complete injury history. As already mentioned, in the next diagnostic step—the examination—there are still enough forgotten injuries in the form of skin lesions, scars, fingernails, and toenails, especially on the dorsal region of the body, to constitute residual injuries.

If all illnesses, operations, and injuries that the patient remembers by way of active assistance from the doctor are documented, the doctor should ask about **general symptoms** that have not yet been assigned a clear diagnosis, since—particularly in the case of chronic diseases—only a single, weakly pronounced symptom that is part of the patient's day-to-day life can become the key to a diagnosis with the corresponding neural therapeutic implications. In order to maintain a clear overview and exhaust all possibilities of the medical history as fully as possible, it is once again advisable to ask specifically about body regions while listing possible symptoms (▶Table 9.1).

▶**Table 9.1** Different symptoms should be queried according to the body region

Body region	Symptoms
Head	• Pain • Dizziness • Feeling of pressure • Fatigue • Difficulty concentrating • Changes in the ability to see, smell, taste, and hear • Speech disturbances
Neck	• Pressure or lumpy feeling • Occasional pain when swallowing • Contraction pains at the ear or in the shoulder–arm region
Thorax and its organs	• Respiration • Recurring cough • Expectoration • Difficulty breathing • Heart sensations • Feeling of pressure • Rhythm disorders
Abdomen and its organs	• Food intolerances • Bloating • Flatulence • Digestion disorders • Recurring pressure at the same location

The medical history of the **maxillodental region** holds a special place in the neural therapeutic medical history. Here, doctors can expect the most inaccurate and sketchy details from the patient. The discrepancy between the patient's knowledge of the condition of their own teeth and jaw and the actual findings relevant to neural diagnostics is widest in this case.

This is surely because neuropathological findings often cause easily overlooked symptoms or no symptoms, and because the difference between the neural diagnostic assessment and dental assessment of the teeth and jaw condition understandably leads to the dentist being given more credibility than the "nondentist."

The patient with a truly unremarkable dental history in the context of neural therapy is more of a rarity; thus, the patient's statement that a localized area in the jaw or an individual tooth sometimes becomes noticeable again is an urgent indication for a tooth/jaw lesion, even if the treating physician found no pathology result. The question of displaced, root-treated, crowned, filled, or pulled teeth cannot be explained solely by the verbal medical history. By already separating the study of the maxillofacial area in medical or dental training, the study of the teeth and jaw regions was separated from general medicine almost simultaneously.

Due to the frequency of chronic inflammatory disorders of the maxillofacial region and the resulting interference field diseases, the cooperation between the neural therapist and the dentist is of crucial importance. he medical history of the maxillofacial region, the examination, the evaluation of X-rays, and the complete description of findings by the dentist and possibly the jaw surgeon are required for assessment of the teeth and jaw, as are examination procedures such as panoramic teeth images or the even more detailed digital volume tomography (DVT).

The recording of the neural therapeutic history is the first diagnostic step which facilitates the decision for therapy on the whole, as well as the decision for **further in-depth examinations by medical specialists.**

Note

In day-to-day neural therapeutic practice, a large portion of patients have previously been extensively examined and have undergone other treatment methods. However, each time it should be newly decided whether diagnostics by specialists are needed to clarify the diagnosis.

This general advice should be followed not only for your own assurance, but also above all for that of the patient, thus contributing simultaneously to the correct classification of the efficiency of the neural therapy treatment method.

Conclusion

In summary, the neural therapeutic medical history is exceptionally important for therapeutic success. Unlike in the traditional medical history, in which only limited reference can be made to obvious direct correlations, such as long-ago joint compression and consequent posttraumatic osteoarthritis, for neural therapy any previous illness or injury can be seen from the viewpoint of a potential interference field possibly related to the current condition to be treated.

9.2 Examination

After taking the medical history as a verbal diagnostic tool, the examination is the next important step in the diagnosis of the current illness. The examination often results in additional findings that can play a decisive role in formulating the framework for the therapy.

Visible and clinically evaluable changes in the skin via the segmental-reflexive pathway can be expected in the case of organ diseases since the supply to the skin—with its adnexa as well as the glands—extends from the sympathetic nervous system. Through focused consideration of the body surface, the posture, and the motion sequence, the examination allows for conclusions about many diseases and functional disorders, such as may be present in the joints, the spine, and the muscles.

9.2.1 Skin

With the patient disrobed, attention should first be given to **scars** of any kind, which should be queried with regard to origin, the healing process, and any possible pain. Especially suspicious as giving rise to interference fields are the scars of infected wounds, furuncles, or scars that may cause discomfort constantly or at intervals. A human's first scar, the navel, should not be underestimated as a possible site for an interference field, particularly in illnesses that have occurred since early childhood. Childhood scars in the periphery of the extremities from abrasions or burns up to second degree often can no longer be seen in adulthood or show discrete pigment alterations and change their localization considerably through the patient's growth. Immunization scars must also be taken into account. The documentation of scars in note form with regard to their localization and origin should be as complete as possible, as they should all be taken into account during interference field testing. The small, non-irritated, and symptom-free vaccination scar can become an interference field in the same way as the large burn scar, which is occasionally itchy in some places.

Trophic disorders of the skin are often found as a segmental reflex response in diseases of body parts not visible to the naked eye. In chronic diseases of the maxillary sinuses or upper jaw, an alternating, slightly edematous swelling of the cheeks and skin of the lower eyelids is frequently observed. In chronic inflammation of the ethmoid cells or frontal sinuses, there is discrete, mostly one-sided edema formation on the upper and lower eyelids, and edema formation on the skin above the mandibular branch in disorders of the inferior teeth. At the same time, there may occasionally be persistent, discrete reddening in this region.

With lumbar sciatica or root irritation of the spinal nerves, **spider veins** (intracutaneous venous ectasias) are often also connected with disk disease in the skin above the spinous process—which then becomes sensitive to percussion—of the diseased segment. Likewise, these venous ectasias can found over the sacrum at level S2–S4 in diseases of the pelvic organs. Sahli described the band-shaped venous ectasia ring at the level of the sixth and seventh ribs in pulmonary emphysema. These are often observed completely encompassing the lower thorax ventrally and laterally in the case of chronic or even lapsed diseases of the liver, whether after hepatitis or severe toxic stress, so that a liver disease must be taken into consideration even if the medical history is blank. This assumption is supported if there is also brownish pigmentation of the eyelids or **xanthelasmas** (intracutaneous cholesterol deposits) in the eyelid area. **Palmar erythema** or **plantar erythema** and **rosacea** of the nose-cheek area are other signs that may indicate liver disease.

9.2.2 Musculoskeletal System

The musculoskeletal system, and the **spine** in particular, often provides examination findings that are early indications of diseases and functional disorders of the joints. The full extent of a disorder is demonstrated only through further functional diagnostics and examination of the range of movement. However, particularly when examining the spine, a functional disorder can already be detected if the physiological lordosis of the cervical and lumbar spine or kyphosis of the thoracic spine is represented with deskewed vertebral sections; in addition, with unilateral hypertension of the paravertebral musculature, there are visible muscle bulges which can occupy large sections of the spine and result in scoliotic deformities of the spine, pelvic obliquity, and functional leg length reduction. This may be due to improper stress on the spine, but also due to diseases of internal organs whose segmental-reflexive innervation via the sympathetic nervous system causes malfunctions of the axial spine organ with all of its functional units, as well as over other interference fields, e.g., tonsils, teeth, and sinuses. Visible muscular atrophy is often the result of a malfunction of the neuromotor units, thus through the demise of motor neurons by decreased stress, e.g., as part of joint degeneration or paralysis.

9.2.3 Oral Cavity and Teeth

Particular attention is necessary during examination of the oral cavity and teeth. Alone through the examination of the teeth, their placement, number, dental care, color, and shape, as well as the inspection of the gums, important indications in the context of neural therapy can be derived with regard to a dental disease or possible focal site. Thus, a beige–gray discolored tooth—even without root treatment—is highly suggestive of devitalization, a mechanically incurred fissure in tooth enamel may indicate a subsequent pulpitis, which can also occur entirely without pain, and a blackened tooth cervix, which is exposed under a crown, is a possible indication of a dentin disorder.

The gum tissue with its possible inflammatory changes can be equally regarded as a focal site in the jaw: for eample, the resulting scar in the jaw after tooth extraction or the irritation of the gums in the case of a bridge can be seen as an indication of chronic jaw osteitis.

A toothless jaw certainly does not rule out a focal site in the jaw, since root remnants, bone sequestrum, or foreign bodies under the nonirritated gum tissue, which do not necessarily cause pain or visible inflammation of the gums, can lie in or on the jaw bone.

> **Note**
>
> **The precise documentation of the dental status is part of the neural therapeutic examination because, from a neural therapeutic perspective, each treated, displaced, or unduly stressed tooth, as well as every empty jaw section resulting from tooth extraction, is potentially a focal site.**

The teeth are assigned a special section in the Chapter ▶ 12 on interference field diagnostics (p. 81) and interference field therapy (p. 82). In addition to confirming statements from the medical history, the inspection as part of the clinical examination provides many additional findings that help to solidify the suspected diagnosis and could be the first possible indications for disease correlations.

9.3 Palpation

Manual examination is also very important for neural therapy, since the findings obtained can be directly applied to the therapy. Selective pressure pain, in addition to resistance, is often the localization for a subsequent injection. The informative capability of “simple” examination with the hands is certainly much underestimated and lengthy training is required to utilize it fully. The opportunity to differentiate by way of palpation is a valuable diagnostic tool. Via the segmental-reflexive pathway, palpation findings can provide diagnostically valuable information on disease correlations, so that more complex tests such as X-ray, MRI, and CT scans can often be avoided.

The subtle palpation of geloses or muscle trigger points as an indication of localized circulatory disorders and the “bonding” of the skin with the subcutaneous tissue can be seen as an areal indication of a segmental disease traveling via the sympathetic conduction arc (viscerocutaneous reflex). Palpable local edema over the spinous processes of one or more vertebrae not only is determined in local vertebra irritation, but also is often an indication of organ or joint disease and can be included directly in the therapy as a valuable diagnostic tool.

> **Note**
>
> **Palpation often reveals findings that were not noticed either in the medical history or in the examination and yet are most important for the therapy.**

Again, the spine and muscles as well as the sacroiliac joints cannot be examined often enough, because they provide decisive findings through palpation for causal therapy. Often, joint diseases of the upper and lower extremities as well as the head are brought to light upon palpation, as there was no information about them provided in the medical history or signs of irritation in these areas when otherwise examined. Only targeted manual examination provides neuraltherapeutically useful findings for pain symptoms in the region of a joint or a previously clinically unapparent organ disease.

> **Note**
>
> **Knowledge of nerve passages or exit points accessible by palpation and their correlation to the corresponding spinal segments or the corresponding cranial nerves is very important for the diagnosis.**

An irritated nerve caused by preexisting stimulus, which does not necessarily provoke subjective symptoms spontaneously, demonstrates its irritation through the additional pressure of the examining finger.

The irritated spinal nerve S1, which does not have to demonstrate the corresponding neurological result of hyperesthesia or hypoesthesia in segment S1 spontaneously, signals itself intensely with isolated finger pressure on the sacral foramen; likewise the peripheral branch of the trigeminal nerve at the level of its discharge points in the facial skull with chronic asymptomatically progressing sinusitis or tooth lesions.

Note

The pressure sensitivity of nerves that can be confirmed in a side-by-side comparison is not sole evidence of nerve irritation, but at the same time may also be evidence of an organ disease or initial evidence of an interference field disease.

Since afferent and efferent fiber portions of the sympathetic nervous system extend all the way to the periphery with all spinal nerves, and since there are also arteries and veins accompanying these nerves as a unit of the neurovascular bundle with their perivascular sympathetic plexus, spinal nerves serve as an orientation for the neural therapeutically relevant sympathetic nervous system which is to be reached by the targeted injection. The injection is usually designated as follows: injection at spinal nerve L5 (for example). A more accurate designation would be: injection at the sympathetic fiber portion of the spinal nerve L5. The same applies to the cranial nerves. To illustrate diagnostic palpation and its significance in the context of a statement relevant to neural therapy, an example which underscores the value of the manual examination should be mentioned.

On examination of the spine, there is percussion sensitivity of the spinous processes T8–T11 and hypertension of the paravertebral musculature which is more pronounced on the right (in lateral comparison) with isolated pressure pain two finger-widths lateral to the spinous processes. In the medical history, there was no information about thoracic spine symptoms. This first finding leads to a palpatory examination of the anterior costal arch, where sharp, selective pressure triggers pain at the level of the nipple. This involves the Vogler pressure point, which represents the anterior intercostal nerve branch 8 as an anatomical substrate extending as a nerve bundle under the costal arch in the direction of the abdominal wall. Lateral comparison at the same location under the left costal arch results in no pressure pain there. The intercostal nerve 8 is segmentally associated with the liver segment. In lateral comparison, the isolated palpation of the nerve exit points of the trigeminal nerve performed henceforth shows right-sided pressure tenderness of the supraorbital nerve and, increasingly, the infraorbital nerve. The clinically relevant finding also indicates a disorder in the area of the liver. The neuroanatomical substrate consists of the afferent connection of the vagus nerve (supply of the liver) with the spinal trigeminal nucleic regions.

Further palpation of the cervical spine results in pressure pain of the spinous processes of C3–C5 with simultaneous pressure pain and slight tension of the right side paravertebral musculature. The neuroanatomical background is formed by the afferent pathways of the phrenic nerve, which supplies the visceral peritoneum of the liver, among others. In terms of neural therapy, this palpation finding indicates urgent suspicion of nerve irritation in the liver, especially if hepatitis, bile duct disorders, toxic liver loads, or an injury was denied in the medical history and there was no pathological finding in the laboratory chemistry. This result from the palpatory exam should be documented in each case, since—in terms of neural therapy—there is suspicion of a liver function disorder, which must then be included in the interference field diagnostics, for example.

It is therefore necessary to correlate the palpation result with the corresponding spinal segment or cranial nerve region via the direct or indirect innervation pathway in order to proceed with a targeted neural diagnostic approach. Palpation findings which extend over the entire side of the body, e.g., right-sided head pressure points, muscular tension on the right side of the cervical spine, functional limitations of the right shoulder, tension of the right-sided thoracic and lumbar paravertebral musculature, and pressure pain in the right lower extremity, are strongly suggestive of a right-sided focal site in the patient. The focal sites are most frequently found in the area of the teeth, the tonsils, the sinuses, or the abdominal organs.

The palpation consists of:

- Manual diagnostics:
  - To evaluate the joints.
  - To determine periarticular edema or the formation of effusion.
- Examination of the major body cavities by means of percussion:
  - To determine the organ borders.
  - To assess the filling of air or fluid in the thoracic and abdominal cavities.
  - To palpate masses, tumors, and tissue gaps as found in torn muscles, tendon ruptures, or hernias.
  - To evaluate vascular pulsation.
  - To evaluate the skin temperature, the surface moisture, and the skin tension.
- Manual examination:
  - To assess range of motion, ligament stability, and capsular stability.
  - To examine muscle groups in side-by-side comparison.

The above comprises the investigational use of hands and fingers in neural therapy and is sufficient for clinical examination in the majority of cases.

9.4 Other Examination Options

The clinical diagnostics described thus far are quite sufficient to the extent that neural diagnostics can follow, via either the segment or the interference field. Neural diagnostics can be understood as the injections or injection series revealed in the medical history, the examination, and the palpation. The actual therapy is derived from this result. The diagnostic approach described above, which can be implemented at any time without tools, can be completed and verified with numerous other studies in case of uncertainties.

Other clinical examination options include auscultation, the measurement of blood pressure and temperature, and illumination of the oral cavity and pharynx, the nose, and the external auditory canal.

Practical Advice

The examination by a medical specialist should be undertaken even when there is little doubt about the self-diagnosis, not only to verify the self-diagnosis, but also above all to protect the patient and not least to document the validity of neural therapy.

Laboratory chemical and bacteriological analysis options help to objectify the clinical diagnosis and to document the neural therapeutic course of treatment. Thus, short-term control of hyperthyroidism, pancreatitis, and pneumonia, to name a few examples, is necessary to assess the course of treatment.

Instrumental diagnostic techniques such as ECG, ultrasound, X-ray, MRI, and endoscopy are available to refine the diagnosis, but one must always take into account potential exposure or harm to the patient. In this case, close collaboration with the appropriate medical specialist is very valuable, as the risks of an examination and the diagnostic value of the techniques, which are sometimes invasive, must be weighed.

Finally, **neural diagnostics** should be explored. Individual targeted injections are made in and at defined tissue structures, whereby the diagnosis can be deduced from the clinical outcome of the injections. This involves a functional diagnosis of the sympathetic nervous system, whose localized impaired function is interrupted by a local anesthetic and can be normalized via autoregulatory processes far beyond the duration of the local anesthetic's effect. Segmental diagnostics (p. 53) and interference field diagnostics (p. 81) are available; these two neural diagnostic options will be described separately in detail. Notable features are the simple implementation, the high diagnostic value in a very short time, and the continuation of the same injections for the treatment in the event of a positive test failure. In neural therapy, diagnosis and treatment are handled with the same technique and without significant expenditure on equipment.

9.5 Documentation

For neural therapy, the detailed recording of the medical history, the findings, and the diagnostic and therapeutic progress is particularly important for the treatment result, since all details that need to be explored in each new treatment must be taken into account. This is mainly due to the treatment tactics being only slightly standardizable which means quite different therapeutic approaches are required to reach similar diagnoses in different patients. In this situation, basically working from memory runs the risk of the practitioner losing the diagnostic and therapeutic thread and thereby thwarting the attainment of therapeutic success.

Note

In addition to precise documentation of symptoms, the exploratory questioning before any new treatment about the reactions to previous treatments is necessary because any new treatment must be tailored to take these reactions into account.

The therapist should assess not only improvement or worsening of the symptomology to be treated, but also the duration of newly occurring symptoms or a change in the initial symptomology Based on the recorded injections, it must be possible to understand the changes that occurred and determine the next injections. This enables follow-up monitoring of a neural therapeutic treatment, from which the disease relationships—the actual etiology—can be deduced. Frequently, diagnostic and therapeutic injections are done in parallel as symptoms of one illness must be treated in order to successfully treat a second disease in the patient, and newly added symptoms can impair the existing therapy plan. If this approach, which determines the neural therapeutic routine, comes primarily from the memories of the therapist and the patient and not from the notes, the success rate will be significantly lower.

The documentation must be done in such a way that the diagnosis, the therapeutic approach based on the injections made, and result achieved remain fully comprehensible, even for a physician not trained in neural therapy. This makes it possible to statistically analyze individual symptomologies and properly classify the efficacy of the method. This is just as important for the individual therapist as it is for the illustration of the treatment method itself. From the clear documentation of the individual case history, it is then possible to identify the following, for example:

- What percentage is due to interference field diseases?
- Where are most of the interference fields localized?
- How variable are the interference field–related diseases despite arising from the same interference field?
- What costs arise through neural therapeutic treatments in comparison to other methods?

For clarity, it may be helpful to choose a medical chart specifically oriented to the neural therapeutic history, examination findings, and the progression. An example is illustrated here (▶ Fig. 9.1).

Neural Therapy

Name: | Date of birth:

Address:

Medical insurance: | Phone number:

Medical history:

Findings:

Drugs: | Allergies:

Diagnosis:

Childhood illnesses:	Operations/injuries	Other illnesses
Gynecological/andrological medical history:		

Tooth status: **X:** Extracted **F:** Filling **C:** Crown **B:** Dental bridge/prosthesis **P:** Pain
C: Cavity **D:** devitalized **Pd:** Parodontitis **I:** Impacted tooth

8	7	6	5	4	3	2	1	1	2	3	4	5	6	7	8
8	7	6	5	4	3	2	1	1	2	3	4	5	6	7	8

Date	Med.	Injection site	Reaction and findings	Number

▶ **Fig. 9.1** Example of a neural therapeutic medical chart and progress sheet.

9.6

Structure of Neural Therapeutic Practice

The material costs for diagnosis and treatment in neural therapy are very low, since the same technique is used for diagnosis and treatment. Injection needles of various lengths are required, which should be as thin as possible and very sharp. The length of the needles should be 2 to 12 cm, measured in 2-cm increments, in order to carry out the injections at different depths. When selecting the needles, the sharpness, good gliding properties, and tight fit on the cone of the syringe are more important than the price. Blunt needles cause more pain on injection, poor gliding poses the risk of incorrect positioning of the injection, and the needle jumping off the syringe may cause unnecessary injuries.

The **5-mL disposable syringe** has been shown to be a valuable tool. Smaller or larger syringes are not as easy to handle. More than 5 mL of local anesthetic is seldom needed for a single injection, so that a change of the syringe in an injection process is rarely required. Injection to the teeth requires a **carpule syringe** as is used for local anesthesia in dentistry. The screwed-on dental needles prevent the needle from jumping off in the oral cavity, futhermore the needle length should not exceed 2 cm since the rear lateral part of the oral cavity is sometimes quite narrow and long needles are too bulky and can snap.

A disadvantage is the addition of **preservatives** to the local anesthetics in the required glass vials. The use of **amide-structured** local anesthetics carries the very low risk of exacerbating existing bacterial infections in the area of infiltration since a slight vasoconstriction which deteriorates tissue perfusion occurs at the injection site. With **ester-structured procaine**, the cleavage product dimethylaminoethanol causes vasodilation and improved tissue perfusion.

A bright source of light is necessary for illuminating the oral and nasal cavities as well as the outer ear. Battery-operated lights with different attachments for use as spatula lights, otoscopes, or rhinoscopes are especially suitable for this purpose.

Practical Advice

The position of the patient is important; relaxed muscles are crucial for the ability to perform the various injections. The first choice is an examination table on which patients can sit or lay comfortably on their back or side.

All possible positions should be reduced to the simplest form, because patients with poor mobility or with severely painful conditions, e.g., those affecting the musculoskeletal system, are not well-suited to special "gymnastics." However, the consistent use of the prone and sitting positions, from which all injections can be made, is of great advantage to the attending physician, since these positions least impair the visualization of the topographic anatomy, in particular for deep injections or injections in the area of the spine. Injections while standing as well as with a non-stabilized head ("free sitting") should be avoided, if only for orthostatic reasons and for injection safety.

For disinfection of the skin (p. 104), the usual disinfectants are sufficient. Injections in joints require sterile disposable gloves, mouth guards, and head covers as well as a room that satisfies the aseptic requirements for joint injections. Lastly, a standardized emergency kit, which is a part of every medical practice, is a necessity.

9.7

Selecting the Neural Therapeutic Agent

As illustrated in detail in the first part of this book, the optimal medication for neural therapy is procaine (p. 37) **in a 1% concentration** without any additives.

Cave

With an existing allergy to procaine, which is very rare, another product must be used, e.g., lidocaine.

General symptoms occasionally described by patients such as persistent nausea and severe discomfort are almost always due to an interference field event and disappear after removal of the interference field effect. For more details on interference field events, see Retrograde Phenomenon (p. 98).

Procaine is most reliable in 5-mL glass vials, as the "rationed" amount in the vial provides a better overview of the total quantity of procaine injected. The possibility of contamination of the procaine with bacteria, or with the patient's blood in the case of repeated refilling of the syringe, is certainly higher when using injection bottles. In addition, in accordance with the Medicines Act, a preservative is added to the procaine in glass bottles, which is undesirable for neural therapy and also means an increased risk of allergies. The warning that fine glass powder may also be taken up when drawing the medicine from glass vials is hardly relevant anymore with today's break-seal ampoules; the claim of the pharmaceutical industry that plastic vials do not bear this risk of a fine glass powder or splinter admixture is certainly true. However, toxic products of the plastic vial (plasticizers) must also be taken into account.

Other preparations that do not have local anesthetic properties can certainly also be used for neural therapy, but only as a "stimulus drug" in wheal therapy. A better effect is not to be expected.

Note

Before using mixed preparations a word of warning: a major advantage of procaine is its good tissue compatibility, which most of the other preparations are lacking, particularly in view of the frequent injections to peripheral nerves.

Other local anesthetics are certainly also suitable for neural therapy. As already explained in detail, the properties of the ester-structured procaine which are important to neural therapy are best combined in this preparation. The amide-structured local anesthetics are more toxic both at the application site and for the entire body. This becomes apparent in the total quantity required for a treatment cycle as well as in the “overdosing” of medication at the injection site itself. In every case, there is an overdose with local irritation on the tissue structures saturated with the local anesthetic, which must lead to a tissue reaction. This is least evident in the case of procaine due to its extremely short half-life; furthermore, procaine is the only local anesthetic whose degradation products **dimethylaminoethanol** and **para-aminobenzoic acid** have a positive tissue effect.

These two properties of procaine also probably contribute to the fact that an infection hardly ever appears at the injection site or that procaine is the only local anesthetic which can be used to infiltrate bacterially infected tissue, whereby it results in accelerated healing of the infection.

Amide-structured local anesthetics are unsuitable for the local treatment of bacterial infections due to their effect on tissue, which is the opposite to that of procaine. The contraindication—from a surgical perspective—of infiltrating bacterial tissue infections with a local anesthetic also reflects this situation, but only applies to amide-structured local anesthetics and not procaine.

10 Segments

10.1 Segment Diagnostics—Segmental Therapy

The segment concept (p. 27) for neural therapy was illustrated in the first part of this book with the aim of showing the extensive innervation relationships that must be taken into account in neural diagnostics and neural therapy. The goal was to illustrate disease correlations that take place purely on the spinal level, even if they seem on first glance to have nothing to do with one another, because the localization of the different illnesses or functional disorders are too far apart. This is reflected in the fact that chronic headaches can be absolutely linked to a liver disorder or a chronic tooth disorder can be connected to heart disease.

The first step of neural diagnostics therefore consists of making an injection locally at the site of the disorder using the information from the medical history (p. 44) and the palpatory examination findings (p. 47). A series of wheals in the area of the disorder and the corresponding dermatome completes this step. In musculoskeletal disorders, the painful pressure points (trigger points), whose associated tissue is partly identifiable by palpation and anatomical visualization, are infiltrated with the neural therapeutic agent, whereby the infiltration should optimally penetrate painful tissue structures such as the following each time:

- Ligament capsule tissue.
- Muscle and tendon attachments.
- Painful pressure points of the muscles.

A few "scale marks worth" of the neural therapeutic agent are quite sufficient for reducing pain. The supplying and outflowing vessels and the efferent–afferent conducting spinal and cranial nerves are structures whose sympathetic nerve fiber content should be reached by the local anesthetic through perivascular and perineural infiltration. Scars in the region, such as in the shoulder, in the shoulder–neck region, and in the arm on the same side should also be infiltrated. The diagnostic approach is based on the fact that significant improvement—up to freedom from symptoms—must occur after treatment in order to ensure that the injections were performed correctly. The previously described process involved neural therapeutic segment diagnostics, since the possible reactions must first be awaited in order to confirm the suspected diagnosis. These reactions are queried at the next neural therapeutic treatment and then the subsequent injections are oriented to this, at first daily for acute conditions, and initially at weekly intervals for chronic conditions.

1. **Potential reaction**: The symptoms to be treated were:
   - Significantly improved or eliminated for 1 day or longer and then reappeared in a less severe form.
   - Significantly improved or eliminated initially for the period that the local anesthesia was used, reappeared at a greater intensity over 1 to 3 days, then occurred only in a diminished form.
   - Significantly and consistently improved or eliminated immediately after the treatment.

In these cases, the suspected diagnosis is confirmed. The therapy consists of repeating the same injections until the patient is free of symptoms. If the symptoms are completely eliminated already after the first treatment, a "prophylactic" repetition of the injections is not required, but only at the recurrence of symptoms.

2. **Potential reaction**: The symptoms to be treated:
   - Improved after the diagnostic injections or were eliminated during the anesthesia period, but then reappeared at the same intensity or worsened temporarily, ultimately achieving the same intensity as before the first diagnostic injection series.
   - Could not be improved with the local infiltrations.
   - Could not be assessed by the patient; the patient could not provide any information about a change in the symptoms.

Practical Advice

After an unsuccessful first treatment, repetition of the diagnostic injections is not indicated since the subsequent identical injections will not lead to a change in the symptomology. Clinical follow-up of the symptomology with comparison to the initial findings should take place in any case so that the therapist can be sure that there has been no change in the findings. If there is an improvement in the clinical examination despite contradictory information provided by the patient, repetition of the injections is indicated.

If the patient is not fully asymptomatic through simple repeated segmental therapy, injections at centrally located sympathetic nervous system structures are indicated in the context of segmental diagnostics and therapy.

Depending on the affected region, the following injections are considered:

- Head:
  - Superior cervical ganglion.
  - – Vertebral artery.
  - – Common carotid artery.
  - Internal carotid artery.
- Eye:
  - Superior cervical and ciliary ganglion.
- Paranasal sinuses and oral-nasopharyngeal space including the upper teeth:
  - Pterygopalatine ganglion.
  - Maxillary artery.
- Ear, parotid gland, tongue, and floor of the mouth:
  - Superior and otic cervical ganglion
- Advanced segment therapy for the neck, thorax and its organs, and upper extremities:
  - Laterally identical stellate ganglion.
- Intra- and extraperitoneal organs:
  - Celiac ganglion (splanchnic nerves, both sides).
- Retroperitoneal kidneys:
  - Renal plexus
- Advanced segment treatment of the lower extremities:
  - Lumbar sympathetic trunk at the level of the third lumbar vertebra.

In the application of the neural therapeutic treatment, both simple and advanced segmental therapy are often necessary. Alternating or combined use must be decided on a case-by-case basis depending on changes in symptomology as treatment progresses. Here, the detailed questioning about the therapeutic effect is particularly valuable, as is the comparison of the results from the individual segmental therapy measures.

Despite extensive segmental therapy, quite often an illness being treated does not completely subside. In these cases, an interference field induced by the residual symptoms must be considered, hence the segmental treatment is temporarily discontinued and interference field diagnostics is carried out (p. 81). It is quite possible that individual symptoms of an illness are supported by an interference field and subside only when the interference field is eliminated, while other symptoms of the same illness can be successfully treated in the segment.

In the diagnosis of an illness from a neural therapeutic perspective as well as in the subsequent therapy, clinical symptoms as well as diagnostically valuable findings which arise on direct or indirect reflex pathways must be recorded. These are the findings that arise from the innervation relationships by way of cranial nerves or spinal nerves, simultaneous innervation by the sympathetic nervous system, the parasympathetic nervous system, and additional partially simultaneous afferent supply by the phrenic nerve. These innervation relationships explain the neurophysiological basis and at the same time the transition from segmental diagnostics to interference field situation. These relationships will be illustrated and justified by way of a clinical example. To this end, **chronic sinusitis** will be regarded as an initial disease and the diagnostic and therapeutic approach will be demonstrated based on the wide range of possible symptoms.

Depending on the focus of the chronic sinusitis, there may be recurrent pressure and pain in the maxilla (maxillary sinus), the forehead (frontal sinus), and eye sockets (ethmoid sinus). Symptoms may be more pronounced on one side. Other frequently found symptoms are alternating nasal obstruction, nasal speech, and alternating secretion from the nose or more often in the nasopharyngeal space, but these symptoms are sometimes so weakly developed that they must first be discussed in detail with the patient. Palpation generally results in pressure-sensitive nerve exit points of the supraorbital nerve, the infraorbital nerve, and, rarely, the mental nerve.

Additional symptoms such as diffuse frontal headache, pulling pain at the ear, occipital headache, cervical pain, shoulder–arm pain, back pain, lumbar ischialgia, joint pain in the upper or lower extremities, pollinosis, and chronic bronchitis up to chronic asthma are no longer as clearly associated with chronic sinusitis since the localization of the concomitant symptoms apparently has no direct connection to the sinuses. This is particularly pronounced when the subjective pain symptoms of the sinus disorder occur in the background or are even missing prior to the occurrence of the concomitant symptoms. The listed concomitant symptoms are already an indication of the effects of the chronic sinusitis which exerts a focal or interference field function.

The innervation relationships for this symptomology determine the localization of the concomitant disease originating from the paranasal sinuses. To this end, it is important to consider the nerve structures supplying the paranasal sinuses as well as their connections at the spinal or diencephalic level:

- As an afferent conducting nerve responsible for mucosal sensitivity, the **trigeminal nerve** has connections to spinal segments C1–C3 via its spinal nucleic regions, which extend up to the three upper neck segments. This results in symptoms in cervical segments C1–C3. In addition, the clinical symptomology can be expanded through the connections of the trigeminal nucleic regions with the **glossopharyngeal nerve**, the **accessory nerve**, and not least the **facial nerve** and the efferent motor portion of the trigeminal nerve.
- The **sympathetic nervous system**, whose afferent pathways flow together with the vessels supplying the mucosa, enables an irritation precisely in these segments through the afferent pathways via its synapse (dorsal root ganglia, superior cervical ganglion) of segments C8–T6 as well as via the sympathetic conduction arc and synapses in area of the dorsal root ganglia.
- The parasympathetic nervous system, whose afferents are partially connected with the spinal nucleic regions of the **trigeminal nerve**, may trigger a response—via the parasympathetic conduction arc—in the supply area of the **vagus nerve**, e.g., in the form of a sinobronchial syndrome, bronchial asthma, or pathological influence on the abdominal organs.
- The connection between the sympathetic and parasympathetic nervous system via the superior cervical ganglion and the inferior ganglion of the vagus nerve as well as the extracranial ganglion of the **glossopharyngeal nerve** via the **jugular nerve** represents an anatomical entity whose function has received little attention. Through this conduction pathway, stimulation of the parasympathetic nervous system (**vagus nerve**) and **glossopharyngeal nerve** is possible via the sympathetic nervous system with the above-mentioned reactions in its supply area. Finally, in the assessment of clinical symptoms, parasympathetic vasodilators originating from the pterygopalatine ganglion and coursing together with the intra- and extracranial vessels must be considered in diseases of the paranasal sinuses with regard to the effects on the brain (circulatory disorders) and the craniofacial skeleton (e.g., trigeminal-autonomic headaches).

Through these innervation relationships, a wealth of symptomatologies originating from the paranasal sinuses is possible. The same neuroanatomical connections exist for the teeth, whose afferent innervation portion is formed by the **trigeminal nerve** and **sympathetic nervous system**.

Overall, these neuroanatomical connections are already at the heart of describing the interference field disease, whose clinical characteristic is based on the fact that the symptomology of the primary disease location is oligosymptomatic or asymptomatic, while the disease evoked on the nerve pathways at another location represents the primary finding.

Starting from the same modalities of the chest and abdominal cavity, the segment diagnostics and therapy get a new defined expanded framework, and the transition in potential interference field diseases is simultaneously demonstrated in terms of neurophysiology.

10.2
Lung Segment

10.2.1 Diagnostics

The lungs as well as the bronchia and the pleura are innervated by the parasympathetic nervous system (vagus nerve) and the sympathetic nervous system (▸Fig. 10.1). The efferent portion of the **parasympathetic nervous system** is responsible for the production of mucous as well as the bronchial muscular tone. Stimulations of the vagus nerve result in increased mucus production and increased tone of the bronchial musculature; severance of the vagus nerve leads to the contrary. The parasympathetic afferents are quickly and slowly adapting lung expansion receptors, which mediate the expansion status of the alveoli and bronchi. The cough reflex also takes place via the parasympathetic afferents. Synaptic connections between the vagal afferent fibers and the spinal nucleic regions of the trigeminal nerve and with the top three cervical segments are important for clinical diagnostics. A stimulation of the parasympathetic fibers can also lead to stimulation of the trigeminal nerve as well as the first three cervical segments, resulting in dysesthesia in the supply region of the trigeminal nerve and the top three neck dermatomes as well as malfunction of the corresponding short neck muscles.

The **sympathetic supply** to the lungs and bronchi regulates their tissue perfusion and microcirculation and causes an effect on the mucous membranes and the bronchial muscles which is opposite to that of the parasympathetic nervous system.

The pathological stimulus of the efferent sympathetic nervous system also leads to a decrease in mucous production (thick mucus) as well as increased bronchial muscle tone through hypoxia of the mucosa and musculature due to impaired perfusion (predominance of parasympathetic

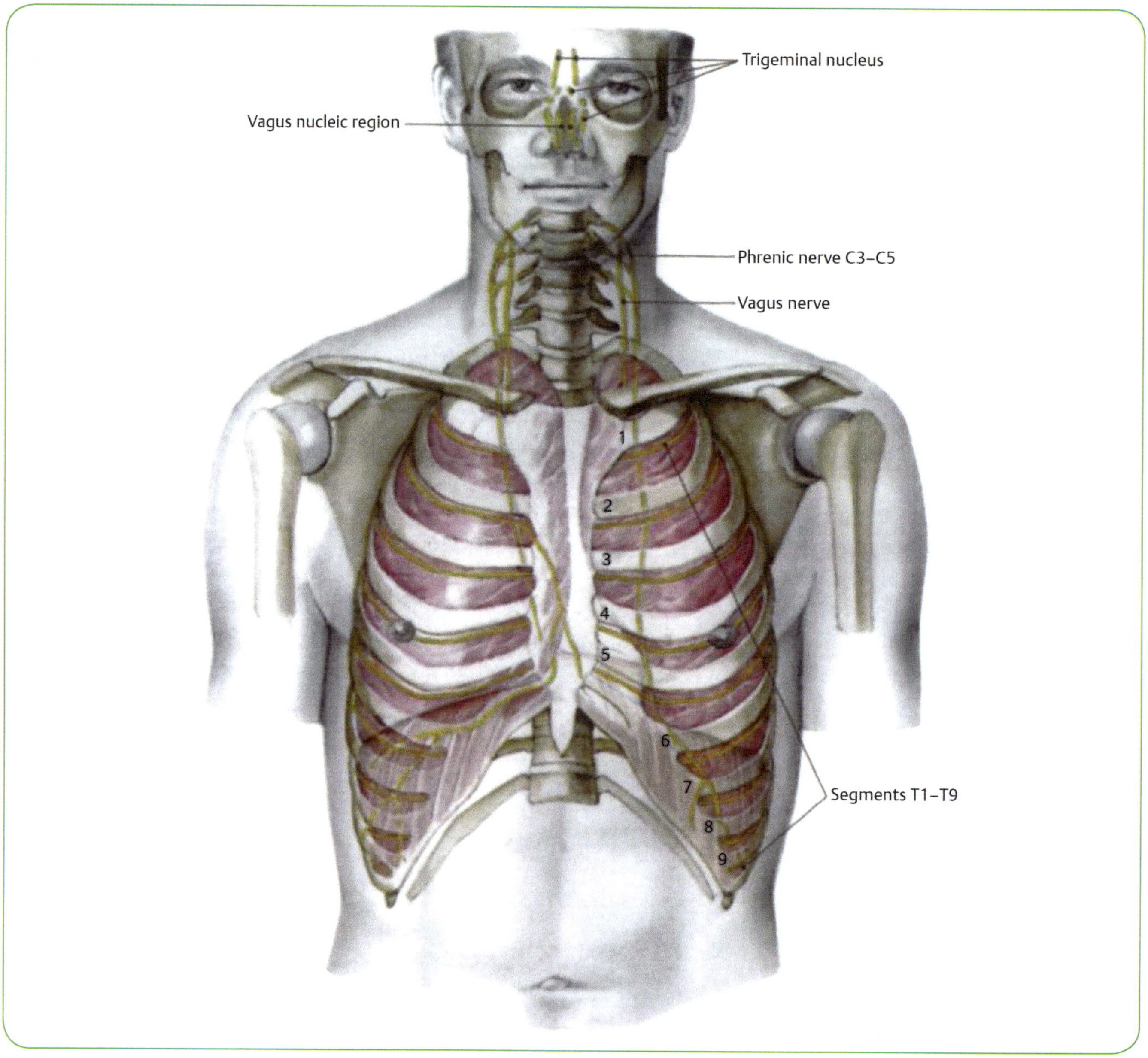

▸**Fig. 10.1** The innervation of the lungs, the bronchia, and the pleura and their relationships.

tone in the muscles). The blocking of the sympathetic nervous system (stellate infiltration) has the opposite effect, a normalizing function (due to the improved perfusion) between the sympathetic and parasympathetic bronchial and lung tissue. The sympathetic afferent fibers mediate, inter alia, pain associated with inflammation or injury of the lung. The core areas of the sympathetic nervous system for the lungs and bronchi are in thoracic segments T1–T4. In the case of lung disorders, segment-reflexive findings are to be expected in the form of sensory disturbances and dysfunction of the muscles as well as changes in skin trophism and subcutaneous tissue (e.g., geloses). "Spider veins" (venulectasias) are often found clinically in the indicated segments as a sign of impaired cutaneous innervation.

With involvement of the pleura in a lung disorder, in addition to the stimulation of the autonomic afferent fibers, there is also stimulation of the phrenic nerve afferent fibers (▶Fig. 10.2), whose sensitive supply area extends, inter alia, to the diaphragmatic mediastinal pleura.

The inputs of the segmental phrenic nerve are in neck segments C3–C5, but often are also lower because the phrenic nerve can be associated with portions of spinal segments C6–C8 as a so-called auxiliary phrenic nerve. Thus, clinical findings for the skin and musculature in the form of sensory disturbances and muscle dysfunction are to be expected.

In diseases of the lungs and the bronchial system, diagnostically usable findings which must be incorporated in the therapy can be expected via the parasympathetic nervous system and the sympathetic nervous system with the trigeminal nerve and the phrenic nerve beyond the lung segment alone. This way, chronic shoulder pain with corresponding motor impairment can be maintained by a subclinically progressing bilaterally identical lung disease. A situation with occipital (C2) or frontal (trigeminal nerve)

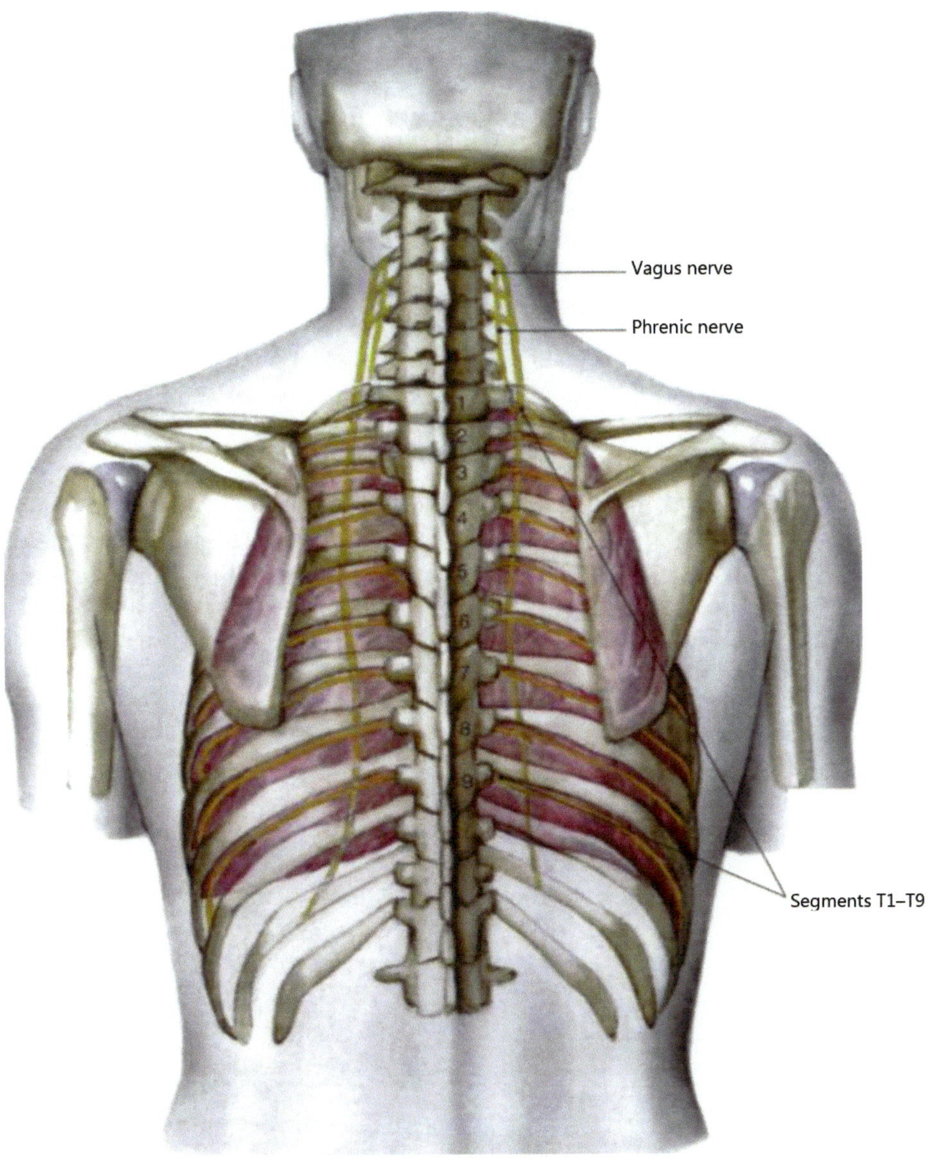

▶**Fig. 10.2** The innervation of the lungs, the bronchia, and the pleura and their relationships.

headache or a disorder of the cervical spine in the C1–C5 region can also be associated with this. In these cases, only primary neural therapeutic treatment of the lungs can resolve concomitant symptoms progressing via the corresponding afferent pathways; however, the treatment of concomitant symptoms will fail because the focal lesion (interference field) is located in the lungs. As part of the lung disease, the stimulation of the sympathetic afferent fibers can operate across segments and lead to disorders of the sympathetic efferent fibers with the effect of trophic dysregulation not only in the lungs, but also at a completely different location. The summation of the pathological impulse outputs gives rise to the disease induced by the interference field.

10.2.2 Therapy

The standard treatment of pulmonary disease (also as an interference field) consists of a series of wheals applied parasternally at the level of the intercostal spaces and two fingerbreadths paravertebrally at the T1-T9 level. level. Tender areas of the ribs, especially at the transition to the costal cartilages, are infiltrated, as are geloses of the subcutis or hypertonic muscle areas. Furthermore, scars of the thorax (also old rib fractures) should be infiltrated.

The further standard treatment of lung and bronchi consists of the infiltration of the stellate ganglion on the right and left alternately, whereby in acute illnesses there should be at least 15 minutes between injections due to possible recurrent anesthesia. The same injections are carried out in interference field diagnostics if the lungs and the bronchial system are suspected as an interference field.

10.2.3 Summary

In diseases of the lungs and bronchi as well as the pleura, a segment-reflexive response originating from the supplying nerves is to be expected:

- Sympathetic nervous system: T1–T4 with sensorimotor reaction of the somatic nervous system.
- Parasympathetic nervous system: reflexive response of the trigeminal nerve, neck segments C1–C3.
- Phrenic nerve: reflexive response of cervical segments C3–C5.

The symptoms of lung, bronchial and pleura disorders can decrease strikingly in comparison to the symptoms of the disease progressing via the reflex pathway.

10.3 Heart Segment

10.3.1 Diagnostics

The afferent innervation of the heart is the basis of clinical symptoms that may occur in the context of heart disease. The corresponding pain symptomology not only is found near the heart, but also appears further away in sections primarily not associated with heart disease. The afferent nerve supply proceeds via the sympathetic nervous system, the parasympathetic system (vagus nerve), and the phrenic nerve starting from the pericardium (▶Fig. 10.3). The efferent supply proceeds only via the sympathetic nervous system and parasympathetic nervous system. The afferent fibers give rise to the clinical symptomology of heart disease, which can be composed of the different individual symptoms.

Symptoms arising from the **sympathetic nervous system** are found directly in the area of the heart in the form of different levels of pain in the precordial, left dorsal region in segments C8–T5 from the area of the spinal nucleic regions of the sympathetic nervous system. Here, the muscles are often hypertonic upon palpation and the spinous processes sensitive to percussion. Particularly in acute myocardial ischemia, pain radiating into the left eighth cervical segment, which can reach up to the fifth finger, is typical. The pathway proceeds from the sympathetic afferents of the heart muscle and the pericardium over the stellate ganglion to the spinal ganglion of C8. From here, it uses a reflexive pathway via the somatosensory connections to produce the pain over the course of cervical segment C8, and this awareness is carried through another conduit to the brain. The pain is interrupted by injecting a local anesthetic to the stellate ganglion. The pain can also be produced by stimulation of the same ganglion.

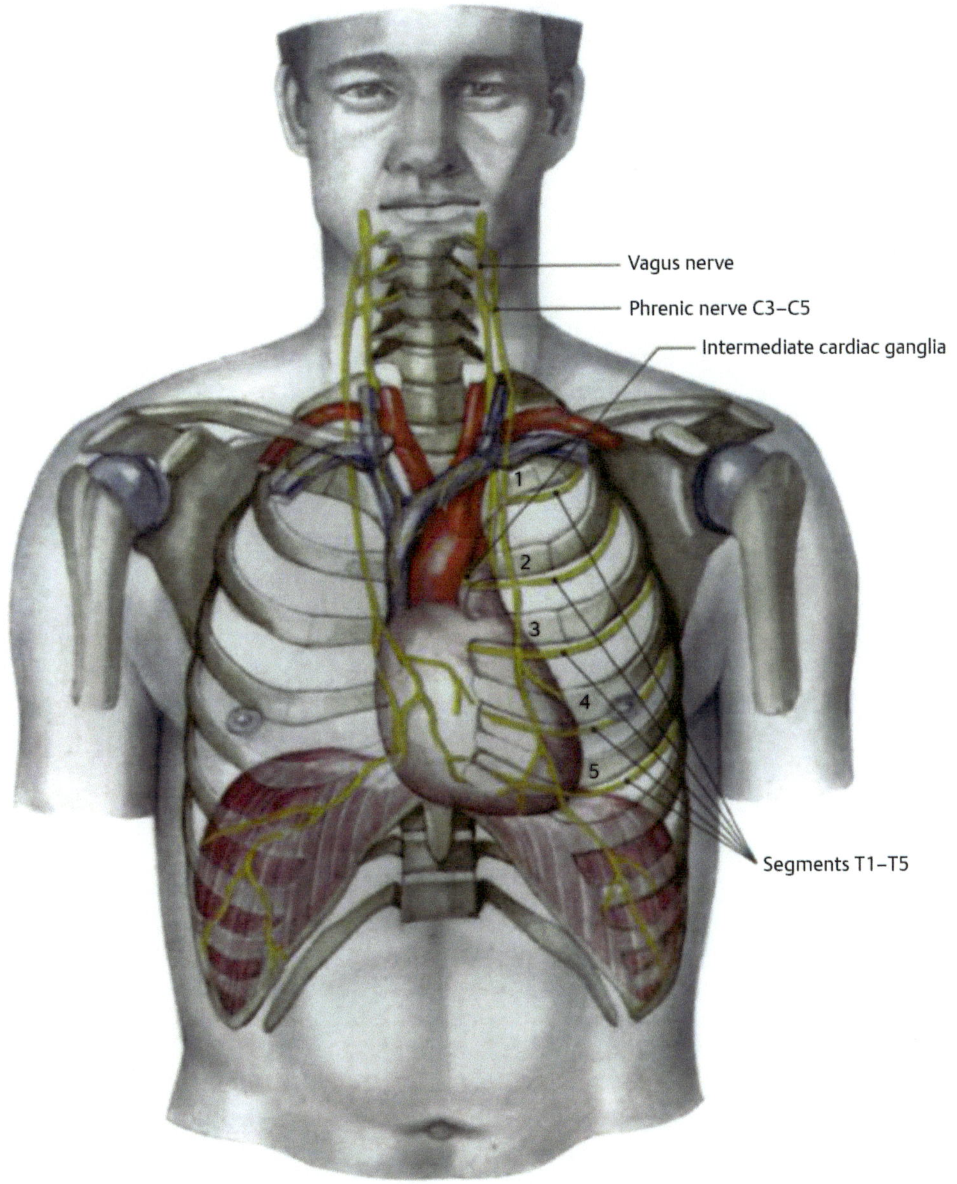

▶**Fig. 10.3** The heart segment and its innervation relationships.

Symptoms arising from the afferent **parasympathetic nervous system** manifest as cardiac asthma, as nausea, or as abdominal symptoms starting with increased bowel or bladder activity. Furthermore, sensory disturbances in the area supplied by the trigeminal nerve are possible on the left side via synaptic connections of the vagal afferent fibers with the spinal nucleic regions of the trigeminal nerve. Through simultaneous connections of the spinal trigeminal nucleic region with the first three cervical spinal segments, there is a possible symptomology of the upper short muscles of the head and neck as well as the greater occipital nerve, and to a lesser extent also the lesser occipital nerve, in the form of occipital pressure or neck pain, mostly focused on the left side.

The afferent fibers of the **phrenic nerve** supply, among others, the pericardium. In spinal segments C3–C5, the nucleic regions of the phrenic nerve (▸Fig. 10.4), enable sensorimotor reflexive symptoms in the area of the middle cervical spine. These can appear in clinical examinations as left-focused neck pain, pressure pain of the spinous processes from C3–C5, and muscular myogelosis as well as dysfunction of the diaphragm muscles, clinically indicated by shortness of breath.

All previously mentioned symptoms can occur in varying degrees depending on the stimulus intensity of the heart disease or remain outside of the subjective sensation, so that these findings can be verified only during manual examination through the additional pressure stimulus of the tactile finger. However, in the absence of cardiac symptoms and chronic left-focused pain in the trigeminal nerve, the back of the head, the cervical spine in segments C1–C5 and C8, and thoracic segments T1–T5, a chronic heart condition that progresses subclinically or a previous heart disease, such as myo-, endo-, or pericarditis, should be considered. In this situation, the heart functions as an interference field.

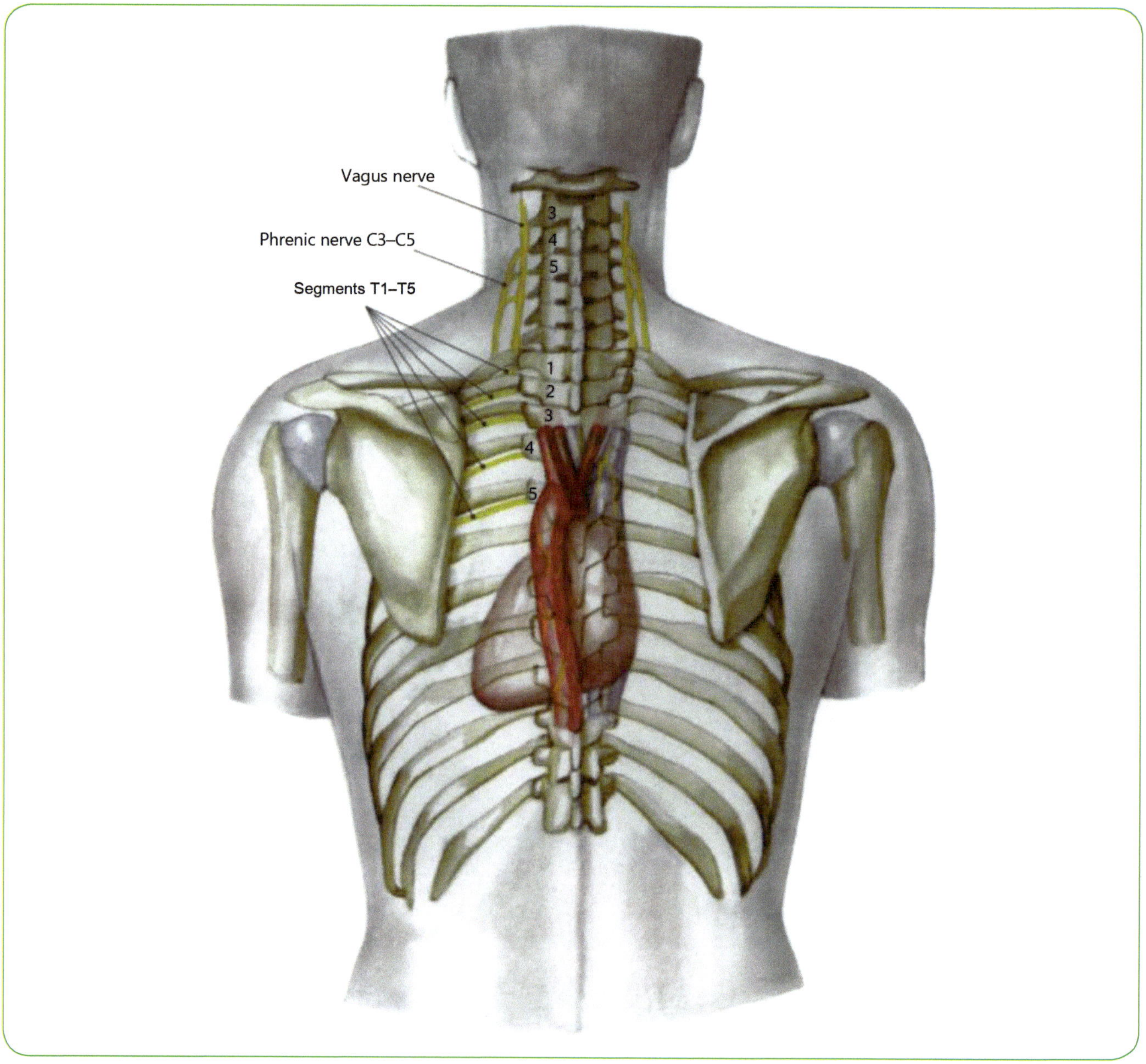

▸**Fig. 10.4** The heart segment and its innervation relationships.

10.3.2 Therapy

The neural therapeutic treatment of heart disease consists of a series of wheals injected left, two fingerbreadths paravertebrally from T1-5 and left parasternally in the intercostal space 1-5. On palpation, there are always maximum pressure pain points, often already indicated by the patient, especially on the front left chest, approximately at the level of the cartilage–bone interface of the ribs and in the area of the mammillary line and anterior axillary line. These points, which lie in the subcutaneous tissue and the major pectoral muscle, are infiltrated with small amounts of local anesthetic. Scars in the region of the left chest, especially in segments T1–T5, must be infiltrated as well, even if these infiltrations already form part of the interference field diagnostics and therapy. Pressure-sensitive spinous processes of the cervical spine at the C2–C5 level and the thoracic spine at T1–T5 should also be infiltrated. If the paravertebral muscles are hypertonic—with emphasis on the left—in the same spinal segments, a few increments of the local anesthetic are injected into the maximum pressure points of these muscle sections.

If, despite one- or twofold repetition, this localized treatment of the heart disease does not lead to a significant improvement of the symptoms, injection to the stellate ganglion, alternating from left to right, is indicated as an additional segmental treatment. Injection to the left stellate ganglion is preferred for conditions based on a myocardial circulation disorder and injections to the right stellate ganglion are preferred in the case of arrhythmias. If this extended segment therapy, which should be performed once to twice weekly, does not lead to a decline in symptoms, interference field diagnostics should be carried out. Specifically in heart disease, the most common interference fields are found in infected tonsils, teeth,[173] and sinuses.

10.3.3 Summary

In addition to the actual heart symptoms, diseases of the heart and pericardium can cause symptoms in completely different areas via a segmental-reflexive pathway. The cause is found in the afferent innervation situation via the sympathetic nervous system, the parasympathetic nervous system, and the phrenic nerve. Sympathetic afferents enable concomitant symptoms in segments C8–T5. Parasympathetic afferent fibers mediate the concomitant symptomology in the area supplied by the trigeminal nerve and neck segments C1 and C3. Afferent fibers of the phrenic nerve can lead to segment exposure of cervical segments C3–C5.

10.4 Hepatobiliary Segment

10.4.1 Diagnostics

The clinical symptomology in diseases of the liver, bile ducts, and gall bladder is characterized by the **afferent innervation** through the sympathetic nervous system, the parasympathetic nervous system, and the afferent fibers of the phrenic nerve (▶Fig. 10.5). The symptoms, mediated by the sympathetic afferent fibers, primarily consist of pain in a variety of nuances, spontaneously felt in the area of the organ below the right costal margin, and less frequently in the epigastrium, or even only with manual pressure on the organ itself. Since the sympathetic efferent fibers that are responsible for controlling the organ perfusion, among other things, have their nucleic areas in T7–T11 and the afferent fibers have the same conduction pathway until reaching the dorsal root ganglia, clinical symptomology of the sensorimotor system is possible in the same segments via sympathetic afferent fibers on a segment-reflexive pathway. This consists of spontaneously painful or pressure-sensitive spinous processes of T7–T11, pronounced paravertebral muscle tension on the right, and spontaneous or pressure-induced pain in the area of the branches of the corresponding right intercostal nerves radiating into the subcutis, with a focus under the right front ribs at the passage of the eighth intercostal nerves; this area corresponds to Vogler's pressure point at the level of the mammillary line.

The liver symptomology mediated by the parasympathetic afferent fibers manifests in a feeling of pressure and general nausea in the case of illness. Through the

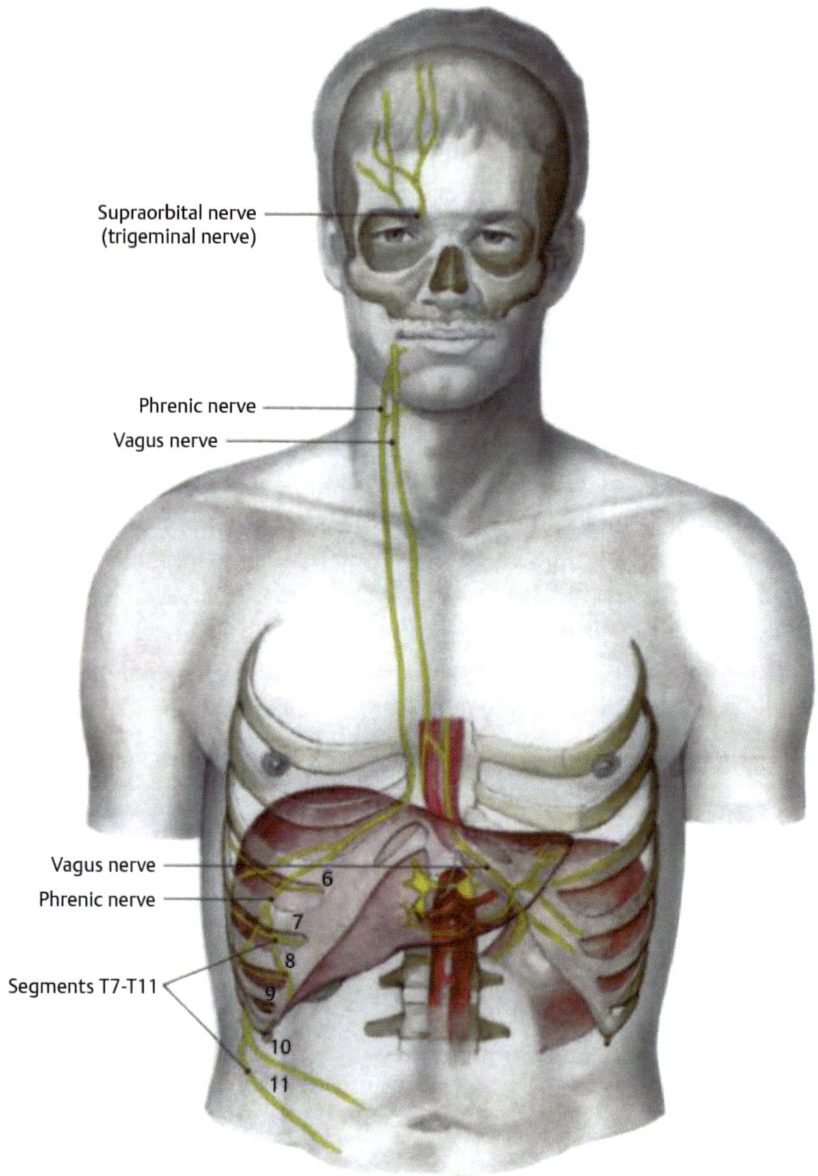

▶**Fig. 10.5** The hepatobiliary segment and its innervation relationships.

connection of the vagus nerve (▸Fig. 10.6) to the spinal nucleic region of the trigeminal nerve, stimulus in the innervation area of the right trigeminal nerve is possible. This arises primarily spontaneously or only on palpation in the form of pain in the right supraorbital/infraorbital nerves.

A cervical-occipital symptomology—more pronounced on the right—is possible via the synaptic connections of the nucleic regions of the trigeminal nerve to the first three neck segments, arising from a disease of the liver and gall bladder.

The symptoms originating from the afferent fibers of the phrenic nerve are characterized by their affiliation to cervical segments C3–C6 with the clinical symptoms of neck and shoulder pain on the right, with right-sided hypertension of the cervical muscles at the same segment height, and an influence on the muscular function of the diaphragm, which, for example, may appear radiographically as an elevated diaphragm on the right in liver or biliary tract disease.

The symptoms of liver/biliary disease are clinically recognized without much effort by their diversity. Some individual symptoms may manifest more intensely, and others will be expressed at a very low intensity.

If all anamnestic or clinical examination findings of the liver segment itself are missing and if the reflexive findings, particularly in the cervical and thoracic area, are also occasionally collected only as individual findings and are not affected locally in therapy, a resolved clinically silent liver disease should always be considered. In this case, the liver takes on an interference field function. If there is also pain in the right shoulder which does not subside with local measures, a resolved or clinically silent liver disease definitely should also be considered as a cause, so that segmental therapy of the

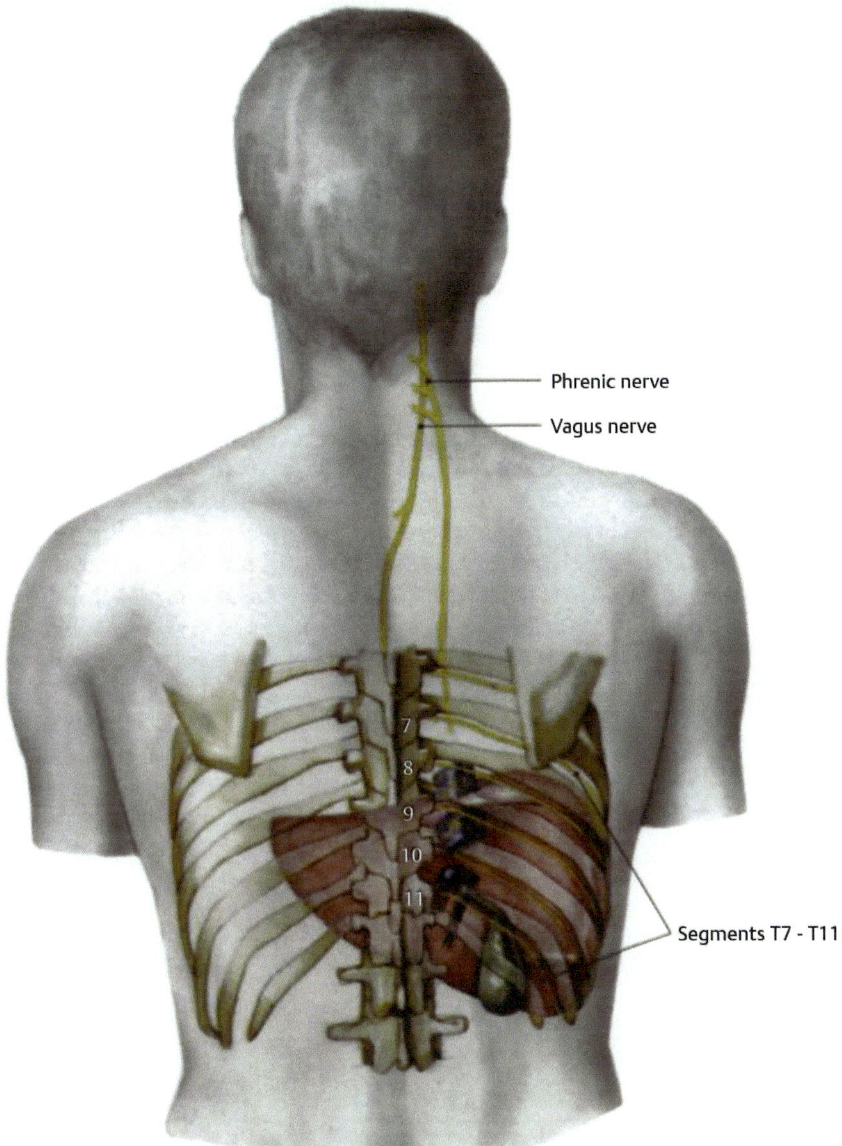

▸**Fig. 10.6** The hepatobiliary segment and its innervation relationships.

liver is diagnostically and therapeutically necessary for treatment of the shoulder pain under suspicion of an interference field.

10.4.2 Therapy

The segmental therapy consists of paravertebral injections of thoracic segments T7–T11 and the infiltration of muscular trigger points and the corresponding intercostal nerves, focusing on the eighth intercostal nerve and the Vogler pressure point below the right costal arch. A series of wheals follows in the right upper abdomen as well as the infiltration of muscular pressure points (detectable through palpation) of the abdominal wall in the respective segments, up to preperitoneal infiltration. Scar infiltrations in the entire segment-related innervation area complete the segmental therapy. The overriding segmental therapy and the most often performed injection for interference field testing of the liver is the injection to the celiac ganglion and the right major and minor splanchnic nerves.

10.4.3 Summary

The clinical symptomology of a liver or bile duct disorder results from the afferent fibers, which originate from this organ region. These are part of the sympathetic nervous system, the parasympathetic nervous system, and the phrenic nerve. The afferent fibers of the sympathetic nervous system enable clinical symptoms of the sensorimotor system in segments T7–T11. Via the nucleic regions of the trigeminal nerve and the first two cervical segments, the parasympathetic afferent fibers mediate a symptomology of the right trigeminal nerve and sensorimotor segments C1–C3. In liver and bile duct disorders, the afferent fibers of the phrenic nerve transfer their stimulus into cervical segments C3–C5, with emphasis on the right, with the corresponding clinical findings of the right-sided shoulder girdle.

10.5 Stomach Segment

10.5.1 Diagnostics

The symptomology of stomach disorders is found not only in the Head zone in the epigastrium and under the left costal arch, but also in the entire supply area of the sympathetic nervous system, parasympathetic nervous system, and the phrenic nerve originating from the afferent fibers of the stomach (▶Fig. 10.7).

The **sympathetic afferent fibers** of the stomach enter via the dorsal root ganglia of thoracic segments T5–T9 on the left, so that subjective symptoms or examination findings of the sensorimotor system are possible in these segments. Examples of the segment-reflexive response of a stomach disorder are hyperesthesia of the dermatomes, tense paravertebral muscles—more pronounced on the left—with possible dysfunction of the spine and respiratory movement of the thorax, and intercostal neuralgias in these segments.

The **afferent fibers of the parasympathetic nervous system**, which directly mediate pressure in the upper abdomen or nausea as clinical symptoms, can lead to symptomology of the left supraorbital nerve and infraorbital nerve simultaneously via the synaptic connections to the spinal trigeminal nuclei, on the one hand, and via connections to the sensorimotor nucleic regions of the first three cervical segments, on the other, and may also lead to

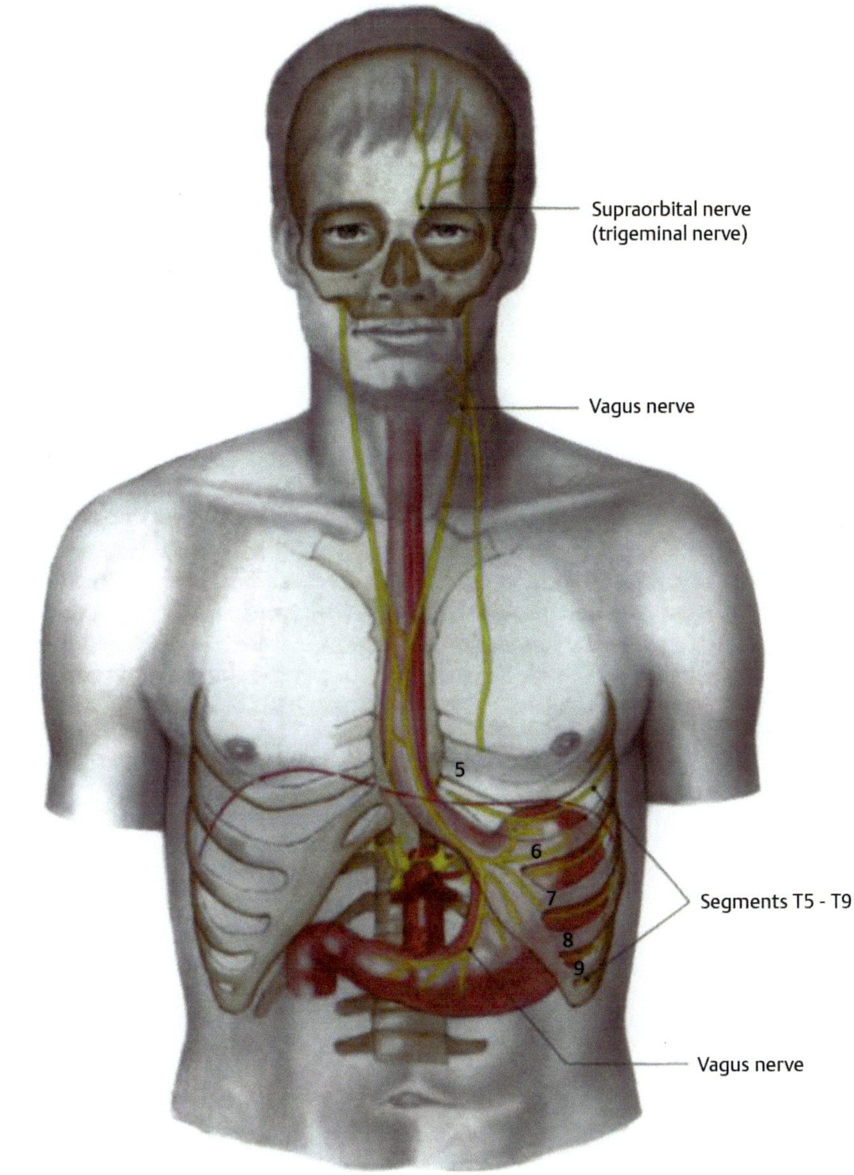

▶**Fig. 10.7** The stomach segment and its innervation relationships.

left-emphasized functional impairment of the first three neck segments, including tenderness or spontaneous pain in the left major and minor occipital nerves.

In the case of stomach disorders, the **afferent fibers of the phrenic nerve** (▸Fig. 10.8) with their inputs in cervical segments C3–C6 can lead to a concomitant functional disorder of the middle cervical spine up to left-sided shoulder pain, comparable with the right-sided shoulder pain in disorders of the hepatobiliary segment. The afferent fibers of the phrenic nerve start in the peritoneal lining of the stomach and are stimulated in the case of stomach disorders with involvement of the visceral peritoneum.

Since the reaction of the nerves depends on the strength of the stimulus, symptoms accompanying a stomach disorder are less pronounced. They can be subjectively missing and are then expressed as pain on palpation. Often, anamnestic findings or findings that only become evident in the examination remain as residuals of a previously resolved disease, such that an incompletely "healed" condition can still be assumed from a neural therapeutic perspective.

Note

If the symptomology of the thoracic and cervical spine, the shoulder, or the left trigeminal nerve predominates, the localized treatment of the sections of the body will fail because the primary cause is an oligosymptomatic or asymptomatic stomach illness.

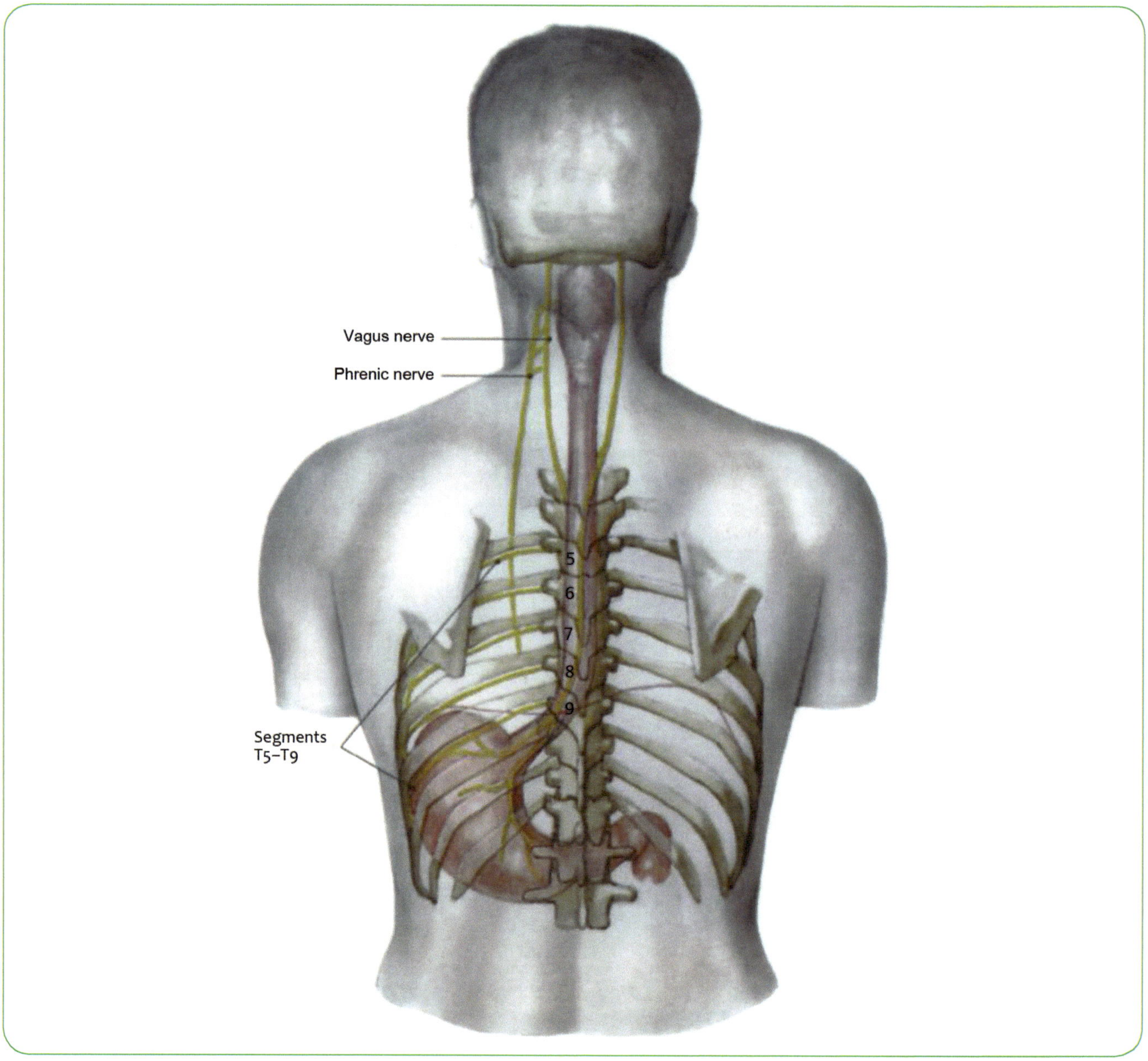

▸**Fig. 10.8** The stomach segment and its innervation relationships.

This can also explain the failure of other therapeutic methods in which the segment is treated. Again, as described above, an interference field disease is present, whereby the stomach represents the interference field in this case.

10.5.2 Therapy

In addition to paravertebral wheals to thoracic segments T5–T9, muscles with pressure pain are also infiltrated up to the intercostal nerves. The Vogler point, which should be infiltrated, is also located ventrally in segment T8 under the left costal arch. The segmental treatment is completed by a series of wheals in the area of the dermatomes T5–T9 on the left, especially ventrally, as well as infiltration of the abdominal wall—in the case of tenderness on palpation—up to the parietal peritoneum. If there is tenderness on palpation of the left supraorbital nerve, this can also be infiltrated. The higher level segmental therapy consists of an injection to the left celiac ganglion and the major and minor splanchnic nerves at the level of L1. Scars in the above-mentioned segments of the sympathetic nervous system should also be infiltrated. With chronic stomach pain, the most frequent interference field locations are in the paranasal sinuses and the maxillary teeth in area 2/4–7.

10.5.3 Summary

The full potential symptomology of a stomach disease is a direct function of phrenic stimulus of the stomach-induced afferent fibers of the sympathetic nervous system, the parasympathetic nervous system, and phrenic nerve. The segment-reflexive symptomology originating from the sympathetic nervous system affects thoracic segments T5–T9 with emphasis on the left. The symptomology originating from the parasympathetic afferent fibers is in the supply area of the left trigeminal nerve and cervical segments C1–C3. Via the afferent fibers of the phrenic nerve, stomach disorder symptomology with involvement of the visceral peritoneum in cervical segments C3–C5 can be maintained.

10.6 Pancreatic Segment

10.6.1 Diagnostics

The symptomology of a pancreatic disease originating from the organ itself is linked to the afferent innervation, which is predefined through the sympathetic nervous system, the parasympathetic nervous system, and the phrenic nerve (▶ Fig. 10.9).

Easily localizable left-sided back pain, with palpatory focus in the Th8 segment, is characteristic of a pancreatic illness (▶ Fig. 10.10). The efferent supply of the sympathetic nervous system originates from this segment, and the **sympathetic afferent fibers** have an entry point in the same spinal segment, such that the sensorimotor reaction can be explained by the autonomic reflex arc. Both with oligosymptomatically or asymptomatically progressing chronic pancreatitis and with a clinically silent previous "healed" pancreatic illness, an irritation of the T8 thoracic segment—detectable through palpation—is definitely possible in the form of a percussion-sensitive spinous process T8, a left paravertebral muscular pressure pain, and the pressure-sensitive Vogler's point under the left costal arch.

The main symptomology derived from the **afferent parasympathetic nervous system** relates to general symptoms such as malaise, nausea, and decreased appetite through stimulation of the parasympathetic afferent fibers.

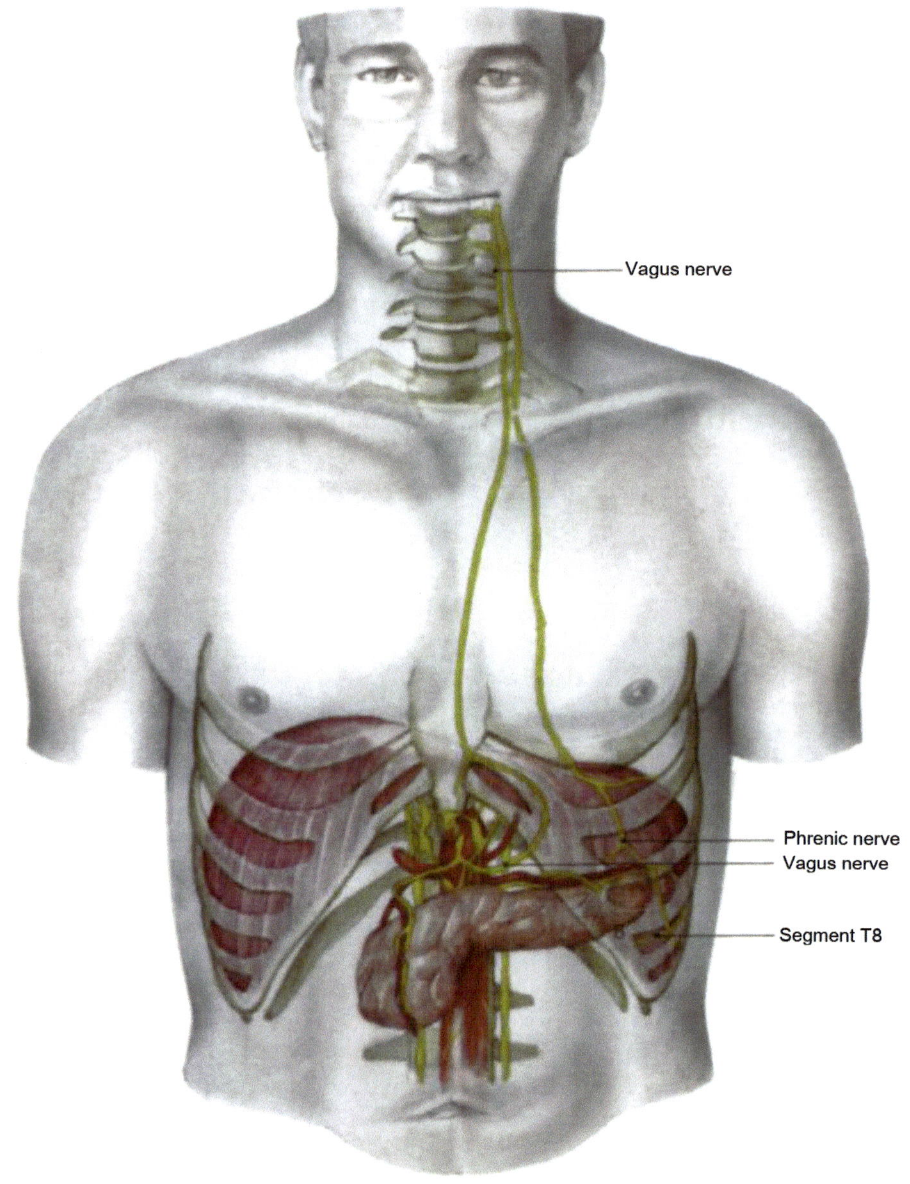

▶ **Fig. 10.9** Relationships and innervation of the pancreas.

Symptomology in the supply area of the left trigeminal nerve and the top three cervical segments is possible through connections between the parasympathetic afferent fibers and the spinal nucleic regions of the trigeminal nerve and, via these, with the first three neck segments.

As illustrated in the previous segment descriptions, involvement of the **afferent fibers of the phrenic nerve** in pancreatic illnesses results in symptoms in cervical segments C3–C5, which may manifest not only as cervical spine pain, but also as left shoulder pain, as in illnesses of the lungs, heart, and stomach.

If the pancreatic symptomology remains clinically silent, e.g., because the illness has subtle progression, then chronic trigeminus, neck, or thoracic spine symptomology is possible, particularly if there are further stimuli originating from other organs and aggravating these segments or if these segments are overloaded. Therefore, an interference field situation originating from the pancreas is present, which can only be illustrated through interference field diagnostics and interference field therapy.

Of note is the autolysis of the organ which occurs in acute pancreatitis and causes a massive inflammation reaction in the surrounding area. Severe conditions of shock, sometimes fatal, can be understood through the topography of the organ and its proximity to the celiac ganglion if this ganglion is captured by the necrotizing inflammation.

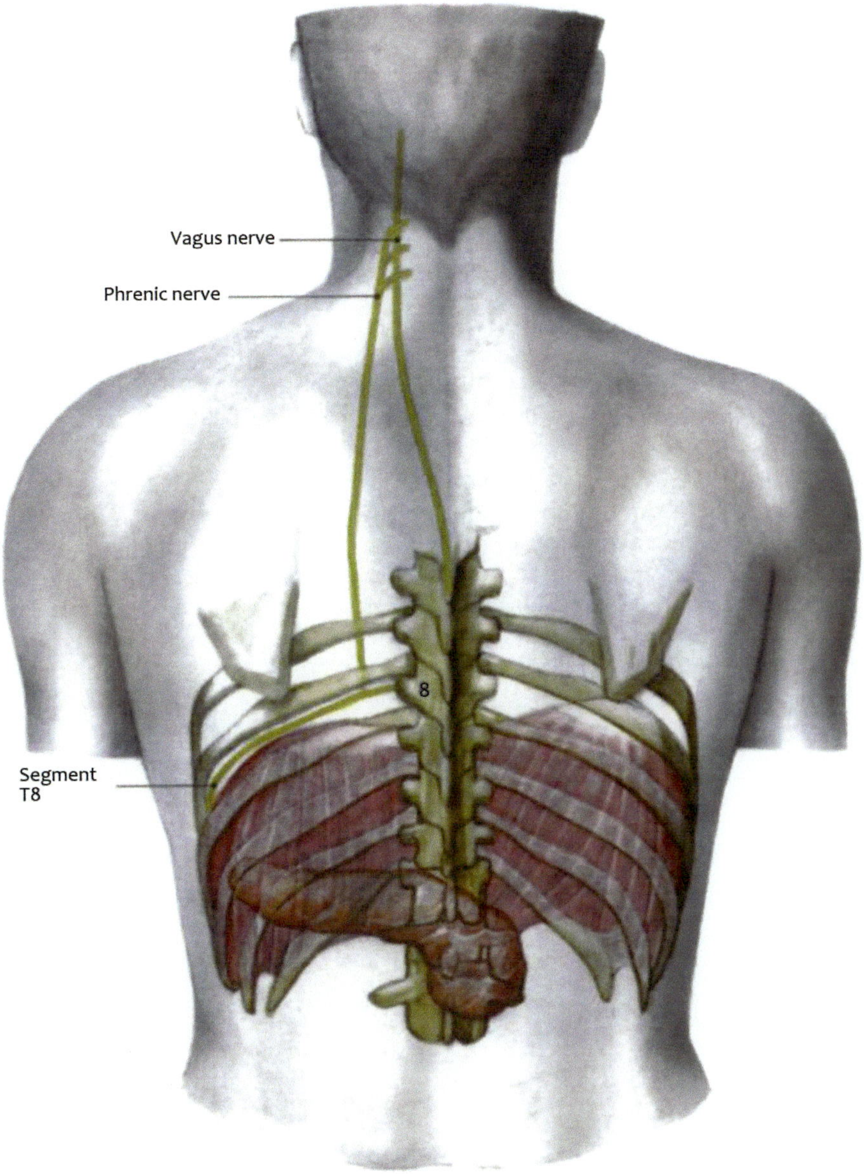

► **Fig. 10.10** Relationships and innervation of the pancreas.

10.6.2 Therapy

Simple segmental therapy for pancreatic illness ranges from the segment-based placement of a wheal series in dermatome T8 and the infiltration of muscular trigger points of the paravertebral musculature to injection to the intercostal nerve T8, particularly in the dorsal section and under the costal arch. Scars in the corresponding dermatome should also be treated. Therapy for pancreatic illness is basically oriented toward the topographic relationships defined by the sympathetic nervous system, since the circulation of the organ is controlled by the sympathetic nervous system. The most effective treatment in chronic recurring and acute pancreatitis is the injection to the celiac ganglion and the major and minor splanchnic nerves. This treatment is superior to all others in terms of its therapeutic effect.

10.6.3 Summary

The segment-reflexive symptomology of the pancreatic illness is dependent on the afferent nerve supply of this organ. The symptoms dependent on the afferent sympathetic nervous system affect the thoracic spinal segment T8. The pain symptomology dependent on the afferent parasympathetic nervous system is characterized by the parasympathetic nervous system itself and the left trigeminal nerve via its spinal nucleic regions and the top three neck segments related to these. The potential symptoms via cervical segments C3–C5 can be traced back to the afferent fibers of the phrenic nerve.

10.7 Intestinal Segment

10.7.1 Diagnostics

The intestinal segment consists of the duodenum, jejunum, ileum, colon, sigmoid colon, and rectum. As with all other organs of the abdominal cavity, the intestine is also innervated via afferent and efferent fibers of the sympathetic nervous system and the parasympathetic nervous system (▶Fig. 10.11). In contrast to the upper abdominal organs, the afferent fibers of phrenic nerve, originating from the visceral peritoneum of the intestine, are not known.

The **sympathetic supply**, and thus the symptomology dependent on the afferent sympathetic nervous system, is in segments T10–L2. The most significantly affected dermatome for the small intestine segment is at the level of the navel (T10) and those of the large intestine are in the middle of the lower abdomen (T11). In addition to percussion-sensitive and spontaneous painful spinous processes of the spinal sections, autochthonous muscle tension is possible, as well as hypertension of the abdominal muscles with hyperesthesia of the abdominal skin. The sympathetic supply of the vermiform appendix is carried out from segments T12 and L1 on the right, and the supply of the descending colon and rectum comes from lumbar segments L1 and L2. The reflexive symptomology via the spinal reflex pathway can be found in the corresponding dermatomes and myotomes of the thoracic and lumbar spine.

In the case of acute appendicitis, the known pressure point according to **McBurney** in the right lower abdomen is probably the most well-known point of pressure pain in the abdominal wall and corresponds to segment T12.

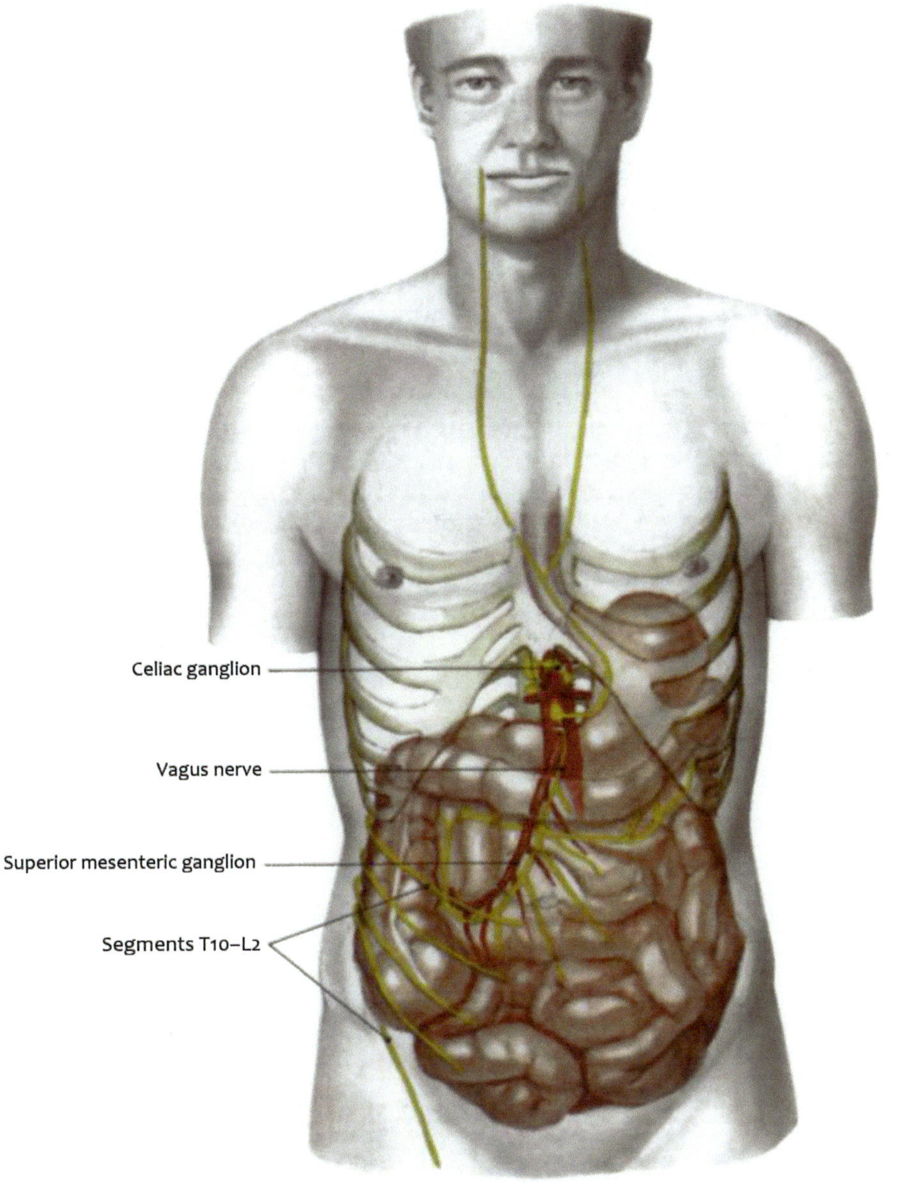

▶**Fig. 10.11** Relationships and innervation of the intestines.

The **parasympathetic** afferent fibers approach various nucleic regions. The entire small intestine, the ascending colon, and half of the transverse colon are supplied by the vagus nerve (▶ Fig. 10.12). The descending colon, sigmoid colon, and rectum are innervated by the afferent and efferent fibers of the sacral parasympathetic nervous system, with nucleic regions in segments S2–S4. Thus, involvement of the trigeminal nerve is possible in intestinal disorders, but less concisely than with disorders of the upper abdominal organs via the parasympathetic afferent fibers in association with the trigeminus nucleic regions, from the duodenum to the transverse colon. The extent to which parasympathetic efferent fibers course together with the branches of spinal nerves S2–S4 cannot be clarified on the basis of the available literature. This is still possible if the distribution pathway of the sympathetic nervous system is used analogously as a basis, whereby the question remains open whether or not these parasympathetic efferent and afferent fibers are involved with the modulation of vascular dilation or cutaneous glands. A remarkable observation is that cutaneous stimulation of segments S2–S4 leads to reflexive increased intestinal activity.

Illnesses of the large intestine sections located further distally have no afferent connection to the trigeminal nerve. However, there must be connections to the sacral sensorimotor system and to the sympathetic nervous system via the sacral parasympathetic afferent fibers. These connections trigger sacrum pain, edema formation over

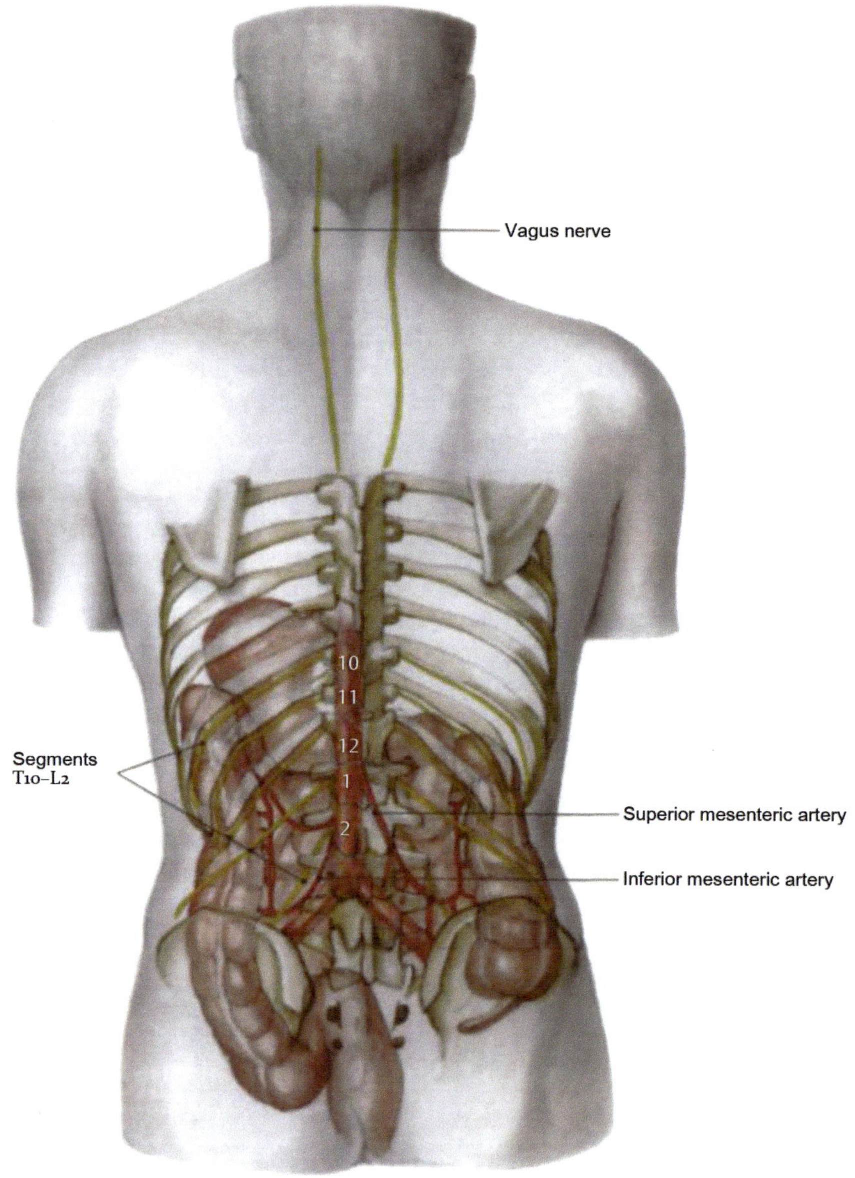

▶ **Fig. 10.12** Relationships and innervation of the intestines.

the sacrum, development of geloses, and painful pressure on sacral segments S2–S4 in the case of disorders of the distal colon, the sigmoid colon, and the rectum.

In the case of an intestinal illness, further symptoms are possible in addition to the abdominal pain experienced by the patients themselves and the pain triggered by palpation. These symptoms affect the supply area of the trigeminal nerve (rare), the top three cervical segments (rare), and the thoracic–lumbar transition from T10–L2, as well as subjective and objectifiable symptoms in the area of the sacrum within segments S2–S4. If a chronic intestinal illness progresses asymptomatically, there may still be a segmental-reflexive disorder in segments C1–C3, T10–L2, and S2–S4 via the predefined afferent innervation pathway of the sympathetic and parasympathetic nervous system. The clinical symptomology of this disorder can vary widely and does not bring to mind a primary illness of the intestine. In this situation, the diseased intestine has an "interference field effect" and the secondary illness can only be eliminated through "segmental therapy" of the intestine.

10.7.2 Therapy

As with other segmental treatments, neural therapeutic segmental treatment of the intestine consists of a series of wheals in the area of dermatomes T10–L2, depending on the section of the intestinal illness and the spinal findings, in infiltrations of the paravertebral musculature with tension or pain on palpation, wheal series in the corresponding dermatomes T10-L2. The exact localization depends on the section of the intestinal illness and the spinal findings. Infiltrations of the paravertebral musculature are indicated in cases of tension or pain on palpation there, with wheal series performed in the corresponding dermatomes of the abdominal wall. If muscular pain presents on pressure there, wheal series are also indicated into the stomach muscles up to the parietal peitoneum.

Note

Disorders requiring surgery, such as acute appendicitis, are excluded from the therapy.

With illnesses of the lower section of the intestine (from the left flexure of the colon), the same treatment is performed in the area of the sacrum. However, the most intensive form of the therapy consists of injection to the celiac ganglion on both sides as well as simultaneous segmental injections from those described above.

10.7.3 Summary

The autonomic afferent fibers of the intestine, along with fibers coming directly from the interior of the stomach and via and via the segmental-reflexive pathway at the spinal level in segments T10–L2, are responsible for the subjective symptoms of an abdominal illness. The segmental-reflexive pathway affects both, the sympathetic afferent fibers (thoracolumbar) and the parasympathetic afferent fibers between S2-S4. Last but not least, "central" disorders such as depression, adynamia, and impaired concentration and sleep are possible due to the direct connection of the vagus nerve to the brain stem region.

10.8 Kidney Segment

10.8.1 Diagnostics

The symptomology of a kidney disease is dependent on the afferent autonomic innervation of this organ, which primarily proceeds via the sympathetic and parasympathetic nervous system and secondly via the segmental-reflexive pathway through the sensorimotor system (▶ Fig. 10.13).

The efferent and afferent **sympathetic nervous system supply** to the kidneys proceeds from the nucleic regions of the sympathetic nervous system of thoracic–lumbar segments T10–L1 via the celiac ganglion and the renal plexus in parallel with the topographical course of the arteries. The afferent fibers follow the same centrally oriented course up to the corresponding spinal ganglia. In addition to direct organ pain, symptoms originating from the sympathetic nervous system are subjective and objectifiable symptoms in the thoracic and lumbar spinal sections T10–L1 in the form of pain in these segments, tension of the paravertebral muscles, spinous processes painful on percussion, or hyperesthesias in the flank over the iliac crest, extending to the groin, corresponding to dermatome L1, the zone according to Head's zone in kidney diseases.

Parasympathetic symptomology in turn consists of general symptoms such as feeling unwell, nausea, and vomiting.

The symptomology in the supply area of the trigeminal nerve or spinal segments C1–C3 in a kidney disorder is likely to be rare in comparison to disorders of the liver-biliary region, the stomach, or the pancreas. This is so despite the afferent connection of the vagus nerve originating from the kidneys, and the oft-mentioned connection of the vagus

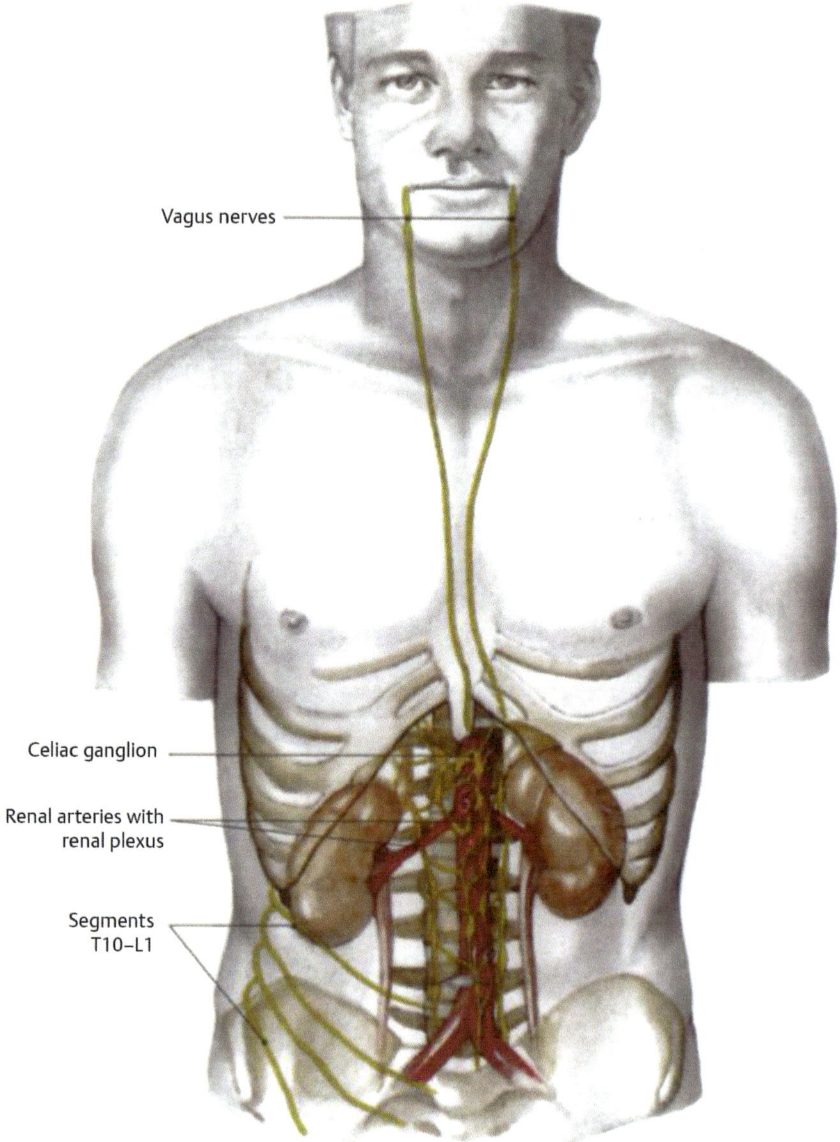

▶ **Fig. 10.13** Relationships and innervation of the kidneys.

nerve with the spinal nucleic regions of the trigeminal nerve and thereby to the top two cervical segments.

The symptoms accompanying a kidney disorder basically originate from the lumbar and flank region, corresponding to segments T10–L1, even with symptom-free progression of the kidney disorder. Therefore, even without knowledge of the innervation relationships owing to the topographical proximity of the thoracic–lumbar transition to the kidneys, there is firm suspicion that the primary cause of chronic thoracic–lumbar pain symptoms is chronic, asymptomatically progressing kidney disease. In this case as well, from a neural therapeutic perspective, an illness induced by an interference field is present in which the chronically ill kidney represents the interference field. The pain symptoms of the spinal column can be eliminated with neural therapeutic interruption of the pathological stimulus from the sympathetic afferent fibers at the primarily diseased organ.

10.8.2 Therapy

The segmental neural therapeutic treatment serves the reflexive pathway via the spinal level in order to exert influence on the kidney disease.

Wheals via the spinous processes T10–L1 as well as paravertebral are used as nonspecific stimulation therapy. The infiltration of the pressure-sensitive spinous processes, muscular trigger points in the course of the paravertebral musculature as well as in the area of the intercostal nerves T10–T12 and the spinal nerves at L1 (▶Fig. 10.14) is also segment-oriented and should incorporate reflexive measures in the case of corresponding tenderness on

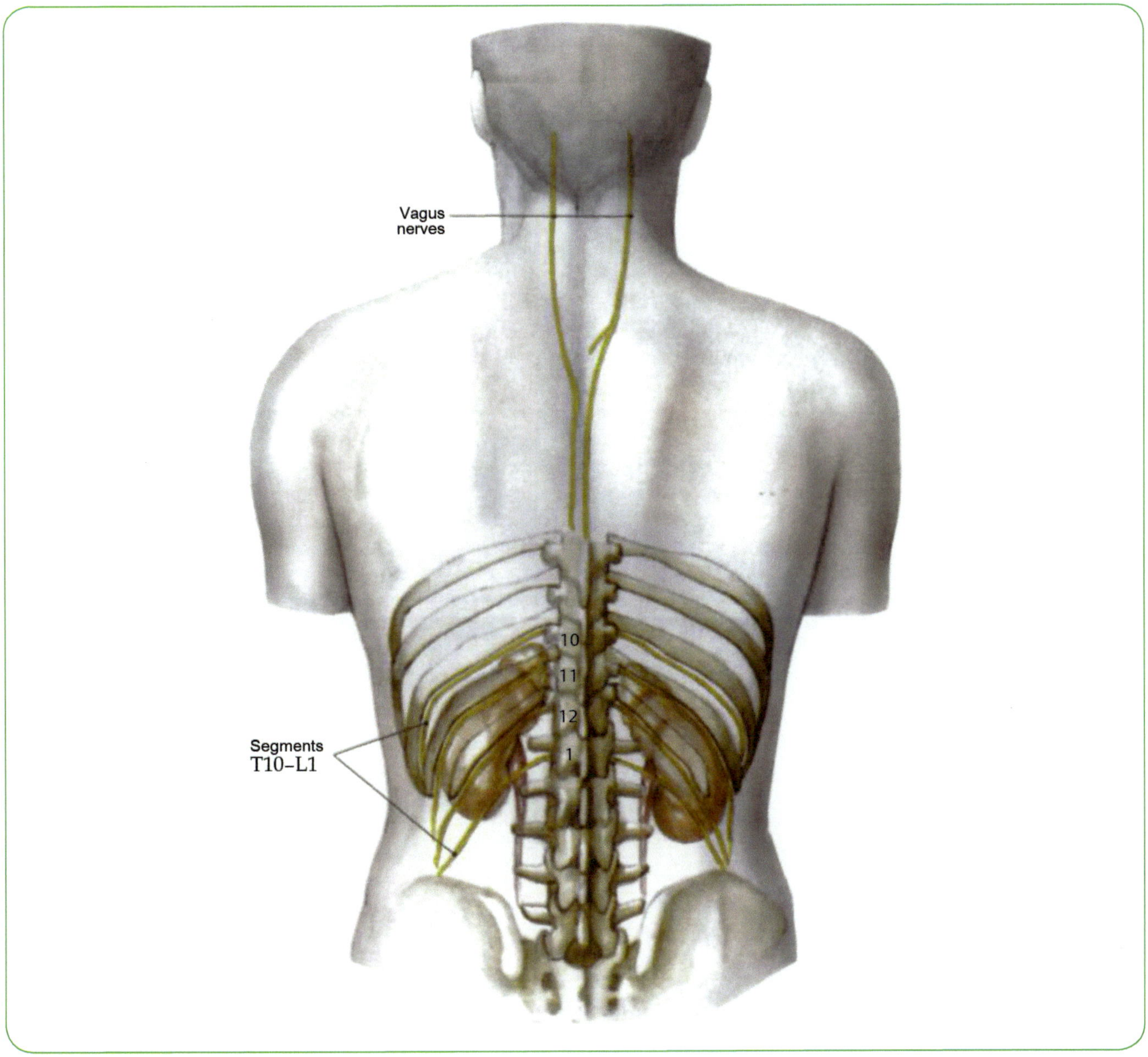

▶**Fig. 10.14** Relationships and innervation of the kidneys.

palpation. Scars in the area of the segments mentioned, particularly hernia repair scars, appendectomy scars, or scars after procedures in the genital area, should also be infiltrated as they are potential nerve irritation sites in the segment.

Following these injections, a notable immediate improvement in the symptomology should occur. With repeated infiltrations, this improvement continues to increase up to permanent symptom-free status. The most intensive form is the injection to the renal plexus, which is to be used particularly in acute illnesses such as renal colic and, above all, pyelonephritis. As long as no significant organ degeneration (kidney insufficiency) has taken place, the acute and chronic symptoms including pathology lab findings subside in a short time if the kidney disorder is not induced by an interference field.

10.8.3 Summary

The clinical symptoms of kidney disease result from the afferent sympathetic and parasympathetic innervation, which enables the involvement of the somatic nervous system through the segmental-reflexive pathway. Symptoms arising via the sympathetic afferent pathways are primarily different pains at the level of the renal bed as well as in segments T10–L1, with reactive changes in skin sensitivity and muscular tension. The parasympathetic afferent fibers contribute to the general symptoms such as feeling unwell, nausea, and vomiting; symptoms in the supply area of the trigeminal nerve as well as in the three upper cervical segments via the vagal connections to the nucleic regions of the trigeminal nerve and the first two neck segments are feasible but rarely observed clinically.

11 Segment Diagnostics

11.1 Tabular Overview

The listed examples of the relationships of organ diseases and the involvement of other sections of the body through the afferent autonomic innervation pathway should explain the variety of symptoms that can occur as part of an organ disease. The differing strengths of the associated symptomologies often blur the causal innervation-dependent relationships, so that only differentiating neural therapeutic segment diagnostics provides some clarity.

The symptomology of primarily diseased organs with impaired afferent nerve supply can definitely appear clinically, which also frequently applies in the case of an acute illness. However, these symptoms can occur subtly or even be missing altogether, which is more common in chronic diseases, so that the pain symptoms occurring on the reflexive pathway become the focal point.

In this situation, it is possible to find the primary disease site from the localization of the secondary symptoms virtually on the reverse reflexive pathway via the innervation relationships. The following tabular illustrations provide an overview of these innervation relationships for segmental diagnostics (▸Fig. 11.1, ▸Fig. 11.2, ▸Fig. 11.3, ▸Fig. 11.4).

Overview of the segmental supply of the internal organs

Organ	Spinal cord segments			
	Sympathetic nervous system	Vagus nerve	Pelvic nerves	Phrenic nerve
Heart and ascending aorta	T_1–T_4 (T_5)	C_2, face		(C_2) C_3, C_4 (C_5)
Lungs and bronchia	(T_1) T_2–T_5 (T_6–T_9)	C_2, face		(C_2) C_3, C_4 (C_5)
Esophagus	T_4, T_5 (T_6)	C_2, face		(C_1) C_3, C_4 (C_5)
Stomach – Cardia	(T_5) T_6, T_7			
Corpus	T_7, T_8	C_2, face		
Pylorus – Pylorus	T_8, T_9			
Small intestine and ascending colon	(T_9) T_{10},–L_1	C_3, face		
Appendix	(T_{12}, L, right)			
Descending colon and rectum	L_1–L_3		S_2–S_5	
Liver and gallbladder	(T_7) T_8–T_{11}	C_2, face		(C_2) C_3, C_4 (C_5)
Pancreas	T_8 (left)			
Kidney	T_{10}–L_1			
Ureter	(T_8) T_9–L_2			
Bladder	T_{11}–L_1 (L_2,L_3)		S_2–S_5	
Testis and epididymis	(T_{11}) T_{12}–L_3			
Ovary and adnexa	(T_{12}) L_1–L_3			
Uterus	(T_{12}) L_1–L_3		S_2–S_5 (?)	
Breast	T_4–T_6			

▸**Fig. 11.1** Overview of the segmental supply of the internal organs.

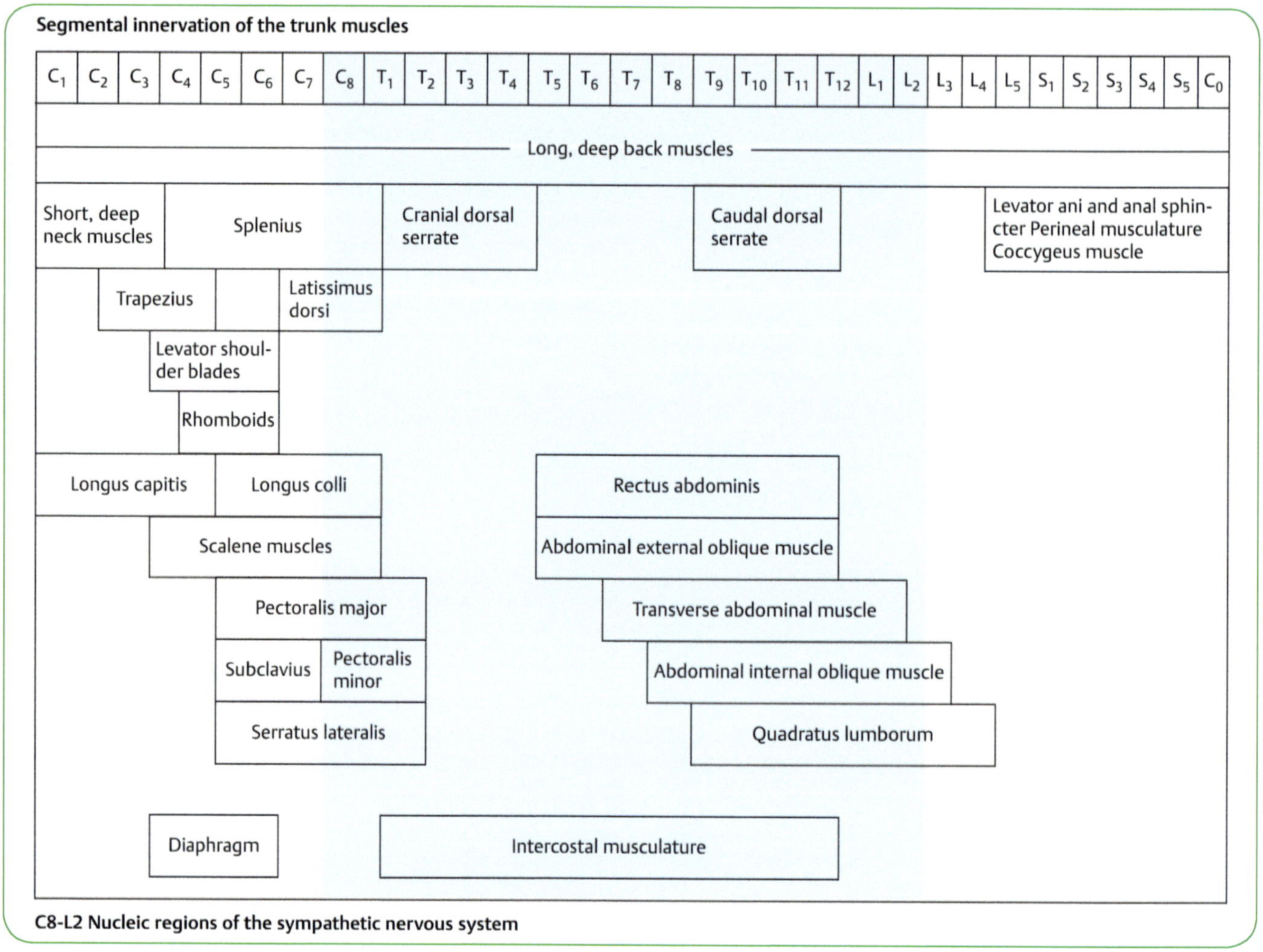

► **Fig. 11.2** Overview of the segmental innervation of the trunk muscles.

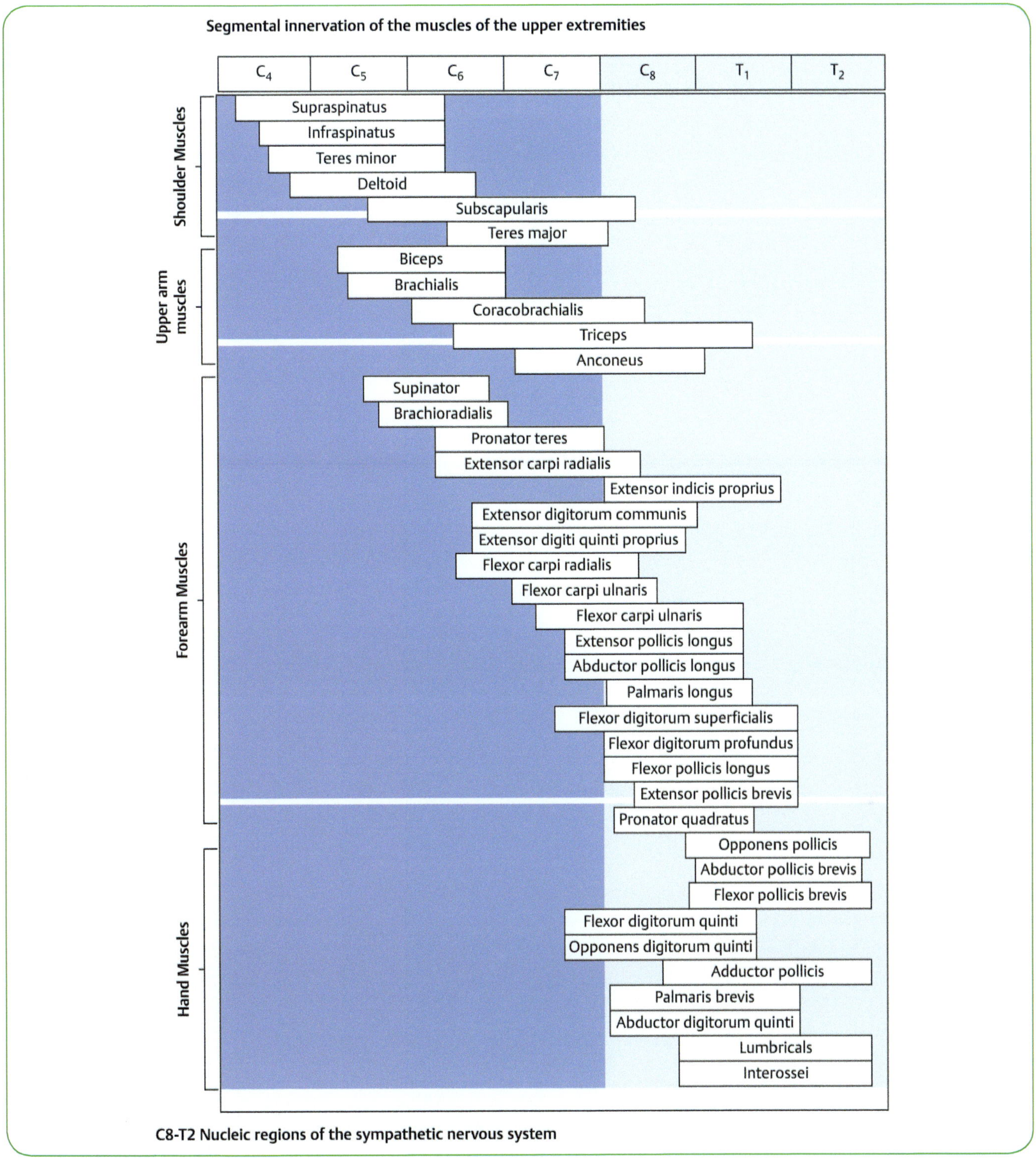

▶ **Fig. 11.3** Overview of the segmental innervation of the muscles of the upper extremities.

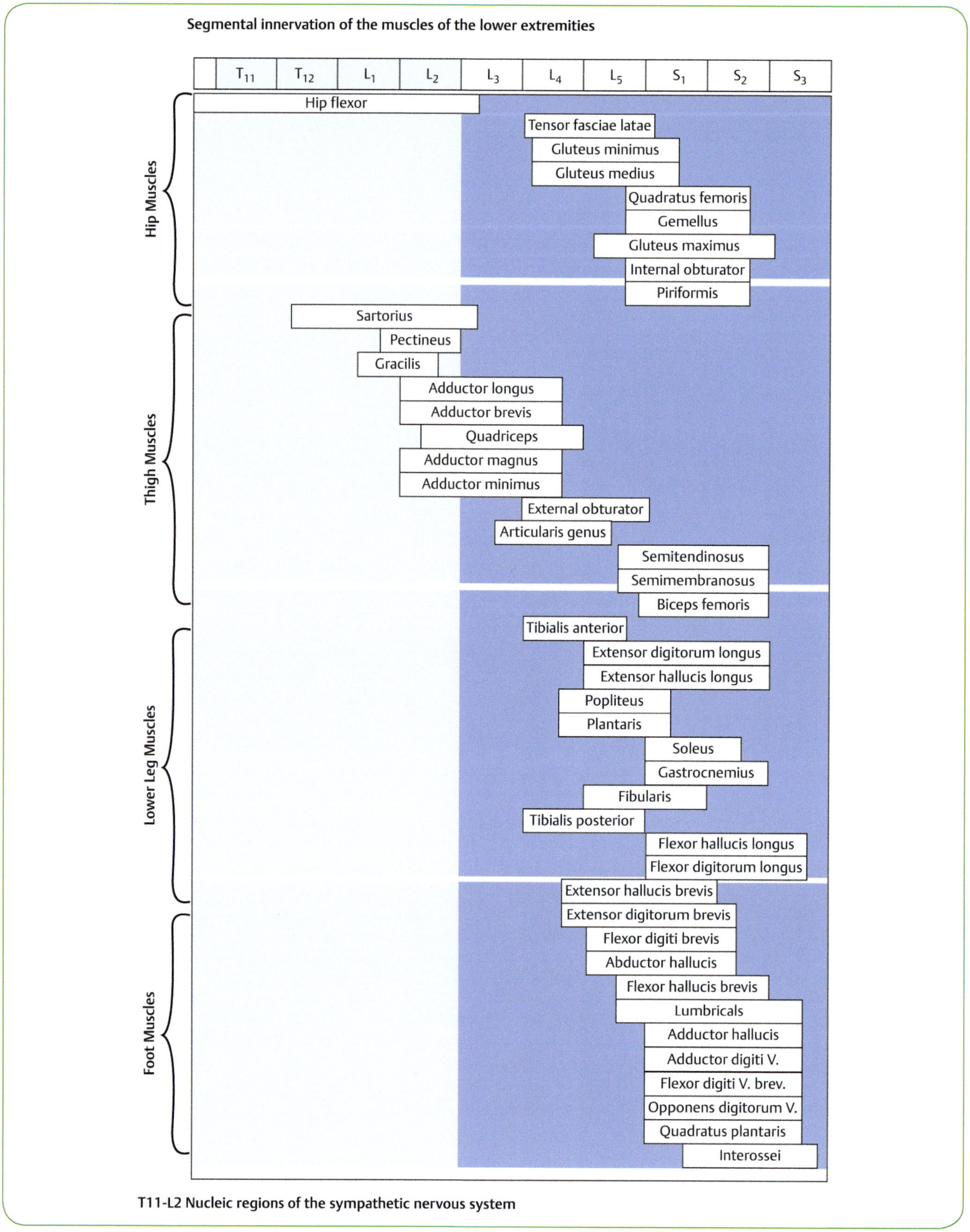

► **Fig. 11.4** Segmental innervation of the muscles of the lower extremities.

12 Interference Field

12.1 Interference Field Diagnostics

The concept of the interference field (p. 29) was described in Part 1 of the book. Interference field diagnostics means infiltrating an initially presumed interference field via corresponding segmental therapy (for organs) or directly with a local anesthetic to await the clinical response of the interference field disorder. Generally, this response occurs in a few seconds, which is why it was named the "second phenomenon" by Huneke (p. 3).

The interference field is then detected when the disorder induced or supported by the interference field is completely suppressed beyond the anesthesia period after the first treatment and subsides with every additional treatment until there is unlimited freedom from symptoms. If the interference field involves the tooth/jaw area, a symptomology originating from one of the teeth must completely subside over a period of at least 8 hours. These requirements are only the framework in which interference field diagnostics and interference field therapy take place in individual cases. As will be shown in due course, however, the interference field–related disease is—at first glance—often much more complex in its correlations and more difficult with regard to the interference field diagnostics in the temporal relationship of the change in the symptomology.

Interference field diagnostics is usually based on unsuccessfully implemented segment diagnostics (p. 53), which means that segment diagnostics in accordance with neural therapy was initially performed without a change in the symptomology. This statement is already possible after one to two treatments. As already mentioned several times, initial evidence of an interference field–related disorder is revealed in the course of segmental diagnostics, particularly if a chronic illness does not improve or even worsens temporarily with segment-oriented diagnostic injections. The worsening of existing symptomology with direct treatment is known not only in neural therapy, but also in all forms of therapy that function via the direct or indirect reflexive pathways.

Likewise, interference field diagnostics means not only testing individual potential interference fields, but possibly also multiple interference fields as part of an individual's treatment. For example, in the injection systematics, all suspicious teeth must be tested in one session; in interference-field testing of scars, all scars should also be infiltrated in one session. In clinical experience, it is often necessary to look for multiple interference fields in one injection series in order to eliminate one single illness in terms of the second phenomenon.

Interference field testing means the injection of a local anesthetic into the suspected interference field, such as any form of scarring, or to the associated autonomic ganglia, nerves, and blood vessels where the tissue that is suspected of being an interference field cannot be reached with the injection needle (e.g., sinuses) or infiltration of the organ (e.g., liver, kidney, pancreas) is ruled out.

12.2 Classification

As previously described, the medical history (p. 37) gives rise to a patient's individual catalog of possible interference fields, represented by all illnesses and injuries that took place before the start of the current, usually chronic illness to be treated. These potential interference fields are tested during interference field diagnostics by way of corresponding injections and the response of the illness to be treated is observed.

The sequence in which the potential interference fields are found varies individually. Ultimately, it is based on experiential values which have evolved in the clinical use of the "interference field by Huneke" since 1940. The goal is to find the evidence of an interference field–related illness through minimal failed injections. In order to approximate this goal, in interference field testing it is useful to incorporate the patient's individually distinguishing information. The additional evidence that the illness to be treated occurred by way of an accident, an operation, a previous illness, or a comparable event is as much a part of this as the evidence of a chronic illness, e.g., sinusitis, recurring appendicitis, tonsillitis, or "irritated" scars in any form or nonspecific "organ signals" after illnesses that have ended, such as liver, lung, stomach, or genital symptoms. Further individual indications are scars of infected wounds, past fractures with delayed bone healing, scars after amputations, or scars following multiple surgical procedures at the same site.

Note

The question recommended by Dosch about the subjectively worst illness or injury outside of the disease being treated can be a key to important evidence of an interference field.

If all interference field options known from the medical history are tested unsuccessfully, interference field testing can also be continued according to experiential values and independently of information from the medical history. Solely due to the clustering of interference fields in the area of the facial bones and the mouth, nose and throat, and the abdomen as well as the small pelvis with the inner genital organs, interference field diagnostics should also be carried out in these areas, even given a blank medical history and unremarkable local findings. Too often, after corresponding interference field testing, the illness being treated becomes symptom-free without there having been any indication of a disorder in these different parts of the body. It is certainly not wrong to perform interference field testing according to body regions in order to keep the number of accidentally overlooked interference fields as small as possible. Too often, clinical practice proves the benefit of unwavering implementation of consistent interference field diagnostics with the successful performance of interference field diagnostics. Clinical practice also shows that patience is more necessary in the patient than in the therapist, especially in chronic diseases which sometimes persist over decades.

As described at the beginning of Part 2, when recording the medical history (p. 44) and during the further course of treatment using neural therapy, monitoring of the symptoms being treated and exact documentation (p. 49) of a change are crucial for the success desired. In particular, the fact that an illness can be supported by multiple interference fields requires the detailed description of the changes in symptoms in order to determine that individual symptoms disappear in the second phenomenon (p. 3) and only the consideration of two or more interference fields in an injection series eliminates all symptoms of an illness. This is more frequently observed in patients with headaches or back pain in particular.

Furthermore, as mentioned in Segment Diagnostics (p. 53), an illness should be eliminated, on the one hand, by way of interference field diagnostics and therapy and, on the other hand, by way of segmental therapy. This should result in the overall reduction of symptoms when tested via segment diagnostics and/or field diagnostics.

12.3 Interference Field Therapy

For interference field therapy, a definite indication of the interference field is necessary, i.e., reproducible initiation of the second phenomenon (p. 3); the therapy consists simply of the continuation of the same injections that were previously used for interference field diagnostics. Again, the ending and frequency of the interference field treatments are individually variable and are oriented toward the symptom-free period, which must be extended from treatment to treatment. It is quite possible that a chronic disease is stopped for the long term with a single injection in the interference field and that repeats are therefore not necessary. However, this is likely an exception. Much more frequently, repeated interference field treatment is necessary. The reason for this can be seen in the strength of the stimulus originating from the interference field, as in the regulation capacity of the organism, above all, which is basically dependent on the condition of the interstitial regulation system. Thus, the question of the number of treatments needed per illness, which often interests patients, can only be answered at the end of therapy. The injection technique for interference field diagnostics and therapy is the same as that used for segment diagnostics (p. 53) and segment therapy.

With interference field therapy, a situation can arise wherein success is temporarily limited despite repetition of the injections, and sustained neutralization of the interference field fails. In this case, it can be assumed that the stimulus of the interference field by means of injections cannot be degraded by the organism. For example, chronically inflamed tonsils whose inflammatory situation cannot be resolved by the organism, a chronically inflamed appendix in the same situation, or teeth with dead roots are possibilities for which a surgical procedure to eliminate the interference field is required. The decision for a surgical procedure should not be made too hastily, i.e., well after the third or fourth neural therapeutic treatment, since nerve-supplying sympathetic ganglia, vessels, and nerves often enable the degradation of the stimulus and therefore the sympathetic nervous system stimulus through repeated interference field infiltration or indirect interference field therapy.

12.4 Basic Principles

The basic principles of interference field diagnostics and therapy are:

- Every chronic illness can be induced and supported by an interference field.
- Any illness or injury can leave behind an interference field. This particularly applies to long-lasting illnesses or injuries with complicated progression.
- Every illness induced by an interference field can only be healed through the elimination of the interference field, by either neural therapy or surgery.
- The identification of the interference field is only possible by way of the second phenomenon (p. 3). The relationship of the interference field with the corresponding illness is reproducible.

12.5 The Most Common Interference Fields

According to decades of experience in neural therapeutic practice, most interference fields are found in the area of the mouth, nose, and throat and in the abdominal organs (intestines, liver). A possible basis for this increased frequency is probably the multiple innervation of this region by the sympathetic nervous system, the parasympathetic nervous system, and cranial nerves, and the close links to the somatic nervous system. This fact is reflected by Huneke's statement that every area in the body can become an interference field after injury or illness.

The teeth should be given a wider berth in the representation of interference field potentials, since the classic diagnostic assessment by the dentist or oral surgeon or the assessment of a dental-maxillary lesion represents the most common cause of miscalculation of the actual interference field situation within the framework of neural therapy. A lesion-free dentition, even when toothless, is a rarity in the treatment of chronic illnesses. Therefore, the neural therapeutic aspect must be especially emphasized when assessing the dental and maxillofacial region because even any minor chronic inflammation in this region may be the cause of symptomology elsewhere.[14] This assessment includes the inspection of the oral cavity and X-ray. This will be detailed in the following by way of a few examples.

13 Maxillodental Region

13.1 Example 1

▶ **Referring diagnosis.** Primary coxarthrosis on the left with slight joint socket dysplasia on both sides.

▶ **From the medical history.** Pain in the left hip joint since age 23 years. Typical clinical and radiological findings for the left hip joint in accordance with advanced coxarthrosis with minor socket joint dysplasia on the left.

▶ **X-ray.** The panoramic image shows the following results (▶ Fig. 13.1):

- Incomplete set of teeth after extraction of teeth 35 and 37.
- Unaligned tooth 31 or 32.
- Extracted tooth 45.
- Multiple fillings in the teeth of the upper and lower jaw.
- Periradicular osteitis at teeth 16 and 26.

▶ **Clinical findings.** The following findings were recorded:

- No subjective tooth pain.
- Slight percussion sensitivity of teeth 16 and 26.
- Slight inflammation of the gums around teeth 26 and 36.

▶ **Assessment**. Repeated neural therapeutic testing of all treated teeth and tooth gaps results in sustained freedom from pain in the left hip joint. Differentiated testing according to panoramic images of the teeth results in the following diagnosis: coxarthrosis on the left with slight joint socket dysplasia by way of lesions on teeth 16 and 26.

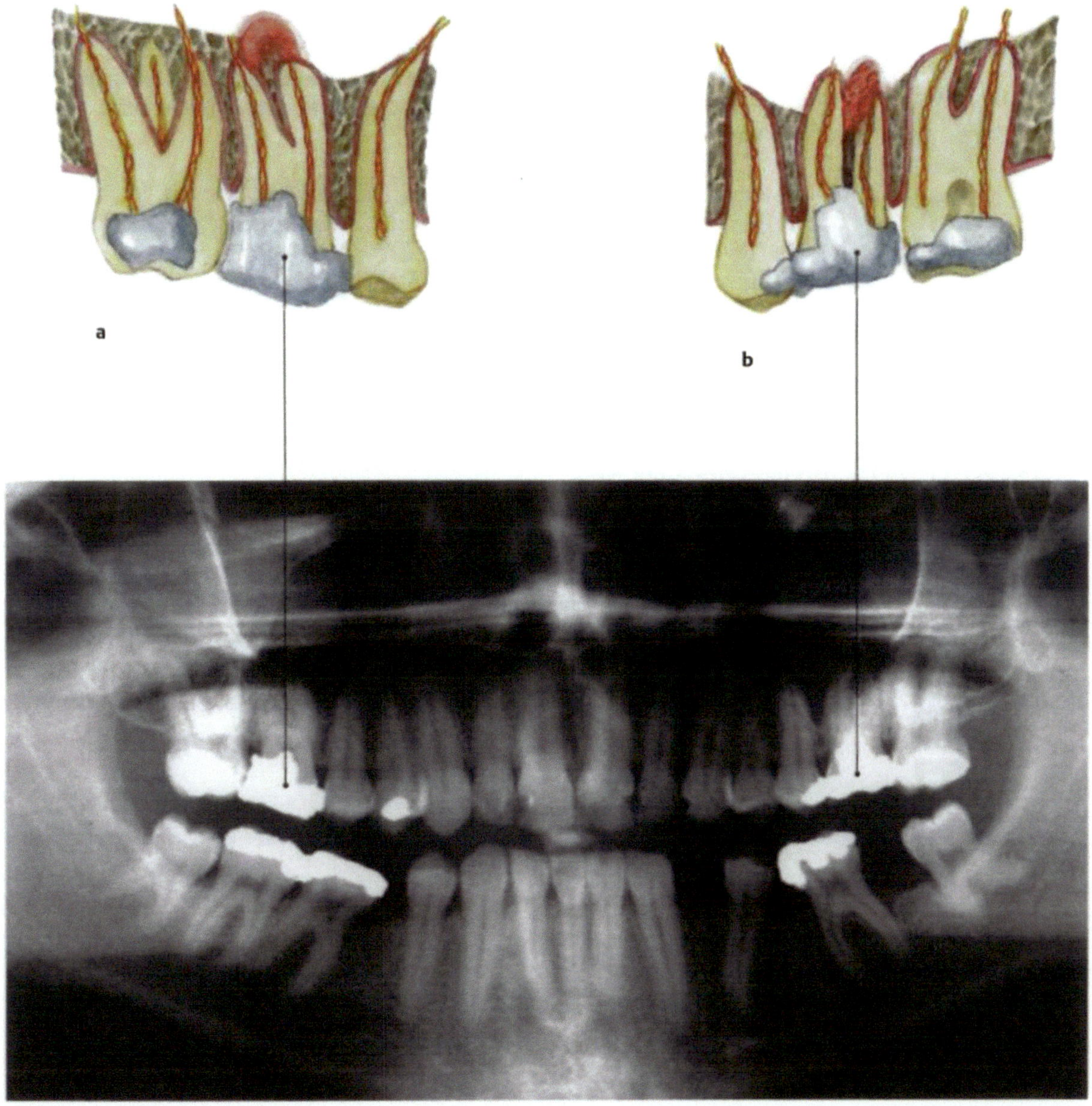

►**Fig. 13.1** Panoramic image of the teeth of a male patient born in 1963. **(a)** Apical osteitis at 16, small cystic inflammation reactions at the right maxillary sinus floor, originating from the roots of tooth 16 with deep amalgam filling. **(b)** Apical interradicular osteitis at 26, originating from incomplete root filling and deep amalgam filling.

13.2
Example 2

►**Referring diagnoses.** Female patient with diverse chronic symptoms of various types and localizations:
- Chronic pansinusitis.
- Dysmenorrhea.
- Migraine.
- Chronic lower back pain.
- Reclus' disease.
- Hypoesthesia of the left corner of the mouth.

►**From the medical history.** Recurring sinusitis since childhood, frequently treated with antibiotics. Dysmenorrhea since onset of period and cycle-related migraines. Lower back pain for many years, improved with movement, no radicular signs. Mastopathy determined radiologically at screening, no symptoms. Hypoesthesia of the left corner of the mouth occurred after tooth treatment in the left lower jaw. There was suspicion of an iatrogenic irritation of the left inferior alveolar nerve.

►**X-ray**. The panoramic image shows the following results (►Fig. 13.2):
- Gapped dentition with missing teeth 36 and 46.
- Root tip resection at tooth 21.
- Fillings in teeth 18, 14, 26, 27, and 34.
- Crowns on teeth 11 and 21.
- Bridges on teeth 17–15, 24 and 25, 35–37, 47–44.
- Osteitis in the area of teeth 16 and 15, 21, 25, 35, and 36, 45, and 44.

►**Clinical findings.** The following findings were recorded:
- Oral mucosa inflammation for all teeth treated with bridges and crowns.
- Pressure and percussion sensitivity at teeth 21 and 34–37.
- Subjective occasional pressure sensation and slight pain at tooth 21.

►**Assessment.** Multiple potential lesions in the dental and maxillofacial region, mainly consisting of inflammatory changes in the periodontal apparatus and jawbone, partially with involvement of the maxillary sinus.

Neural therapeutic treatment of the dental and maxillofacial area resulted in:
- Cessation of migraines.
- Elimination of the hypoesthesia of the left lower lip.
- Cessation of dysmenorrhea.
- According to neural therapeutic experience, the patient's various symptomologies cannot be remedied without restoration of the dental and maxillofacial region in the long term without removal of all inflammatory lesions.

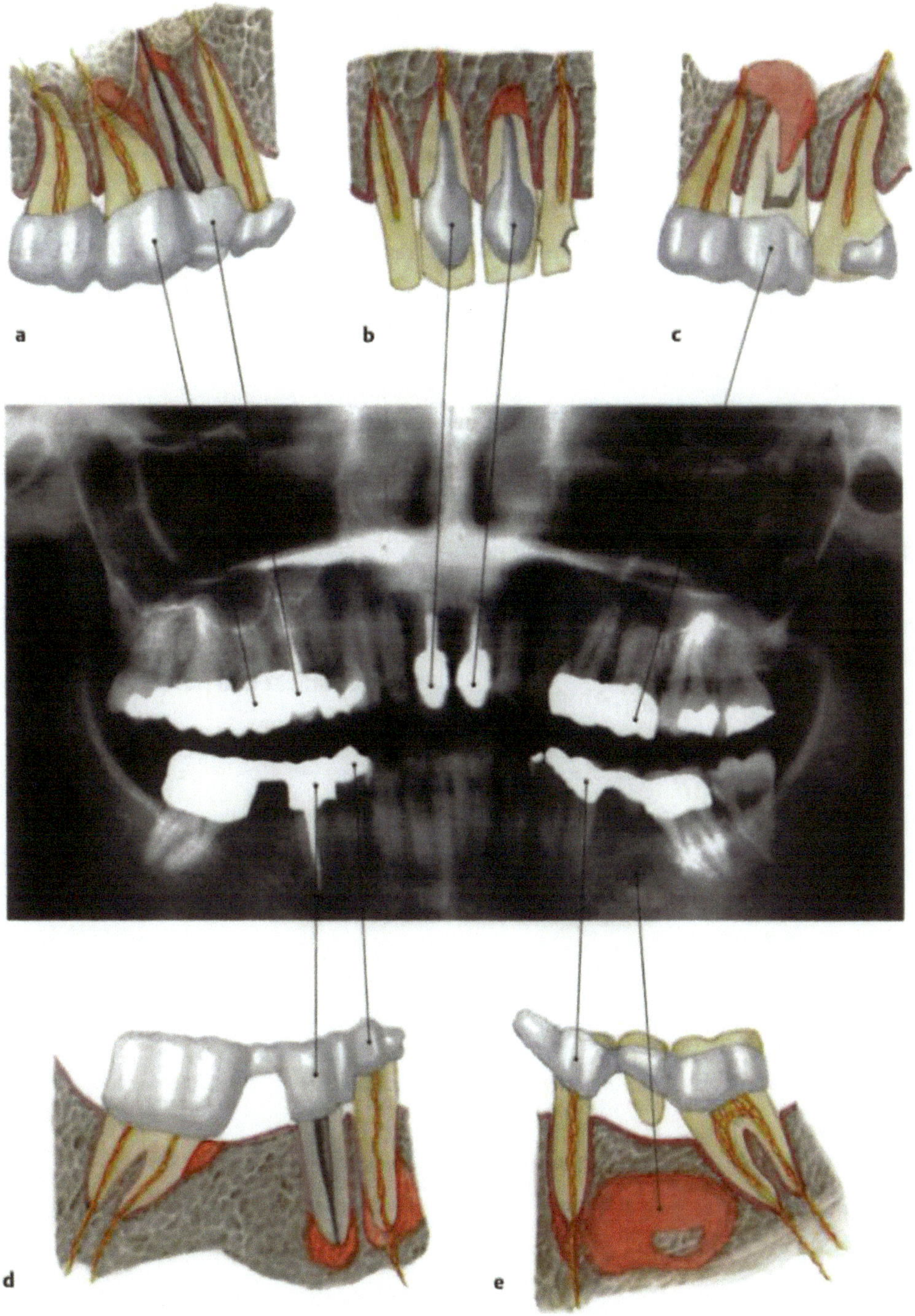

►**Fig. 13.2** Panoramic image of the teeth of a female patient born in 1958. **(a)** Region 17–14: Overfilled root 15 with apical osteitis and concomitant inflammation of the maxillary sinus floor, osteitis in the area of root 16. **(b)** Region 11 and 21–22: incomplete root filling at 11 without significant reaction in the alveolar region, root filling at 12 and subsequent root tip resection and osteitis. **(c)** Region 24–26: crowning of teeth 24 and 25 by two-part bridge, periapical osteitis at tooth 25 with involvement of the floor of the maxillary sinus. **(d)** Region 47–44: four-part bridge with root treatment at 45, periradicular osteitis at 45 and 44, marginal periodontitis at 47. **(e)** Region 35–37: periapical osteitis at 35, residual osteitis in the alveolar region.

13.3 Example 3

▶ **Referring diagnosis.** Varus gonarthrosis on both sides, more pronounced on the left. Status post renal cell carcinoma surgery on the right. The patient also has chronic lower back pain.

▶ **From the medical history**. Repeated lower back pain for many years, conservatively treated. Gradually increasing knee pain on both sides, more pronounced on the left. The X-ray examination shows bilateral varus gonarthrosis. Conservative treatments only with limited improvement of pain. Right nephrectomy due to renal cell carcinoma without metastasis. Inpatient admission for implantation of a knee joint prosthesis on the left.

▶ **X-ray.** The panoramic image shows the following results (▶ Fig. 13.3):

- Gapped dentition with extracted teeth 36 and 46.
- Fillings in teeth 18, 27 and 28, 37, and 47.
- Osteitis in the area of root tips 16, 37, 41, and 47.
- Deep cavity at 41.
- Periodontitis in upper and lower jaw with horizontal bone loss.

▶ **Clinical findings**. The following findings were recorded:

- Slight percussion sensitivity of teeth 16 and 41.
- Gums with chronic inflammatory changes around all teeth.
- Untreated cavity at 41 and brownish discoloration of the tooth as a sign of impaired vitality.

▶ **Assessment**. According to the panoramic image of the teeth, there are multiple potential lesions in the dental and maxillofacial region that should be removed. The neural therapeutic testing of the teeth was negative, so that a causal relationship of the tooth lesions with the referring diagnoses could not be established, but also could not be definitely ruled out. This statement is only possible after tooth extraction and neural therapeutic follow-up treatment of the emerging wounds and scars.

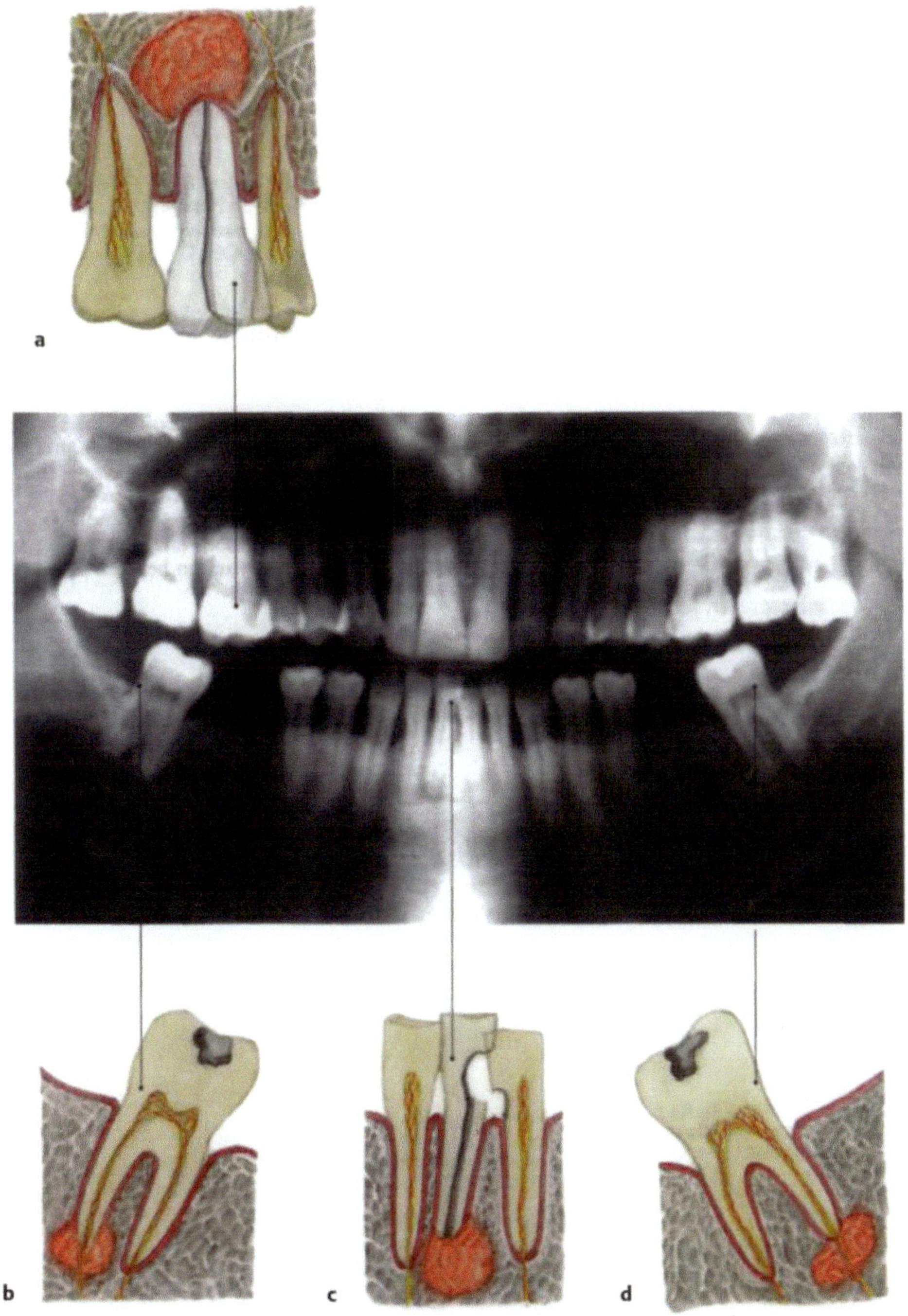

►**Fig. 13.3** Panoramic image of the teeth of the patient born in 1941. (a) Region 16: vitality-impaired tooth with inflamed root region, periapical osteitis involving the right maxillary sinus floor and polypoid mucosal changes. **(b)** Region 47: periapical osteitis with sclerotization lines as an indication of chronic inflammation. **(c)** Region 42 and 41, 31: advanced deep cavity with opening of the pulp and reactive periapical osteitis and severely impaired vitality. Suspected loss of vitality. **(d)** Region 37: periapical osteitis with moderate sclerotization lines as an indication of a chronic illness.

13.4
Example 4

▸**Referring diagnosis.** Left shoulder pain of unclear origin:

- Status post left shoulder joint luxation and left clavicle fracture in 1962.
- Painful functional impairment of the left shoulder joint as of 1980.
- Cycle-related migraines.
- Postcholecystectomy syndrome after cholecystectomy in 1986.

▸**From the medical history.** After falling on the left shoulder in 1963, luxation of the shoulder joint and fracture of the left clavicle. Largely pain-free after repositioning and osseous knitting of the clavicle fracture. As of 1980, gradually increasing pain in the left shoulder and increasing limitation of movement. No degenerative changes in the left shoulder joint were found in radiology. Conservative treated was attempted without success. Furthermore, the patient has cycle-related migraines as well as functional upper abdominal pain after cholecystectomy.

▸**X-ray.** The panoramic image shows the following results (▸Fig. 13.4):

- Gapped dentition with missing teeth 18 and 17, 15 and 14.
- Fillings in teeth 16, 13, 12, 16, 21, 22, 26, and 27.
- Bridges for 35–37 and 47–45.
- Osteitic lesions at 21–24, 36, and 46.
- Massive shadowing of the left maxillary sinus.
- Horizontal bone loss in the maxillary dental arch, also to a lesser extent in the anterior mandible.

▸**Clinical findings.** The following findings were recorded:

- Gapped dentition.
- Moderate periodontitis of the upper and lower jaw.
- No spontaneous pain in the teeth.
- Slight percussion sensitivity of teeth 23, 34, 35, and 37.

▸**Assessment.** Multilocular osteitis of the dental and maxillofacial region. The first neural therapeutic tooth test resulted in improvement of the left shoulder pain, strong upper abdominal pain on the right, and subsequent numbness throughout the left side of the body for several hours. After the first removal in region 36 through mandibular surgery, there was an improvement in the left shoulder pain. Complete restoration of the left upper and lower jaw is necessary in order to eliminate the various conditions.

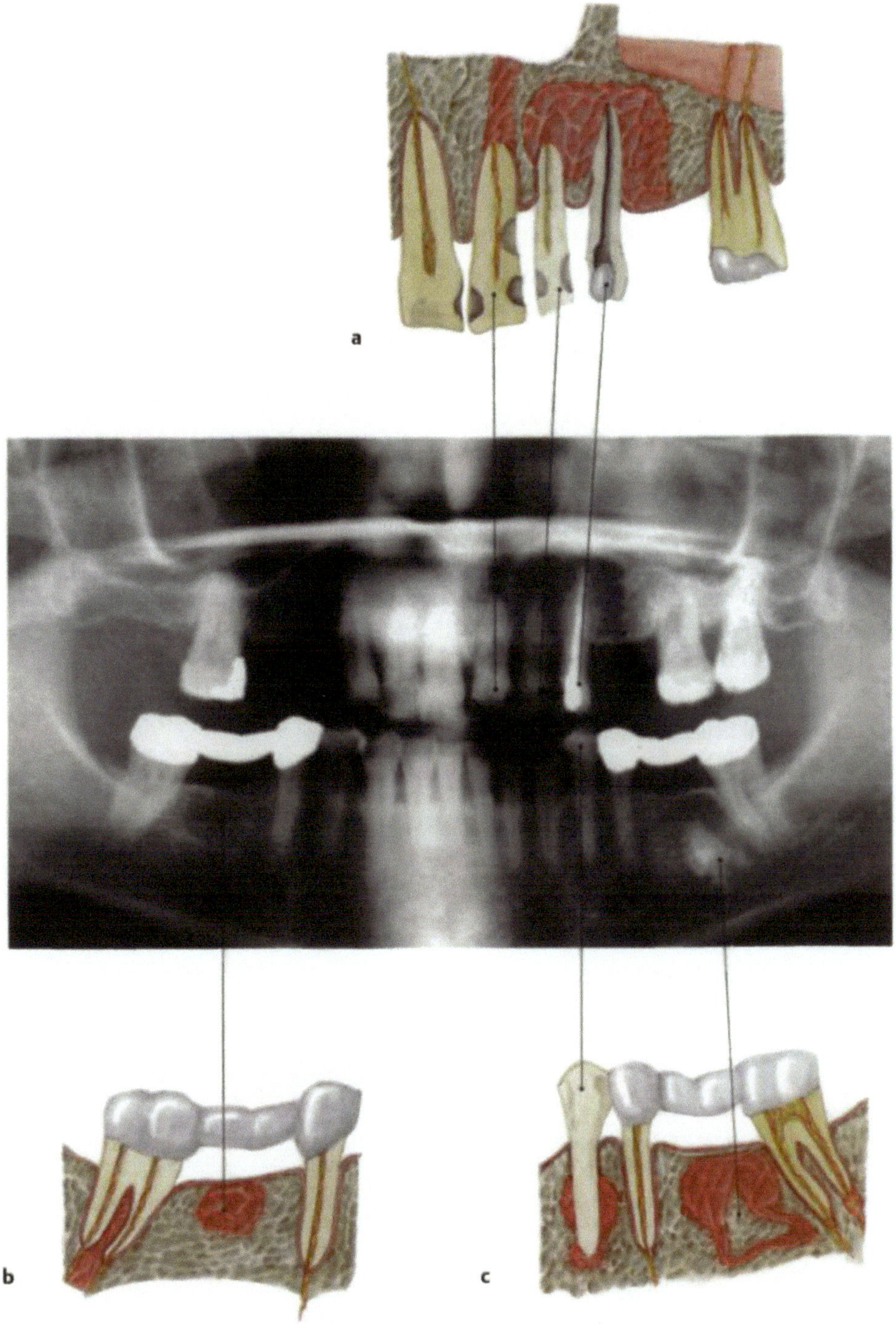

▶**Fig. 13.4** Panoramic image of the teeth of a female patient born in 1942. **(a)** Region 21–26: apical osteitis at 21 due to deep caries, periradicular osteitis at 22 and 23, suspected vitality disorder in 22, root filling at 23 with sclerosing periradicular osteitis, status post extraction of 24 and 25, massive concomitant shadowing of the left maxillary sinus. **(b)** Region 46 and 45: residual osteitis in area 46 at the level of the root region with rarefication of the spongiosa structure. **(c)** Region 34–37: extensive residual osteitis in root area 36 with sclerosing island as a sign of chronic osteitis, periradicular osteitis in region 34, and apical osteitis of the same tooth.

13.5 Example 5

► **Referring diagnosis.** Coxarthrosis on both sides, left more than right.

► **From the medical history.** Gradually increasing strain-related groin and buttock pain for about 5 years, more pronounced on the left than the right. Bilateral idiopathic coxarthrosis was determined after X-ray examination. Due to unsuccessful conservative treatment, implantation of a total left hip prosthesis is planned.

► **X-ray** The panoramic image shows the following results (► Fig. 13.5):

- Residual dentition, in which the five remaining teeth serve as supports for a maxillary and mandibular prosthesis.
- Capping of teeth 14 and 13, 25, 32, and 43.
- Inflammatory changes of the upper and lower jaw bone of region 13 and 47–45, 42, 32, and 36 with tooth root residue and involvement of the left maxillary sinus in the form of polypoid mucosal inflammation.
- Significant horizontal bone loss in the maxilla.
- Slightly swollen zone in region 48 with a lack of sponginess and low-bone zones vertically below this at the level of the mandibular canal (possibly a radicular cyst at 48, the patient does not recall a tooth extraction in this area).

► **Clinical findings**. The following findings were recorded:

- Chronic gum inflammation in the area of the five remaining teeth.
- No percussion or pressure sensitivity of the teeth.
- The single standing tooth at 25 shows painless significant mobility as a response to pressure.

► **Assessment**. Significant inflammatory foci of the dental and maxillofacial region with residual dentition. Pain symptoms occurring at tooth 36 after dental testing were remedied through jaw surgery and the residual root was removed. Repeated dental testing did not result in improvement in the hip joint pain symptoms. Thus, clear evidence of an interference field could not be detected.

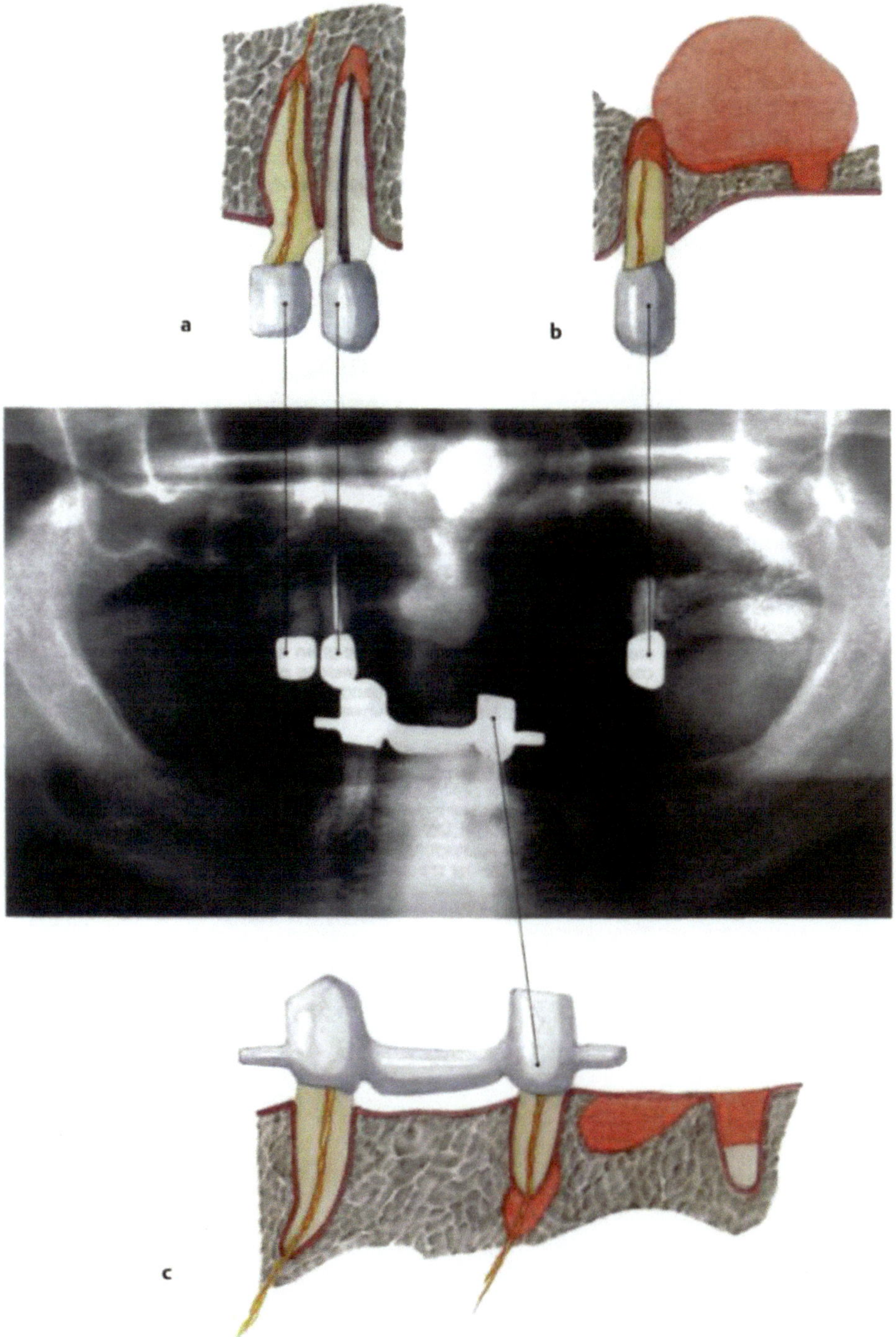

► **Fig. 13.5** Panoramic image of the teeth of the patient, born in 1929. (a) Region 14 and 13: apical osteitis for crowned teeth and root treatment of tooth 13. The teeth serve as supports for a maxillary prosthesis, suspicion of impaired vitality in tooth 14. (b) Region 25–27: apical osteitis of a crowned tooth (25) with probable vitality impairment and serving as a support for a maxillary prosthesis. From this and from a residual stenosis originating at 27, there is polypoid mucosal inflammation in the left maxillary sinus. (c) Region 32–36: apical osteitis at 32, residual osteitis after tooth extraction at 34 and 35, and residual osteitis at 36 with remaining tooth root residue.

13.6
Example 6

▶**Referring diagnosis** Highly advanced ankylosing coxarthrosis on the right, planned implantation of a total hip prosthesis.

▶**From the medical history** First hip pains at age 19. Right-sided coxarthrosis was determined after X-ray examination. Conservative treatment unsuccessful. At age 23 years, varus displacement osteotomy of the right hip with the subsequent worsening of the symptoms and the X-ray findings. After tooth removal, further worsening of the symptoms. Inpatient admission for implantation of a knee joint prosthesis on the left.

▶**X-ray** The panoramic image shows the following results (▶Fig. 13.6):

- Gapped dentition with inflammatory changes in region 16, 15, 13, 12 and 22, 23, and 26.
- X-ray evidence of impaired vitality in teeth 17, 15, 24, 25, 27, and 47.
- Wisdom teeth were not inherent, according to information from the patient.

▶**Clinical findings** The following findings were recorded:
- No subjective tooth pain.
- Teeth 16 and 26 sensitive to percussion.
- Gingivitis in the area of all crowned teeth.

▶**Assessment** Considerable lesions in the right and left maxillary region after bridge work. In the second phenomenon (p. 3), neural therapeutic testing of the teeth results in a pain-free right hip joint. Long-lasting freedom from pain after radical dental treatment. Significant improvement in agility, observation period of 10 years. The implantation of a hip joint prosthesis is not necessary.

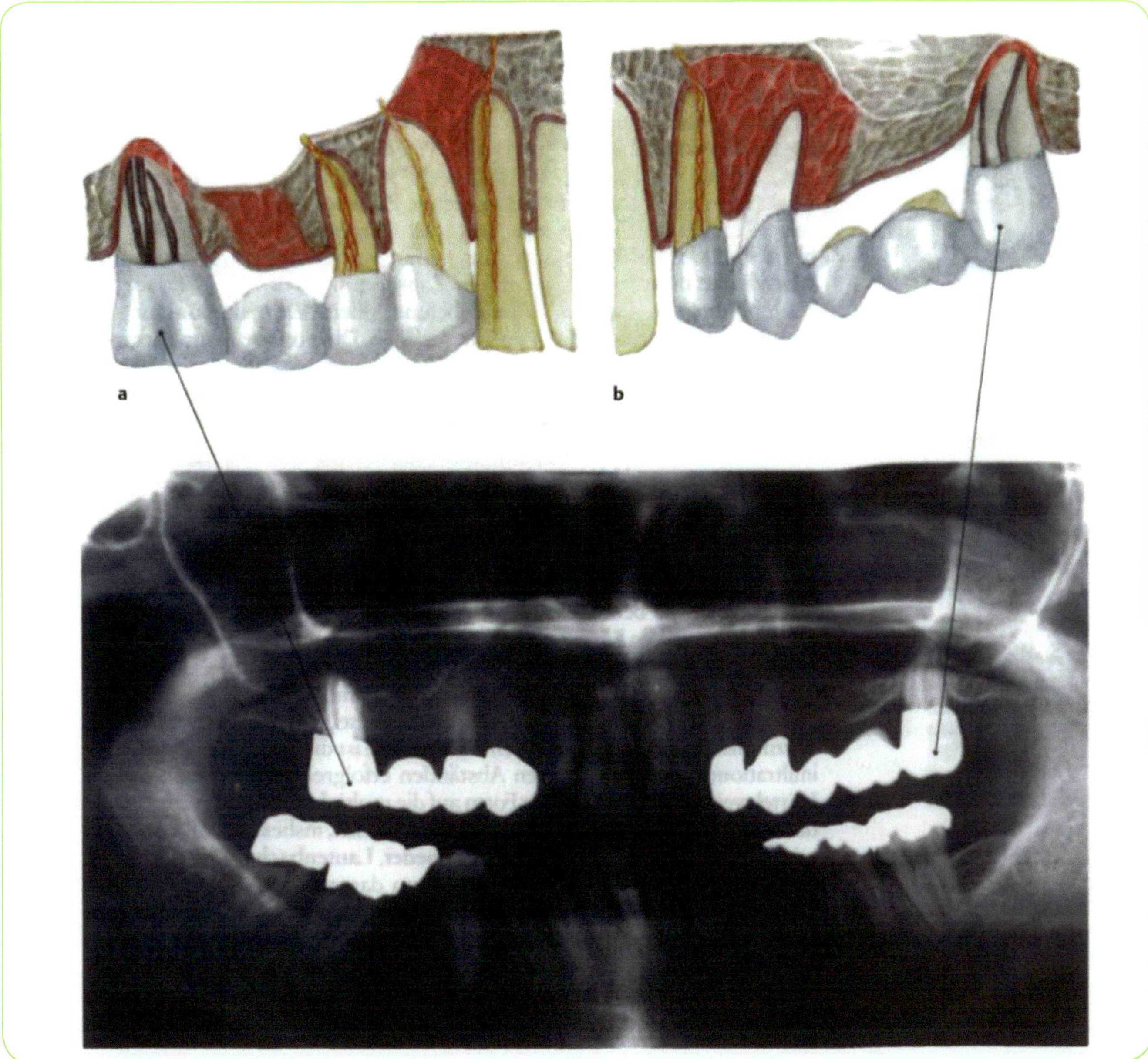

▸ **Fig. 13.6** Panoramic image of the teeth of the female patient born in 1955. **(a)** Region 16–12: periradicular osteitis in the area of teeth 13 and 12. Striking is the low radiation density of tooth 13, which is used together with tooth 14 as a bridge abutment. There is suspicion of impaired vitality in tooth 13. There is residual osteitis in former dental bearing 15. The root tip of tooth 16, which has had a root canal treatment and is used as a support, lacks a bony covering to the maxillary sinus, which can be assessed as evidence of chronic osteitis. At the junction of the crown's rear portion to the tooth, there is defective dentin as an indication of tooth decay. **(b)** Region 22–26: teeth 22 and 23, which serve as supports, do not provide much contrast in the X-rays; impaired vitality can also be assumed here. Under a strong light source, a significant reduction in the spongiosa as radiographic evidence of osteitis is reflected in the entire root area of 21 and 22. Tooth 26, which also serves as a support, shows an expanded periodontal gap as well as wedge-shaped mesial bone loss as a sign of chronic inflammation. Next there is punctiform defect formation mesially and centrally just below the crown as an indication of carious change.

13.7 Summary

The subtle diagnosis of the dental and maxillofacial region as well as the restoration that is usually necessary represents a problem that is often underestimated.The patient experiences severe changes in the dentition, which also must not be trivialized, especially in terms of the psychological impact. The collaboration with the attending dentist or oral surgeon often becomes a problem because of differences in evaluating the occurrence of an interference field, resulting in only "half-hearted" maxillofacial restoration. Furthermore, neural therapeutic dental testing results in a false-negative about 30 to 40% of the time, although clinical findings, X-ray findings, and any subjective pain provide clear evidence. Positive neural therapeutic dental testing easily convinces the patient to agree to tooth extraction. Tooth extraction which is performed as an interference field elimination after a negative neural therapeutic test in order to eliminate a chronic health issue arguably causes difficulties from a medical perspective, primarily if the desired result of ending the chronic illness fails after tooth extraction.

It is important that the resulting scars in each tooth extraction are re-treated by way of repeated infiltration or, even better, provided with neural therapeutic care during wound healing. In this case, painless and irritation-free healing is observed. The medication of choice for this is procaine 1%. In individual cases, it is worthwhile to repeat the neural therapeutic dental testing several times, as that can sometimes postpone dental extraction considerably. With inflammatory diseases of the gums, repeated neural therapeutic treatment must be provided prior to surgical treatment. In the majority of cases, the inflammation is successfully eliminated by way of procaine infiltration at weekly intervals.

Härtel convincingly explains the multiple potentials for lesions in the maxillofacial region.[190] The anatomical and especially the neuroanatomical conditions are described in relevant dentistry textbooks and are part of the standard knowledge of dentistry.

Voll, along with **Kramer,** compiled relationships originating from electroacupuncture diagnostics between dental lesions and possible organ disease in a clear table (▶Fig. 13.7).[530] From a neural therapeutic perspective, this table is valuable as an additional diagnostic overview. However, according to neural therapeutic experience, there is no definite diagnostic/therapeutic reliability.

The energetic interactions between the maxillofacial area and the rest of the body

The chart below shows the energetic relationships between pathological changes in dental, oral and jaw area and the rest of the body.

The relationships were determined by R. Voll, MD, from Plochingen, Germany, on the basis of many measurement results from electro-acupuncture diagnostics using a diatherapy puncture device. The chart was compiled by Ms. Kramer, DDS, Nuremberg, Germany. It should especially help to facilitate the diagnosis of patients with lesions or suspected lesions and thereby improve therapy.

Definitions in the chart:

C 5-Th 1	=	Brachial plexus
Th 1-Th 4	=	Upper intercostal nerves
Th 5-Th 7	=	Middle intercostal nerves
Th 8-Th 10	=	Lower intercostal nerves
Th 11-Th 12	=	Lowermost intercostal nerves
Th 12 - L 3	=	Lumbar plexus
L4-S3	=	Sacral plexus = sciatic plexus
S4-S5	=	Pudenal plexus
S 5-Co	=	Coccygeal plexus

The muscles belonging to the individual odontons were described by Voll in the 4th special edition of the International Association of Electro-acupuncture **"Interrelationships of odontogenic lesions to organs and tissue systems"**, Med. Lit. Publishers, Uelzen.

The relationship between the odonton of the upper jaw to the body.																	
Sensory organs		Inner ear	Maxillary sinuses		Ethmoidal cells		Eye	Frontal sinus		Frontal sinus		Eye	Ethmoidal cells		Maxillary sinuses		Inner ear
Joints		Shoulder Elbow	Jaw		Shoulder Elbow		Posterior knee			Posterior knee			Shoulder Elbow		Jaw		Shoulder Elbow
		Ulnar hand Foot Plantar toes and 1*	Anterior knee		Radial hand Foot Big toe		Hip	Sacrococcygeal bone		Sacrococcygeal bone		Hip	Radial hand Foot Big toe		Anterior knee		Ulnar hand Foot Plantar toes and 1*
							Foot			Foot							
Spinal cord segments		Th 1 C8 Th 7 Th 6 Th 5 S 3 S 2 S 1	Th 12 Th 11 L 1		C 7 C 6 C 5 Th 4 Th 3 Th 2 L 5 L 4		Th 8 Th 9 Th 10	L 2 L 2 Co S5 S4		L 2 L 3 S 4 S 5 Co		Th 8 Th 9 Th 10	C 5 C 6 C 7 Th 2 Th 3 Th 4 L 4 L 5		Th 11 Th 12 L1		C 8 Th 1 Th 5 Th 6 Th 7 S 1 S 2 S 3
Vertebrae		B 1 H 7 B 6 B 5 S 2 S 1	B 12 B 11 L 1		H 7 H 6 H 5 B 4 B 3 L 5 L 4		B 9 B 10	L 3 L 2 Co S 5 S 4 S 3		L 2 L 3 S 3 S 4 S 5 Co		B 9 B 10	H 5 H 6 H 7 B 3 B 4 L 4 L 5		B 11 B 12 L 1		H 7 B 1 B 5 B 6 S 1 S 2
Organs	**Yin**	Right heart	Pancreas		Right lung		Right liver	Right kidney		Left kidney		Left liver	Left lung		Spleen		Left heart
	Yang	Duodenum	Left stomach		Right large intestine		Gall bladder	Right bladder urogenital region		Left bladder urogenital region		Bile **ducts, left**	Left large intestine		Left stomach		Jejunum Left ileum
Endocrine Glands		Pituitary gland anterior lobe	Para-adenoid gland	Adenoid gland	Thymus	Pituitary gland posterior lobe		Epiphysis		Epiphysis		Pituitary gland posterior lobe		Thymus	Adenoid gland	Para-adenoid gland	Anterior
		Central nervous system	Right mammary gland												Left mammary gland		Central nervous system mind
New nomenclature for the teeth of the upper jaw		18	17	16	15	14	13	12	11	21	22	23	24	25	26	27	28
Lesions: = very severe = significant = weak	X = missing C = crown B = bridge unit	8+	7+	6+	5+	4+	3+	2+	1+	+1	+2	+3	+4	+5	+6	+7	+8
		8-	7-	6-	5-	4-	3-	2-	1-	-1	-2	-3	-4	-5	-6	-7	-8
New nomenclature for the teeth of the lower jaw		48	47	46	45	44	43	42	41	31	32	33	34	35	36	37	38
The relationship between the odonton of the lower jaw to the rest of the body.																	
Other		Energy balance			Mammary gland right								Mammary gland left				Energy balance
Endocrines of the tissue system		Peripheral Nerves	Arteries	Veins	Lymph vessels	Gonads		Adrenal gland		Adrenal gland		Gonads		Lymph vessels	Veins	Arteries	Peripheral Nerves
Organs	**Yang**	Right ileum Ileocecum	Right large intestine and area		Right stomach Pylorus		Gall bladder	Right bladder urogenital region		Left bladder urogenital region		Left bile ducts	Left stomach		Left large intestine		Jejunum Left ileum
	Yin	Right heart	Right lung		Pancreas			Right kidney		Left kidney			Spleen		Left lung		Left heart
Vertebrae		B 1 H 7 B 6 B 5 S2 S 1	H 7 H 6 H 5 B 4 B 3 L 5 L 4		B 12 B 11 L 1		B 9 B 10	L3 L 2 Co S 5 S 4 S 3		L 2 L 3 S 4 S 5 Co		B 9 B 10	B 11 B 12 L 1		H 5 H 6 H 7 B 3 B 4 L 4 L 5		H 7 B 1 B 5 B 6 S 1 S 2
Spinal cord segments		Th 1 C 8 Th 7 Th 6 Th 5 S 3 S 2 S 1	C 7 C 6 C 5 Th 4 Th 3 Th 2 L 5 L 4		Th 12 Th 11 L 1		Th 8 Th 9 Th 10	L 3 L 2 Co S5 S4		L 2 L 3 S4 S5 Co		Th 8 Th 9 Th 10	Th 11 Th 12 L 1		C 5 C 6 C 7 Th 2 Th 3 Th 4 L 4 L 5		C 8 Th 1 Th 5 Th 6 Th 7 S 1 S 2 S 3
Joints		Shoulder - Elbow			Anterior knee		Posterior knee			Posterior knee			Anterior knee		Shoulder - Elbow		
		Ulnar hand Foot Plantar toes and 1*	Radial hand Foot Big toe				Hip	Sacrococcygeal bone		Sacrococcygeal bone		Hip			Radial hand Foot Big toe		Ulnar hand Foot Plantar toes and 1*
					Jaw		Foot			Foot			Jaw				
Sensory organs		Ear	Ethmoidal cells		Maxillary Sinuses		Eye	Frontal sinus		Frontal sinus		Eye	Maxillary Sinuses		Ethmoidal cells		Ear

1* = Sacroiliac joint (part of the 8th odonton)

Distributed by: Internat. Association for Electro-acupuncture (Reg. Assoc.), Office 73207 Plochingen/Neckar, Richard-Wagner-Straße 5, Phone 071 53/279 42
Published by: Dr. Fritz Kramer, 90482 Nuremberg, Ostendstraße 161, Phone 0911/57 13 26 Printed by: Karl Pfeiffer's Book Printing and Publishing oHG, 91217 Hersbruck. P.O. Box 440 Order no. form EAV/1

▶**Fig. 13.7** The energetic interactions between the maxillofacial area and the rest of the body.

14 Neural Therapeutic Phenomena

14.1 Neural Therapeutic Phenomena and Types of Reactions

The assessment of the reactions in accordance with neural therapeutic treatment determines the therapeutic approach. Therefore, it is crucial to correctly classify the following types of reactions in order to exhaust all possibilities for consequent treatment of an illness.

14.1.1 Segment Phenomenon

This phenomenon was the first neural therapeutic reaction form that was initially observed over 100 years ago and was the reason for using local anesthesia for therapeutic purposes. The infiltration of a local anesthetic in painful areas or pressure points often resulted in improvement in symptoms and elimination of the symptoms after repeated infiltration. The concept of segmental therapy was developed on the basis of this individual observation.[223,302,446,469,470,471]

The full utilization of injections in segmental therapy marks the beginning of each neural therapeutic treatment. In many cases, painful illnesses or nonpainful organ function disorders (e.g., hormonal dysregulation) are eliminated with repeated injections. In segment diagnostics, particularly in the first treatment, there can be a temporary increase in symptoms with subsequent improvement. This worsening of symptoms no longer occurs in the successive treatments. The symptomology can be eliminated by continuing the segmental therapy. In the case of unsuccessful segmental therapy, interference field diagnostics (p. 81) are performed.

14.1.2 Reaction Phenomenon (According to Hopfer)

The reaction phenomenon is a special type of reaction occurring in segment diagnostics (p. 53). It involves a worsening of the treated illness over the course of 1 to 3 days after neural therapeutic segment treatment. After this worsening of symptoms, the symptoms decrease back to baseline. In segment diagnostics, the reaction phenomenon is the clearest indication of an interference field illness. The reaction phenomenon is therefore connected to interference field diagnostics (p. 81); the continuation of segmental treatment remains unsuccessful.

14.1.3 Retrograde Phenomenon (According to Hopfer)

Direct Retrograde Phenomenon

Under segmental treatment, symptoms that were previously not present occur at another location in the form of pain, inflammatory reactions, or organ function disorders. After initial local treatment of the lumbar spine, the patient may report, for example, tonsillitislike symptoms or variable itching of a scar. By addressing these new pain symptoms in the form of injection to the tonsils or infiltration of the newly itchy scar, the initially treated pain symptoms in the lumbar spine are often eliminated by way of the second phenomenon (p. 3). The interpretation of this treatment pathway shows that the responsible interference field is signaled under segmental treatment.

The conditions are similar when patients repeatedly report nausea, belching, bloating, or changes in digestion after a treatment. These symptoms should not be interpreted primarily as an intolerance reaction to the local anesthetic used, but quite possibly as a message from the relevant interference field, in this case the stomach, liver, or intestine. Accordingly, the neural therapeutic treatment would be focused on these organs in order to treat the actual primary disease.

Indirect Retrograde Phenomenon

As with the direct retrograde phenomenon, symptoms in another location occur with neural therapeutic segmental treatment or interference field treatment, whereby addressing these new findings under suspicion of an interference field function does not eliminate the symptomology initially to be treated. In the course of the first neural therapeutic treatment, a previously asymptomatically occurring regional disorder of the body appears, which has been enabled by the preceding neural therapeutic measures. It is important to address this new symptomology with neural therapy anyway, because the previously unsuccessful segmental treatment of the initial symptoms may have positive progression after normalization of these additional symptoms.

In this case, the newly occurring disorder acted as a blocking element.

14.1.4 Second Phenomenon (Huneke's Phenomenon)

This is surely the most interesting phenomenon in neural therapy. Its observation and implementation in a therapeutic concept were made possible by the Huneke brothers and opened up new possibilities in therapy. The basis is formed by the neural interference field, from which an illness is triggered and maintained by way of the autonomic nervous system.

The reaction sequence is designated the second phenomenon, whereupon a disorder subsides "in a second" after infiltration of an interference field, as long as the anatomical conditions allow it, and the normalization of the function is restored. Thus, a joint with severe degenerative changes remains restricted in its function but is movable without pain. It is important that the initial pain-free state lasts more than 1 day and that repeated interference field infiltration after reappearance of the old symptoms leads to permanent freedom from symptoms.

The second phenomenon is still the most impressive phenomenon in neural therapy and documents the strong dysregulatory effect the interference field can exert on the organism. The clinical evidence continuously shows that chronic illnesses can very frequently be traced back to an interference field. Examples include the rapid normalization of hyperthyroidism, the cessation of bronchial asthma, the painless lumbar spine in chronic low back pain, or pain-free advanced coxarthrosis despite unchanged radiological findings. Modification of the second phenomenon reveals further phenomena related to the interference field.

14.1.5 Delayed Second Phenomenon

In this case, symptomology is not normalized in matter of a second after infiltration of the interference field, but over a few hours, sometimes days. Thus, a chronic headache disorder related to a toxically exposed liver through an interference field is not eliminated seconds after injection to the right celiac ganglion including "liver segment therapy," but only after hours, or in some cases only after a few days. The interpretation of this slowed regulation process suggests that impaired liver function takes a longer time to normalize than an infected scar or the tonsils, for example. Compared to the normal second phenomenon, a delayed second phenomenon requires a bit more patience and a potentially prolonged, repeated interference field therapy.

14.1.6 Incomplete Second Phenomenon

In the normal second phenomenon, all symptoms must subside completely within seconds. This is not the case with the incomplete second phenomenon. Instead, only certain symptoms of an illness subside, while others remain unaffected. Observation of the incomplete second phenomenon requires particular attentiveness on the part of the therapist and the patient, and precise documentation of symptoms. It is important to record the individual symptoms of an illness in order to detect the cessation of individual symptoms after the interference field treatment. Diffuse abdominal pain, numerous headache disorders, polyarthralgia, or spinal disorders often fall into this category. The remaining symptoms can then often degrade via segmental therapy or via other interference fields until the patient is entirely symptom-free. This documents the possibility that an illness can be triggered and maintained by multiple interference fields.

14.1.7 "Silent" Second Phenomenon

This phenomenon requires more patience than the other types of reactions that can occur in neural therapy. After unsuccessful segmental therapy and thorough, equally unsuccessful exploration of the interference field, it has been proven that segmental therapy should be restarted, even if this initially resulted in no improvement in the symptoms. Symptomology can often be eliminated with a second round of segmental therapy, so to speak. The reason for this phenomenon is likely that one or more interference fields impair the body's autoregulation through general autonomic exposure without exerting a direct effect on the diseased organ structure.

This blockade is removed with "blind" interference field therapy, so that simple segmental treatment can then be successful.

Conclusion

In summary, knowledge of the body's different modes of reaction during neural therapeutic treatment is critical to success, as some reactions are obvious and others are rather obscured. The informed and attentive patient facilitates the course of treatment significantly, whereby sufficient patience from the doctor and patient is necessary.

14.2 Tactical Approach

Neural therapeutic treatment basically starts with segment diagnostics (p. 53) and segmental therapy (p. 53). Thus, a minimal number of targeted injections are performed and the first reaction is awaited. With experience, however, the interference field (p. 81) may be initially used if the patient reports earlier unsuccessful treatments in the segment or even worsening of symptoms with this treatment, or if suspicion of an interference field is virtually obligatory owing to the medical history, e.g., with cycle-related migraines or chronic constipation immediately after hepatitis. Depending on the type of illness, the indicated symptoms are often significantly improved or eliminated immediately after treatment with the correct injection technique. The patient's next appointment should be dependent on the pain symptomology. In the case of acute pain, the patient should be called in 1 to 2 days later, and after 1 week in the case of a chronic illness. The next treatment often already shows whether the selected segmental treatment path was correct, whether it must be continued only with the same injections or expanded, or if there is suspicion of an interference field induction.

If the segmental treatment can be continued, the initial injections can be continued until the patient is symptom-free, whereby the treatment intervals are significantly lengthened. Once free of symptoms, the patient can be discharged with instructions to return if the old symptomology reoccurs. Prophylactic treatment should be rejected because it results in no advantage for the patient.

Interference field diagnostics are initiated if the result after the first two to three treatments shows that the illness is likely induced by an interference field. In this case, one should focus on the interference field potentials in the medical history. If these have been exhausted, and even in the absence of a medical history, interference field diagnostics are continued from "head to toe" accordingly to likelihood. Due to the incidence of interference fields in the tooth–jaw area and the restricted examination-based and palpatory diagnostics, a dental panoramic image—and possibly also a digital volume tomography (DVT)—should be performed in order to capture the focal situation as fully as possible.

If there is a diagnosis of an **interference field** or multiple interference fields which are the cause of the treated illness, the corresponding injections are continued over increasingly longer intervals until the patient is symptom-free. If the symptomology cannot be consistently resolved through subtle interference field treatment, but only for variable, shorter periods, it is possible that the interference fields cannot be eliminated with neural therapeutic measures alone. Thus, it must be considered whether a surgical removal of the interference field is required. Here, too, the tooth–jaw area is shown to have the most interference field localization.

Surgical removal of an interference field should be accompanied by repeated neural therapeutic infiltration of the resulting wounds and scars, not only to achieve safe, nonirritated wound healing, but also to prevent the formation of renewed interference fields from the newly formed scars. Especially in the treatment of fresh wounds, it is recommended to use only the ester-structured procaine since optimal perfusion ratios are achieved through the vasodilatory effect of the cleavage product diethylaminoethanol at the site of injection.

If the treated illness cannot be normalized after interference field treatment, possible surgical removal of foci, and a reattempt at segmental treatment, a **general regulatory disorder** should be suspected, which cannot be resolved with neural therapeutic measures alone. The neural therapeutic treatment already carried out, particularly the interference field treatment, should by no means be considered useless, since interference fields only restrict the function of the interstitial regulation system via the autonomic branch. Other **processes in regulatory medicine**, which are also initiated in the interstitial regulation system, would then come into play.

14.3 Side Effects

As with any treatment method, side effects are also possible in neural therapy according to Huneke. By using a local anesthetic, all general side effects typical of this medication as well as side effects from the injection procedure are possible. They are dependent on the dose and the location of the injection. As illustrated in detail in Part 1, the optimal medication for neural therapy is procaine 1% (p. 37) without any additives.

Note

Given the quantity of procaine administered per session, which is far below the toxic maximum dose, no toxic side effects are to be expected with proper injection technique.

Possible side effects are frequently mild dizziness, rarely a metal taste on the tongue, slight internal trembling, and sweating. These side effects caused by procaine subsided after a few minutes without further treatment. In no way do they indicate "allergic" reactions to the local anesthetic. As already described, these are far below the allergy rate of other products.

Side effects that are not due to the local anesthetic but can be traced back to the nervous system, particularly the autonomic nervous system, as the body's reaction to the therapeutic intervention, are described in the chapter Neural Therapeutic Phenomena and Types of Reactions (p. 98). This involves diagnostically valuable and therapeutically viable reactions of the body, which are very important for the therapy process. These should be classified as "undesirable effects" since they have no harmful character.

The risks of neural therapy (p. 105) according to Huneke, which arise from injection therapy as an invasive procedure, are described in detail in Part 3. Possible risks and errors in the case of deeper injections, and especially injections in the head-neck area, will be discussed separately. Overall, all injections in clinical practice are regularly performed and repeatedly evaluated for possible risks, and amended in their implementation in a straightforward way so that they can be easily learned.

It is always important that the therapist has a clear understanding of the goal with each injection, focuses on each injection, and performs them in a calm manner. Comparing the trauma of neural therapy with other procedures sometimes used only for diagnostic procedures, such as organ biopsies, endovascular catheter examinations, and the various endoscopy procedures applied to diagnostics and therapy, the trauma from neural therapy is fairly low, as is the risk of iatrogenic injury.

Practical Advice

Complications that occur should be documented in detail in order to enable proper processing and information (e.g., Central Register of Neural Therapy Associations). This way, every complication can serve as a piece of the puzzle for further practical improvement of neural therapy and thereby help reduce the risks for patients. Assessment tasks are hereby more objectively possible and improve the quality of management.

14.4 Failure of Neural Therapy

14.4.1 Causes

Despite the very wide range of applications of neural therapy, which extends over almost all disciplines of medicine, not every neural therapeutic treatment can be successfully completed. On the one hand, the reasons for this may lie with the therapists themselves if an individual fails to recognize all disorders of the body which can be addressed with neural therapy. On the other hand, incomplete medical history data from the patient can lead to failure of neural therapeutic efforts. Furthermore, there may be blockages by the body which cannot be reached through neural therapy but are easily accessible by other therapy methods. These include blockages of the ground regulations system from:

- Toxins from the food chain.
- Heavy metal exposure.
- Residues from elapsed viral, bacterial, or fungoid infectious diseases.
- Dysbioses of the intestine.

14.4.2 Further Diagnostic and Therapeutic Possibilities

Diagnostic and therapeutic methods such as electroacupuncture, Vega test procedures, or bioresonance are sometimes able to detect these blockages and initiate therapeutic steps. In the presence of dysbiosis of the intestine (differentiated bacteriological examination of the intestinal flora is necessary), targeted intestinal cleansing is essential. Other generally effective transitional procedures, such as autologous blood therapy and therapeutic fasting, to name just two examples, are quite capable of improving existing restrictions on regulatory capacity to the extent that they can eliminate a chronic disease alone or after another subsequent neural therapeutic treatment attempt.

Part 3
Injection Technique and Indications

15 General Information

15.1 Introduction

The third part of this book describes the injection techniques used in neural therapy. They are the tools of this treatment method which is performed via the autonomic system. The different forms of injection originate from all specialties in medicine and were changed somewhat to increase the safety of the injections.

The injection techniques illustrated for different regions of the body are those which are most often performed in practice. The range of possible injections can certainly be expanded. After learning the listed injections, it is easily possible to administer all injections and make adjustments for individual anatomical requirements.

Practical Advice

A comprehensive anatomical textbook and a human skeleton model have proven useful for repeatedly studying, feeling, and understanding the topographical conditions.

The anatomical drawings in this textbook were reworked in order to individually emphasize the palpable structures (e.g., bones) and the structures associated with the sympathetic nervous system such as the spinal nerves, vessels, and ganglia. The photographs facilitate the practical orientation to palpable structures by way of "body painting." This should provide the most seamless possible transition from the patients to the anatomical structures relevant to neural therapy.

15.2 Positioning of the Patient

For every injection treatment, the patient should be in a relaxed yet secure position so that the injections can be performed safely. The patient should be positioned in such a way that does not require repositioning for each injection or cause any unease that may inhibit the patient's relaxation. For the therapist, it is fundamentally important to use "standardized" positioning as much as possible for the injections and therefore achieve better "accuracy." Thus, the supine position is favorable for all injections in the ventral and lateral regions of the body. A relaxed sitting position on the lounger has proven effective for injections in the dorsal region of the body from the head to the coccyx. Positioning on the side is favorable for injections to the dorsal sections of the lower extremities. In principle, the patient's position should be kept as simple as possible in order to enable the therapist to perform the work with a clear overview. Furthermore, every patient—even those with poor mobility—can easily receive the injections.

15.3 Disinfection

Basically, the skin should be disinfected before each injection, whereby the exposure time of the (usually) alcoholic disinfectant should not be less than 3 minutes. Due to the pharmacological effect (p. 38) of procaine described above, the experiences in working with procaine show that there is no increased occurrence of injection-related infections when the "disinfection time" is not complied with.

Note

Injections in joints and in the epidural space, with the low risk of dura injury, should be performed under strict aseptic conditions.

The infection risk with the use of procaine is negligibly low depending on the suitability of the tissue. To this end, it should be reiterated that procaine is highly valuable as a sole local anesthetic for localized treatment of viral—and above all, bacterial—infections.

The injection of amide-structured local anesthetic in bacterially infected tissue is **contraindicated**. Unlike the ester-structured local anesthetics, there is a vasoconstriction at the site of injection due to stimulus of the sympathetic nervous system, which causes a decline in the tissue trophism with the risk of spread of the infection.

15.4 Injection Method

Each injection should be safe, as painless as possible, and precise in its localization. It is advisable to make each injection with a firmly positioned and supported hand. Hands-free injection carries a risk of incorrect injection and unnecessary injury to the patient due to possible evasive movements. In order to get a feeling for the various types of tissue that must be penetrated, sometimes to considerable depth, to reach the actual injection site (e.g., paravertebral sympathetic chain, prevertebral ganglia, retroperitoneal space in the pelvis), the needle should be advanced slowly with light pressure on the plunger, i.e., with less simultaneous infiltration, which is more painless for the patient. For this purpose, the use of sharp, extremely thin disposable needles is necessary. These must be changed often. Sometimes, particularly in epidural injection, the free hand is used to support the needle, holding the cone which must be advanced extremely slowly through the coarse yellow ligament in order to reach the epidural space, which is just 2 to 3 mm wide, without injuring the spinal dura mater.

One-handed operation of the syringe and needle must be learned. It may sound trite, but it has been shown to be the cause of unsteady injections in neural therapeutic practice. The simple tool is not only for the application of the local anesthetic to the defined anatomic structure, but also simultaneously the "feeler" for the various tissue structures during a subtle injection technique. Frequent practice is required to master one-handed aspiration, turning the needle 180°, and the reaspiration that must be done before each deeper infiltration. The "one-handed technique" is necessary in cases where the second hand must be used for fixation, e.g., with injection to the stellate ganglion (p. 154) or for holding the spatula light, e.g., for injections to the tonsils.

15.5 Briefing

It is important to brief the patient about the purpose of the injections and not only about the risks. It has proven useful to brief the patient **before every** treatment:

- About expected reactions after every treatment.
- The possible side effects (p. 101) of the procedure.
- The possible risks of the injections.

This way, the documentation of the briefing in the medical chart is easy and understandable. The legally correct requirement for a **one-time** general briefing on the methodology at the beginning of therapy, describing efficacy, side effects, and risks of the method, usually overwhelms the patient and does not satisfy the objective purpose of the briefing. In any case, the patient should be able to turn to the therapist directly at any time if unclear symptoms occur after treatment.

Injection-related pain, e.g., the occasional flash of pain during injections to peripheral nerves, should be reported, as well as the contracting pain in the bladder and perineal region during injection to the branches of the uterovaginal plexus, which are used to check the correct position of the needle. When injecting, the therapist should also be mindful of the patient's reports of pain, since they could be an indication of incorrect needle positioning.

Note

Severe pain should not occur with any injection. If this happens, the injection must be interrupted and the needle position checked and corrected.

After a neural therapeutic treatment, each patient should remain under medical supervision, if possible for the duration of the local anesthetic's action; not only should expected reactions such as dizziness, slightly impaired sensory function, or sensitive or motor paralysis be resolved, but also, very rarely, unexpected reactions in the circulation (e.g., after injection to the celiac ganglion) or early allergic reactions can also occur, which may require treatment,.

15.6 Complications, Risks, and Errors

Despite control of the injection technique and the utmost care during the injection itself, complications can never be completely ruled out. Every complication occurring in the treatment should be documented, not only for in-house control, but also to better understand the complications and learn from them. Situationally correct behavior toward the patient is always essential.

> **Cave**
>
> **The inadvertent injection of a local anesthetic into an artery directed toward the brain, with the attendant consequences, is the most severe, albeit rare, complication that requires intensive care.**

The principal cause is the incorrectly performed two-time aspiration with 180° turning of the needle.

> **Cave**
>
> **The very rare case of anaphylaxis, which differs from intoxication in the absence of convulsions, is independent of the injection technique and requires intensive medical treatment under inpatient conditions.**

Hematomas are among the less avoidable complications that can be treated conservatively or (rarely) with surgery, depending on the localization and extent. Conservative neural therapeutic treatment of a hematoma involves the earliest possible, if necessary repeated, infiltration with procaine for fast absorption and infection prophylaxis through improvement of the tissue blood flow. **Organ damage** from a needlestick (e.g., lungs, kidneys, liver) generally does not have surgical consequences, but in case of doubt it should be monitored under inpatient conditions for the patient's safety. Besides errors in the injection technique, anatomical and topographical anomalies are definitely a possible cause.

The mistaken **puncture** of the **spinal dura mater** in epidural infiltration is a rare complication which often results in "postspinal headache" in the patient for several days. This can be reliably prevented by pulling the needle back into the epidural space after determining the intrathecal needle position (CSF aspiration), infiltrating 2 to 3 mL there to eliminate or reduce the stimulus which generates the CSF in the epidural space. Afterward, the injection must also be made to the occipital nerves. These injections are also very helpful for existing postspinal headaches after spinal anesthesia was given for a surgical procedure.

15.7 Dosage of the Local Anesthetic

For extravascular application, the maximum dose of 1% procaine is 500 mg. This corresponds to a volume of 50 mL for the 1% solution. This amount is never needed in the context of an extensive neural therapeutic treatment. A maximum amount of 30 mL is the upper limit per session and does not need to be exceeded. If this is unavoidable in an isolated case, there must be a break of 30 minutes to 1 hour between the first and second injection series.

> **Note**
>
> **For each treatment, the aim should be to manage with the smallest amounts of procaine and deliver the drug to the diseased structure through subtle injection technique. Extensive "flooding" of the tissue should not be performed.**

15.8 Frequent Injections

15.8.1 The Wheal

The **intracutaneous application** of a drug produces a firm swelling of the cutis with a skin surface similar to an "orange peel skin." This is not quite correctly referred to as a "wheal" (▶Fig. 15.1). The true wheal consists of a lifting of the corium of the cutis, as in a cutaneous allergic reaction, for example; plasma can be found in this small space. The neural therapeutic wheal does not produce this cavity, but is an infiltration which extends through all layers of the skin. Wheal therapy is a nonspecific stimulation treatment which is designed to have a therapeutic effect on diseases in the same segment via the segmental-reflexive pathway which, inter alia, leads to an improved circulation in this segment. Wheals are used before numerous other neural therapeutic injections at the beginning in order to use the skin as a strongly sympathetic innervated organ, as do many other physical therapy measures. Thus, a wheal series is obligatory for the paravertebral region, around joints, and around diffuse painful or edematous changes in skin areas.

The intradermal injection of neural therapy wheal is performed with a needle 2 cm long, 0.4 mm-thick and primarily produces a short burning pain by stimulating the somatosensory and sympathetic afferent fibers. The pain is followed by anesthesia of the skin over the region of the wheal.

In spite of this minimal treatment, the result is often a noticeable improvement in the preexisting ailments; 0.2 mL procaine is adequate per injection.

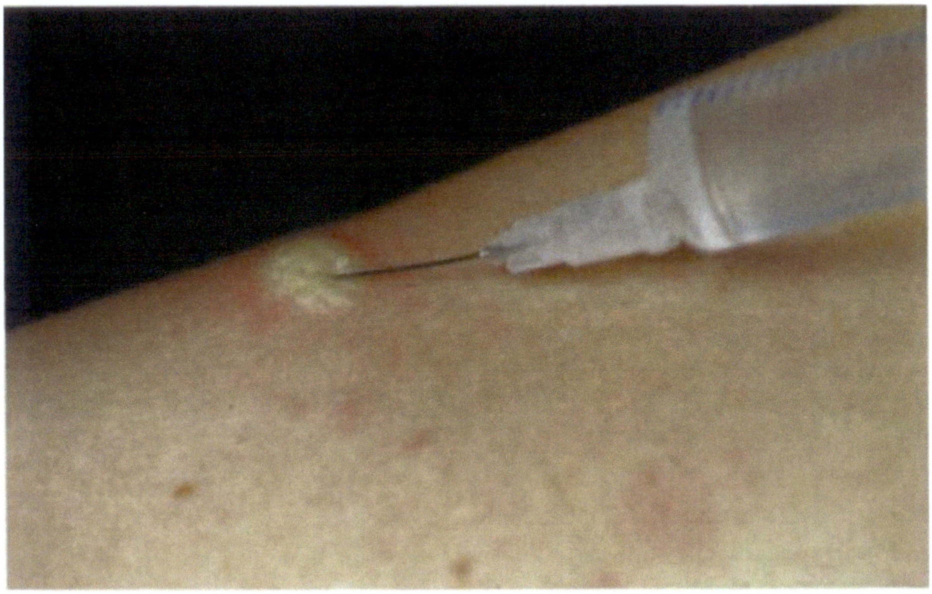

▶ **Fig. 15.1** Representation of the wheal (intracutaneous infiltration) immediately after infiltration with procaine.

Note

A reddening of the wheal when using procaine should not be misdiagnosed as an allergic reaction, but is an expression of intradermal vasodilation caused by the cleavage product of procaine, viz. diethylaminoethanol.

15.8.2 Infiltration of Geloses

A gelosis is a region of tissue that can be defined as a soft tumor localized in the interstitial connective tissue. The cause is assumed to be a circumscribed disorder in the tissue perfusion which is associated with localized edema of the connective tissue and, according to **Ricker**, is induced by a distinct slowing of the blood flow (prestasis) through stimulation of the perivascular sympathetic nervous system. The position of the gelosis can be easily felt in the subcutis; it is somewhat more difficult to detect in the muscle. The term “**myogelosis**” is used here.

The gelosis is easily overlooked in deeper tissue layers. As a segmental-reflexive autonomic response, the geloses are found, for example, in the reflexive region of the inner organs, such as over the sacrum in disorders of the pelvic retroperitoneum or in the abdominal wall in the case of abdominal organ diseases.

Note

Geloses should not be confused with lipomas which can be easily and painlessly shifted and are generally bigger than geloses.

Depending on the depth, 0.5 mL of procaine is repeatedly infiltrated with a 2- to 4-cm needle under manual control. The gelosis becomes significantly smaller and ultimately disappears as the symptoms are reduced.

15.8.3 Injection in Muscular Trigger Points and Muscle Insertions

The few-millimeter, small edematous, indurated “triggers” in the muscles are often observed as a response of the sensorimotor system in internal diseases or functional overloading of the musculoskeletal system. In these tight muscles, subtle palpation reveals small areas with strikingly severe pressure pain; the same “maximum points” detectable through palpation can be found in the area of the corresponding muscle origin or root. Here, a 2- to 6-cm needle is used to infiltrate 0.5 mL procaine, resulting in long-lasting normalization of the muscle tone and corresponding reduction in the symptomology.

15.8.4 Infiltration of Trigger Points

A trigger point is a point in any part of the body that is easily located through selective pressure pain. The digital compression of the pressure point strengthens the presence of the symptoms.

A clearly palpable tissue change is not detected. The patient often shows these points to the examiner and reports experiencing temporary relief from the symptoms when a point is lightly massaged. A trigger point is an irritated bundle of nerves in the peripheral somatic nerve systems passing through muscle fascia or subcutaneous fascia. These nerve structures are generally accompanied by an arterial vessel and veins. These trigger points very often correspond to acupuncture points.

Targeted infiltration with a 2- to 4-cm needle using 0.5 mL procaine improves the treated symptomology immediately, whereby the patient reports a feeling of warmth in the area of infiltration. The irritation, and therefore the pressure pain, can be eliminated over the long term or significantly reduced; this also applies to the treated corresponding symptomology. The treatment approach proceeds via the segmental-reflexive pathway with substantial involvement of the vascular sympathetic nervous system progressing along with the spinal nerves.

15.8.5 Infiltration of Scars

Since each scar—via persistent stimulation of the afferent sympathetic nervous system—can potentially represent a general overload of the sympathetic nervous system, up to an interference field function, the infiltration of the scar has major diagnostic and therapeutic significance. This not only refers to cutaneous scars (▶ Fig. 15.2), but also the scars from previously injured or inflamed tissue structures, i.e., scars of the following:

- Subcutis.
- Musculature.
- Nerves.
- Vessels.
- Bones.
- Peritoneum as well as pleura.
- All organs.

Except for the organs that can be reached via the responsible vessels and autonomic ganglia, the scar of the corresponding tissue is infiltrated directly with the 6-cm-long needle. The amount of procaine to be used is highly variable and depends on the extent of the scar. Areal scars after burns or skin grafts often require dilution of procaine to 0.5 or 0.25% with saline or fractional infiltration into two or three sections with breaks of 30 minutes each. Coarse scars can be infiltrated more easily with an unscrewed cannula, e.g., with the carpule syringe.

Infiltration of scar tissue has a twofold effect. With regard to afferent stimulus interruption and the associated interruption of the interference field, the infiltration of a local anesthetic has an effect via the sympathetic nervous system on the entire body or on the interference field–induced illness of the "target organ" via the second phenomenon.

Thus, chronic low back pain or osteoarthritis can become symptom-free through the infiltration of a cutaneous scar from a boil in the neck. The causal component of the scar

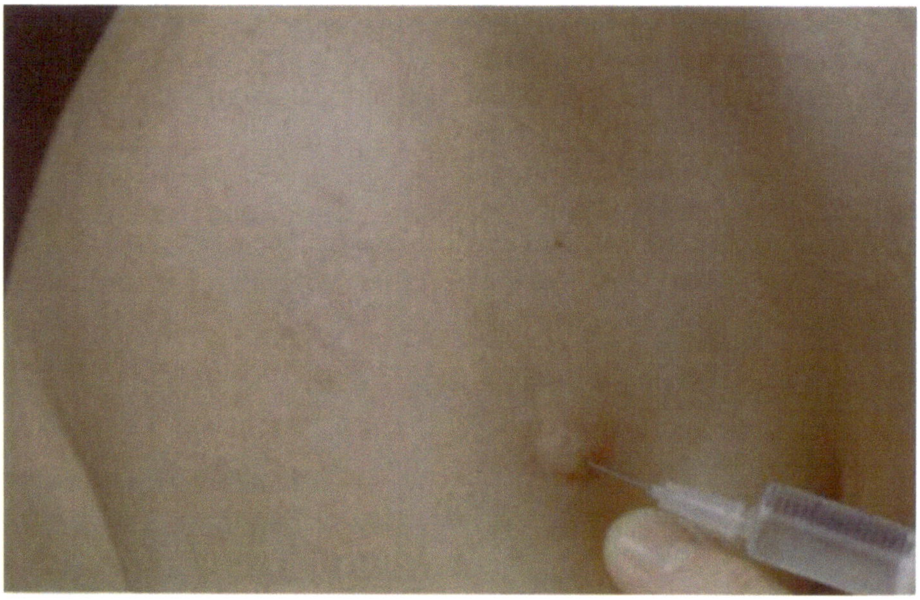

▶ **Fig. 15.2** Intracutaneous and subcutaneous scar infiltration as exemplified by the smallpox vaccination scar.

interference field—the actual stimulus—in the form of a local, nonspecific inflammation progressing without symptoms, initially briefly loses its effect on the sympathetic nervous system from the infiltration of the scar, with the repetition certainly also sustained when the stimulus can be eliminated from the body. Otherwise, the surgical removal of the stimulus through excision of the scar would be considered.

The second effect of scar infiltration relates to the scar itself. Through the medicinal effect of procaine and its degradation products (para-aminobenzoic acid and diethylaminoethanol), there is often a macroscopic change in the scar tissue. Therefore, with repeated scar infiltration, a change in the consistency of the scar can be observed:

- The scar becomes soft.
- Particularly keloidlike changes become normalized.
- Abnormal sensations subside, even from very old scars.
- Paresthesias disappear.

The rough scar strands of the palmar aponeuroses with their mechanical impact on the flexor tendons of the fingers in Dupuytren's contracture are often made significantly softer on palpation with improvement in the stretch function of the fingers involved.

Neural therapeutic infiltration of scar tissue has major significance for diagnostics and therapy. Since every human body has at least one scar—the navel—infiltration of the navel is possible at every age after birth.

Note

The size of the scar is not related to the possible interference field effect. Thus, the lancet stitch scar, often made immediately after birth to obtain a drop of blood, can become an interference field, just like the areal scar after a burn.

Invisible scars, e.g., second degree burns on the hands from early childhood, change their localization through length growth in the proximal direction. The aim is to infiltrate all existing scars in one neural therapy session. This may prove a challenge if there are too many scars or large-area scars. However, infiltration should still be attempted, since an interference field effect can also originate from the sum of all scars or there can be interactions between the scars. Should injecting all scars in one session not be possible, a "fractional" approach should be used.

15.8.6 The Intravenous Injection

One of the standard injections in neural therapy is the intravenous application of1% procaine as a bolus of 1 to 2 mL in the cubital vein. Hahn-Godeffroy has researched the general effects of 1% procaine for many years, collated the range of efficacy for this pharmaceutical, and confirmed and expanded the "endoanesthetic effect" as described by Zipf. Since procaine infusion therapy is being increasingly performed along with neural therapy, the clinically relevant effects of procaine have become clearer. In particular, the stress-equalizing effect through the inhibition of dopamine, serotonin, and norepinephrine reuptake within the central nervous system lead to a psychoanaleptic effect and thus to a better general condition.[194,195] Lidocaine lacks these effects. Via the sympatholytic effect with impaired perfusion and microcirculation, procaine has an anti-inflammatory and thus pain-relieving, spasmolytic, and antihistamine effect. Furthermore, there are attenuating effects on vessel receptors (mechano- and chemoreceptors) as well as on organ receptors (heart, lung, intestine). However, replacing neural therapy with the sole intravenous application of procaine is not allowed.

16 Head

16.1 Injection under the Scalp

16.1.1 Indications

The indications given are only a sample of those possible:
- Skull/brain injury.
- Posttraumatic headache.
- Postapoplectic symptoms.
- Cerebral circulation disorders.
- Vertigo.
- Tinnitus.
- Impaired concentration.
- Postmeningitis and postencephalitic symptoms.
- Cranium as interference field (posttraumatic, post -infec- tious).

The expected success depends, among other things, on the the patient's "interference field situation."

16.1.2 Anatomy and Neurophysiology

The subgaleatic injection reaches the peripheral sensory nervous system (trigeminal nerve, occipital nerves) at the same time as the sympathetic nervous system coursing alongside the vessels and nerves of the brain and spine. Circulation in the scalp is improved through efferent peripheral sympatholysis and intracranial circulation is improved through the afferent reflexive pathway. The arterial anastomoses between the internal and external carotid artery are present over the facial artery, and superficial temporal artery to the ophthalmic artery, and from the occipital artery to the vertebral artery (▶Fig. 16.1). Furthermore, the vascular nerve bundles verified by Heine connect the intracranial and extracranial space transosseously, particularly in the area of the cranial seams, and form the anatomical and neurophysiological substrate of the indication for injection under the scalp.

16.1.3 Injection Technique

An examination must be performed before every new injection treatment (▶Fig. 16.2). It includes:
- Thorough palpation of the skullcap.
- Exploration of painful pressure points and infiltration of these.
- Taking into account scars, attachment points (coup, contrecoup), and personal pressure points.

The injection should be subgaleatic, not subperiosteal.

Note

Be careful with open fontanelles or bone defects (e.g., after skull surgery); aspirate if in doubt!

16.1.4 Material

Required:
- 5-mL syringe.
- 0.4 × 20 mm cannula.
- 1% Procaine, 0.2 to 0.5 mL per injection.

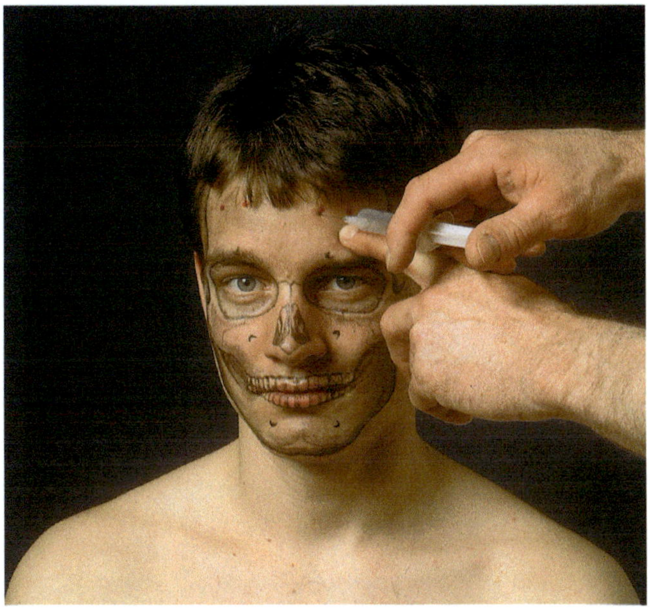

► **Fig. 16.1** Injection under the scalp.

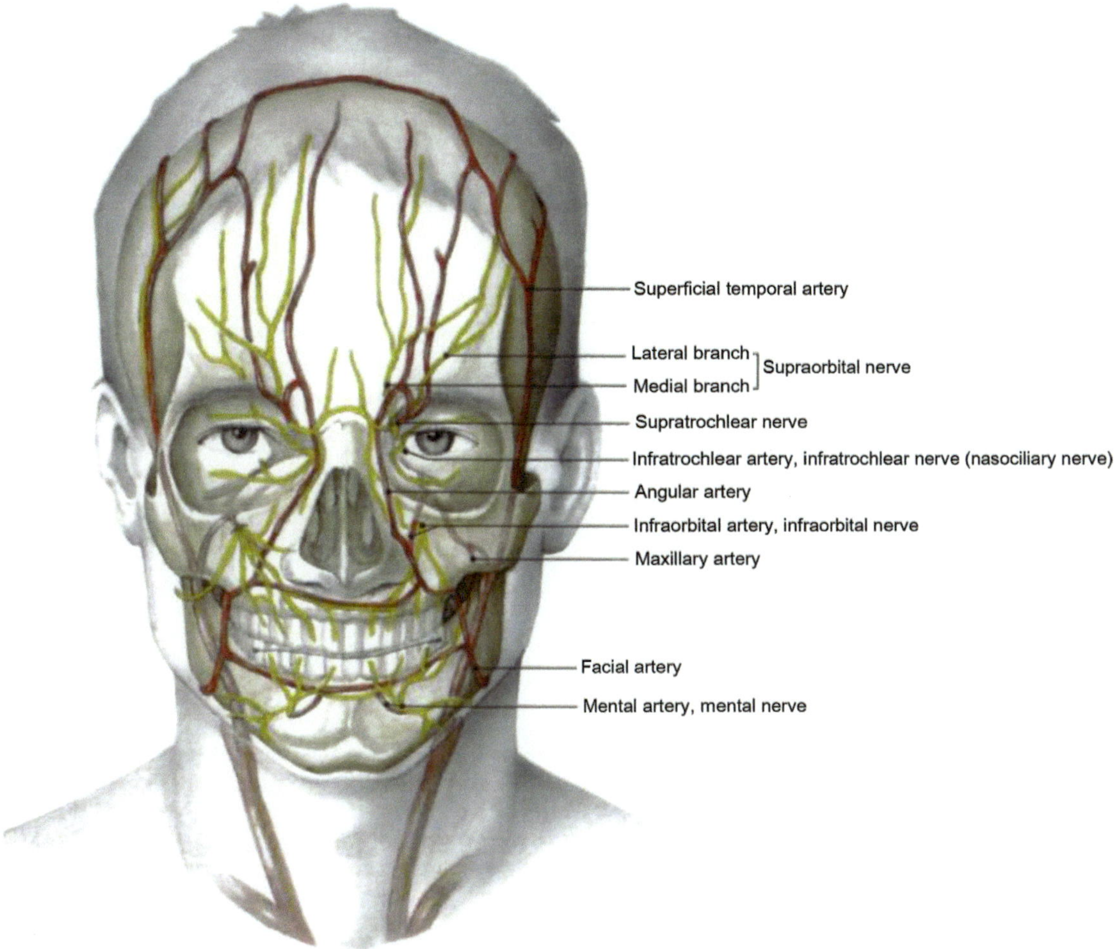

► **Fig. 16.2** Topography of the arterial vessels of the skull, connection between internal and external carotid artery (angular artery).

16.2 Injection to the Branches of the Trigeminal Nerve

16.2.1 Indications

The indications given are only a sample of the possible indications:

- Neuralgias of the three trigeminal branches.
- Facial pain.
- Herpes zoster in the supply area of the trigeminal nerve.
- Forehead, eye, and jaw pain.
- Boils in the supply area of the trigeminal nerve.
- Acne.
- Ozena.
- Anosmia.
- Rhinitis sicca.
- Allergic rhinitis.
- Acute and chronic inflammation of the sinuses.
- Allergic disorders of the sinuses and paranasal sinuses.
- Paranasal sinuses as an interference field.

The expected success depends, among other things, on the the patient's "interference field situation."

16.2.2 Anatomy and Neurophysiology

The injection to the three trigeminal branches—the ophthalmic nerve, the maxillary nerve, and the mandibular nerve—proceeds further peripherally at the level of the nerve exit point of the facial skull (▸Fig. 16.3, ▸Fig. 16.4). The first and second trigeminal branches are purely sensory, and the third branch is sensory and motor (chewing muscles). Important to neural therapy is the parallel coursing of sympathetic nerve fibers for supplying the vessels, the sweat glands, and, in particular, the mucosa of the sinuses, the paranasal sinuses, and mucosal coating of the oral cavity. The peripheral trigeminal branches at the level of the nerve exit points accompany the trigeminal arteries with the afferent and efferent periarterial sympathetic nerve plexus. In addition to the local anesthesia at the trigeminal branch, injection to the nerve exit points also triggers sympatholysis, which leads reflexively in the efferent peripheral direction and the afferent central direction to improve arterial circulation of the corresponding supply areas. This reflexive mechanism represents the actual neural therapeutic effect.

Of significance is the afferent and efferent connection of the nucleic regions of the trigeminal nerve to one of the nucleic regions of the vagus nerve, glossopharyngeal nerve, facial nerve, and the accessory nerve via the reticular formation as well as via the same pathway with the somatosensory and somatomotor systems. This can explain, for example, the muscular tension of the upper cervical spine up to C3 as well as the always-detectable irritation of the major and minor occipital nerves up to neuralgia as a motor-sensory response to a trigeminal stimulus with chronic inflammation of the paranasal sinuses. The distal portion of the trigeminal nucleus extends up to the level of the cervical segment C3 and has a synaptic connection with it.

A further example of the connection of the trigeminal nucleic region with the nucleic regions of the vagus nerve is found in ear-nose-throat medicine as a sub-bronchial syndrome with chronic inflammations of the paranasal sinuses through stimulation of the vagus nucleic region with existing sinusitis, which supplies the bronchial mucosa, among others. The fact that a tooth disease can trigger and maintain chronic sinusitis is demonstrated in the everyday practice of ear-nose-throat medicine, since the teeth and the paranasal sinuses are innervated by the trigeminal nerve. The frequently observed occurrence of diarrhea during the emergence of baby teeth is reflected neurophysiologically in the same neurological relationships.

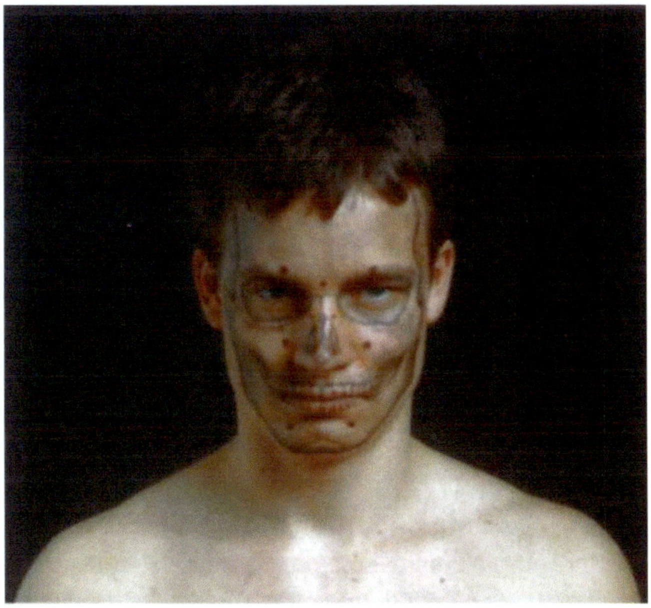

►**Fig. 16.3** Injection to the branches of the trigeminal nerve.

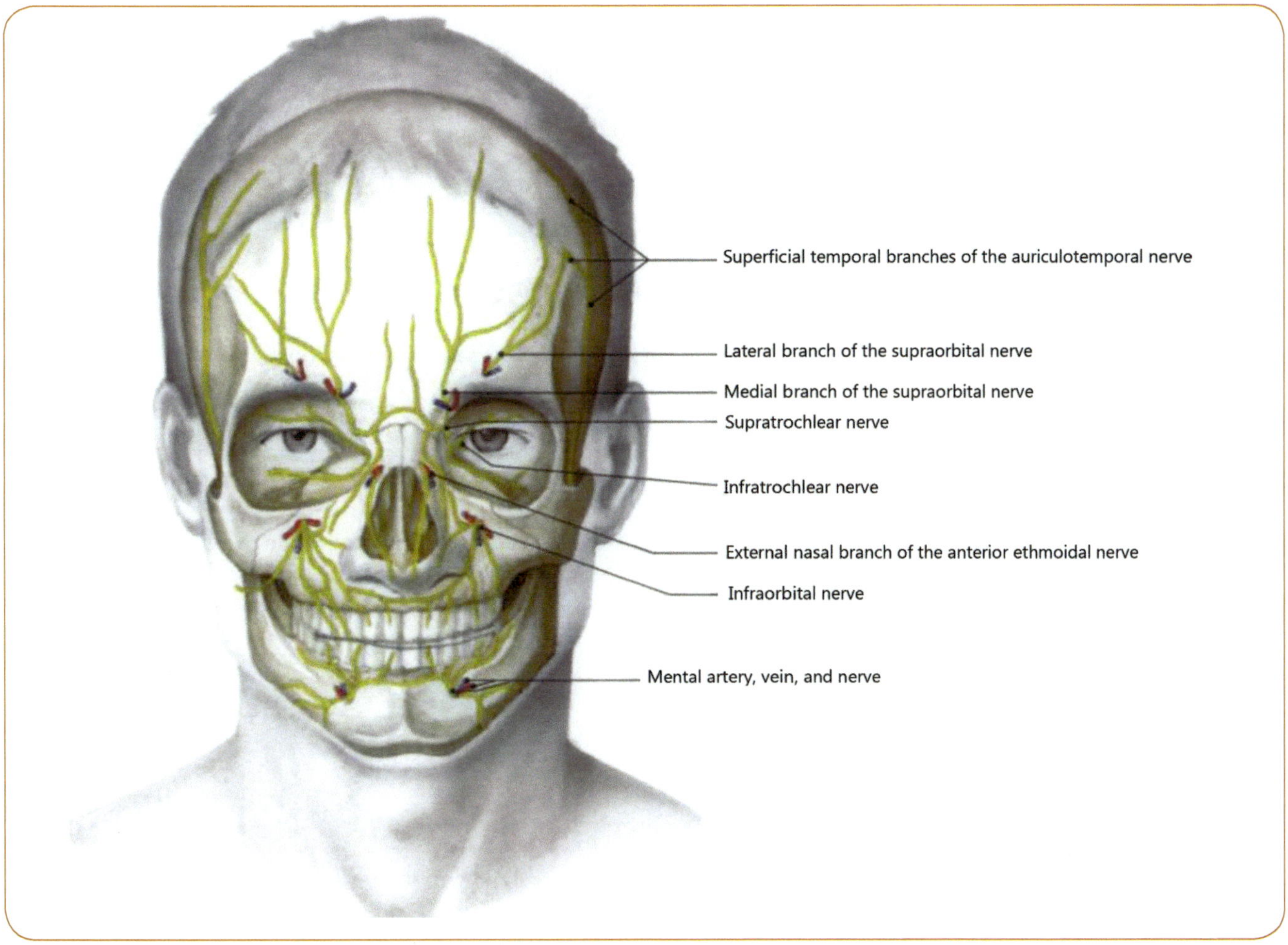

►**Fig. 16.4** Topography for injection to the branches of the trigeminal nerve.

16.2.3 Injection Technique

▶**Supraorbital nerve.** Palpation of the supraorbital foramen somewhat medial from the middle of the upper edge of the orbit, subcutaneous infiltration of 0.5 mL procaine 1% (▶Fig. 16.5a), distribution of the medication through slight finger pressure.

> **Cave**
>
> **Due to the risk of vessel–nerve damage, avoid inserting the needle in the supraorbital foramen.**

▶**Supratrochlear nerve.** At the level of the nasal bridge, subcutaneous infiltration of 0.5 mL procaine 1% (▶Fig. 16.5b), which is distributed right and left with slight finger pressure.

▶**External nasal branch of the nasociliary nerve.** Palpation of the cartilage–bone edge at the level of the proximal half of the nose. Subcutaneous infiltration of 0.5 mL procaine 1% (▶Fig. 16.5c) in the distal quarter of the nasal bone about 1 cm lateral to the center of the nasal bridge.

▶**Infraorbital nerve.** Palpation of the infraorbital foramen about 0.5 to 1 cm below and somewhat medial to the middle of the lower edge of the orbit. Subcutaneous infiltration of 0.5 mL procaine 1% (▶Fig. 16.5d), distribution of the medication through slight finger pressure.

A second option is the enoral injection (▶Fig. 16.5e):

- Raising the upper lip.
- Injection at the level of the vestibular fold between the third and fourth upper teeth.
- Insertion of the 20-gauge needle by 1.5 to 2 cm in the direction of the lower edge of the orbit.
- Submucosal infiltration of 0.5 to 1 mL procaine 1%.

To avoid vessel–nerve damage, the infraorbital foramen should not be penetrated.

▶**Mental nerve.** Palpation of the mental foramen in the center of the lower jaw branch at the level of the third to fourth lower tooth. Subcutaneous infiltration of 0.5-mL procaine 1% (▶Fig. 16.5f) in the nerve exit point.

16.2.4 Complications

Hematoma formation from vessel injury can be avoided through digital compression. Puncture of a nerve causes lightening sharp pain. In this case, the needle should be pulled back about 1 mm before the injection.

16.2.5 Material

Required:

- 5-mL syringe.
- 20-gauge needle.
- Procaine 1%, 0.5 to 1 mL per injection.

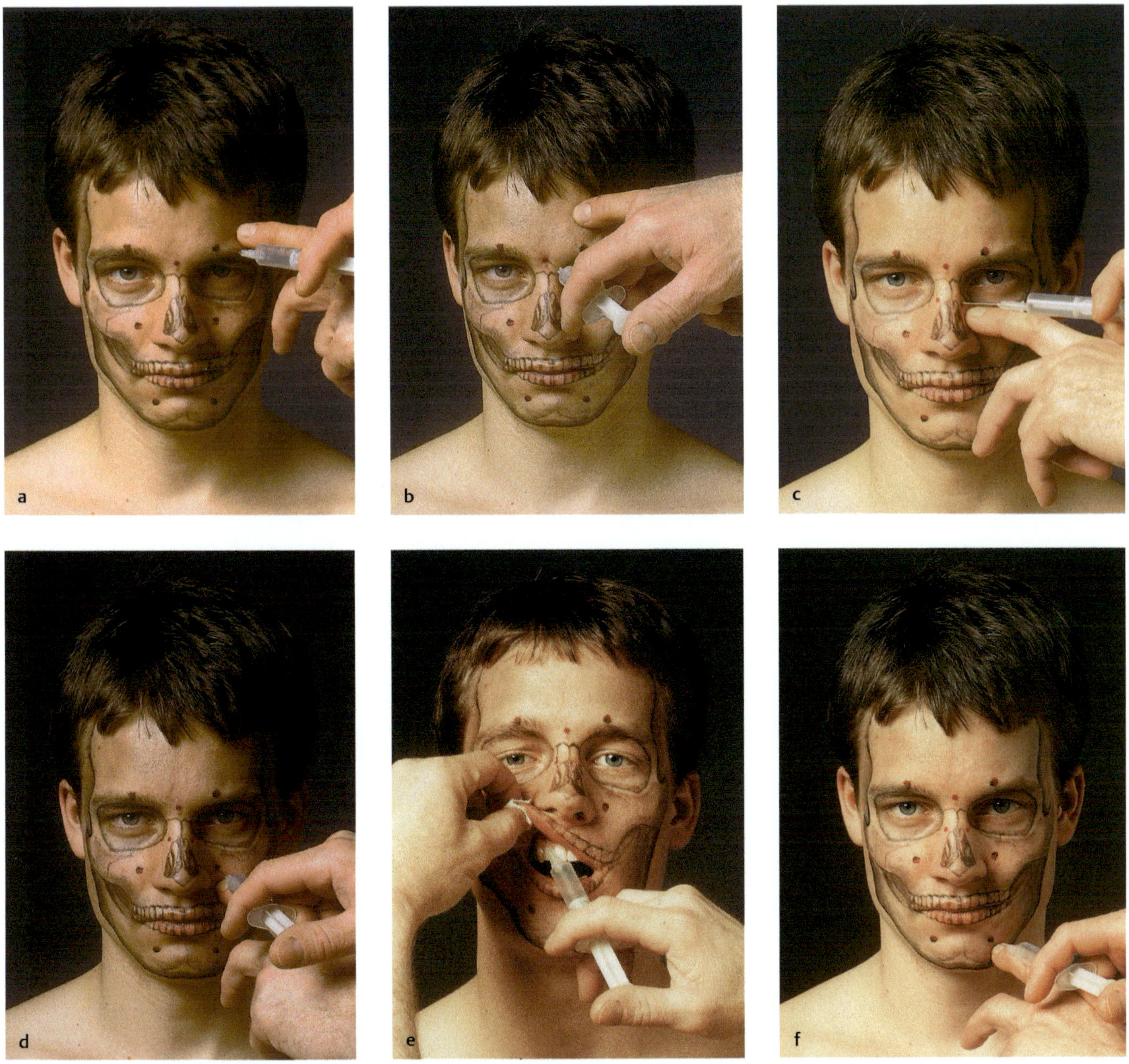

► **Fig. 16.5** **(a)** Injection to the supraorbital nerve. **(b)** Injection to the supratrochlear nerve. **(c)** Injection to the external branch of the nasociliary nerve. **(d)** Injection to the infraorbital nerve, outer version. **(e)** Injection to the infraorbital nerve, enoral version. **(f)** Injection to the mental nerve.

16.3 Injection to the Mastoid

16.3.1 Indications

The indications given are only a sample of those possible:
- Otitis media (acute and chronic).
- Otogenic dizziness.
- Tinnitus.
- Hypoacusis and hyperacusis.
- “Travel sickness”.
- Otitis externa.
- Inner ear as interference field.

The expected success depends, among other things, on the the patient’s “interference field situation.”

16.3.2 Anatomy and Neurophysiology

Sympatholysis of the periarterial nerve plexus of the mastoid branch of the occipital artery from the external carotid artery leads to improved blood circulation in the supply area of the mastoid cells through the efferent pathway and the reflexive afferent pathway. The mastoid occipital artery branch emerging through the mastoid foramen supplies the diploid and dura mater. The auricular artery, which branches off from the external carotid artery at the level of the mastoid peak, and which proceeds along the styloid process between the mastoid process and the ear, supplies the middle and inner ear, the eardrum, the stapedius muscle, the auricle, and the ear muscles. The corresponding perivascular sympathetic plexus is the anatomical structure through which the circulation of the outer and inner ear can be improved.[69]

It is **important** to note that the outer ear, including the eardrum, is supplied by numerous nerves:
- Sympathetic nervous system (perivascular plexus, cranial nerves, spinal nerve portion).
- Vagus nerve.
- Trigeminal nerve.
- Intermediate branch of the facial nerve.
- Glossopharyngeal nerve.
- Great auricular nerve.

The capillary sealing effect of procaine leads to improved regional lymph drainage and thereby supports improved microcirculation.

16.3.3 Injection Technique

Palpation of the mastoid process 1 cm cranial to the mastoid peak; the 20-gauge needle is used to subcutaneously infiltrate 0.5 to 1 mL procaine 1% each into the mastoid anterior edge, which is the entry point of the posterior auricular artery, and the mastoid posterior edge, which is the entry point of the mastoid branch of the occipital artery (► Fig. 16.6, ► Fig. 16.7). Scars of the auricle and the mastoid should also be infiltrated along with this.

16.3.4 Material

Required:
- 5-mL syringe.
- 20-gauge needle.
- Procaine 1%, 0.5 to 1 mL per injection.

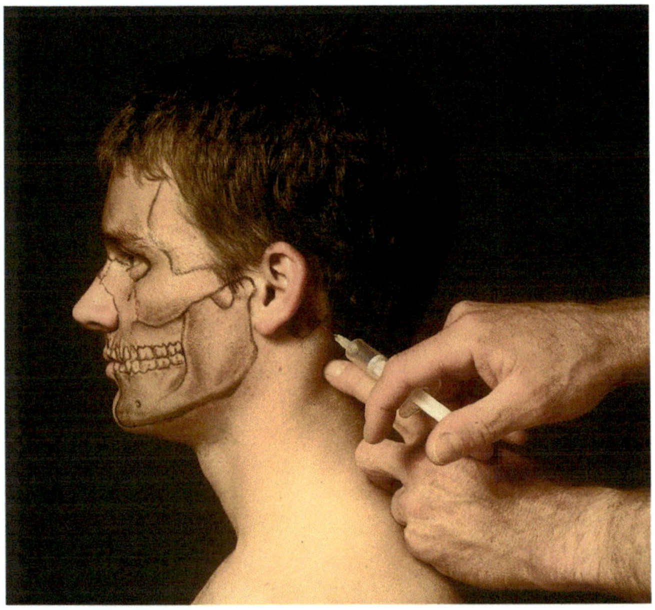

►**Fig. 16.6** Injection to the mastoid.

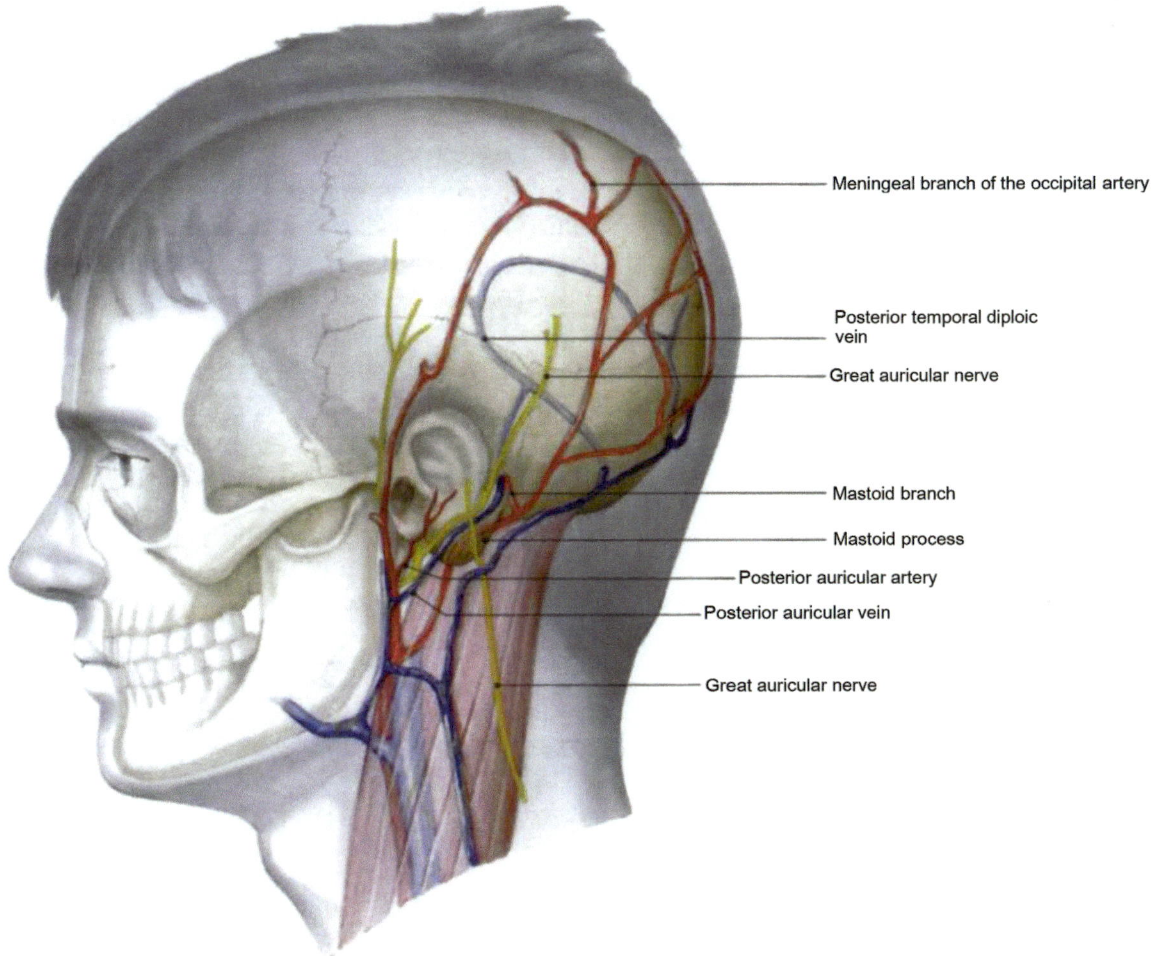

►**Fig. 16.7** Topography for injection to the mastoid.

16.4 Injection to the Facial Artery, Superficial Temporal Artery, and Auriculotemporal Nerve (from the Mandibular Nerve/ Trigeminal Nerve)

16.4.1 Indications

The indications given are only a sample of those possible:

- Temporal arteritis.
- Diffuse facial-head pain in the supply area of the superficial temporal artery and the facial artery.
- Herpes zoster.
- Migraine.
- Cerebral circulation disorders.
- Postapoplectic symptoms.
- Neuralgia of the auriculotemporal nerve.

The expected success depends, among other things, on the patient's "interference field situation."

16.4.2 Anatomy and Neurophysiology

The area to be reached is the sympathetic perivascular nerve plexus, which not only is responsible for vascular function, but also provides efferent and afferent support of the sympathetic nervous system supply to the bones, the periosteum, the muscles, the adenoids, the skin, and skin appendages. Through dilation of the supplying vessels, sympatholysis causes improved circulation with consecutive improvement in the tissue trophics. Since afferent conducting sympathetic pain fibers progress along with the arteries, the perivascular infiltration of procaine can interrupt this pain-conducting afferent effect.

16.4.3 Injection Technique

▶**Superficial temporal artery.** Palpation of the artery at the zygomatic arch near the ear. Subcutaneous perivascular infiltration of 1 mL procaine 1% (▶Fig. 16.8, ▶Fig. 16.9).

Note

Aspirate before the injection!

▶**Facial artery**. Palpation of the artery at the lower jaw branch about 1 cm before the parotid gland. Perivascular infiltration of 1 mL procaine 1%.

▶**Auriculotemporal nerve**. Palpation of the superficial temporal artery at the zygomatic arch near the ear. The auriculotemporal nerve proceeds directly behind the superficial temporal artery (▶Fig. 16.8, ▶Fig. 16.9). The injection made dorsal to the palpable artery at about 0.5 to 1 cm depth, infiltration of 1 mL procaine 1%. The periarterial infiltration should be done before the intra-arterial, since the essential portion of the accompanying sympathetic plexus proceeds perivascular.

In normal anatomical conditions, the arterial blood flow—dependent on a low pressure gradient of the external carotid system—is always directed toward the external carotid system, compared to the internal carotid system via the ana stomoses in the region of the angular artery / ophthalmic artery. With deep occlusions of the internal carotid system, however, flow reversal can occur, so that the intra-arterial injection in the temporal superficial artery becomes an injection in a vessel pulling toward the direction of the brain, which should be avoided in all cases.

16.4.4 Material

Required:

- 5-mL syringe.
- 20-gauge needle.
- Procaine 1%, 1 mL per injection.

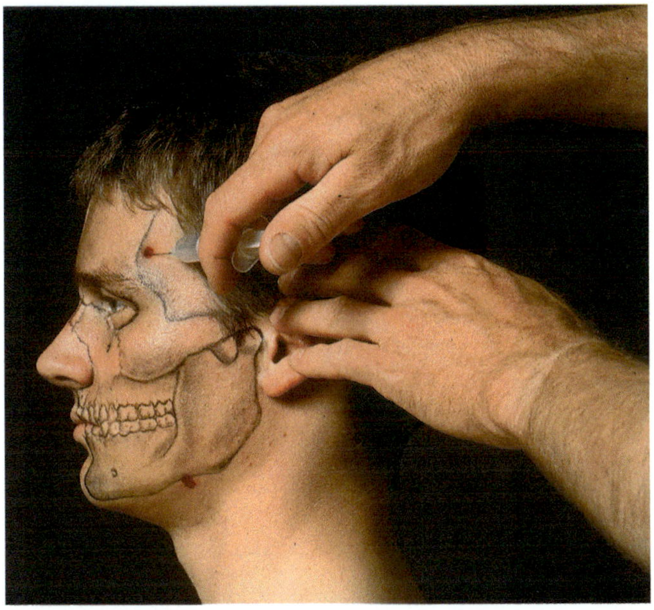

▶ **Fig. 16.8** Injection to the frontal branch of the superficial temporal artery, the facial artery, and the auriculotemporal artery.

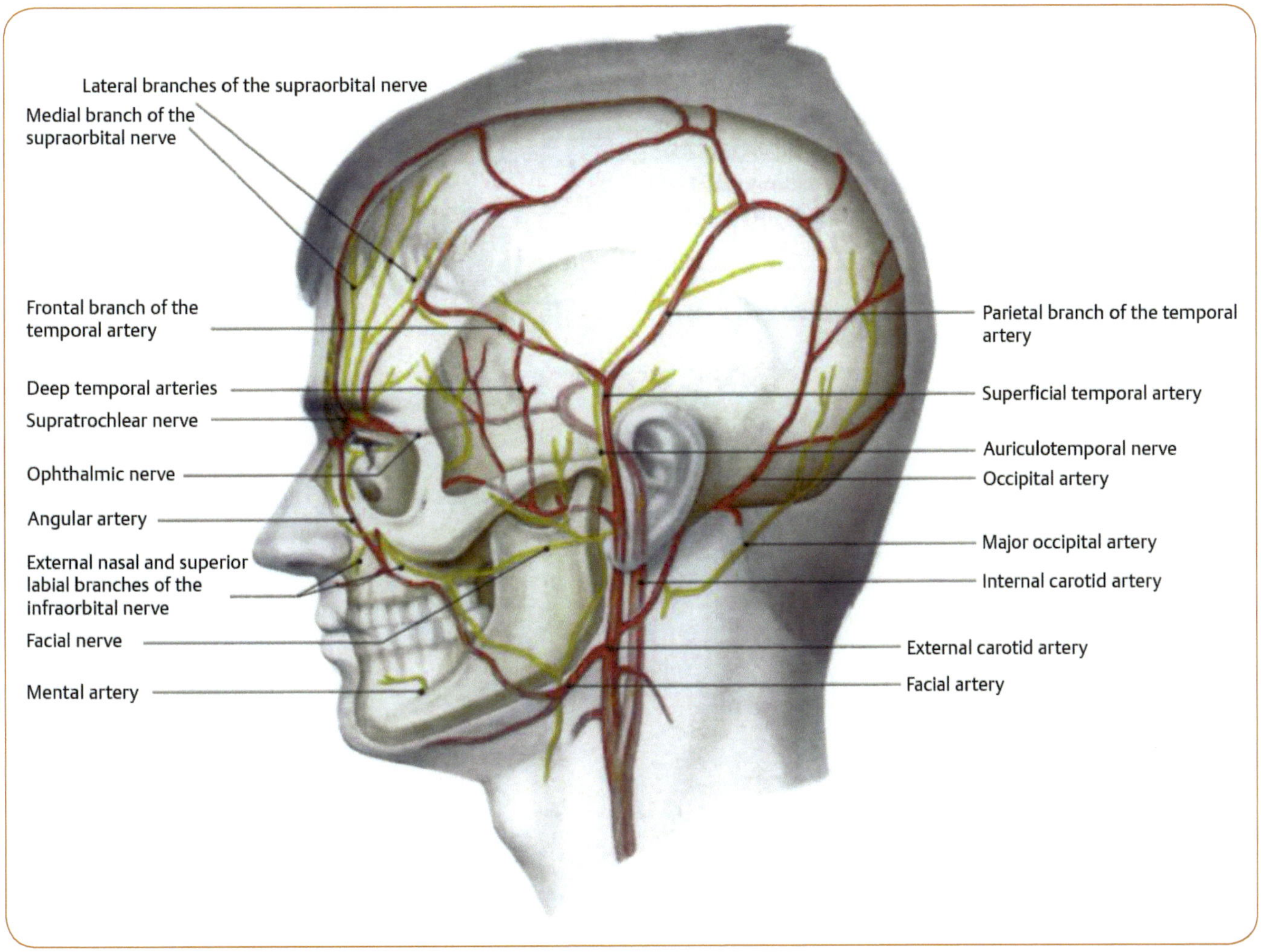

▶ **Fig. 16.9** Topography of the outer arterial and neural supply to the head.

16.5 Injection at and in the Parotid Gland

16.5.1 Indications

The indications given are only a sample of those possible:

- Epidemic parotitis.
- Unspecific parotitis.
- Parotid hyperplasia.
- Unexplained pain in the parotid region.
- Sialadenitis and sialolithiasis research.
- Sialorrhea.
- Sialosis.
- Parotid as interference field (e.g., after mumps).

The expected success depends, among other things, on the patient's particular "interference field situation."

16.5.2 Anatomy and Neurophysiology

The parotid gland is found above the angle of the jaw, encompassing it superficially, and halfway overlaying the masseter muscle. The arterial supply and thus sympathetic innervation proceed via the side branches of the superficial temporal artery. The gland function itself is controlled by the parasympathetic nervous system. The preganglionic fibers emerge from the medulla oblongata, coming from the inferior salivatory nucleus with the glossopharyngeal nerve. With the minor petrosal nerve, the parasympathetic fibers travel toward the otic ganglion, are switched there to the second neuron, and thereby travel toward the parotid gland with the auriculotemporal nerve. By interrupting the sympathetic efferent fibers, infiltration of the parotid gland with procaine 1% leads to vasodilation with reactive improvement in circulation of the glandular tissue and, at the same time, leads to interruption of the afferent sympathetic pain conduction. Interrupting the parasympathetic efferent fibers leads to reduced production of secretion as well as a reduction in inflammation, swelling, and pain in the glandular tissue through localized action of the local anesthetic in accordance with membrane stabilization and an increase in microcirculation, which is dependent on the sympathetic nervous system.

16.5.3 Injection Technique

Palpation of the parotid gland on the mandibular branch; 1 to 2 mL procaine 1% is infiltrated at 1 cm depth 2 cm in the facial direction from the jaw angle and 2 cm in the cranial direction from the mandible (► Fig. 16.10, ► Fig. 16.11).

16.5.4 Material

Required:

- 5-mL syringe.
- 20-gauge needle.
- Procaine 1%, 1 to 2 mL per injection.

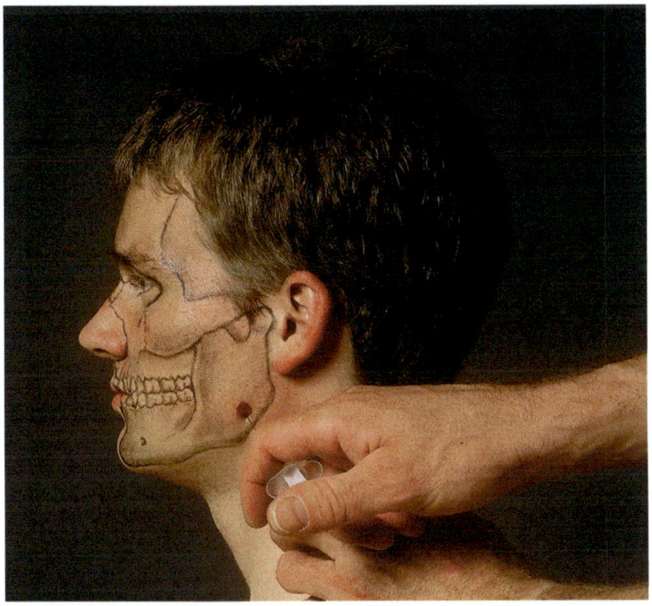

►**Fig. 16.10** Injection in the parotid gland.

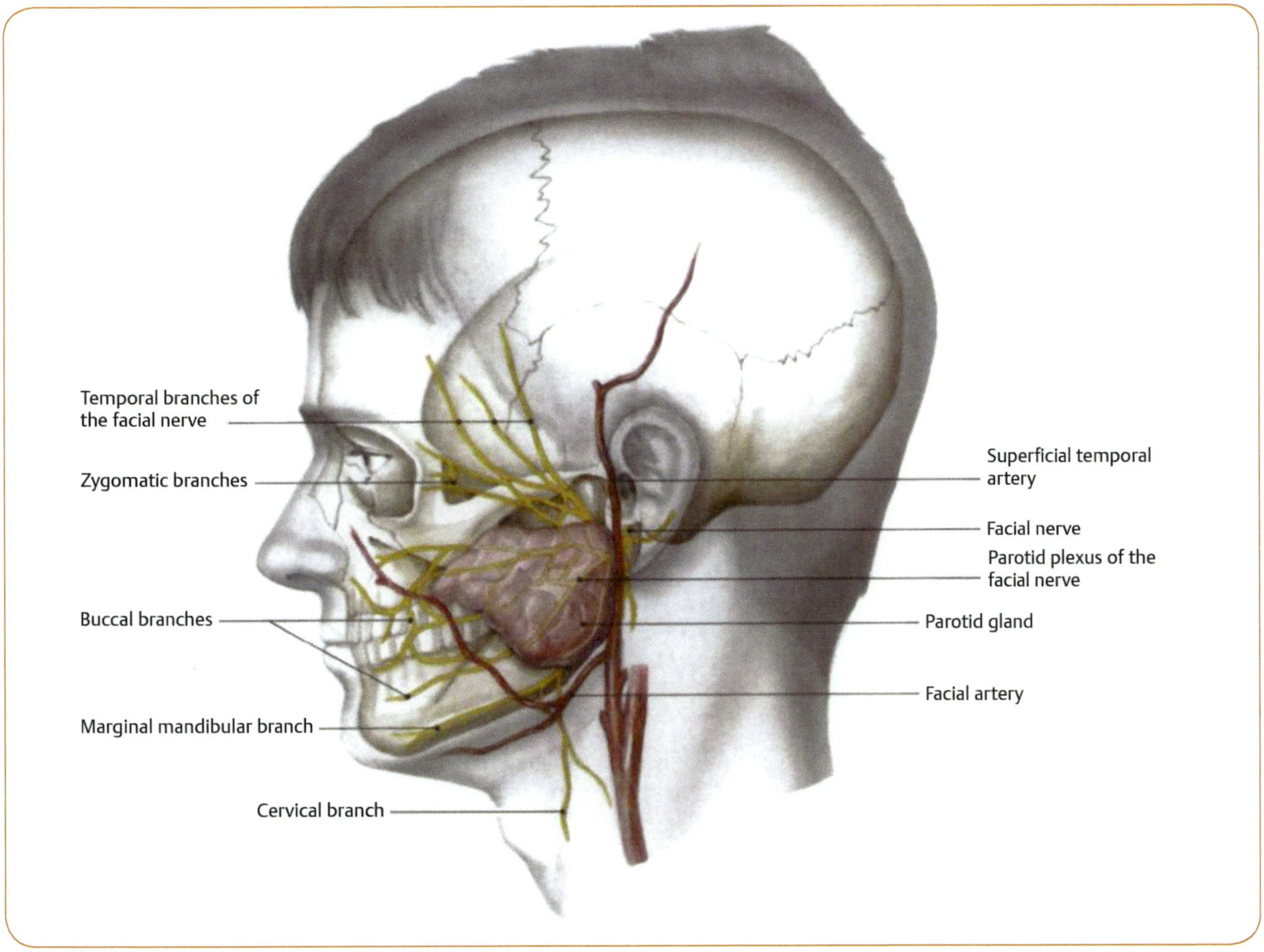

►**Fig. 16.11** Topography for injection in the parotid gland.

16.6 Injection at the Jaw Joint

16.6.1 Indications

The indications given are only a sample of those possible:

- Degenerative diseases of the jaw joint.
- Posttraumatic symptoms after luxation or fracture of the condyloid process.
- Unexplained symptoms in the area of the ear and the auriculotemporal nerve.
- Jaw joint as interference field.

The expected success depends, among other things, on the patient's particular "interference field situation."

16.6.2 Anatomy and Neurophysiology

The jaw joint is a sliding joint with an articulated disk that divides the joint into two chambers, and a ligament structure that enables sliding in the anterior–posterior direction as well as laterally. The vascular supply occurs via the temporal superficial artery and the sensory innervation of the capsule and the joint occurs via the auriculotemporal nerve from the third trigeminal branch. Both the supplying artery and the supplying branch of the trigeminal nerve conduct afferent and efferent sympathetic fibers which represent the anatomical substrate to be reached by the infiltration. The fine tuning of the jaw movements is controlled by the trigeminal nerve whose third branch innervates the masticatory muscles simultaneously. Inflammatory or physical disorders of the tooth–jaw area (teeth, paranasal sinuses) can certainly take effect at the jaw joint solely at the nerve level of the trigeminal nerve, but also via the portions of the sympathetic nervous system progressing with the trigeminal and arterial vessels, so that a "segmental disorder" as well as an "interference field disorder" of the jaw is possible via the sympathetic nervous system.

16.6.3 Injection Technique

Palpation of the jaw joint before the ear and below the cheek bone. The movement of the lower jaw shows the glide path and thus the size of the jaw joint. Puncture directly at the level of the mandible neck. At 1 to 1.5 cm depth, 1 to 2 mL procaine 1% is infiltrated ventrally and dorsally around the jaw joint (▶ Fig. 16.12). Due to the vascular nerve supply of the joint sections, periarticular injection is more effective than intra-articular injection (▶ Fig. 16.13).

16.6.4 Material

Required:

- 5-mL syringe.
- 20-gauge needle.
- Procaine 1%, 1 to 2 mL per injection.

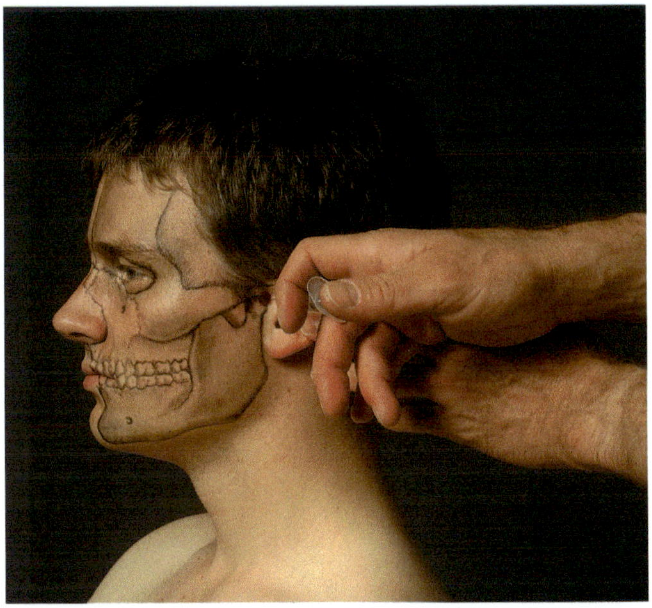

► **Fig. 16.12** Injection to the jaw joint.

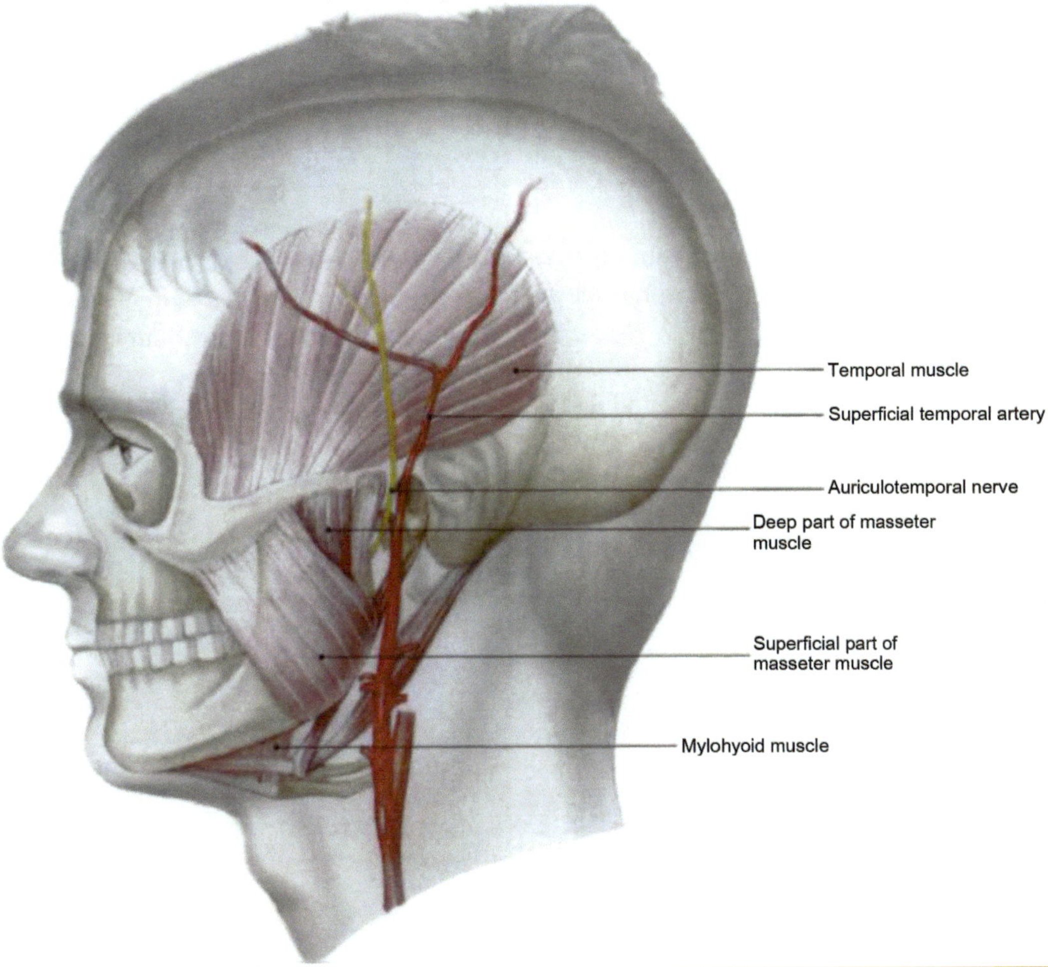

► **Fig. 16.13** Topography for injection to the jaw joint.

16.7 Injection to the Ciliary Ganglion (Retrobulbar Injection)

16.7.1 Indications

The indications given are only a sample of those possible:

- Chronic and acute glaucoma.
- Macular degeneration (moist, dry).
- All forms of inflammation of the eye, the eye vessels, and nerves supplying the eye.
- Eye injuries without indication for surgery.
- Posttraumatic eye symptoms (also surgery-related).
- The eye as an interference field.

The expected success depends, among other things, on the patient's paticular "interference field situation."

16.7.2 Anatomy and Neurophysiology

The ciliary ganglion, which is about 2 mm large, is positioned at the transition from the middle to the posterior third of the orbit (▶Fig. 16.14, ▶Fig. 16.15) between the lateral side of the optical fasciculus and the lateral rectus muscle. The ciliary ganglion consists of:

- A sensory portion from the nasociliary nerve (first trigeminal branch) for supply of the choroid, iris, ciliary body, sclera and cornea.
- A parasympathetic portion which enters the orbit with the oculomotor nerve and supplies the sphincter muscle of the pupil as well as the ciliary muscle.
- A sympathetic portion which enters the orbit with the ophthalmic artery and supplies the eye vessels and the dilator muscle of the pupil, the tarsal muscle, and the orbital muscle.

An additional nerve branch (orbital branch) from the pterygopalatine ganglion generates sensory fibers to the eye from the second trigeminal branch as well as sympathetic and parasympathetic fibers which partially supply the mucosa of the posterior ethmoid cells and sphenoid sinus.

Basically, the sympathetic portion is responsible for the nutrition of the eye, in such a way that the increased stimulus of the sympathetic nervous system triggers vascular constriction and thus poorer trophism of the eye, while decreased stimulus triggers improved trophism. Injection to the ciliary ganglion (retrobulbar injection) means:

- A pain-free eye.
- Increased muscle function of the pupil sphincter muscle and ciliary muscle.
- Increased muscle function of the pupil dilator muscle, tarsal muscle, and orbital muscle.

This causes the pupil to occupy a central position and, above all through vasodilation of the arteries, results in improved eye circulation and thus improved tissue trophism. In contrast to the selective suppression of the sympathetic nervous system via injection to the stellate ganglion, which triggers a temporary increase in the inner eye pressure (according to Monnier), the simultaneous suppression of parasympathetic and sympathetic nerves through injection to the ciliary ganglion causes significant reduction in the inner eye pressure after 20 to 30 minutes, probably through improved aqueous outflow and/or lower aqueous humor production at the same time. In surgical ophthalmology, this effect is called "soft eye" and is used in the operation technique.

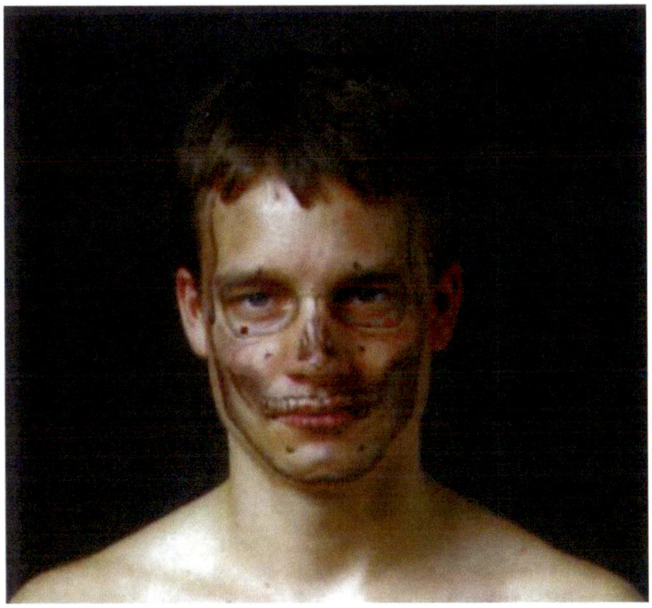

►**Fig. 16.14** Puncture points (red) for injection to the ciliary ganglion.

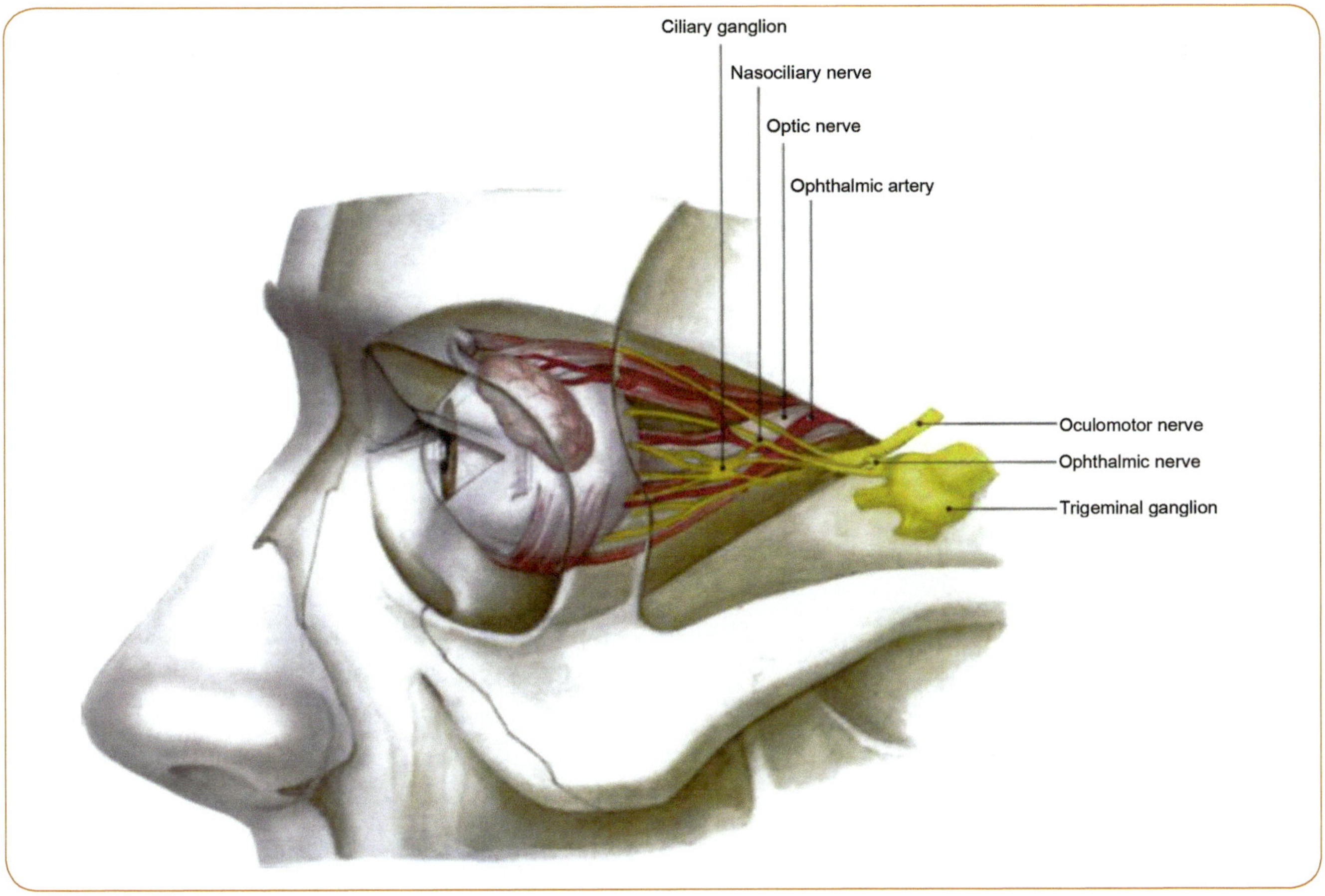

►**Fig. 16.15** Topography of the eye socket and the ciliary ganglion.

16.7.3 Injection Technique

With the head stabilized—better in the prone position than sitting position—the lower edge of the orbit is palpated. The 4 cm long and 0.4 mm thick needle is inserted on the right at 7 o'clock position and on the left at 5 o'clock position (▶ Fig. 16.16). The eye should be looking up and in the opposite direction; with a free finger, the bulb can be lightly pushed away in the craniomedial direction. The direction of the needle puncture is first slightly oriented toward the orbital floor (2–3°) under the bulb (▶ Fig. 16.17). In case of contact with bone, lightly pull back the needle and simultaneously raise the needle tip from the orbital floor to push forward only a maximum of 1 cm (no further). After aspiration, slowly infiltrate 2 to 3 mL procaine 1%. This prevents injury to the bulb. After injection, the medication can be distributed through light massaging/ pumping pressure around the closed eye.

16.7.4 Complications

A lower lid hematoma and retrobulbar hematoma with exophthalmos can be prevented with 3 to 5 minutes of light compression.

16.7.5 Material

Required:

- 5-mL syringe.
- 4 cm long needle (0.4 × 40 mm).
- Procaine 1%, 2 to 3 mL per injection.

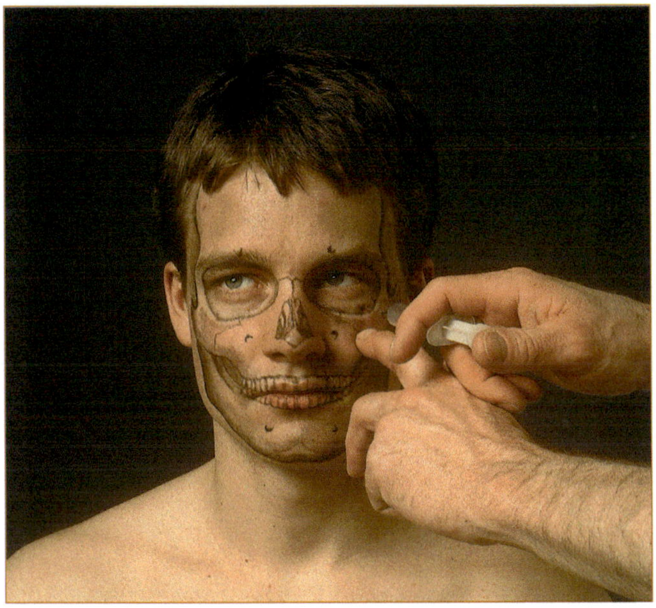

▶ **Fig. 16.16** Injection to the ciliary ganglion.

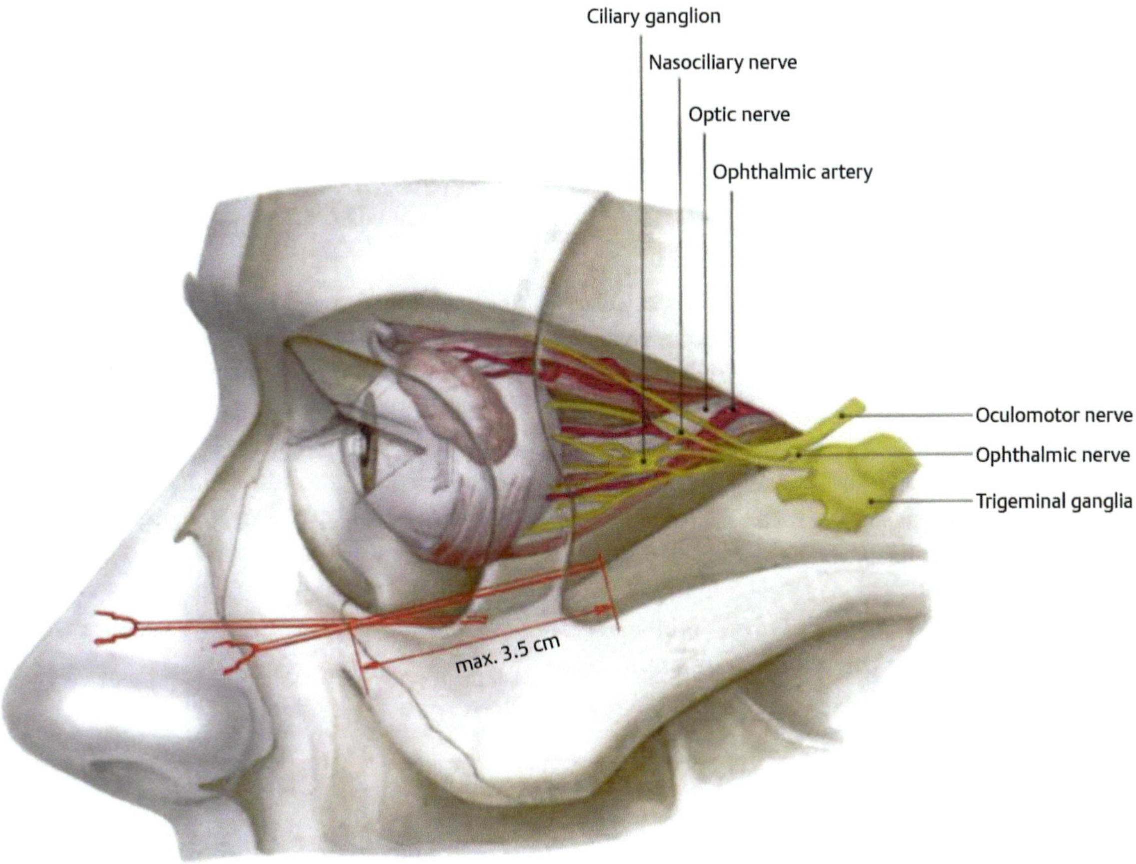

▶ **Fig. 16.17** Topography of the orbit and the needle position.

16.8 Injection to the Pterygopalatine Ganglion, the Maxillary Nerve, and Maxillary Artery

16.8.1 Indications

The indications given are only a sample of those possible:

- Acute and chronic sinusitis.
- Cluster headache (neuralgia of the pterygopalatine ganglion).
- Neuralgia of the maxillary nerve.
- Vasomotor rhinitis.
- Anosmia.
- Ozena research.
- Rhinitis sicca.
- Nasal obstruction after tumor exclusion.
- Unexplained pain in the supply region of the maxillary nerve (nose, maxillary sinus, hard palate, upper jaw).
- Hay fever.
- Allergic diathesis.
- Nonspecific inflammatory eye disorders.
- Degenerative/inflammatory brain disorders.
- Paranasal sinuses as an interference field.

The expected success depends, among other things, on the patient's particular "interference field situation."

16.8.2 Anatomy and Neurophysiology

▶**Pterygopalatine ganglion.** The parasympathetic pterygopalatine ganglion is in the pterygopalatine pit, somewhat underneath the maxillary nerve (second trigeminal branch; ▶Fig. 16.18, ▶Fig. 16.19). Four neurological components can be differentiated:

- Sensory branch; consists of the pterygopalatine nerves.
- Parasympathetic portion from the major petrosal nerve; the root cells are in the parasympathetic upper salivary nucleus.
- Sympathetic portion from the deep petrosal nerve; the fibers come from the internal carotid plexus parasympathetic neurons (vasodilators) of the cerebral vessels.[491,490,506,558]

The sensory and sympathetic portions pass through the pterygopalatine ganglion; the parasympathetic portion is switched to the second neuron. The nerve branches emerging from the pterygopalatine ganglion supply the nose, gum, and sinus regions. This way, each nerve branch contains a sensory portion from the second trigeminal branch and a parasympathetic as well as sympathetic portion. These nerve branches supply the nasal mucosa including the nasal septum, the mucosa of the hard and soft palate, the maxillary sinuses, the posterior portion of the ethmoid cells, and sphenoid sinuses.

Zhu et al described parasympathetic fibers exiting from the pterygopalatine ganglion as vasodilators of cerebral vessels in rabbits.[558] When the same parasympathetic vasomotors are also present in humans, injection to this ganglion would be relevant from a neural therapeutic perspective with regard to modulation of cerebral circulation. Interruption of the trigeminal nerve alone will not bring about complete freedom from pain, since part of the sensory fibers proceeds via the pterygopalatine ganglion and the arterial vessels.

▶**Maxillary nerve.** The maxillary nerve is divided into three branches:

- Pterygopalatine nerves, which flow to the pterygopalatine ganglion.
- The infraorbital nerve, which supplies the teeth of the upper jaw, parts of the tooth mucosa, the maxillary sinuses as well as the skin of the lower lid, the corner of the eye, the nostril, and the skin and mucous membranes up to the respective corner of the mouth.
- The zygomatic nerve, which supplies the skin over the cheekbone, the lateral forehead, and the anterior temporal area.

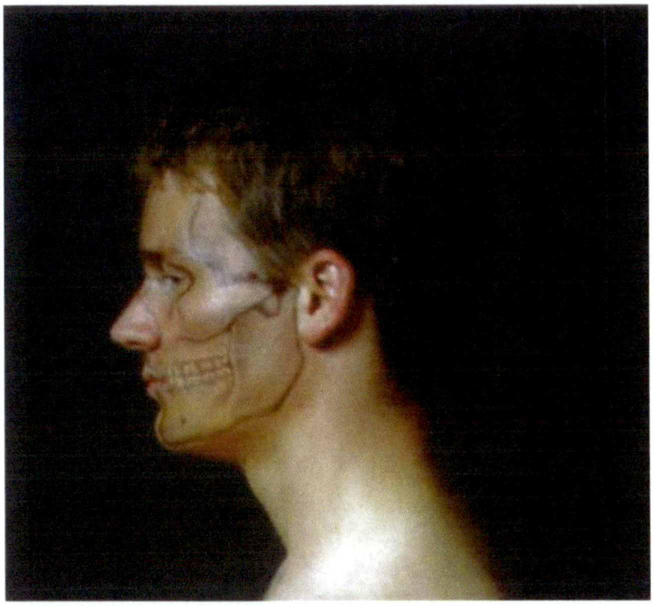

► **Fig. 16.18** Puncture point for injection to the pterygopalatine ganglion.

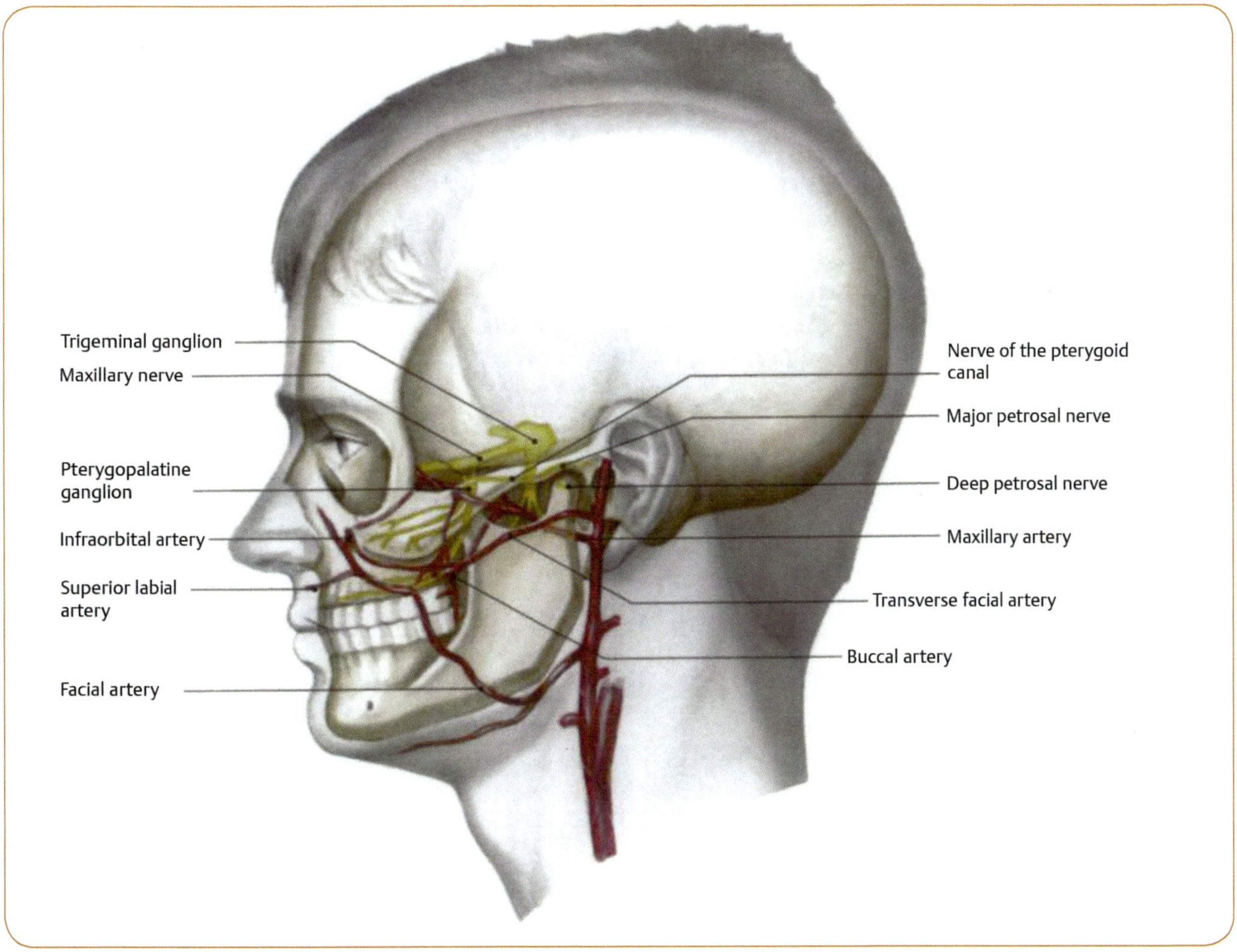

► **Fig. 16.19** Topography for injection to the pterygopalatine ganglion.

▸**Maxillary artery.** The maxillary artery appears as a stronger terminal branch of the external carotid artery behind the mandible and through the jaw muscles into the infratemporal fossa. The maxillary artery supplies the jaw joint, the outer ear canal, and the mucous membrane of the tympanic cavity up to the eardrum, the teeth, the periodontal apparatus from the upper and lower jaw, the tympanic cavity, the orbit, the anterior and middle cranial fossa, and the trigeminal ganglion.

Injection to the maxillary nerve, the pterygopalatine ganglion, and the maxillary artery results in sensitivity failure in the indicated skin and mucus membrane area and improved circulation in the indicated supply area of the artery through suppression of the sympathetic fibers.

16.8.3 Injection Technique

Palpation of the cheekbone. The puncture is made with the 4 cm long, 0.4 mm gauge needle at the upper edge of the cheekbone center (▸Fig. 16.20, ▸Fig. 16.21). The 4-cm needle is advantageous because the risk of injury to the maxillary artery is lower. For this reason, the required injection quantity of the local anesthetic is larger in order to reach the pterygopalatine ganglion, the maxillary nerve, and maxillary artery. After placement of a wheal, the full length of the needle is slowly pushed forward and down in the direction of the seventh to eighth tooth of the opposite side of the upper jaw. Depending on the size of the skull, the pterygopalatine fossa and the pterygopalatine ganglion are at a depth of 4.5 to 5.5 cm. After two-time aspiration with 180° rotation of the needle, 3 mL procaine is infiltrated slowly.

Cave

If shooting pain occurs in the upper jaw or nostril before injection, the maxillary nerve has become irritated. If blood appears during aspiration, it originates from the pterygoid venous plexus or the maxillary artery. In this case, the needle should be pulled back by 1 mm before injection.

16.8.4 Complications

A hematoma can be caused by injury to the pterygoid venous plexus or the maxillary artery. The expansion of the hematoma can be curbed by digital compression of the mouth by placing one finger between the upper jaw and cheekbone at the level of the wisdom tooth. The unpleasant feeling of pressure, particularly when chewing and speaking, subsides after repeated immediate injection of 2 to 3 mL procaine in accordance with the above technique, whereby this time the needle is only pushed forward about 3.5 cm.

16.8.5 Material

Required:

- 5-mL syringe.
- 4 cm long needle, 0.4 × 40 mm.
- Procaine 1%, 3 mL per injection.

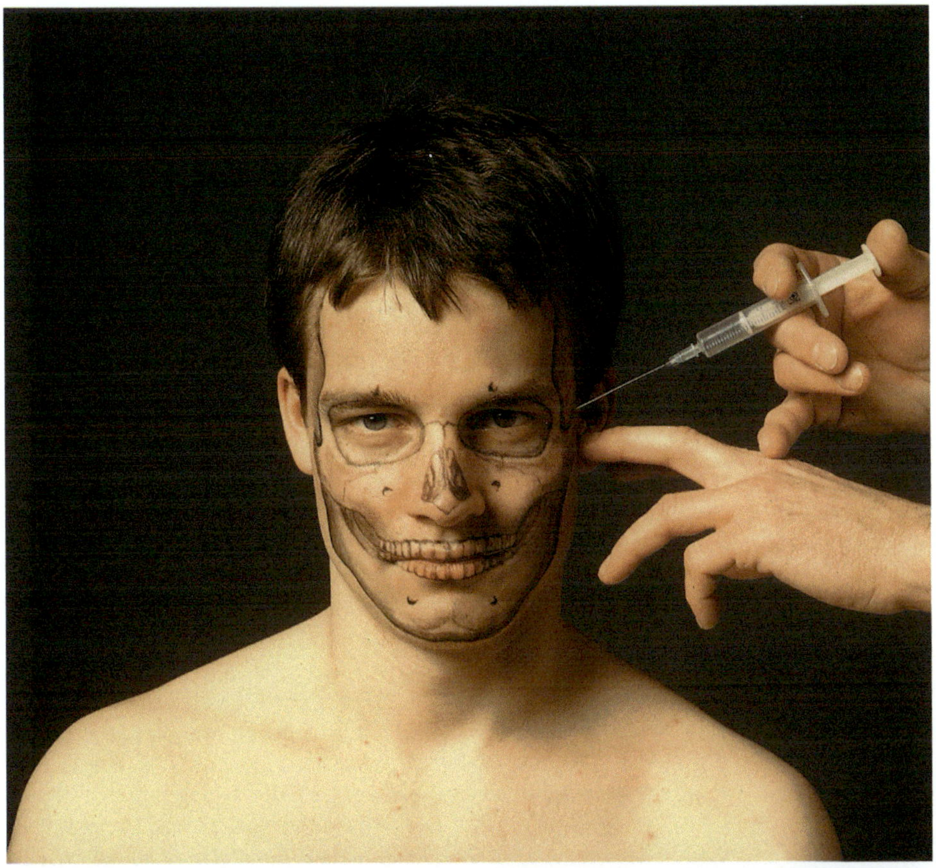

▸ **Fig. 16.20** Puncture direction to the pterygopalatine ganglion, ventral view.

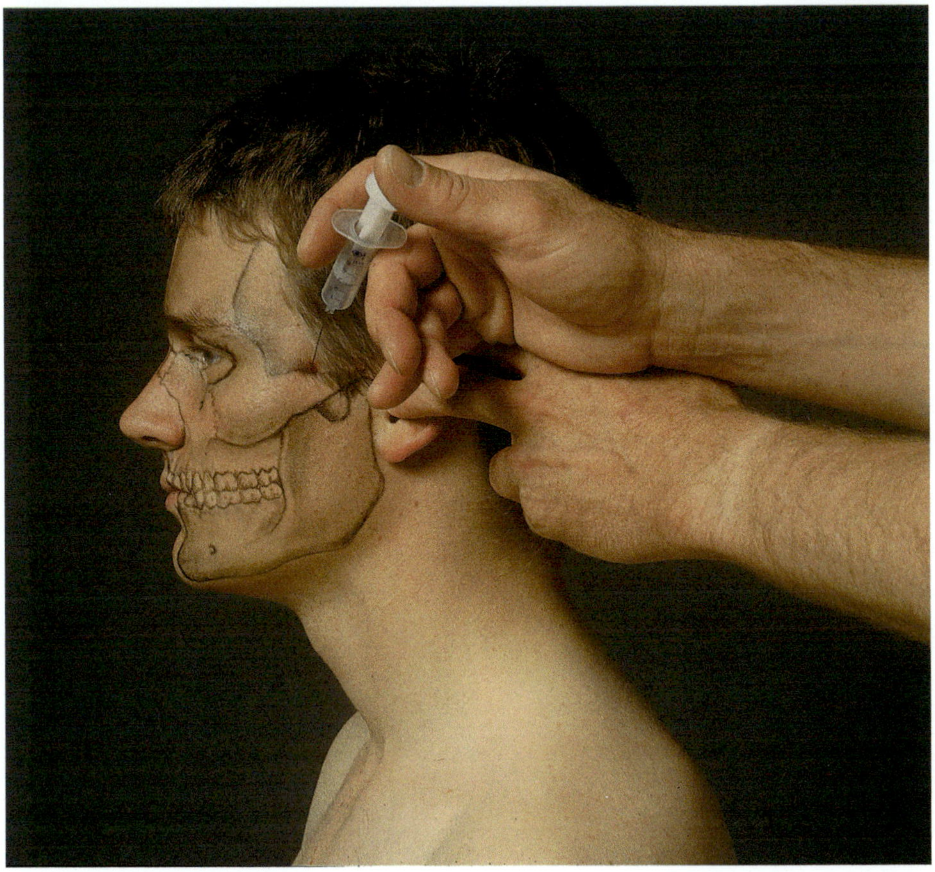

▸ **Fig. 16.21** Puncture direction to the pterygopalatine ganglion, side view.

16.9
Injection to the Otic Ganglion and the Mandibular Nerve

16.9.1 Indications

The indications given are only a sample of those possible:

- Neuralgia of the third trigeminal branch.
- Jaw joint pain.
- Impaired function of the chewing muscles.
- Inflammatory and benign tumorous diseases of the parotid gland.
- Unexplained pain in the supply region of the mandibular nerve.
- Otalgia.

The expected success depends, among other things, on the patient's particular "interference field situation."

16.9.2 Anatomy and Neurophysiology

▶Otic ganglion. The parasympathetic otic ganglion is before the foramen ovale in the temporal fossa directly medial to the mandibular nerve (▶Fig. 16.22, ▶Fig. 16.23). It consists of three neurological components:

- The sensory portion from the mandibular nerve.
- The parasympathetic portion from the superficial petrosal nerve originating from the tympanic nerve of the glossopharyngeal nerve.
- The sympathetic portion, which courses alongside the medial meningeal artery arises from the internal carotid artery.

The sensory and sympathetic portions pass through the otic ganglion; the parasympathetic portion is switched to the second neuron. The nerve branches emerging from the ganglion provide parasympathetic supply of the parotid gland and mucosal glands of the cheek mucous membranes. Further, the otic ganglion receives fibers from the chorda tympani, which provide motor supply to the levator veli palatini muscle by crossing the pterygopalatine ganglion. From the otic ganglion, the tensor tympani nerve reaches the tensor tympani muscle and controls the tension of the eardrum.

▶**Mandibular nerve.** The mandibular nerve is the third branch of the trigeminal nerve. It conducts sensory fibers for supply of the dura mater, the skin of the chin, the lower lip, the lower half of the cheek, the temporal region, the ventral pinna, and the external auditory canal to a narrow edge of the outside of the eardrum (residual innervation by the vagus nerve), as well as the mucosa of the cheek, floor of the mouth, and the proximal two-thirds of the tongue, gums, all the mandibular teeth, and the jaw joint. It also conducts motor fibers for the chewing muscles (temporal muscle, masseter muscle, medial and lateral pterygoid muscles), the mylohyoid muscle, the biventer muscle, and the tensor tympani.

The injection to the otic ganglion and the mandibular nerve for therapeutic purposes results in sensitivity failure in the indicated skin and mucous membrane areas of the mandibular nerve, transient paralysis of the chewing muscles, and anesthesia of the jaw joint. Important to neural therapy is the interruption of the parasympathetic–sympathetic innervated glandular function of the parotid gland, the submandibular gland, and the sublingual gland as well as the mucosa and vessels of the same region supplied by the sympathetic nervous system. The injection certainly reaches a portion of the sympathetic perivascular plexus of the maxillary artery and medial meningeal artery (from the external carotid artery) with the result of improved arterial circulation of this supply region through vasodilation.

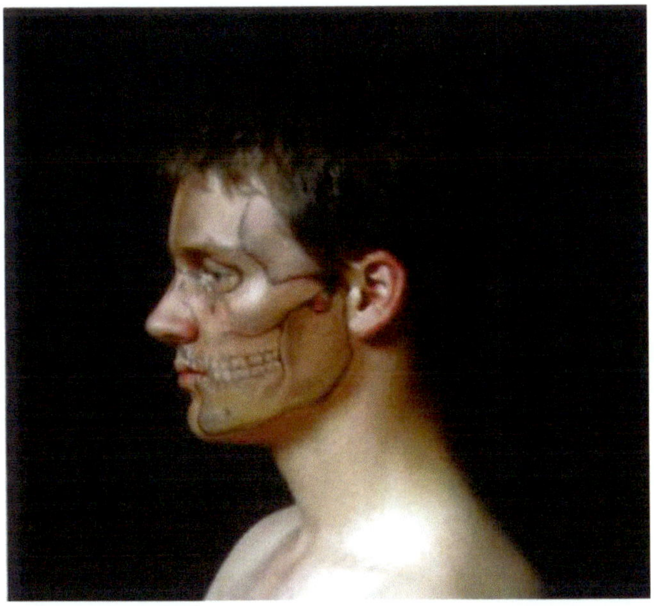

► **Fig. 16.22** Injection point for injection to the otic ganglion.

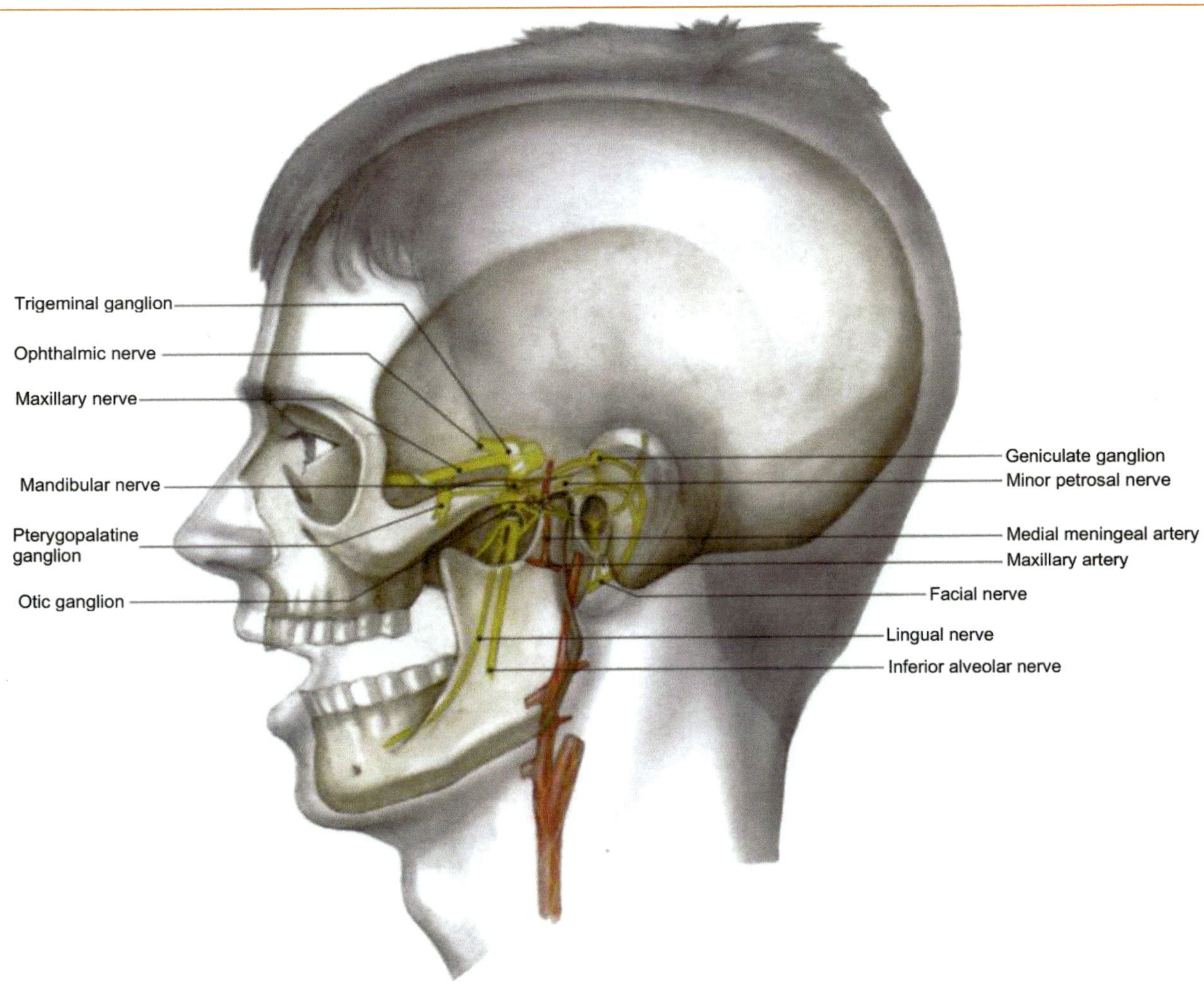

► **Fig. 16.23** Topography for injection to the otic ganglion.

16.9.3 Injection Technique (According to Hauberrisser)

Palpation of the cheekbone. With the mouth slightly opened, the 4 cm long needle is inserted about 3 cm before the external auditory meatus below the cheekbone (►Fig. 16.24, ►Fig. 16.25). After wheal and subcutaneous infiltration, push the needle horizontally and strictly laterally between the coronoid process and the condyloid process (mandibular notch) until the lateral lamina of the pterygoid process is encountered at about 4 cm depth. Pull back the needle by about 2 cm. Turn the needle tip horizontally by 10 to 20° dorsally and reinsert the needle about 2 cm. Now the needle tip is directly in front of the mandibular nerve which indicates any possible sensations in the lower jaw. After two-time aspiration, 2 to 3 mL anasthetic is slowly infiltrated.

The neural therapeutic effect is not in the complete interruption of the stimulus conduction of the mandibular nerve, but rather in the interruption of the sympathetic and parasympathetic limbs .

> **Note**
>
> **It is important that the needle is not pushed further forward, is not pointed in the cranial direction, and that the two-time aspiration definitely rules out intravascular or intrathecal needle positioning (possible dura protrusion in the area of the foramen ovale).**

16.9.4 Material

Required:

- 5-mL syringe.
- 0.4 × 40 mm needle.
- Procaine 1%, 3 mL per injection.

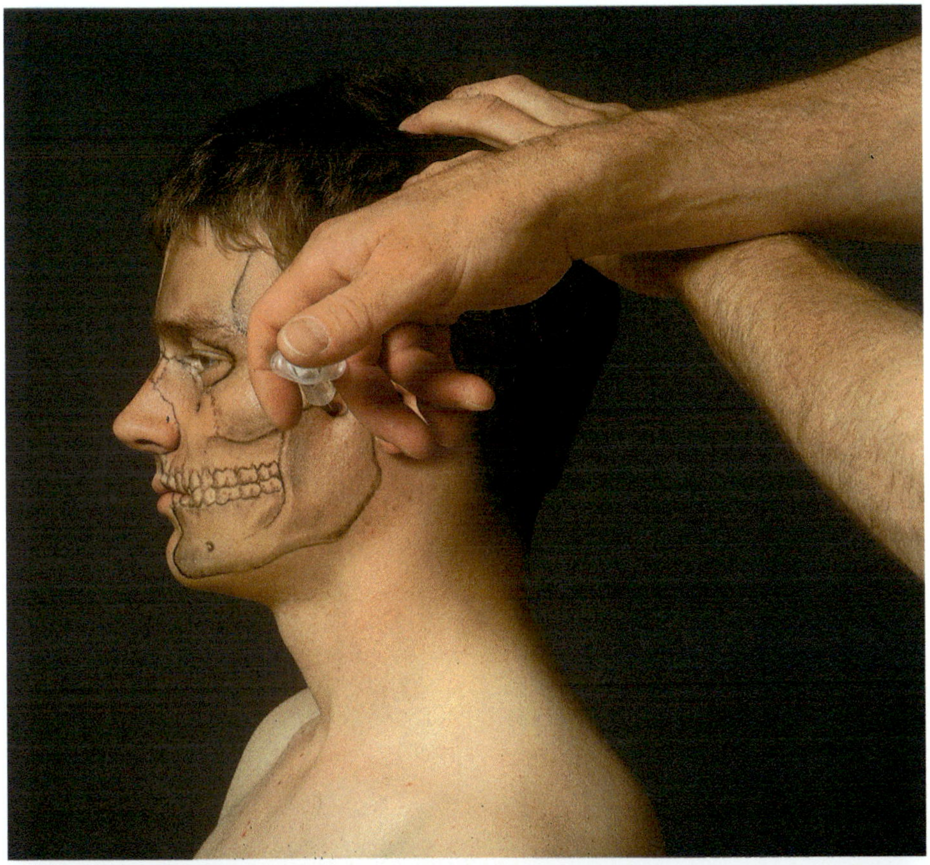

►**Fig. 16.24** Injection to the otic ganglion, side view.

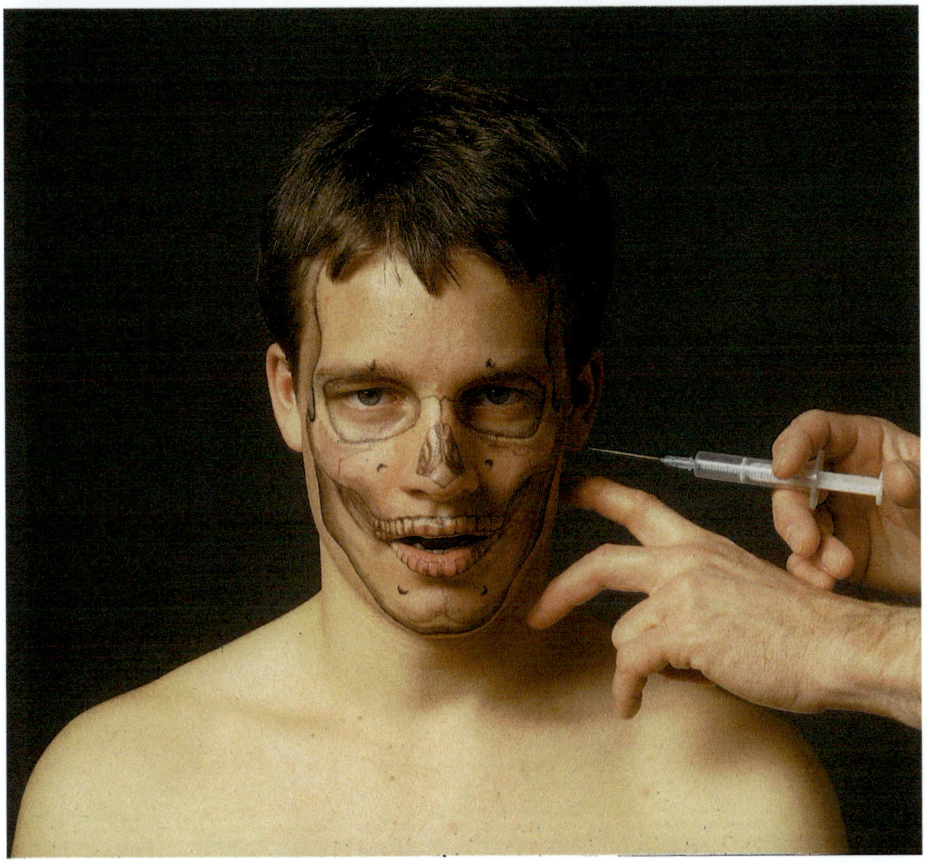

►**Fig. 16.25** Injection to the otic ganglion, front view.

16.10

Injection to the Major Occipital Nerve, Occipital Artery, and Minor Occipital Nerve

16.10.1 Indications

The indications given are only a sample of those possible:

- Neuralgia of the major occipital nerve.
- Occipital headache.
- Whiplash injury.
- Disorders in the supply area of the trigeminal nerve and vagus nerve.
- Cervical migraines.
- Difficulty concentrating.
- Burning eyes with subjective impaired vision.
- Vertebral weakness.

The expected success depends, among other things, on the patient's particular "interference field situation."

16.10.2 Anatomy and Neurophysiology

The major occipital nerve from C2 is the strongest sensory branch of the cervical spinal nerves. It provides sensory supply of the back of the head and sideways to the temporal region. There are connections to the dorsal branch from segment C1 as well as segment C3. The connection of the second cervical segment via the rear column with the terminal nuclei of the trigeminal nerve and afferent fibers of the vagus nerve is important. These connections topographically and neurophysiologically reflect the repeatedly observed clinical finding of occipital neuralgia with diseases in the supply area of the trigeminal nerve, particularly the first two branches, as well as in diseases in the supply area of the vagus nerve. The sympathetic fiber portions of the major occipital nerve as well as the sympathetic supply of the occipital artery originate from the superior cervical ganglion, so that a therapeutic effect can be exerted on the microcirculation of the upper cervical spine, the skull, and cerebral vessels in addition to the segmental-reflexive treatment via the sympathetic nervous system. Chronic sinusitis is also able to maintain occipital pain conditions, as is cholecystitis.

16.10.3 Injection Technique

▶**Major occipital nerve and occipital artery.** The occipital artery is palpable about 4 cm lateral from the center line. The major occipital nerve runs directly medial to this. With the 20-gauge needle, 0.5 to 1 mL anesthetic is infiltrated perineural to about 1 to 1.5 cm depth (▶Fig. 16.26, ▶Fig. 16.27). Anesthesia of the occipital scalp and a feeling of warmth, based on sympatholysis of the perivascular plexus of the occipital artery, indicate the correct positioning of the injection.

▶**Minor occipital nerve.** Palpation of the rear edge of the mastoid process. The sternocleidomastoid muscle branches of the lesser occipital nerve extend about one finger-width in medial direction and are disseminated in occipital direction. These branches are pressure sensitive when irritated. After insertion of a wheal, 1 mL anesthetic is infiltrated subcutaneously at about 0.5 to 1 cm depth. As second injection site, the lesser occipital nerve is reached at the Erb point.

16.10.4 Material

Required:

- 5-mL syringe.
- 0.4 × 20 mm needle.

Procaine 1%, 0.5 to 1 mL per injection.

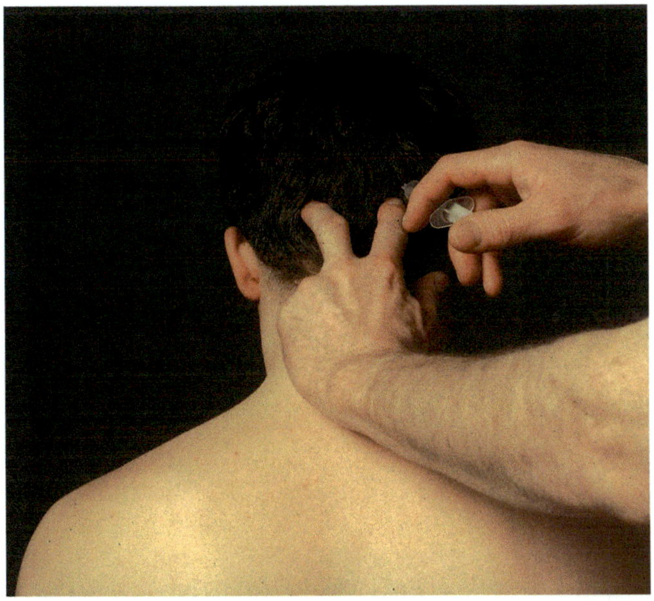

►**Fig. 16.26** Injection to the occipital nerves and the occipital artery.

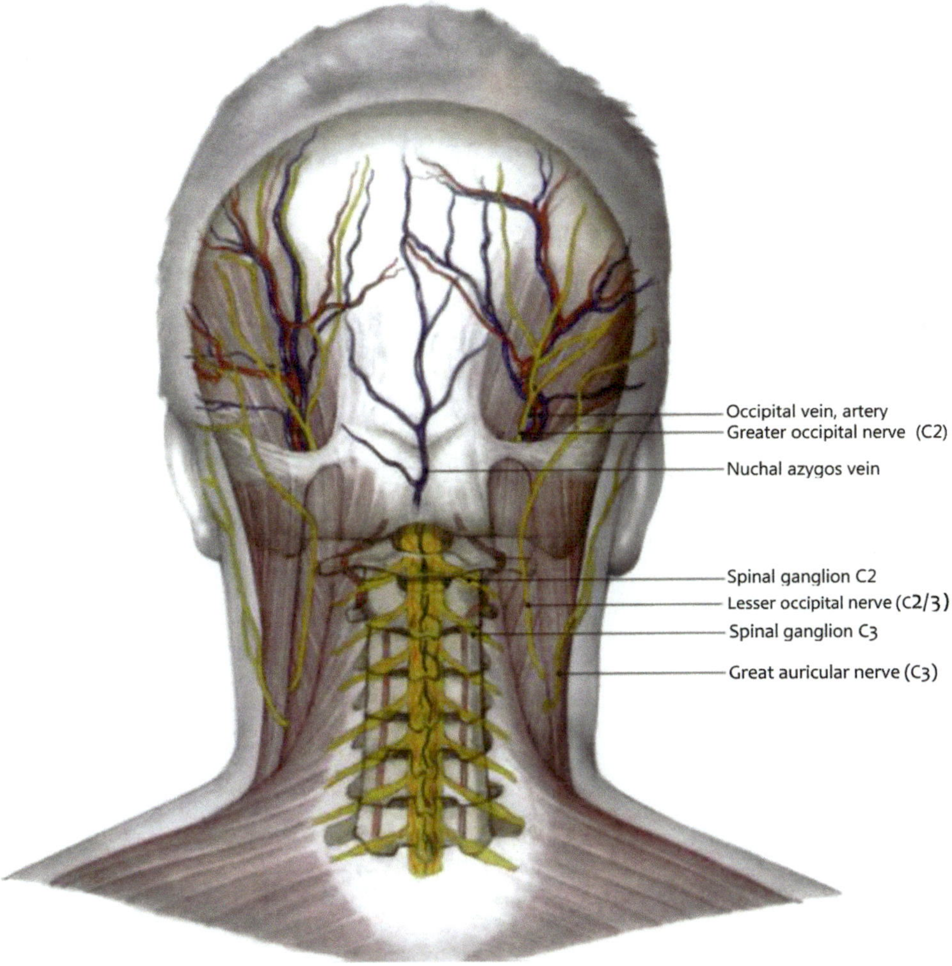

►**Fig. 16.27** Topography for injection to the occipital nerves and the occipital arteries.

16.11 Injection into the Lymphatic Drainage Area of the Facial Skull

16.11.1 Indications

The indications given are only a sample of those possible:

- Sinusitis.
- Tonsillitis.
- Mastoiditis.
- Otitis media.
- Inflammatory disorders of the eye.
- Inflammation of the oral cavity and the teeth.
- Bacterial and viral infections of the skin of the head and face.

The expected success depends, among other things, on the the patient's "interference field situation."

16.11.2 Anatomy and Neurophysiology

The lymphatic drainage from the facial skull basically flows in the direction of the jaw angle, whereby the lymph nodes are oriented to the venous drainage system. The superficial drainage is via the superficial lymph node in line with the external jugular vein, and deep drainage is in line with the internal jugular vein. The lymph stations, which are easily reached for neural therapeutic treatment, are in the area of the jaw angle (lymphatic node of the deep parotid gland) and the lower jaw (lymphatic submandibular node). The lymph node drainage flows from the eyes, the paranasal sinuses, the teeth, the mouth/throat area, the tonsils, and the tympanic cavity.

Clinical experience shows that existing inflammations in the above-named regions subside faster through the apparently improved lymph drainage, and thus the lymphatic edema as well as the pain which often accompanies the inflammation. Particularly with acute inflammation, this injection shows a clear immediate effect lasting far beyond the anesthesia time. The physiological basis is the capillary sealing effect of procaine as well as the improved microcirculation of the lymph nodes through sympatholysis.

16.11.3 Injection Technique

Palpation of the jaw angle. At about 1 cm depth, 0.5 mL anesthetic is subcutaneously infiltrated into this area (▸Fig. 16.28, ▸Fig. 16.29). Further subcutaneous injections are made to the anterior edge of the sternocleidomastoid muscle at about 1 to 1.5 cm depth as well as in the area of the lower jaw branch of the facial nerve. Before each injection, two-time aspiration is performed to document the extravascular needle position.

16.11.4 Material

Required:

- 5-mL syringe.
- 0.4 × 20 mm needle.
- Procaine 1%, 0.5 mL per injection.

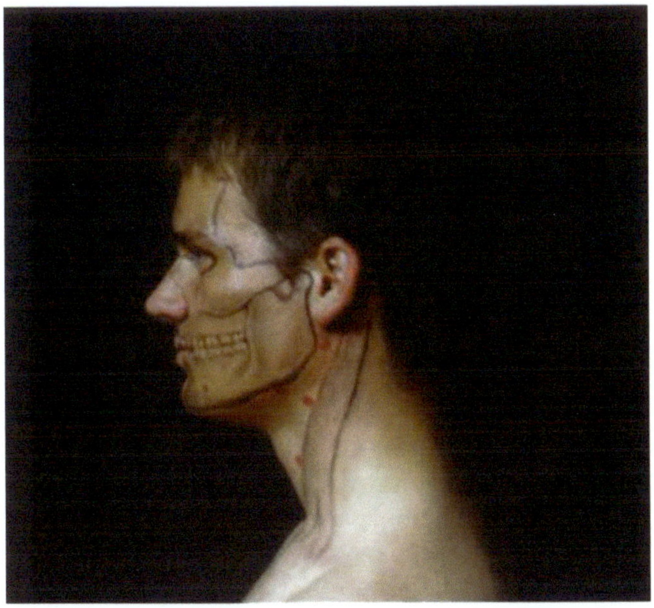

▶ **Fig. 16.28** Injection points in the lymphatic drainage area of the facial skull.

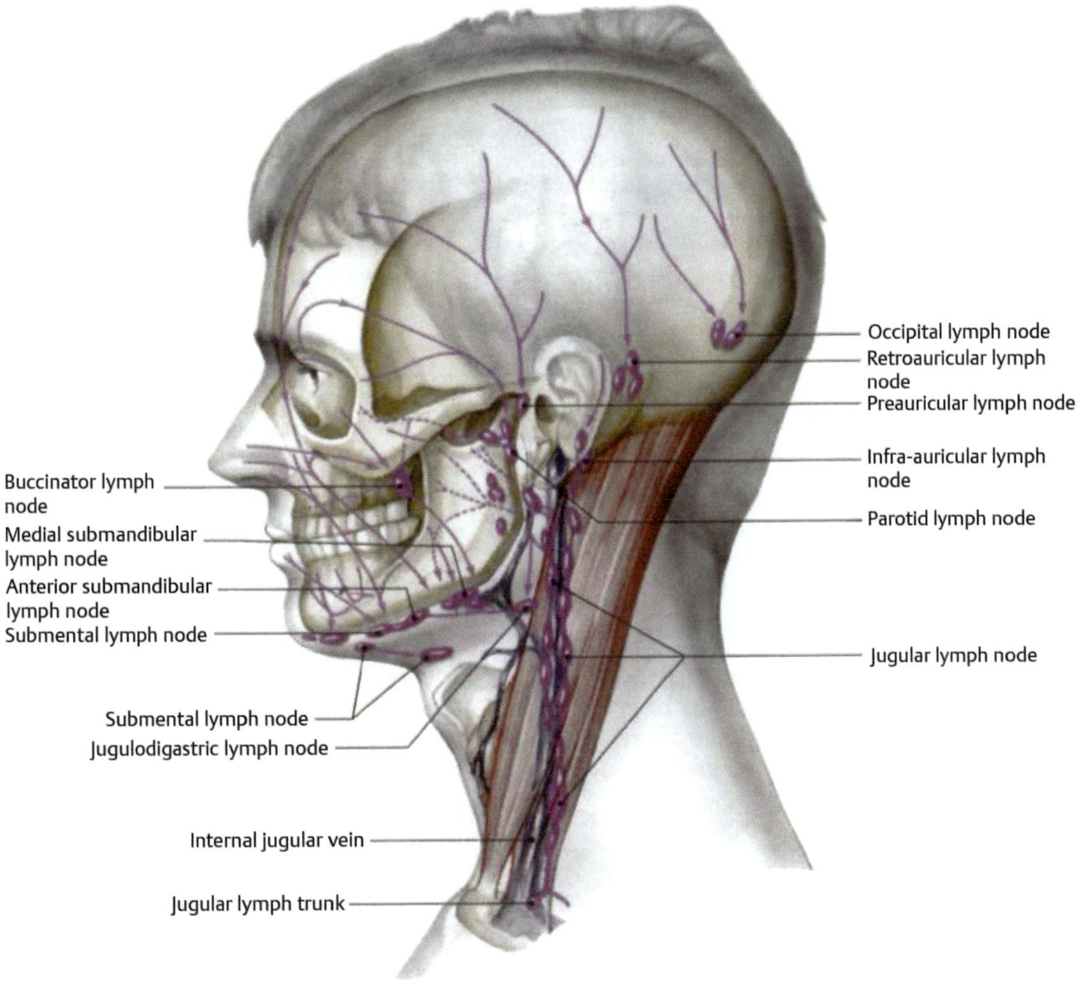

▶ **Fig. 16.29** Topography of lymphatic drainage from the facial skull.

16.12 Injection to the Tonsils

16.12.1 Indications

The indications given are only a sample of those possible:

- Chronic and acute tonsillitis.
- Recurring infections of the nose and throat region.
- Tonsil hyperplasia.
- Recurring lateral funiculus angina after tonsillectomy (injection in the tonsillectomy scars).
- Tonsils as interference field.

The expected success depends, among other things, on the the patient's "interference field situation."

16.12.2 Anatomy and Neurophysiology

During examination of the pharynx, the palatine tonsils are seen as an approximately almond-sized formation embedded between the anterior palatoglossal arch and the posterior palatopharyngeal arch in alignment with the lower row of teeth which is pulled further in the dorsal direction (▶Fig. 16.30, ▶Fig. 16.31). The pharyngeal tonsil is at the pharyngeal fornix at the posterior nasal pharyngeal wall and is covered by the soft palate.

The paired palatine tonsils belonging to the lymphatic pharyngeal ring (gum, pharynx, tongue, and eustachian tonsils) are supplied by the arteries and thus simultaneously by the ascending palatine artery from the facial artery (external carotid artery). The sensory supply proceeds via the tonsillar branch of the glossopharyngeal nerve.

The autonomic supply appears to be very important. The palatine tonsils are in the supply area of the pharyngeal plexus, a nerve plexus formed of fibers from the glossopharyngeal nerve, the vagus nerve, and the sympathetic cervical trunk (superior cervical ganglion). Apparently, this parasympathetic and sympathetic innervation of the tonsillar region and the short afferent conduction pathways to the parasympathetic inferior ganglion of the vagus nerve and to the sympathetic superior cervical ganglion plays the dominant role in concomitant illness in other organs and organ systems with primary disease of the tonsils. The interference field effect of the tonsils, which plays a remarkably frequent role in neural therapy, is easily explained using the topographical situation between the lymphatic tonsil organ and the sympathetic and parasympathetic system. The two autonomic ganglia act as interfaces in the efferent autonomic system with an effect on the whole body. Thus, injection to the tonsils in neural therapy is one of the most frequent and important injections ever performed.

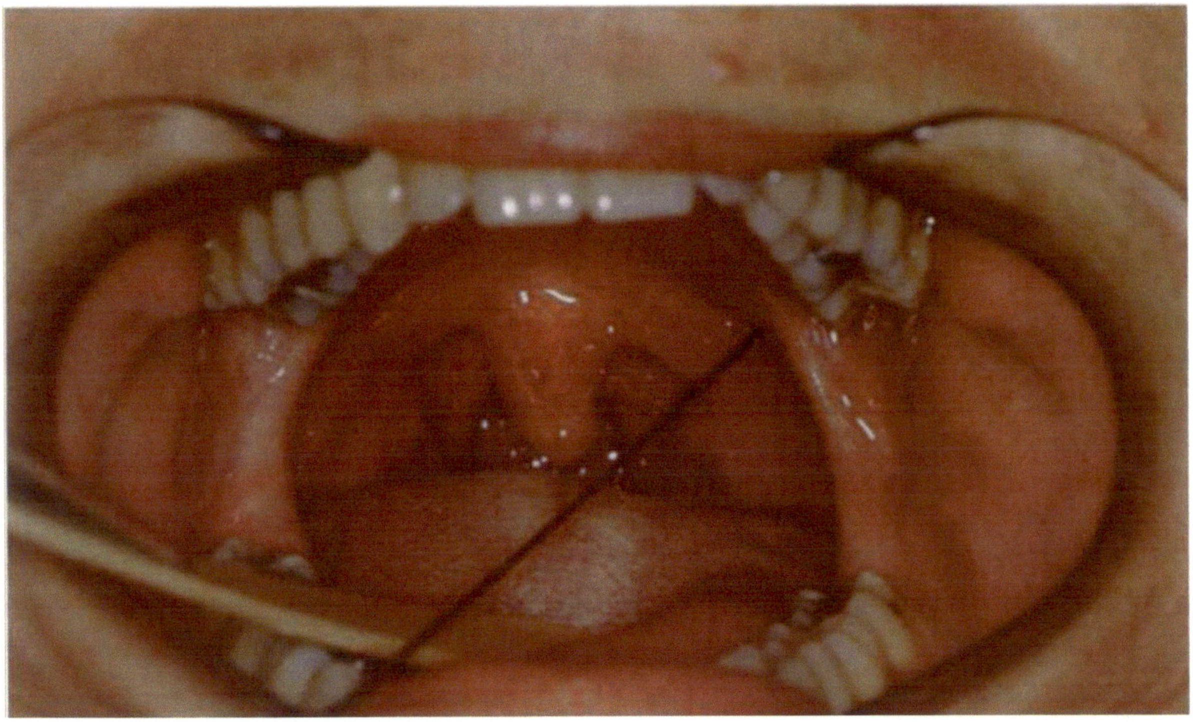

▸**Fig. 16.30** View of the pharynx for injection to the tonsils (injection at the top left tonsil pole).

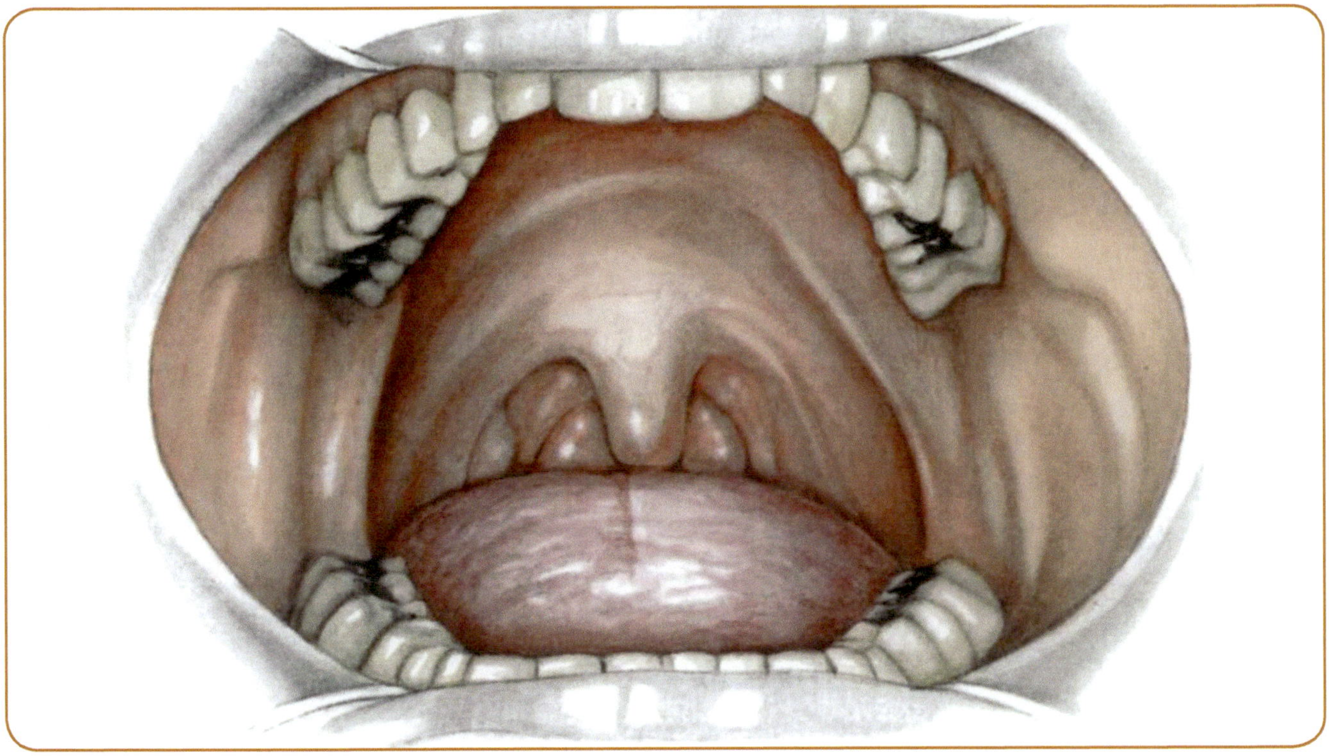

▸**Fig. 16.31** Topography for injection to the tonsils.

16.12.3 Injection Technique

▶ **Palatine tonsils.** Inspection of the pharynx of a wide open mouth. The patient should only breathe through the mouth since the tongue is pressed toward the cranium when breathing through the nose. With a well-lit mouth–pharyngeal space (tongue depressor light), the tonsils can be found behind the palatoglossal arch. Using a depressor, the tongue is very carefully pushed down. Puncture with the 6-to 8-cm-long needle directly above the upper tonsil pole through the base of the palatoglossal arch (▶ Fig. 16.32, ▶ Fig. 16.33). 0.5 mL procaine 1% is infiltrated submucosal at a 1 to 2 mm depth. The injection is performed visually in order to see the swelling of the mucosa during the injection process and thereby rule out an intravascular needle position. Without a clear view during the injection process, aspiration should be performed in any case. Afterward, the same injection is made in the same way to the lower tonsil pole.

▶ **Pharyngeal tonsil and the sphenoid sinuses.** This is performed through the soft palate (▶ Fig. 16.32, ▶ Fig. 16.33), approximately 1 cm dorsal to the boundary between the hard and soft palate, 1 to 2 mm lateral to the midline. The 6- to 8-cm-long needle, which is bent 40° in the cranial direction 4 cm before the needle tip, encounters the floor of the sphenoid bone in direct proximity before the pharyngeal tonsil about 2 to 3 cm after penetration through the soft palate. After negative aspiration, 0.5 mL procaine 1% is infiltrated.

In tonsillectomy patients, the injection is carried out with the same technique in the scar tissue after prior aspiration.

16.12.4 Material

Required:
- 5-mL syringe.
- 0.6 × 60 to 80 mm long needle, bent 40° in the cranial direction 4 cm before the needle tip.
- Procaine 1%, 0.5 mL per injection.

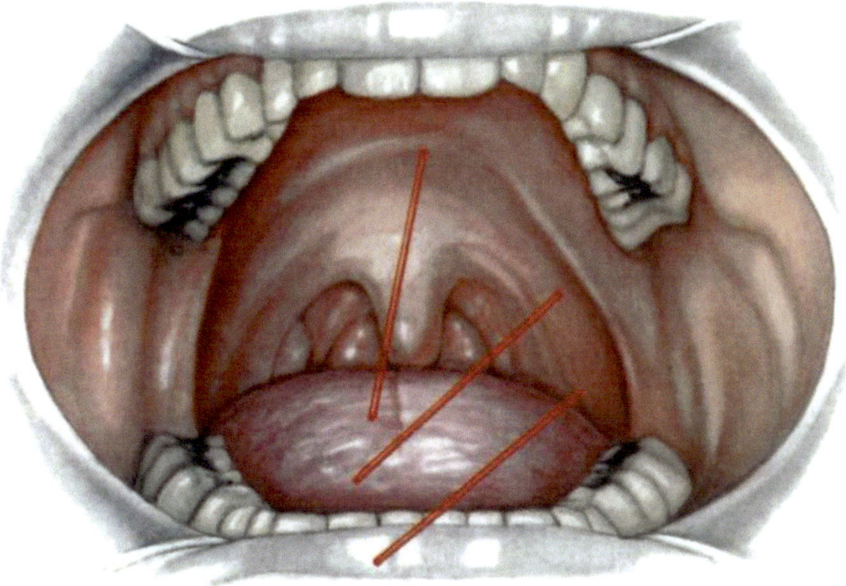

▶ **Fig. 16.32** Injection to the palatine tonsils and the pharyngeal tonsils.

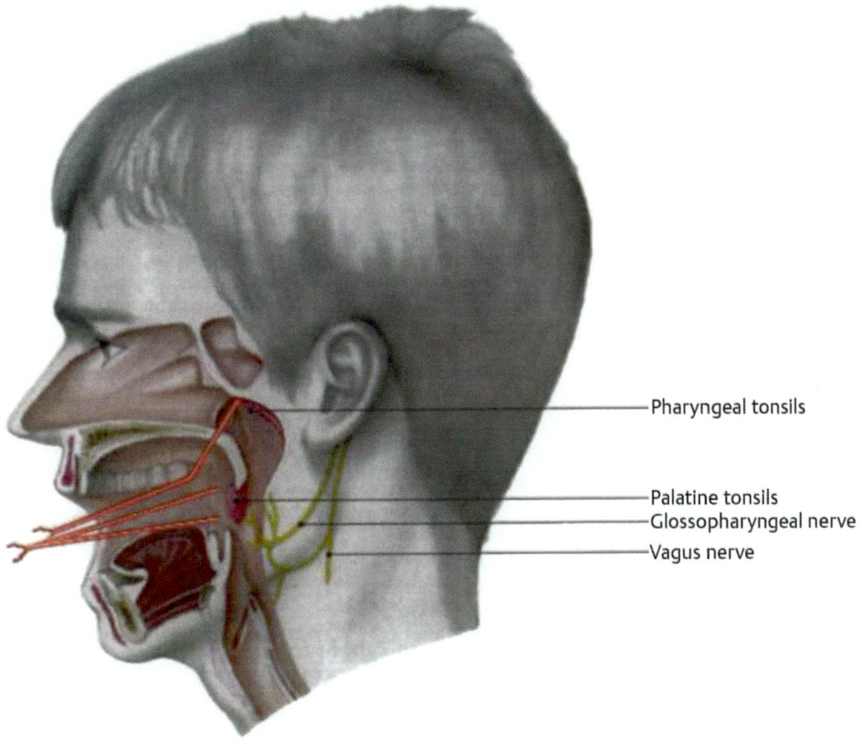

▶ **Fig. 16.33** Topography for injection to the tonsils.

16.13 Injection to the Teeth

16.13.1 Indications

The indications given are only a sample of those possible:

- Periodontitis.
- Paradontosis.
- Unexplained tooth pain or tooth symptoms (above all after dental treatments of any kind).
- Pain in the dentition.
- Unexplained jaw pain after tooth extraction.
- Neuralgias in the supply area of the trigeminal nerve.
- Teeth as an interference field.

Note

If an interference field is suspected, all distinct teeth as well as all empty spaces in the jaw (scars) must be tested in a session.

The injection of the maxillary or mandibular nerve to circumvent neural therapeutic dental testing—which is somewhat unpleasant for the patient—has not been successful, because only part of the sympathetic nervous system proceeds with the trigeminal branches, and the other part proceeds with the vessels. The diagnostic/therapeutic value of the injections is in the immediacy of the injection at the disease site (interference field).

16.13.2 Anatomy and Neurophysiology

The number of teeth in an adult is 32, or between 28 and 31 if the wisdom teeth are missing. A child's mouth generally has 20 teeth. The dentition starts with the sixth month of life (+1–2 months) and is completed at the end of the second year of life (±6 months). In the sixth year of life (+1–9 months), the first molar emerges (first permanent tooth), such that a child's mouth can comprise 24 teeth during this time. The continued dentition of the permanent teeth proceeds from front to back, lower jaw before upper jaw, and earlier in girls than in boys.

The tooth consists mostly of dentin, which is coated in enamel in the visible portion of the oral cavity. In the dental cavity, the dentin contains the tooth pulp consisting of loose connective tissue, vessels (arterial, venous, lymphatic), and nerves (trigeminal nerve, end formation of the sympathetic nervous system) which are responsible for the circulation and sensitivity of the tooth. The tooth is suspended in the jaw bone via the periodontium, whereby the periodontal ligament represents the very powerful connective tissue link between dentin and alveolar bone. The periodontal ligament is also rich in vessels and nerves, i.e., responsible for circulation and sensory supply of the periodontium. The vascular nerve bundle which provides nutrients to the tooth emerges into or exits the tooth through the apical dental foramen (see ▸Fig. 16.34). The sensory supply of the tooth proceeds via the trigeminal nerve (second and third branch), the arterial supply via the mandibular artery and the maxillary artery, and the sympathetic supply via the perivascular plexus of the same arteries emerging from the superior cervical ganglion.▸

In neural therapeutic practice, injection to the teeth is done for diagnostic purposes, i.e. during interference field exploration with a suspected interference field in the tooth/jaw area, as well as for primarily therapeutic purposes in tooth disease.[14,107,173]

The interference field localization in the dental and maxillofacial region is frequently classified similarly to that of the tonsils. On the one hand, this is because of the double innervation by the sympathetic nervous system and trigeminal nerve and its connections to other cranial nerves and the segments C1–C3. On the other hand, this frequency is an indirect result of the current dental treatment options. Subtle tooth restoration, root canal treatment, and root resection treatment have emerged in place of early tooth extraction. This way, the "diseased" tooth is "preserved" for a longer time and can continue its mechanical function of the mastication of food. However, refined tooth preservation to avoid premature tooth replacement, by bridges, partial, or full dentures, at the same time increases the risk of chronic inflammation in the dental and maxillofacial region. While this causes the patient no local or only occasional pain, there are significant consequences for the whole body.[14,107,173,176,208]

Outside of the more likely local disorder in the area of the trigeminal nerve, whose second and third branch is responsible for the sensory supply of the tooth, in the form of trigeminal neuralgias in various categories or chronic sinusitis, there are chronic functional disorders of the spine with somewhat significant degeneration, degenerative-inflammatory joint disorders of single or multiple joints, systemic illnesses, e.g., forms of rheumatism, or heart-circulatory disorders, which can only be interrupted after radical tooth extraction. The organ damage which has already occurred is only partially or no longer reparable depending on the body's ability to regenerate.

The previously mentioned possible disease correlations between dental and maxillofacial areas and the rest of the body are only a small excerpt of the actual range of disease correlations which can be demonstrated in the clinical application of neural therapy. It should also be noted that a lesion of the teeth or jawbone does not necessarily lead to a disorder causing pain at another site. Apparently, there is variable compensation for the interference field effect on the body which proceeds via the sympathetic nervous system. In every case, the goal should be a nonirritated tooth/jaw region in order to prevent potential negative effects on the whole body.

The concept of a lesion not only means bacterial infection of the tooth or jaw, but any kind of particularly chronic nonspecific inflammation which can also maintain such a chronic local irritation of the nerve system supplying the teeth (trigeminal and sympathetic nervous system).

If one follows the regional stimulus on its afferent pathway toward the center, many initially incomprehensible disease relationships, which have their origin in the dental and maxillofacial region, become clear. The afferent impulses emerging from the periphery of the trigeminal nerve reach the mesencephalic and spinal nucleic regions of the trigeminal nerve, which reach up to the level of spinal segment C3 and can reflexively maintain a neuralgia of the greater and lesser occipital nerves, as well as the muscular tension of the short neck muscles between C1 and C3. Therefore, an inflammation-induced stimulation of the trigeminal nerve in the context of an eye disease or reactive inflammation of the jawbone not only results in stimulus of the trigeminal nucleic regions, but also can be further conducted through the reticular formation to the nucleic regions of the **vagus nerve**, the **glossopharyngeal nerve**, **facial nerve**, and **accessory nerve** in the brain stem as well as the corresponding somatosensory and somatomotor spinal nucleic regions (C1–T6).

The result is the occurrence of illnesses in the form of various disorders in the range of the cranial nerves listed above as well as in different spinal segments. Thus, the conduction of chronic pathological stimulus of the trigeminal nerve toward the center not only causes awareness of stimulus in the form of pain or pressure sensation in a circumscribed spot in the craniofacial or teeth/jaw region. When considering the topography of the nucleic regions of the trigeminal nerve and related synaptic connections to other nucleic regions of the brain stem, it is not surprising that chronic disorders in the supply area of the trigeminal nerve can have such a complex impact on other locations of the body. The clinical response to this neurophysiological basis comes from the experience that the most common interference field localization is found in the area of the facial skull, teeth, and throat and the abdominal organs supplied by the autonomic nervous system.

To date, only the effects of irritation on the peripheral trigeminal branch were considered, which may occur in a chronic disorder of the dental and maxillofacial region. The vessels entering the tooth through the root canal not only are responsible for the circulation of the tooth, but also are carriers and guides for the peripheral sympathetic nerve plexus—not only for the efferent limb progressing to the nucleic regions of the sympathetic nervous system, but also for the afferent. The nerves proceed via the maxillary artery or mandibular artery, the external carotid artery via the ganglia chain of the cervical sympathetic trunk, up to the nucleic regions of the cervical sympathetic nervous system from segment C8–T6.

The chronic stimulation of the afferent sympathetic nervous system in a chronic disorder of the tooth/jaw region inevitably leads to increased stimulation of the efferent sympathetic system resulting in a disturbance of the vasomotor function regionally as well as across regions, depending on the duration of the stimulus effect. Depending on the site of onset, chronic vasomotor disruption in microcirculation results in inflammation or degeneration of this organ section with corresponding impaired function. The clinical corollary for this can be found in the aforementioned disease relationships, which can be identified with interference field therapy. The reproducible interference field effect of the tooth/jaw area on other sections of the body can be explained with the above-listed topographical and neurophysiological principles and confirmed by the also reproducible suppression of the interference field effect using injection to the teeth, which will be demonstrated below.

16.13.3 Injection Technique

As a tool, the normal 5 mL syringe is not very well suited, since the necessary injection pressure is too high and the injection needle disengages from the syringe. Using the carpule syringe with a screwed-on dental needle, 0.1 to 0.2 mL each is infiltrated from the buccal (▶ Fig. 16.35) and palatal (▶ Fig. 16.36) regions, respectively, at the level of the root of the tested tooth.

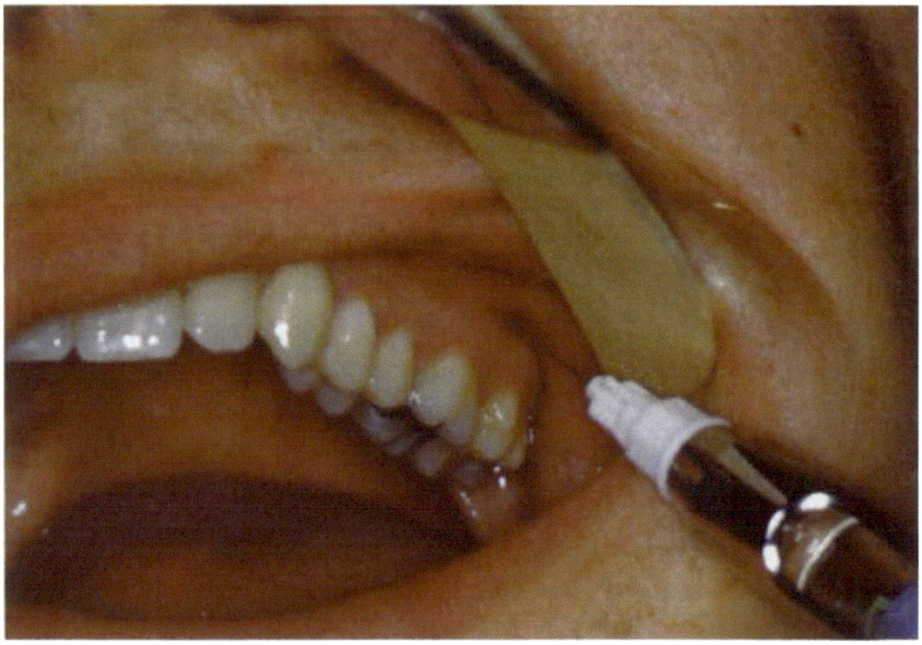

▶ **Fig. 16.34** Injection to the teeth from buccal region.

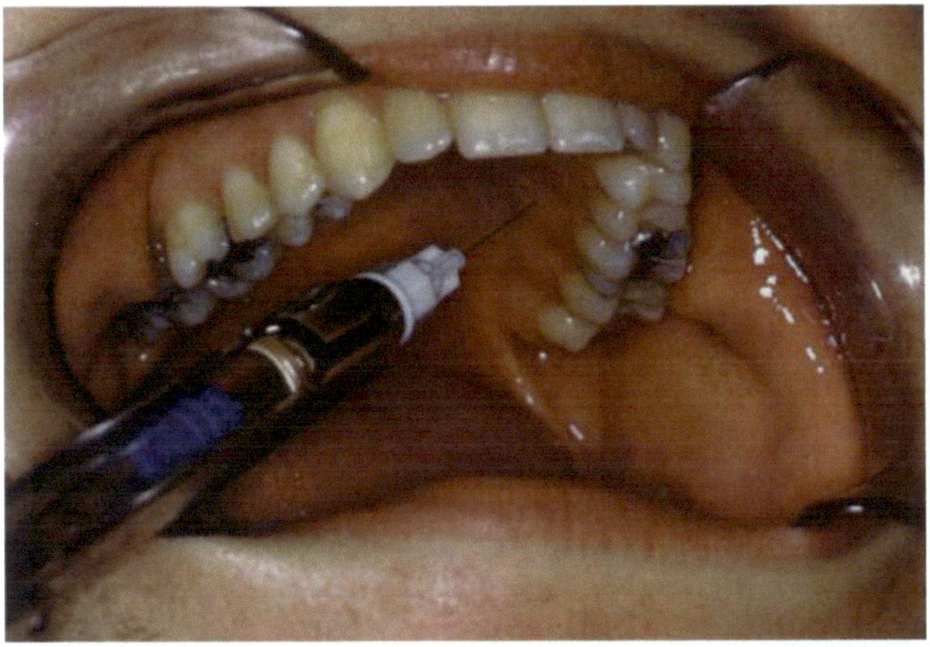

▸**Fig. 16.35** Injection to the teeth from palatal region.

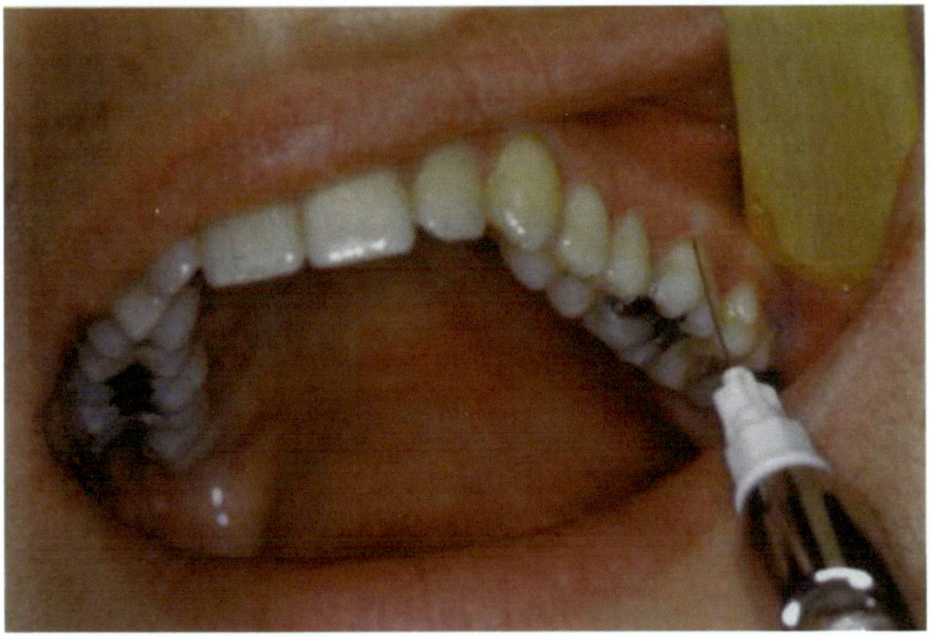

▸**Fig. 16.36** Intraligamental injection.

Intraligamental injection should be performed on teeth with root canal treatment and root tip resections (► Fig. 16.37). The intraligamental injection should be performed very slowly so that there is no pain during the injection procedure. The intraligamental injection can be performed from the buccal direction. With several adjacent potentially infected teeth, injection between the teeth in the area of the lingula has proven effective since two teeth can be reached with one injection.►

In neural therapeutic interference field testing, all prominent teeth should be tested, including empty areas of the jaw and **always the four wisdom teeth regions**. A panoramic image created before dental testing shows additional radiology findings that are hidden during a simple examination of the oral cavity (jaw osteitis, root remnants, displaced teeth, foreign bodies).

The following are relevant to neural therapy:

- Stained teeth.
- All teeth that previously underwent dental treatment (fillings, crowns, half-crowns, root canal treatment or root tip resections as well as bridges).
- Misaligned or stressed teeth.
- Implants.
- Pathological radiology findings in the tooth/jaw region.

Time and a "fine touch" are necessary in dental testing.

16.13.4 Material

Required:

- Carpule syringe.
- Dental needle; not larger than 0.3 mm, <25 mm long.
- Tongue depressor light.
- Procaine 1 to 2%.

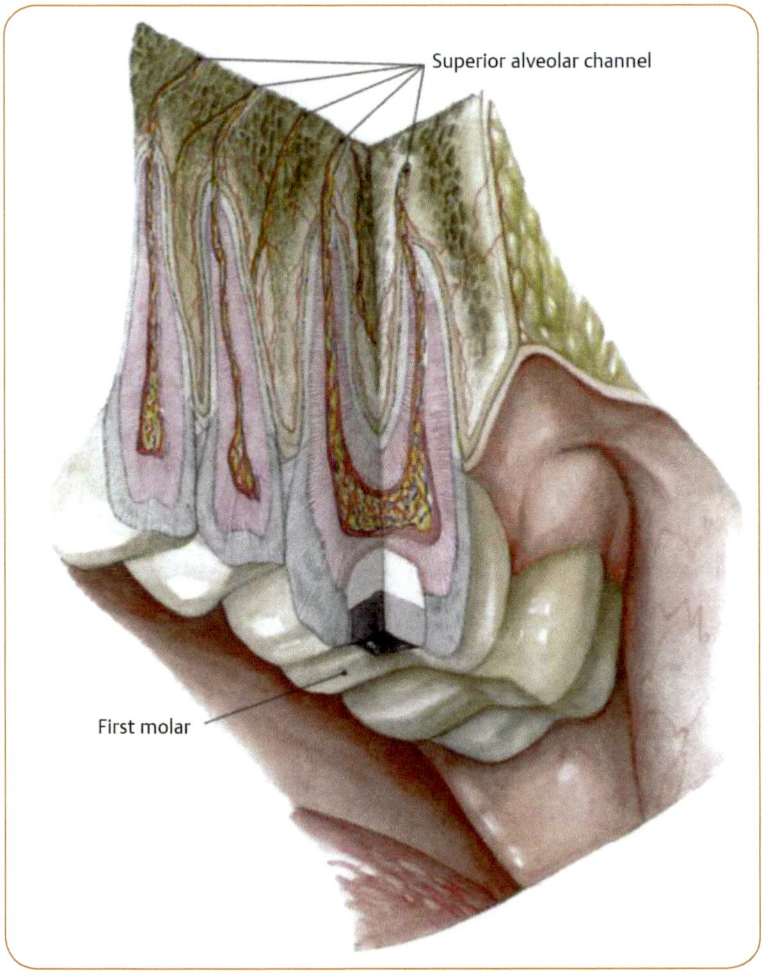

► **Fig. 16.37 Anatomy of the** tooth and the periodontal apparatus.

17 Neck

17.1 Injection in the Thyroid Gland

17.1.1 Indications

The indications given are only a sample of those possible:

- Manifest and clinical hyperthyroidism.
- Hyperthyroidism.
- Goiter.
- Grave's disease.
- Sleep disorders.
- Depression.
- Anxiety disorders.
- Change of life (male, female).
- Psychovegetative imbalance.
- Sensation of a lump.
- Cycle disorders.
- Osteoporosis.
- Recurring miscarriage.
- Unexplained fever.
- Hyperhidrosis.
- Headaches with stress or distress.
- Thyroid gland as an interference field (after infections or operations).

The expected success depends, among other things, on the the patient's "interference field situation."

Contraindications:

- **Hashimoto's thyroiditis (interference field disease).**
- **Period within 6 weeks after a scintigraphy of the thyroid.**

17.1.2 Anatomy and Neurophysiology

The thyroid gland is a hormone-producing organ in a paired structure on either side of the trachea at the level of the seventh cervical vertebra and the first thoracic vertebra. Both thyroid lobes are connected through the isthmus of the thyroid gland which contracts over the trachea. The function of the thyroid is the production of thyroxine, which has a general metabolism-boosting effect, as well as the hormone calcitonin, which reduces the serum calcium level. The vascular supply is arterial via the superior thyroid artery from the external carotid artery and the inferior thyroid artery from the thyrocervical trunk.

The nervous autonomic supply is from the sympathetic nervous system via the periarterial plexus of the superior and inferior thyroid artery as well as via the superior cervical ganglion which delivers secreting fibers for the thyroid. Further sympathetic branches to the thyroid originate from the common carotid plexus emerging from the medium cervical ganglion. Via the stellate ganglion there are sympathetic connections to the caudal thyroid plexus of the thyroid. The parasympathetic supply is via the pharyngeal plexus, a mixed nerve plexus with conduits from the sympathetic nervous system (superior cervical ganglion, glossopharyngeal nerve, vagus nerve). This is the same nerve plexus through which the palatine tonsils are also supplied. The hormone production, dependent on the releasing factor thyroid stimulating hormone (TSH) which is transported by the bloodstream, is also influenced by the sympathetic and parasympathetic nervous system which innervates the thyroid.

Injection in the thyroid gland leads to partial interruption of afferent and efferent impulses of the neurovegetative end formation and to stabilization of the parenchyma cell membrane. Clinically, repeated injection in the thyroid leads to normalization of the symptoms triggered by it, if the thyroid function disorder is not induced by an interference field.

17.1.3 Injection Technique

Palpation of the thyroid lobes on either side of the trachea approximately two fingers above the jugular with slightly dorsal flexion of the cervical spine. About 2 cm lateral to the median, insert the 20-gauge needle 1 to 1.5 cm deep in the sagittal direction (▶Fig. 17.1, ▶Fig .17.2). After negative aspiration, infiltrate 1 mL procaine per thyroid lobe. In the case of an enlarged isthmus, this is also infiltrated with 0.5 mL.

17.1.4 Material

Required:

- 5-mL syringe.
- 0.4 × 20 mm needle.
- Procaine 1%, 0.5 to 1 mL per injection.

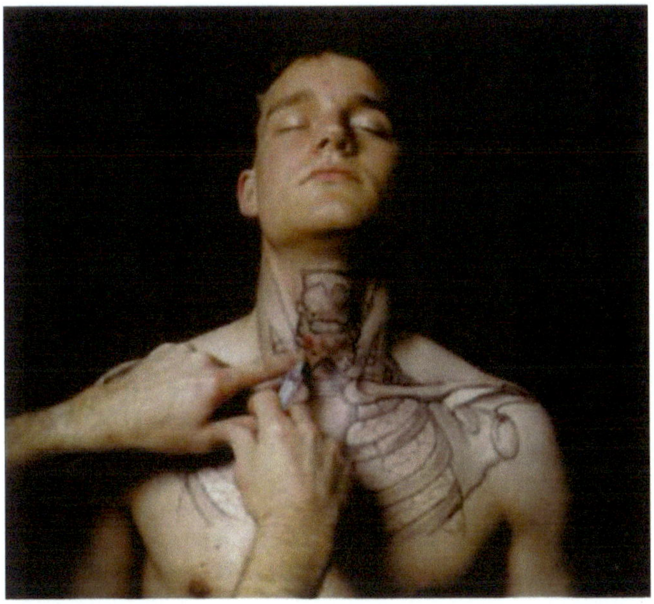

►**Fig. 17.1** Injection in the thyroid gland.

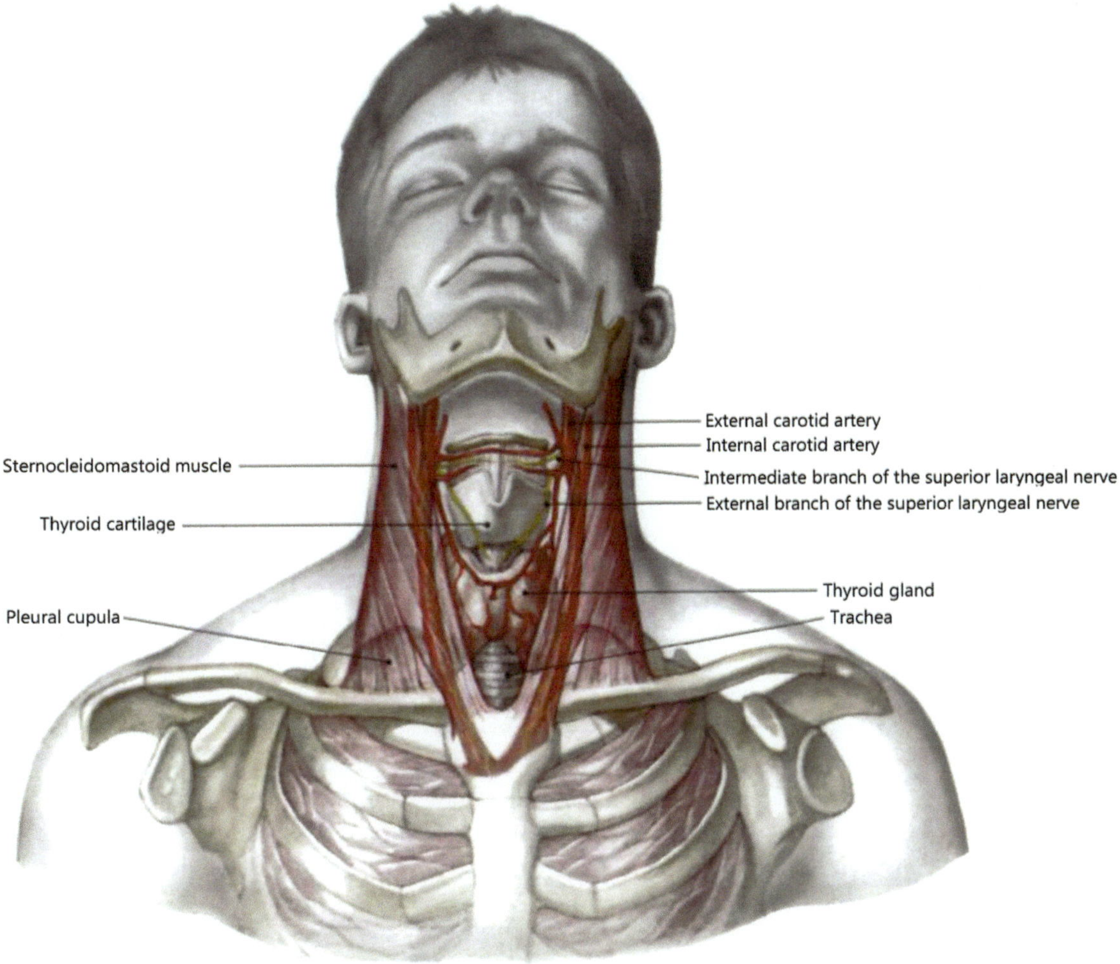

►**Fig. 17.2** Topography for injection in the thyroid gland.

17.2 Injection to the Superior Laryngeal Nerve

17.2.1 Indications

The indications given are only a sample of those possible:
- Chronic hoarseness.
- Sensation of a lump.
- Chronic laryngitis.
- Neuritis of the superior laryngeal nerve.
- Malignant pain of the larynx.

The expected success depends, among other things, on the the patient's "interference field situation."

17.2.2 Anatomy and Neurophysiology

The superior laryngeal nerve originates from the vagus nerve, which it exits at the level of the superior ganglion. After taking up sympathetic fibers from the superior cervical ganglion, it divides itself into two branches for supplying the larynx:
- The external branch, which supplies the cricothyroid muscle (all remaining larynx muscles are supplied by the recurrent laryngeal nerve).
- The internal branch, which supplies sensory function to the mucosa of the larynx.

Furthermore, the internal branch conducts taste fibers for the area of the epiglottis and parasympathetic fibers for the mucous glands. The entry point of the internal branch of the superior laryngeal nerve is simultaneously the site of the superior laryngeal artery whose sympathetic plexus supplies the mucosa of the larynx. Injection to the superior laryngeal nerve leads to transient paresis of the cricothyroid, reduced mucous secretion, and improved blood flow to the laryngeal mucosa through sympatholysis of the superior laryngeal artery.

17.2.3 Injection Technique

Palpation of the lateral upper edge of the thyroid cartilage. The superior laryngeal nerve is in the subcutaneous tissue between the hyoid bone and the thyroid cartilage, before the more significant internal branch enters the larynx. Here, 1 mL procaine is infiltrated subcutaneously with the 20-gauge needle (▶Fig. 17.3, ▶Fig. 17.4) and distributed using slight massage. The injection is repeated on the opposite side.

17.2.4 Material

Required:
- 5-mL syringe.
- 0.4 × 20 mm needle.
- Procaine 1%, 1 mL per injection.

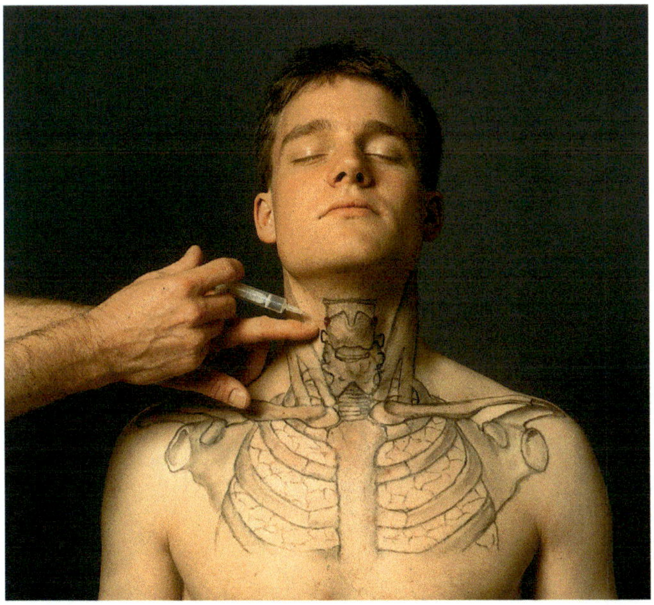

►**Fig. 17.3** Injection to the superior laryngeal nerve.

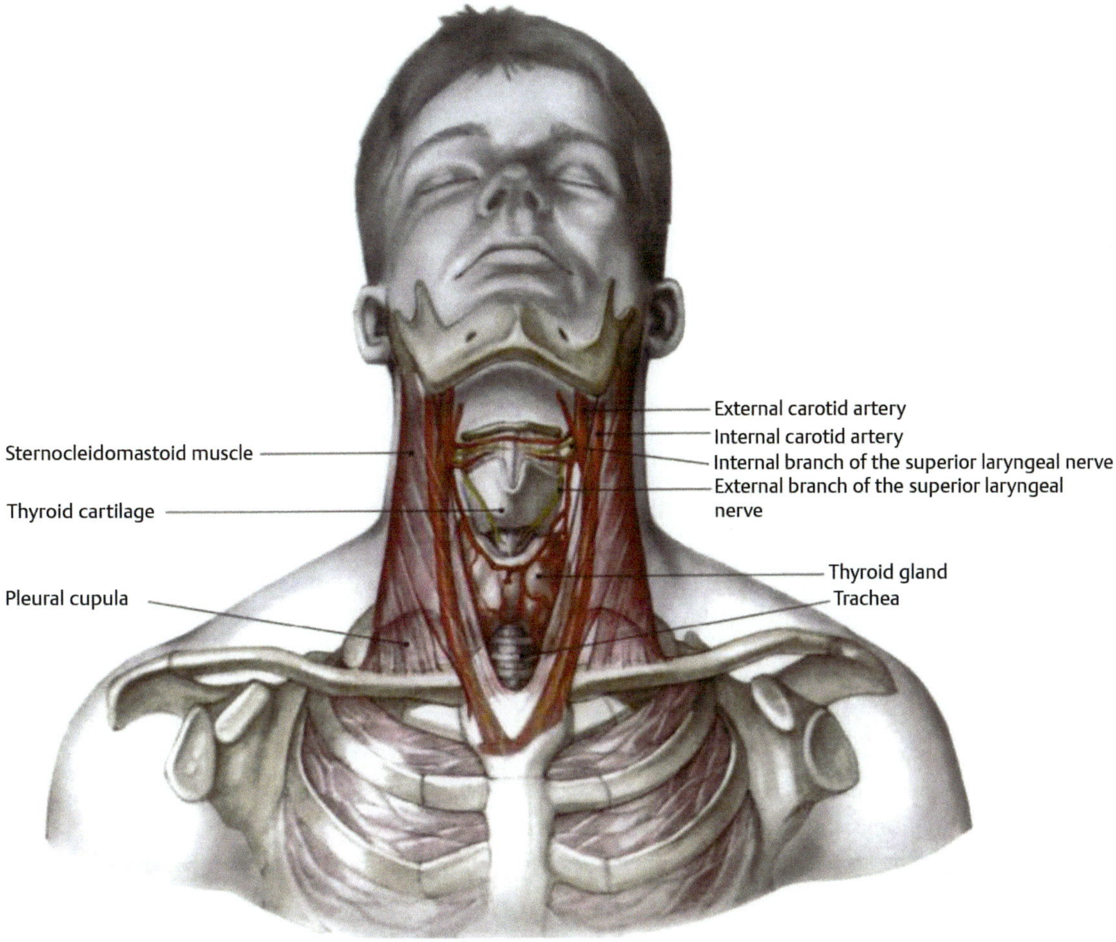

►**Fig. 17.4** Topography for injection to the superior laryngeal nerve.

17.3

Injection to the Stellate Ganglion (Cervical Thoracic Ganglion)

The injection to the stellate ganglion is among the most important injections in neural therapy. The reason for this is explained in the following. From this point, the sympathetic nervous system takes up an expansive nerve connection to the entire upper half of the body, i.e., the head, neck, upper extremities, and the entire chest area. Via the stellate ganglion and indirectly via the superior cervical ganglion, there are connections to the cranial nerves, the vagus nerve, glossopharyngeal nerve, hypoglossal nerve, and the phrenic nerve of the spinal nerves. A significant proportion of the interference fields are located in the region of the head, so that injection to the stellate ganglion indirectly enables an influence of the interference fields in the head region. The indications for injection to the stellate ganglion therefore primarily concern disorders of the head, neck, the upper extremities, and the chest area.

17.3.1 Indications

Disorders of the Head and Its Organs

The indications given are only a sample of those possible:
- Cerebral circulation disorders.
- Apoplectic insult (new, old).
- Chronic recurring or persistent headache.
- Cerebral dizziness.
- First- to fourth-degree skull/brain injury.
- Posttraumatic head symptoms including epilepsy.
- Postoperative symptoms including edema formation.
- Bacterial and viral disorders of the cranial and facial skull.
- Malignant pain of the head.
- Neuritis and neuralgia of the cranial nerves (e.g., trigeminal nerve).
- Arterial and venous circulation disorders of the eye.
- Bacterial, viral, and nonspecific inflammation of the eye and eye socket.
- Arterial circulation disorders of the ear and balance organs (e.g., sudden deafness, otogenic dizziness, tinnitus, Meniere's disease).
- Research on chronic recurring otitis.
- Disorders of the nose, the paranasal sinuses, and the oral cavity with failed local treatment.

The expected success depends, among other things, on the the patient's "interference field situation."

Disorders of the Neck and Its Organs

The indications given are only a sample of those possible:
- Painful degenerative diseases of the cervical spine and neck muscles.
- Neuralgias in the supply area of the cervical spine (cervical plexus).
- Whiplash injury.
- Thyroiditis.
- Vertebral dizziness.
- Postoperative swelling.
- Tracheomalacia research.
- Bacterial and viral infections of the larynx, trachea, and pharynx.
- Pain from malignant diseases of the neck.

The expected success depends, among other things, on the the patient's "interference field situation."

Disorders of the Shoulder Girdle and Upper Extremity

The indications given are only a sample of those possible:
- Cervicobrachialgia.
- "Frozen shoulder."
- Painful shoulder syndrome.
- Root irritation between C5 and T6.
- Degenerative-inflammatory disorders of the shoulder girdle joints and the upper extremity.
- Plexus neuralgia and neuritis of the brachial plexus.
- Traumatic plexus lesions.
- Chronic root tendinopathy of the shoulder girdle and arm muscles.
- Chronic tendovaginitis.
- Arterial circulation disorders of the upper extremities (Raynaud's disease, arteritis nodosa. arteritis obliterans).
- Lymphedema of the upper extremities, also after lymphadenectomy.
- Malignant pain of the shoulder girdle and upper extremities.
- Sudeck's atrophy (CRPS) of the upper extremity.

The expected success depends, among other things, on the the patient's "interference field situation."

Disorders of the Thorax and Its Organs

The indications given are only a sample of those possible:
- Chronic degenerative disease of the thoracic vertebrae segments T1–T6.
- Bacterial, viral, and nonspecific pleuritis.
- Pneumonia.
- Lung emphysema with dyspnea.
- Bronchial asthma.
- Chronic bronchitis.
- Interstitial edema.
- Adjuvant in pulmonary embolism (stellate infiltration on both sides with an interval of 30 minutes).[299]
- Research on chronic cough with unexplained origin.
- Pain from inoperable tumor diseases.
- Coronary heart disease.
- Cardiac pain after bypass, stent, or dilatation.
- Cardiac asthma.
- As supplemental therapy for myocarditis.

- Congestive heart failure.
- Heart rhythm disorders.
- As supplemental therapy for mediastinitis.

The expected success depends, among other things, on the the patient's "interference field situation."

17.3.2 Anatomy and Neurophysiology

As a 1- to 3-cm elongate structure on the longus colli muscle, the stellate ganglion is at the level of the C7 transverse process and the first rib head behind the initial part of the subclavian artery from the last cervical (C8) and the first thoracic ganglion (T1). The efferent preganglionic sympathetic influx comes from spinal segments C8–T5, and the afferent influx converges in this ganglion and further in the dorsal spinal roots C8–T5. As an interface from the first to the second neuron, branches pull from the stellate ganglion to the phrenic nerve, the vagus nerve, and recurring laryngeal nerve as well as the vascular branches to the subclavian artery and its further branches. Emerging from these vascular branches, networks form for the subclavian artery, the inferior thyroid artery, the vertebral artery, and the internal thoracic artery. Further nerve branches from the stellate ganglion (independent of the vascular pathway) are the visceral branches in the form of the inferior cardiac nerve, which travels to the cardiac plexus, as well as small branches for the sympathetic supply of the thyroid and parathyroid.

Via the cardiac plexus, there is a direct connection to parasympathetic fibers provided to this plexus by the vagus nerve. The function of the cardiac plexus is to modulate the parasympathetic and sympathetic innervation of the heart. The stimulation of the sympathetic portion results in an increase in the heart rate, the contraction strength, the stimulus conduction speed, and excitability. Stimulation of the parasympathetic nervous system causes the opposite effect. In healthy patients, there is a balanced interplay between the sympathetic and parasympathetic nervous system, depending on situational needs, whereby the basic tone is determined by the parasympathetic nervous system. In addition to overworking the heart muscle, chronic sympathetic stress can cause "silent inflammation" via the vascular system due to a lack of recovery periods and thus result in myocardial disease (including neuromodulatory sympathetic stimulation [interference field] through chronic inflammation, e.g., the teeth,[14] the tonsils, or intestines).

Accordingly, the complete sympathetic innervation of the respective upper body quadrants takes place via the stellate ganglion. Sympathetic efferent nerve fibers start from the stellate ganglion or pass through the ganglion to the medium cervical ganglion and to the superior cervical ganglion. Typical of the sympathetic nervous system, from these two ganglia there is also innervation of the bilaterally identical upper body quadrants—though with different areas of focus—in order to "secure" the sympathetic nervous system function. The medium cervical ganglion, which also may not be present, provides nerve branches to the recurring laryngeal nerve, to the phrenic nerve, to the arterial vessels from the common carotid artery, to the thyroid, and the cardiac plexus. The supply via the superior cervical ganglion (p. 188) is discussed separately since this ganglion also has other areas of focus for nervous connection which are significant for the study of neural therapy.

Particular attention is required by the sympathetic connection of the cervical sympathetic trunk to the vagus nerve. Under general neurophysiological considerations, increased stimulus of the sympathetic nervous system—in the case of positive stimulus transfer—should result in increased stimulus of the vagus nerve. In fact, clinical observation shows, for example, a quickly occurring stress situation of cumulative typical sympathetic symptoms (increased heart rate, sweating, skin reddening) as well as a simultaneously occurring increased activity of the parasympathetic nervous system (tenesmus of the abdomen, nausea, later diarrhea, possible circulatory depression). Further clinical observation supports these correlations. Injection to the stellate ganglion, that is, partial one-sided interruption of the sympathetic efferent pathway, leads to a clinically impressive reduction in bronchospasm in asthmatics, at least for the period of medicinal sympatholysis. Since the bronchial musculature is innervated by the parasympathetic nervous system, and there is increased parasympathetic stimulus of the bronchial musculature in the case of bronchospasm, sympatholysis alone should cause an increase in bronchospasm for asthmatics. The neuroanatomical and neurophysiological basis is in the above-mentioned connections of the stellate ganglion to the vagus nerve, and in the neural connection between the superior cervical ganglion and the superior ganglion of the vagus nerve via the jugular nerve.

Injection to the stellate ganglion triggers a partial incomplete interruption of the sympathetic efferent and afferent stimulus conduction in the bilaterally equal upper body quadrants from the head to the diaphragm, whereby the parasympathetic "recovery phase" is enabled at the same time. This way, the illness or symptoms to be treated, which are always accompanied by a pathological regional stimulus of the sympathetic nervous system, can be interrupted via the "sympathetic collecting point." In pathological stimulus, sympathetically induced hypoxia also leads to a hypoxic stress response in all perfused tissue sections: spasm in the bronchial musculature and reduced mucosal secretion in the bronchial mucosa (thicker mucous for asthmatics). In this way, sympatholysis can become therapeutically effective via the stellate ganglion.

Clinical experience shows that after the pharmacological interruption of the stellate ganglion function subsides, the former disease or symptoms do not immediately recur, but often can be interrupted entirely at a later time and with a repetition of the injection. The prerequisite is that an interference field disease is not involved. To date, the cause of this universal neural therapeutic phenomenon has been clarified only in theory; experimental studies and results are lacking.

17.3.3 Injection Technique

Injection to the stellate ganglion is of major importance to neural therapy owing to the far-reaching effect on the bilaterally equal upper body quadrants. The injection is essentially just performed in pain therapy and, above all, in neural therapeutic practice. The main reasons for this are the numerous and rather different techniques, the lack of knowledge about the range of indications, the little-known precise topographic and anatomical conditions, and the overemphasis on partially serious complications due to the injection technique. The injection technique described here, based on Leriche and De Seze, was further simplified by Dosch and represents the lowest risk compared to other techniques:

- The injection is performed on a patient in the sitting or prone position, whereby the head must be supported (▶Fig. 17.5, ▶Fig. 17.6). The therapist stands to the side and performs the injection from there. The patient's head is turned to the opposite side and slightly reclined, whereby the ventral neck muscles must remain relaxed (▶Fig. 17.7, ▶Fig. 17.8).
- Depending on the length of the neck, palpate the transverse process of C6 about two fingers width above the clavicle behind the sternocleidomastoid muscle, which is pushed in medial direction, whereby the frequently palpable carotid tubercle on the C6 transverse process can serve as an orientation point (▶Fig. 17.9, ▶Fig. 17.10). The palpating finger is used to push away the sternocleidomastoid muscle and the common carotid artery and internal jugular vein behind it.
- The palpating finger remains on the transverse process during the entire injection time. Directly above the palpating finger, the injection is made with the 0.5 × 40 mm needle, which is converged about 30° and pushed forward on the transverse process.
- Depending on the thickness of the neck, the depth of the injection is between 1 and 3 cm. The needle should maintain slight bone contact with the transverse process. The first aspiration is performed, rotating the needle by 180° with further aspiration.
- This one-handed rotation of the syringe should be practiced beforehand. If no blood or CSF is aspirated, start slow infiltration of 0.2 to 0.4 mL procaine 1%. If the

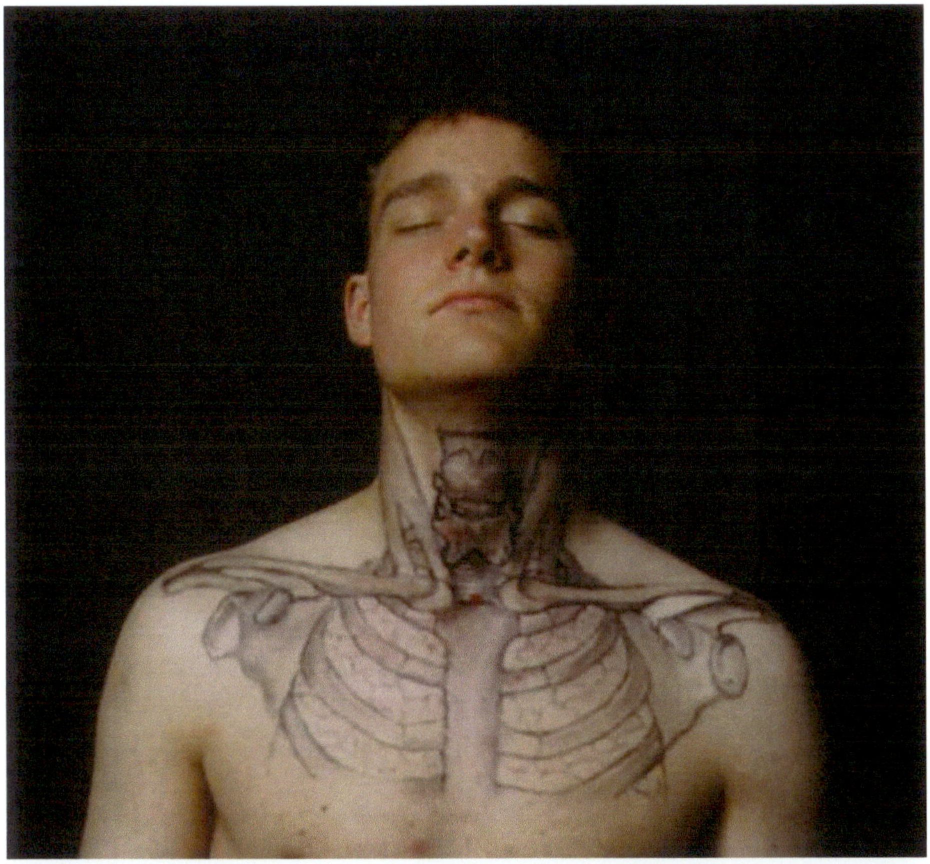

▸**Fig. 17.5** Front neck view with palpable structures for injection to the stellate ganglion.

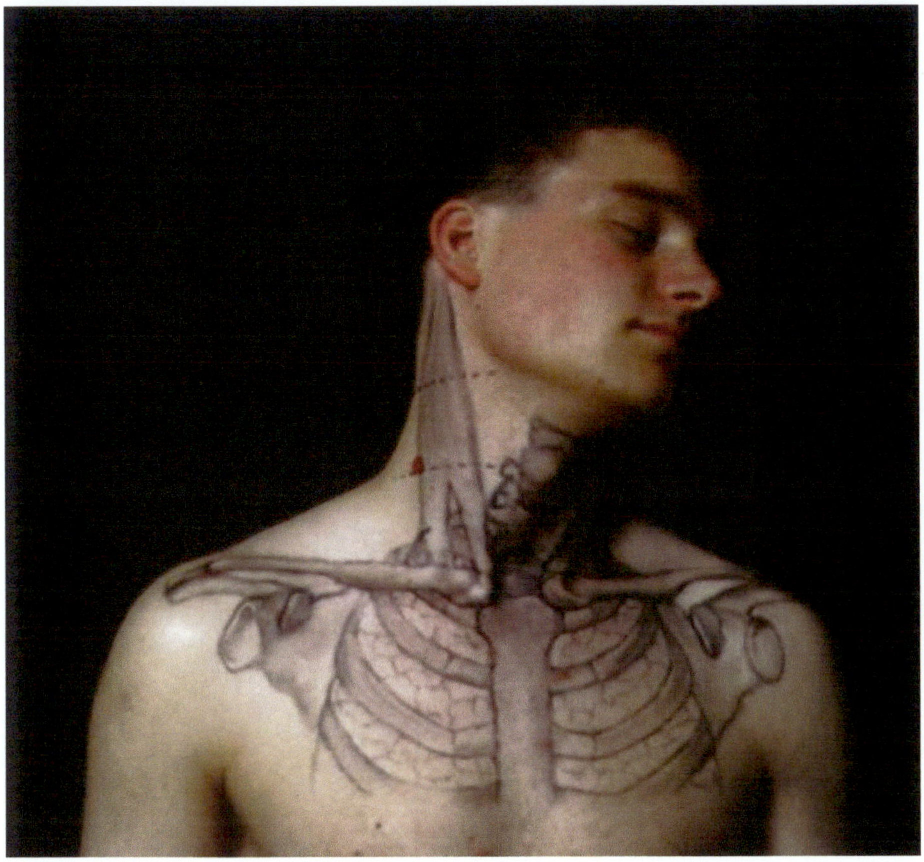

▸**Fig. 17.6** Positioning of the head and neck section before injection to the stellate ganglion.

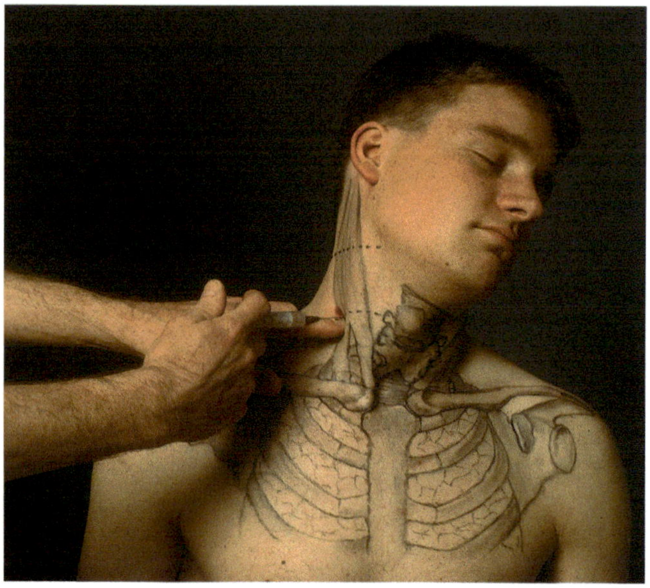

▶ **Fig. 17.7** Injection to the stellate ganglion.

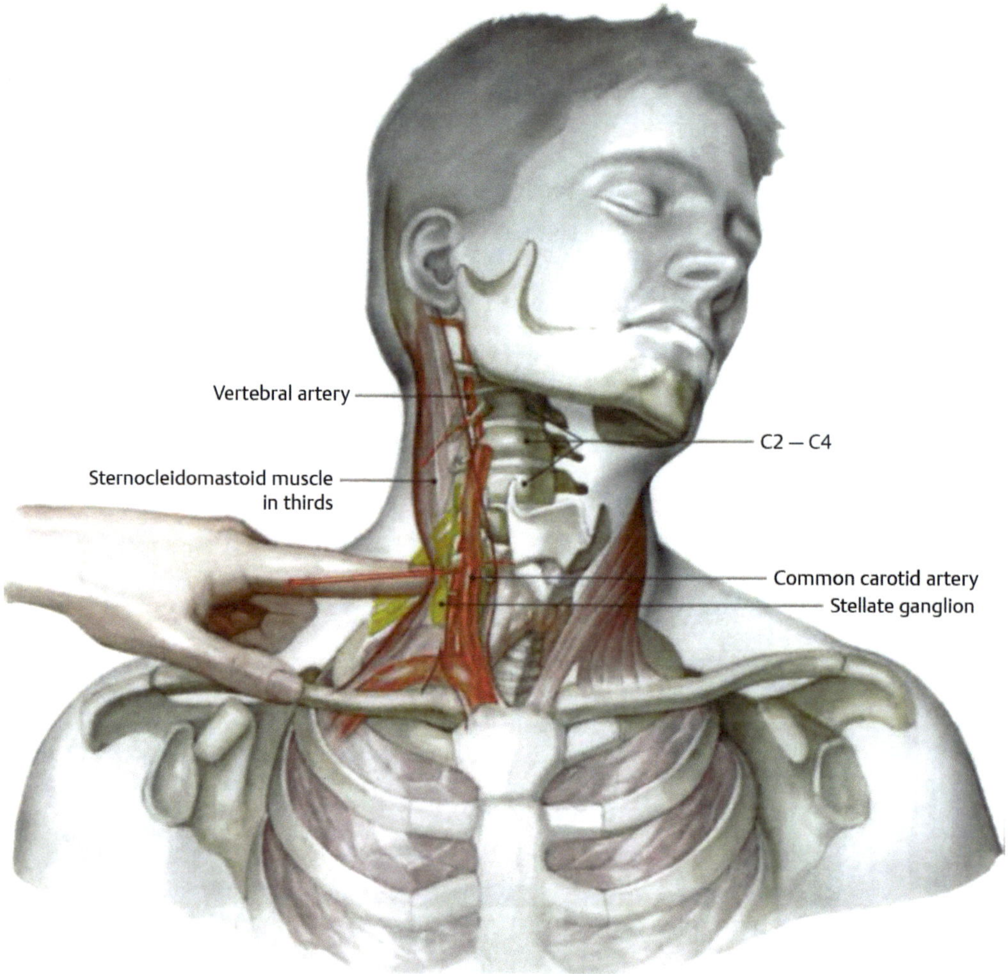

▶ **Fig. 17.8** Topography for injection to the stellate ganglion.

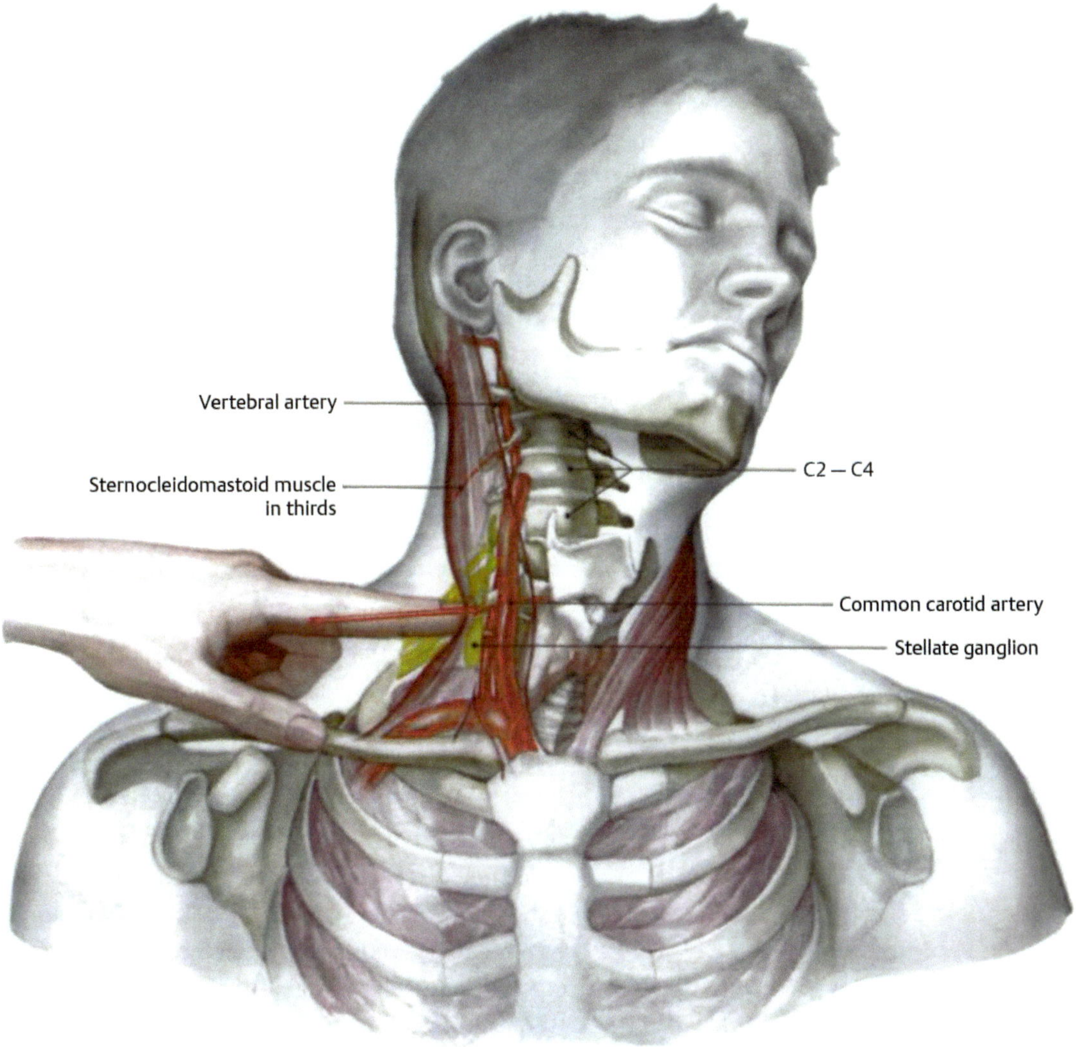

► **Fig. 17.9** Topography for injection to the stellate ganglion.

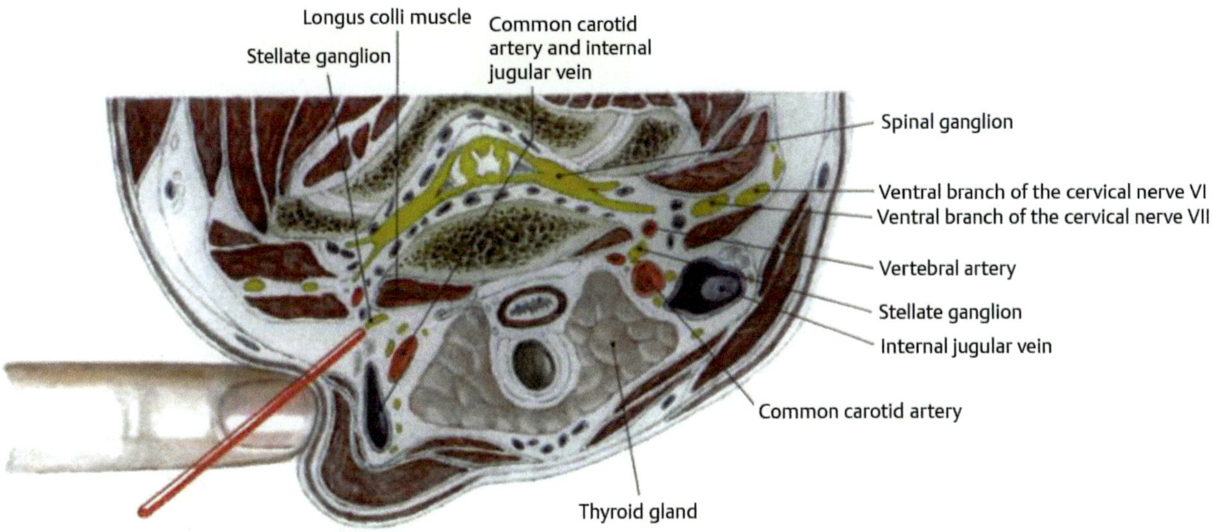

► **Fig. 17.10** Topography for injection to the stellate ganglion, transverse section at the level of C6/7.

patient does not indicate any symptoms (pain, eye flashes, dizziness), another 2 mL procaine 1% is slowly infiltrated. With the correct needle position, the medication distributes itself in the craniocaudal direction over 2 to 4 cm (fascia progression of the longus colli muscle) and thus reaches the cervical sympathetic trunk and the stellate ganglion. Thus, the injection is an injection to the sympathetic trunk and ganglia. Generally, after about 1 to 4 minutes, the Horner symptom complex (myosis, ptosis, enophthalmos) indicates the proper injection.
- The remaining palpating finger prevents injury to the pleura during the injection and inadvertent intra-arterial injection (common carotid artery; ▶Fig. 17.10).

Through feedback, double aspiration ensures extravascular and extrathecal placement of the needle. Bone contact to the transverse process of the sixth or seventh cervical vertebra prevents an accidental change in the needle position.

Note

The simple-sounding instruction to always perform the entire injection procedure slowly, from palpation to removal of the needle, is actually very important. The few seconds gained with a quick injection to the stellate ganglion never outweigh the potential increase in injection errors associated with this!

Risks

Risks associated with noncompliance with the described injection technique:
- Intra-arterial injection (common carotid artery) with centralized toxic reaction (p. 38).
- Intrathecal injection (high spinal anesthesia).
- Pleura injury with occurrence of pneumothorax.

General Clinical Symptoms

The following can occur with injection to the stellate ganglion:
- Initial slight circulatory depression and slight slowing of the pulse.
- Slight dizziness.
- Congested feeling in the half of the nose on the same side (Guttmann's sign).
- Horner's symptom complex (ptosis, myosis, enophthal -mus).
- Increased vascularity of the sclera.
- Feeling of warmth in the half of the head on the same side, the upper extremity, and the chest area.

The description of other techniques for injection at the stellate ganglion will be omitted because these techniques are difficult, partly unpleasant for the patient, and more risky. In addition to verifying the correct injection performance through the presence of the Horner symptom complex, it is very important to observe the treated symptomology after injection to the stellate ganglion.

If there is no Horner's symptom complex and no change in the symptomology (even beyond the anesthesia time of the procaine), the procaine has not reached the stellate ganglion or the sympathetic cervical trunk. The injection should be repeated without delay. If there is no complex of symptoms, but the treated symptoms are improved or eliminated beyond the anesthesia period of the procaine, repeated injection until the symptomology subsides is indicated. The same procedure applies with the occurrence of the symptom complex with improvement or cessation of the symptomology. If the Horner symptom complex occurs without a change in the treated symptomology beyond the anesthesia time, further injections to the stellate ganglion are not therapeutically indicated. The same applies to temporary worsening or subsequent improvement of the treated symptomology. In such patients, the presence of an interference field disease is highly likely.

17.3.4 Material

Required:
- 5-mL syringe.
- 0.5 × 40 mm needle.
- Procaine 1%, 2 to 3 mL per injection.

17.4 Injection to the Superior Cervical Ganglion

17.4.1 Indications

The indications given are only a sample of those possible:
- Chronic headache.
- Cerebral circulation disorders.
- Postapoplectic symptoms.
- Vertigo.
- Depression after brain disease or injury.
- Cognitive brain disorders (e.g., onset of dementia).
- Tinnitus.
- Meniere's disease.
- Hearing loss research.
- Ozena research.
- Chronic sinus infections.
- Allergic disposition.
- Polyvalent allergies with sinusitis.
- Chronic inflammatory disorders of the eye, ears, and throat.

The expected success depends, among other things, on the the patient's "interference field situation."

17.4.2 Anatomy and Neurophysiology

Isolated injection of a local anesthetic to the superior cervical ganglion is not technically possible. The reason for this is the dense proximity to other nerves and vessels as well as the direct interganglionic connection to these. Therefore, this injection also reaches other important structures.

As a proximal sympathetic trunk ganglion of the neck, the superior cervical ganglion is before the second to fourth cervical vertebra transverse process on the longus capitis muscle, mediodorsal to the internal carotid artery and the vagus nerve (▶Fig. 17.11, ▶Fig. 17.12). The preganglionic fibers from C8–T6 arising from the corresponding sympathetic nuclei regions of the bone marrow are switched to the second neuron in this ganglion and basically supply the head, the vascular system of the brain, the neck to C4, the neck organs, and the heart. On the one hand, the preganglionic fibers proceed with the spinal nerves (C1–C4) and vessels (internal carotid artery, external carotid artery) to the target organs. On the other hand, they proceed as the superior cardiac nerve freely to the right brachiocephalic trunk and left common carotid artery in order to reach the cardiac plexus with these vessels.

Note

Particularly in the context of neural therapy, the direct sympathetic connection to the vagus nerve along with the connection to the hypoglossal nerve appears to be very important for vasomotor function of the tongue.

This connection exists between the superior cervical ganglion to the superior ganglion of the vagus nerve as well as the inferior ganglion of the glossopharyngeal nerve via the jugular nerve. The sympathetic interganglionic connection to the vagus nerve suggests that increased or reduced sympathetic activity results in simultaneous linear changes in the activity of the parasympathetic nervous system. Clinical indications so far suggest this, as the stellate sympathetic trunk blockade in asthmatics causes immediate bronchospasmolysis and reduced secretion, both of which are activities of the parasympathetic nervous system. Since the stellate blockade performed according to the neural therapy technique at the level of C6–C7 definitely rules out simultaneous suppression of the vagus nerve, the elimination or significant reduction in asthmatic symptoms can only be explained by sympatholysis, predetermined through the interganglionic connection between the superior cervical ganglion and the superior ganglion of the vagus nerve through the jugular nerve. Without this interganglionic connection, the stellate blockade would lead to an intensification of asthma symptoms since the activity of the parasympathetic nervous system would predominate.

Based on the neural connection between the sympathetic nervous system and the parasympathetic nervous system, injection to the superior cervical ganglion is the strongest form of regulating influence on the autonomic system. As mentioned, the infiltration is made to the superior cervical ganglion with simultaneous infiltration of the vagus nerve or the inferior ganglion of the vagus nerve, i.e., a one-step reduction of the sympathetic and vagus function.

This is probably also the reason for the injection's very positive effect (▶Fig. 17.13, ▶Fig. 17.14) on pulmonary diseases, namely, bronchial asthma as well as allergic disorders without particular consideration of the allergen.[77] Certainly, in the case of asthma, not only is bronchodilation via reduced parasympathetic activity to be seen as an effect of the infiltration to the superior cervical ganglion, but also the simultaneous improvement (through sympatholysis) of the overall perfusion in the range of the cervical sympathetic nervous system. The affected organs are, among others, the hormone-producing pituitary gland, the pineal gland, and the neurotransmitter-producing hypothalamus region.

Using the example of bronchial asthma in connection with an injection to the superior cervical ganglion, an attempt will be made to show the regulatory effect of this injection. The list of indications is certainly not complete, since this injection is not well known and experimental results are only available to a small extent. However, when considering the neural structure with its function in the body and the many possible disorders associated with different diseases, the therapeutic benefit has certainly not been fully exploited yet.

The following are the results of an injection in the area of the superior cervical ganglion and the subsequent interruption of the neural structure present here:

- Superior cervical ganglion (sympathetic nervous system): Horner's symptom complex (myosis, ptosis, enophthalmus), Guttmann's sign, feeling of warmth in the half of the head on the same side, slight dizziness.
- Inferior ganglion of the vagus nerves: Hyperesthesia or anesthesia of the posterior pharyngeal wall, the tongue base, the larynx, a portion of the ear canal, rarely unilateral vocal cord paresis (recurrent laryngeal nerve), slight acceleration of the pulse and increase in blood pressure, and reduced activity of the pharynx muscle, the esophagus, and gastrointestinal tract

Note

It is important to note that suppression of the right or left vagus nerve can cause various reactions in the heart (vagus asymmetry).

The interruption of the vagus function on the right results in slight tachycardia since it controls the sinus node function (carotid-sinus reflex). The left vagus nerve controls the function of the atrioventricular node (nodus atrioventricularis). Pharmacological interruption of this nerve causes slight, reversible prolongation of the AV time. These reactions of the right or left vagus blockade do not elapse as clearly, since the sympathetic nervous system function is reduced in the heart.

Other nerves reached with the injection are:

- Glossopharyngeal nerve: Hyperesthesia or anesthesia of the mucous membrane of the pharynx, the tonsils, the

posterior third of the tongue, the epiglottis, and paralysis of the soft palate. A feeling of a lump occurs in the throat, along with an urge to swallow this lump. Due to the loss of sensitivity in the epiglottis, neither liquid nor food should be consumed until the nerve interruption has subsided.
- Hypoglossal nerve: Partial paralysis of the tongue musculature (one-sided) occurs.
- Perivascular sympathetic plexus of the internal carotid artery, sometimes also the external carotid artery: Through sympatholysis, vasodilation occurs in the supply area of the two arteries with corresponding improvement in circulation.
- Superior cervical ganglion: The improved perfusion of the ganglion alone is certainly therapeutically valuable, since the metabolism of this neuronal structure is crucial to the function, e.g., in the case of Raynaud's disease or collagenosis, in which there is a ganglionic degenerative-inflammatory disorder of the ganglion.[488]

17.4.3 Injection Technique

The technique for injection to the superior cervical ganglion is relatively simple, with the two different methods described in the following:
1. The injection, modified according to Orsoni, corresponds to retrostyloid infiltration, the same technique with which the glossopharyngeal nerve and vagus nerve can be reached. Since the superior cervical ganglion is farthest from the puncture point in this technique, the infiltration depth is greater, as is the infiltration quantity (3–5 mL).
2. The technique in the direction of the retropharyngeal space comes from ear-nose-throat medicine and the practice of tonsillectomy under local anesthesia.

Technique According to Orsoni

Palpation of the styloid process between the posterior lower edge of the jaw and edge of the mastoid. With the patient's mouth closed, insertion of the 4 cm long needle at the intersection of the front edge line of the mastoid with the lower edge of the mandible (▶Fig. 17.15). At about 3 to 4 cm depth, the needle strikes the transverse process of C2. After slightly pulling back the needle, it is pushed further forward another 0.5 cm directly ventral to the transverse process. The tip of the needle is now in front of the longus capitis muscle and laterally behind the vascular nerve bundle (internal carotid artery, internal jugular vein, vagus nerve, glossopharyngeal nerve, superior cervical ganglion, hypoglossal nerve) in the retropharyngeal space. Aspiration with 180° rotation of the needle is performed. If blood or CSF is aspirated, start slow infiltration of 0.2 to 0.5 mL procaine 1%. If neither pain nor flashes in front of the eyes occur, another 3 to 4 mL procaine is slowly infiltrated and the needle is removed.

Technique According to Göbel

Visualize the back wall of the throat by opening the patient's mouth wide and slightly pushing down the tongue with the tongue depressor. The line connecting the upper and lower poles of the tonsils indicates the position of the second cervical vertebra, whose transverse processes are in the same horizontal plane. The puncture point is about 0.5 cm from the medial tonsil edge at the level of the center of the tonsils. The 8 cm long needle is inserted about 1.5 cm deep diagonally in the lateral direction, approximately at an angle of 20°, and slid past the C2 vertebra (▶Fig. 17.16). The needle tip is now in the retropharyngeal space immediately before the vascular nerve bundle, directly at the level of the superior cervical ganglion. The proximal end of the needle is at the level of the third to fourth tooth on the opposite side of the lower jaw. After two-time negative aspiration with rotation of the needle by 180°, 0.2 to 0.4 mL procaine 1% is infiltrated. If the patient indicates no symptoms, 2 mL procaine is slowly injected and the needle is removed. An intrathecal needle position is not possible with this injection technique.

Cave

The injection to the superior cervical ganglion should only be performed on one side per day. With simultaneous bilateral injection, bilateral recurrent nerve paresis with respiratory distress can occur along with circulatory dysregulation.

17.4.4 Material

Required:
- Technique according to Orsoni:
  - 5-mL syringe.
  - 0.4 × 40 mm needle.
  - Procaine 1%, 3 to 5 mL per injection.
- Technique according to Göbel:
  - 5-mL syringe.
  - 0.6 × 80 mm needle.
  - Procaine 1%, 2 mL per injection.

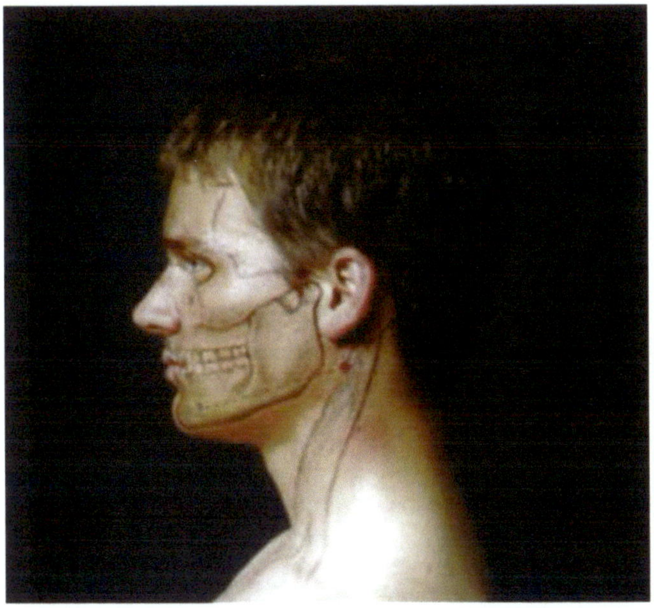

► **Fig. 17.11** Puncture point for injection to the superior cervical ganglion.

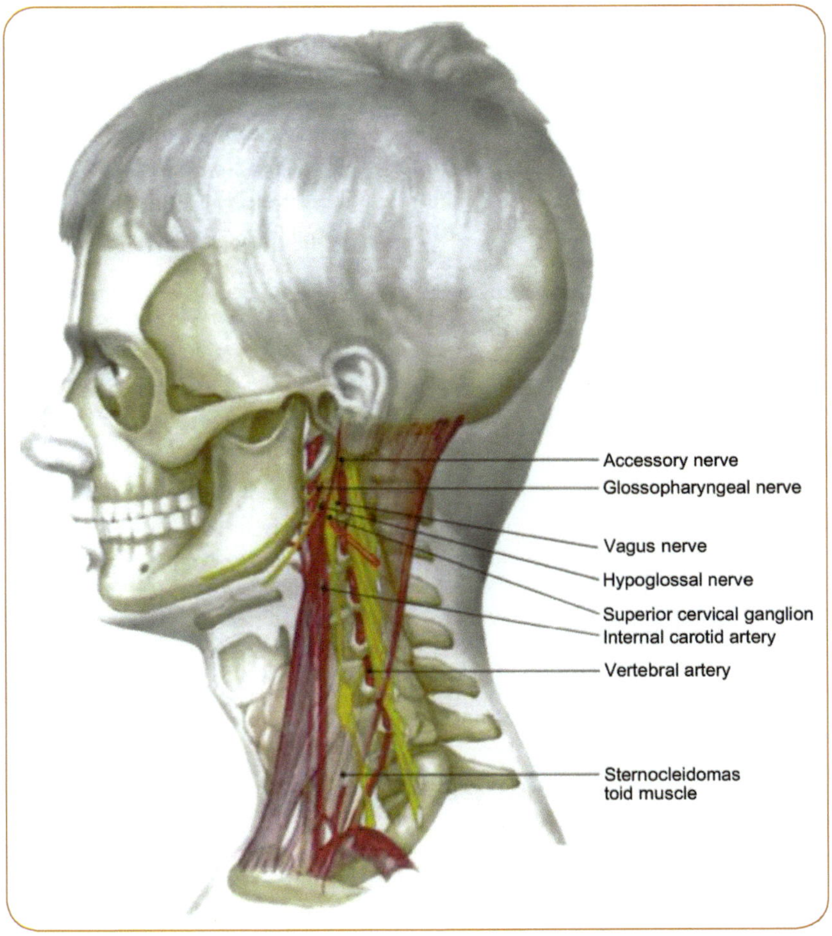

► **Fig. 17.12** Topography of the superior cervical ganglion, side view.

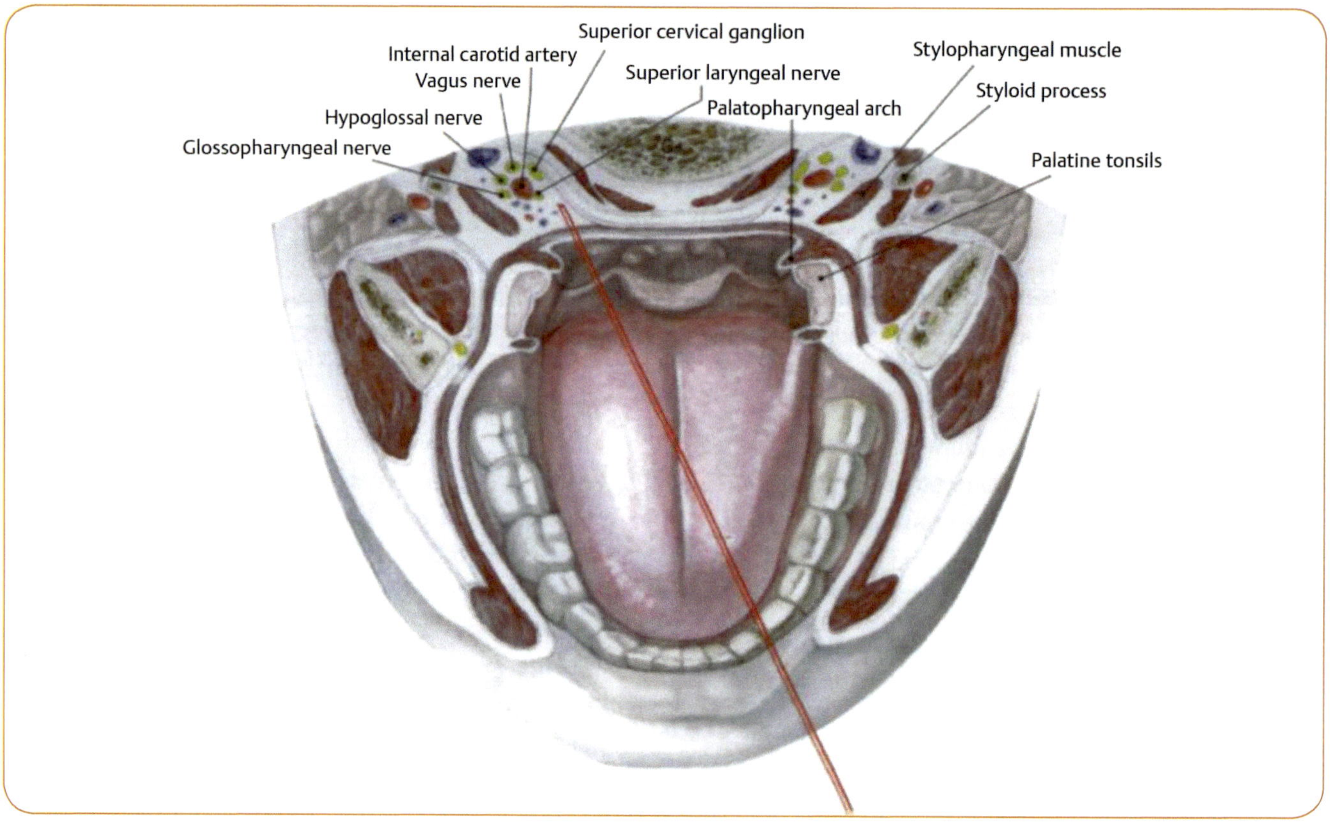

► **Fig. 17.13** Topography for injection to the superior cervical ganglion.

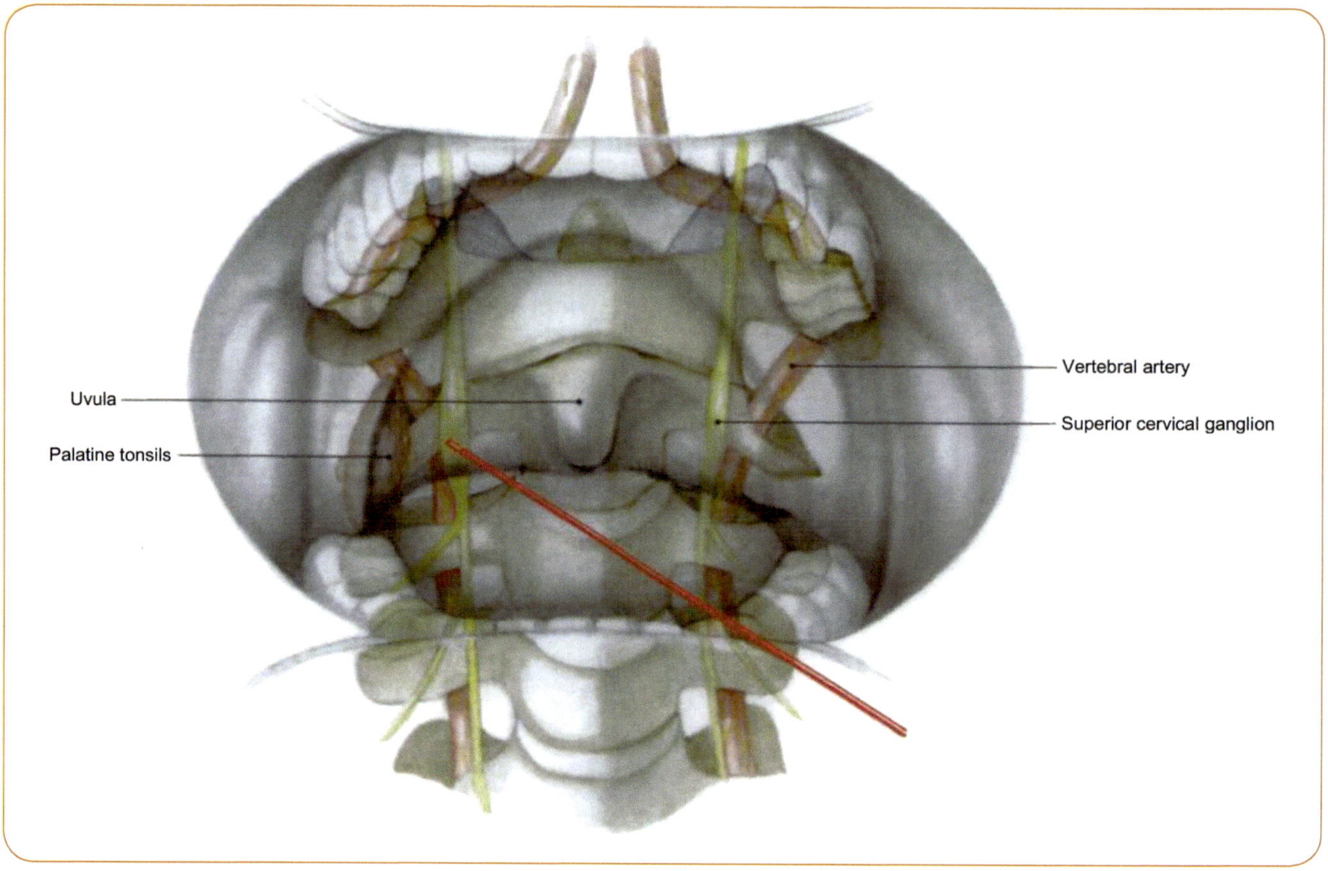

► **Fig. 17.14** Transparent topography for injection to the superior cervical ganglion (according to Göbel).

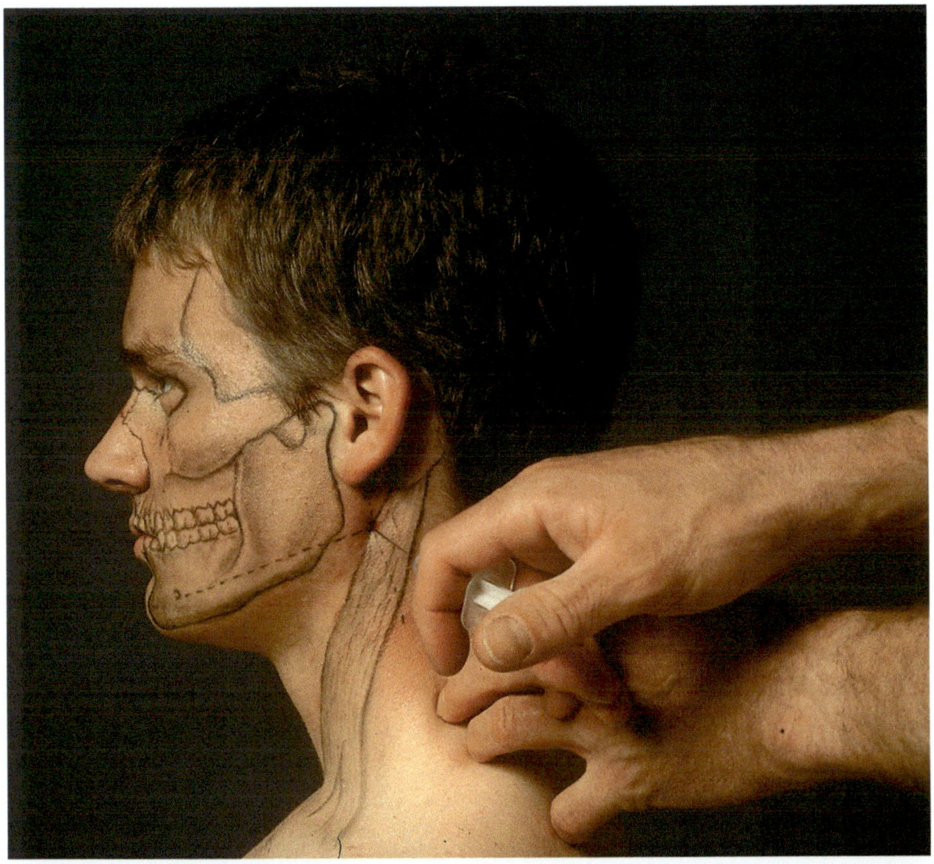

► **Fig. 17.15** Injection to the left superior cervical ganglion (retrostyloid space, technique according to Orsoni).

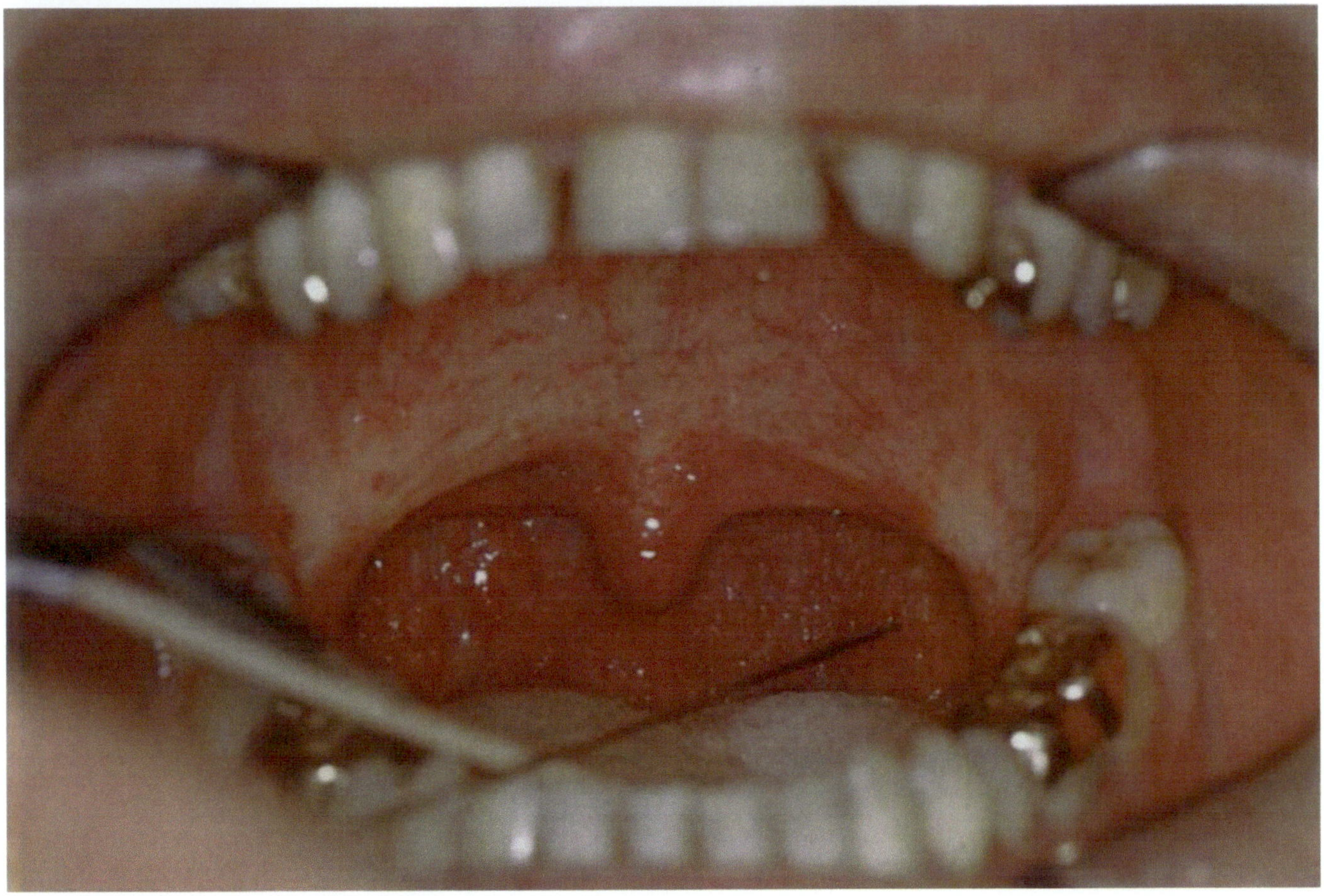

► **Fig. 17.16** Injection to the left superior cervical ganglion (technique according to Göbel).

17.5 Injection to the Accessory Nerve, Great Auricular Nerve, Transverse Cervical Nerve, and Lesser Occipital Nerve (Punctum Nervosum)

17.5.1 Indications

The indications given are only a sample of those possible:

- Neuralgia of the great auricular nerve, transverse cervical nerve, cervical loop of the facial nerve, and the lesser occipital nerve.
- Unexplained pain in the region of the ear, the mandibular angle, and the lateral occiput.
- Spasmodic torticollis.
- Dizziness.

The expected success depends, among other things, on the the patient's "interference field situation."

17.5.2 Anatomy and Neurophysiology

The anatomical term "punctum nervosum" indicates the point in the middle of the posterior edge of the sternocleidomastoid muscle. Cervical nerves from segments C2 and C3 as well as the accessory nerve (11th cranial nerve)—whose root area stretches from the caudal third of the olive to cervical segment C6—spread out from the sternocleidomastoid muscle into the further periphery. Part of the accessory nerve finer bundle (internal branch) connects to the vagus nerve and distributes itself further via the pharyngeal branches, the laryngeal branches, and the cardiac branches. The external branch of the accessory nerve comes from the spinal nucleic region of this cranial nerve, has purely motor function, and supplies the major portion of the sternocleidomastoid muscle and the middle and lower part of the trapezius muscle. The upper portion of the trapezius muscle is also supplied from cervical segments C3 and C4.

The great auricular nerve (C3), lesser occipital nerve (C2 and C3), and transverse cervical nerve (C2 and C3) provide sensory supply to the skin of the chin, the neck, the ear, and the neck and shoulder region. Like all remaining spinal nerves, the spinal nerves from the cervical plexus (C1–C4) contain less myelinated and nonmyelinated fibers from the cervical sympathetic trunk. Sympathetic fibers proceed with the spinal nerves in the periphery and supply the skin, the vessels, and the cutaneous glands.

Therefore, infiltration of the punctum nervosum with a local anesthetic triggers not only motor paralysis (accessory nerve) and anesthesia (great auricular nerve, lesser occipital nerve, transverse cervical nerve) in the corresponding skin region. Sympatholysis results in improved circulation in the tissue section supplied by the spinal nerves and the cranial nerves, which is demonstrated by a feeling of warmth in the region.

17.5.3 Injection Technique

Palpation of the posterior edge of the sternocleidomastoid muscle. The injection is made at the level of the muscle bisector (▶Fig. 17.17, ▶Fig. 17.18). After two-time aspiration, 2 to 3 mL procaine is infiltrated at a depth of 1 to 1.5 cm. Correct injection is indicated by a feeling of warmth in the lateral neck region, hyperesthesia to anesthesia of the skin, and relaxation of the sternocleidomastoid muscle and trapezius muscle.

17.5.4 Material

Required:

- 5-mL syringe.
- 0.4 × 40 mm needle.
- Procaine 1%, 2 to 3 mL per injection.

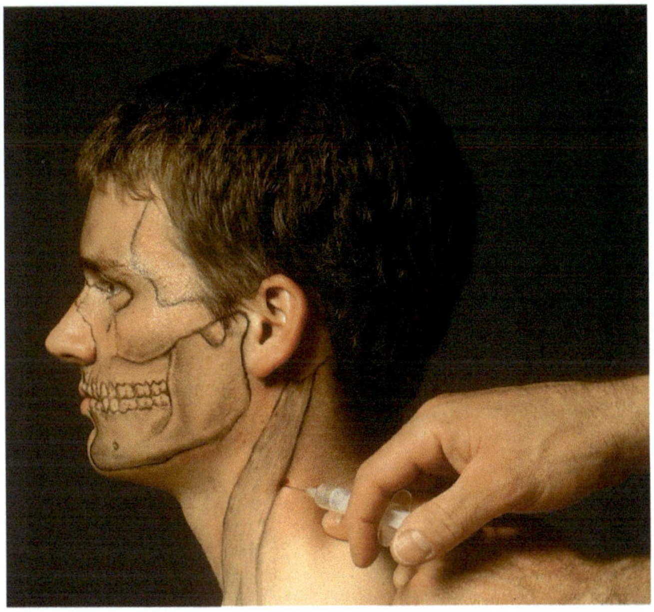

► **Fig. 17.17** Puncture point (punctum nervosum).

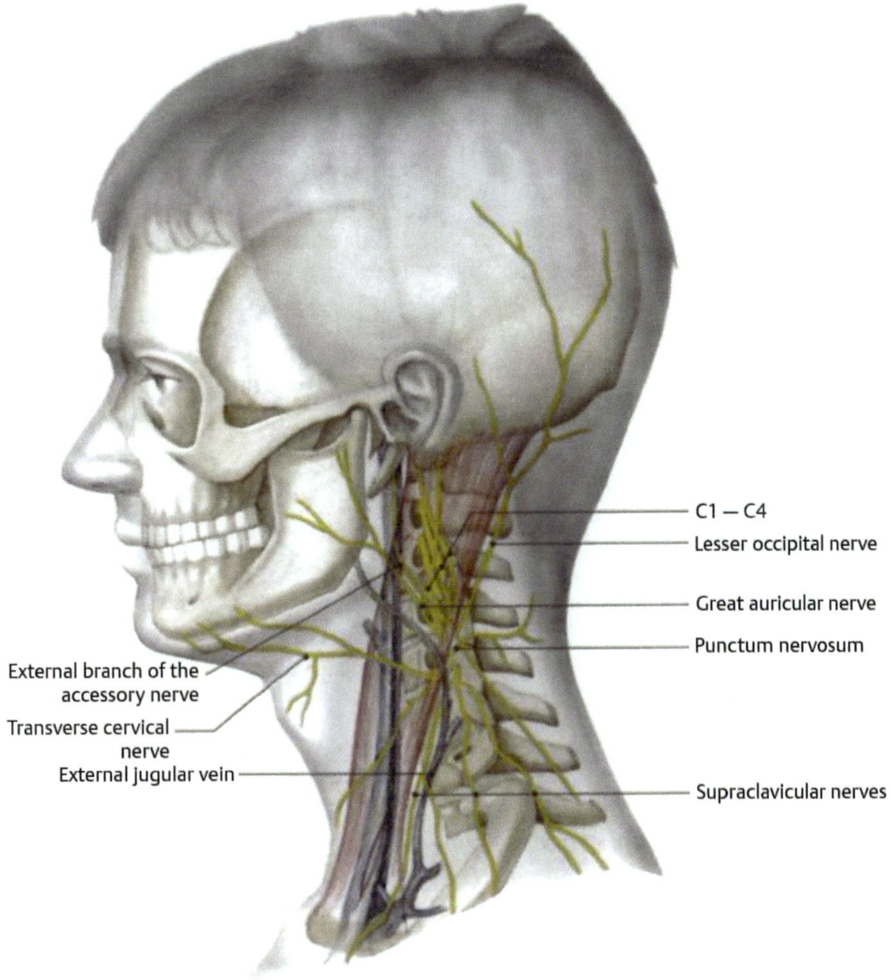

► **Fig. 17.18** Topography of the "punctum nervosum."

18 Spine

18.1 Information on Diagnostics

In order to understand the neural therapeutic treatment of the spine, some explanation is required regarding both the anatomy and especially the nerve supply of the spine and its structures controlling static and dynamic functions, i.e., ligament, joint capsule, and the muscles. Disregarding the central control mechanisms, we will discuss only the innervation relationships at the spinal level in order to demonstrate the neurophysiological background of neural therapeutic treatment. In particular, each injection of a local anesthetic to an anatomically defined structure, e.g., to the spinous processes, the vertebral joints, the ligaments, muscles, and spinal nerves, is only therapeutically significant if the injection reaches the sympathetic nervous system at the same time. Otherwise, the result would be only temporary local anesthesia or muscle paralysis.

The spinal nervous system is divided segmentally, which is indicated by the nomenclature of the nerves. Segment L5, for example, refers to the spinal nerve and its innervation area which originates in the fifth lumbar segment of the spinal cord. The spinous process of the fifth lumbar vertebra serves as a clinical point of orientation, although the topographical position of the fifth lumbar spinal cord segment is at the level of the twelfth thoracic vertebra. The spinal nervous system comprises 8 cervical segments, 12 thoracic segments, 5 lumbar segments, 5 sacral segments, and a coccygeal segment.

The sympathetic nervous system has its root areas in segments C8–L3 and is not strictly segmentally split in its further peripheral distribution. According to the divergence principle, one sympathetic nucleic region supplies multiple spinal segments. The distribution of the sympathetic nervous system in the periphery is relevant to neural therapy. Sympathetic nerves, in fact the efferent as well as the afferent nerves, proceed together with the spinal nerves and the vessels in order to reach their supply area. This explains why each tissue structure with spinal innervation and arterial supply always has sympathetic innervation as well. The vessel or the spinal nerve, like all other tissue structures, are chosen from a neural therapeutic perspective only for the purpose of reaching the sympathetic nervous system. The afferent fibers of the sympathetic nervous system proceed—exactly like the remaining afferent fibers—via the dorsal root of the spinal cord. The nerve cells for this are in the spinal ganglia and the sympathetic trunk ganglia. Reflex arcs on the spinal level require the synaptic connection between afferent and efferent neurons, namely in the form of monosynaptic (direct) and polysynaptic (indirect) reflex pathways via switching neurons, regardless of the affiliation to the somatic or visceral nervous system. Intrasegmentally as well as intersegmentally, i.e., via multiple segment levels, the interneurons conduct the impulses arriving via the afferent fibers. This includes, among others, the switching cells, the association cells, and the commissural cells. This can help us to understand the known viscerovisceral, viscerosomatic, and somatovisceral reflexes, e.g., hyperesthesias of the skin and hypertension of the corresponding segmentally supplied muscle in diseases of the thoracic and abdominal organs. The clinically derived experiences of Mackenzie and Head may serve as evidence of these relationships.[317]

Taking into account the previous statements, the segmentally structured spine "axis organ" is interesting with regard to three aspects of neural therapy:

1. The orthopaedic treatment of the spine, the joints, the ligaments, and the musculature is possible via the sympathetic nervous system.
2. Disorders of the extremities with their joints, ligament structures, vessels, nerves, and musculature can be reached through neural therapy.
3. Internal disorders of the chest and abdominal space as well as gynecological, urological, and andrological disorders can be treated via the corresponding segments. This is accomplished by the clinically detectable, somatic changes of the skin, the musculature, and the spinal cord function, which occur reflexively via the stimuli of the afferent sympathetic nervous system.

18.2 Information on Therapy

The neural therapeutic treatment of the spine and the reflexively progressing disorder is based on the targeted infiltration of a local anesthetic in and to the diseased segment. Initially, a series of wheals is injected on both sides of the spinal cord section, at intervals of 3 to 4 cm lateral to the spinous process line, as well as above and between the spinous processes of the spinous process sequence itself. Geloses of the subcutis are easily palpated and infiltrated with the local anesthetic. With subtle palpation, the paravertebral musculature exhibits hypertonic, strandlike areas sensitive to pressure, which are also infiltrated at the site of maximum pressure pain with a small quantity of the local anesthetic. The infiltration of the ligament and capsular structure is detailed in the following, as well as the injection to the spinal nerves and the sympathetic trunk, since the technique for this is somewhat more complicated.

The basic goal of the treatment is to use stimulus therapy through a wheal series to reach each irritated tissue structure through the reflexive pathway—precisely and with small amounts of the local anesthetic—in order to eliminate "on-site" the impaired tissue perfusion progressing via stimulus to the sympathetic nervous system.

18.3 Injection to the Cervical Spine

18.3.1 Indications

The indications given are only a sample of those possible:

- Painful restricted movement of the cervical spine after trauma.
- Pseudoradicular discomfort of the upper extremity and shoulder girdle.
- Root irritation of the cervical plexus and brachial plexus.
- Myotendinoses.
- Periarthropathy of the upper extremity.
- Spondylodiscitis.
- Cervicobrachialgia.

The expected success depends, among other things, on the the patient's "interference field situation."

18.3.2 Anatomy and Neurophysiology

The cervical spine consisting of seven vertebrae is the osseous basis for the connection of the head to the torso (▶ Fig. 18.1, ▶ Fig. 18.2a,b). In addition to this static function, it enables head movements at three levels, consisting of flexion, rotation, and lateral bending. Problem-free operation of these functions requires undisturbed interaction of the capsular ligament system and the muscles. The static and dynamic functions of the cervical spine are controlled primarily on afferent–efferent pathways via the spinal nerve system. Proper functioning is further bound to the unimpaired and necessary microcirculation of the individual tissue components of the cervical spine, including the spinal nervous system, which in turn is directly related to the unimpaired function of the sympathetic nervous system.

The spinal nerve system and the sympathetic nervous system are connected to each other via intra- and intersegmental pathways, so that stimulation of the spinal nerve system causes stimulation of the sympathetic nervous system, while stimulation of the sympathetic nervous system causes stimulation of the spinal nerve system.

Of further clinical significance is the synaptic connection between the upper two to three cervical spinal segments and the spinal nucleic region of the trigeminal nerve, which reaches up to the level of C2–C3. Thus, in disorders of the trigeminal nerve, especially in the teeth and sinuses, irritation in segments C1–C3 is regularly detectable. With longstanding chronic diseases, muscle tension, "blocked" vertebral joints, and root irritation can be found in deeper sections.

Since parts of the glossopharyngeal nerve, which supplies the palatine tonsils, are connected directly to the spinal root of the trigeminal nerve as well as the root areas of the accessory nerve (sternocleidomastoid muscle, trapezius muscle) reaching C1–C6, reflexive tensions of the cervical muscles and functional disorders of the cervical spine are understandable with chronic diseases of the tonsils.[69] In this case, neural therapeutic treatment of the tonsils is causal, and therapy of the cervical spine is futile.

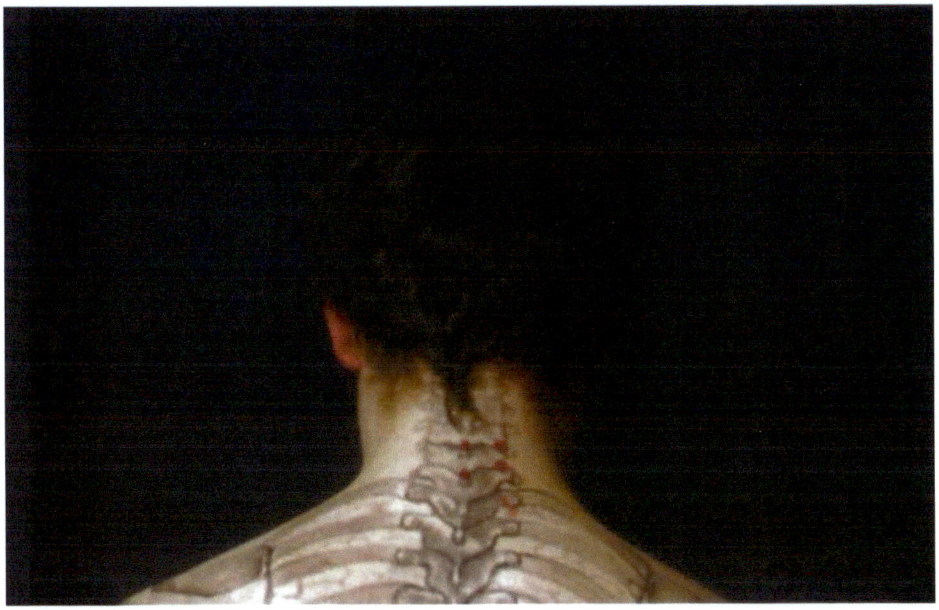

▸**Fig. 18.1** Injection to vertebral joints and spinous processes of the cervical spine.

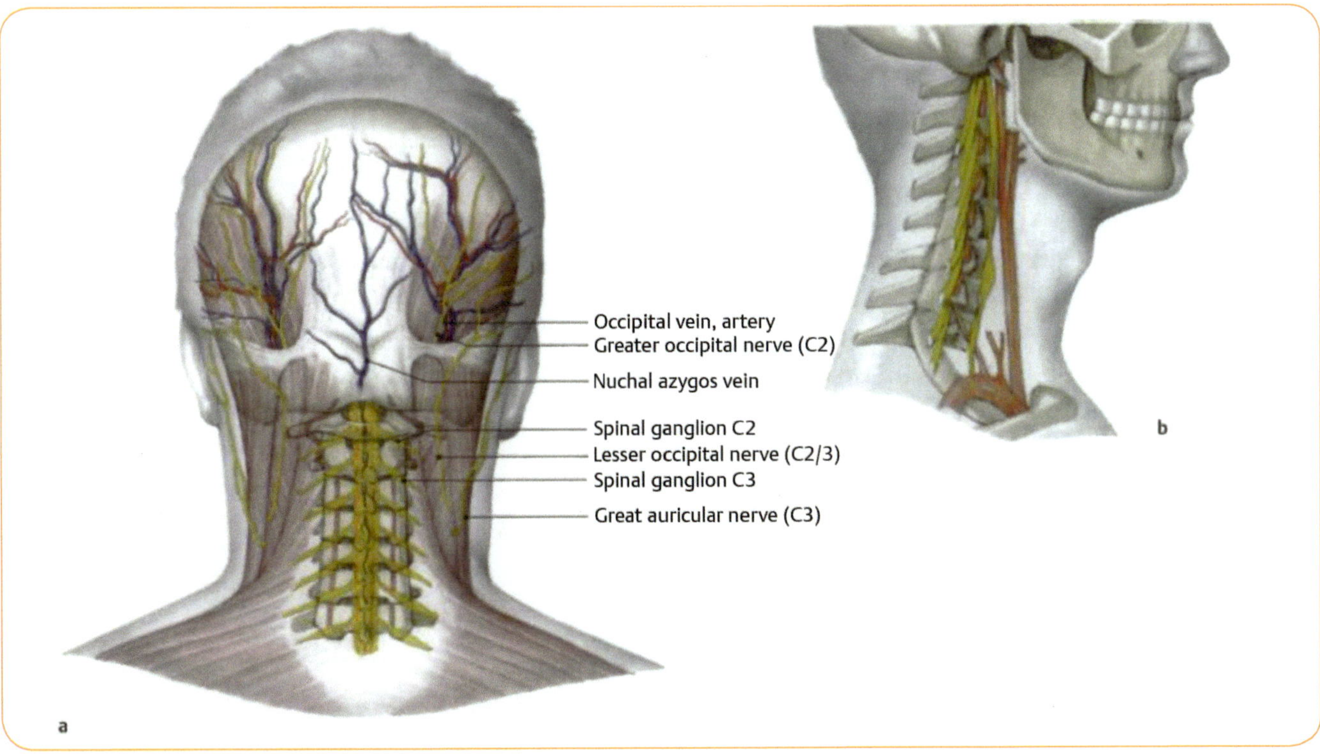

▸**Fig. 18.2** **(a)** Topography for injection to the cervical spine. **(b)** Lateral view of the cervical spine with exit of the spinal nerves, cervical sympathetic trunk, carotid artery, and vertebral artery.

18.3.3 Injection Technique

▶**Spinous processes.** At the start of the treatment, a series of wheals should be injected over the spinous processes of the cervical spine as well as paravertebral with an interval of 3 cm each at the level of the spinous processes. Depending on palpation findings, local subcutaneous geloses or hypertonic muscle strands are infiltrated with 0.2 to 0.5 mL procaine at the point of maximum pressure pain.

Note

Except in the case of the wheal, the extravascular and extrathecal needle position must be ensured by aspiration before each infiltration.

The spinous processes of the spine are the only definitely palpable bony structures of the spine for the differentiation of the vertebra, which can be taken as reference points for all injections in the spine. The irritated structure is usually painful upon pressure. Starting with the spinous process C2, which is palpable in the suboccipital region as the first prominent spinous process down to the next readily palpable spinous process C7 (vertebra prominens) and the spinous process of the sixth cervical vertebrae. The target of the injection is the spinous process with pressure pain (▶Fig. 18.3) and the interspinous space. After digital identification of the spinous process, and with a slightly antiflected head, the 12-gauge needle is inserted with light infiltration between the spinous processes up to a 1 to 2 cm depth. Aspiration with 180° rotation of the needle is performed. After a negative suction test, 0.5 to 1 mL is infiltrated.

▶**Vertebral joints.** The vertebral joints of the cervical spine are at the level of the spinous processes, each 2 cm lateral to the spinous process line. Here, the puncture site is perpendicular to the skin (▶Fig. 18.4). Advance the 4-cm-long needle until it makes contact with the bone at a depth of 2.5 to 3.5 cm. After aspiration in two levels and a negative suction test, slowly infiltrate 1 mL.

▶**Spinal nerves C5–C8** (**brachial plexus**). Palpation of the spinous processes and identification of the spinous process with pressure pain by counting down from C2 and upward from C7. The needle is inserted—with the patient's head slightly bent forward—2 cm lateral to the spinous process line and level with the lower edge of the spinous process (▶Fig. 18.5). The 6-cm-long needle is inserted vertically to the skin and advanced to bone contact (vertebral joints). Retraction of the needle into the subcutis and re-advancement with slightly lateral needle direction, at a maximum of 1 cm deeper than the skin–vertebral joint distance specifies. Aspiration with 180° rotation of the needle and slow infiltration of 2 to 3 mL with negative suction test are performed. Intravascular and intrathecal needle position must always be ruled out by aspiration.

18.3.4 Material

Required:

- Needle length: 4 cm (spinous processes), 4 cm (vertebral joints), 6 cm (spinal nerves C5–C8).
- 5-mL syringe.
- Procaine 1%, per injection:
  - To the spinous processes: 0.5 to 1 mL.
  - To the vertebral joints: 1 mL.
  - To spinal nerves C5–C8: 2 to 3 mL.

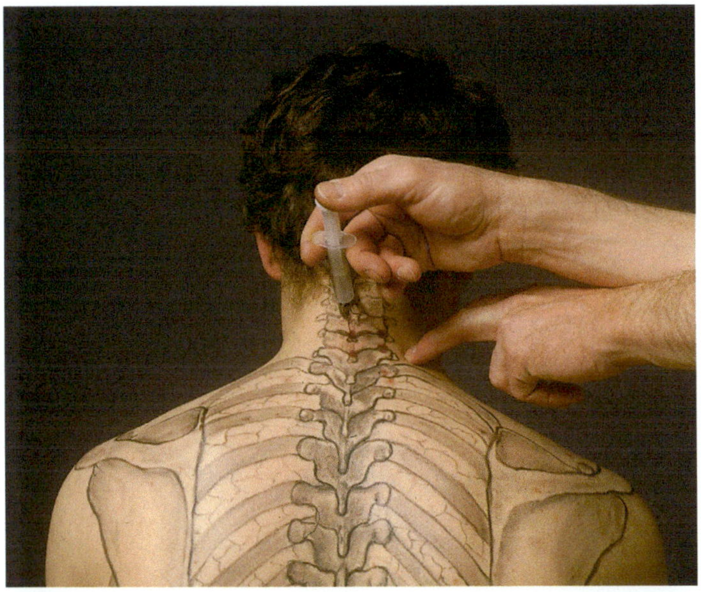

►**Fig. 18.3** Injection to the spinous processes of the cervical spine.

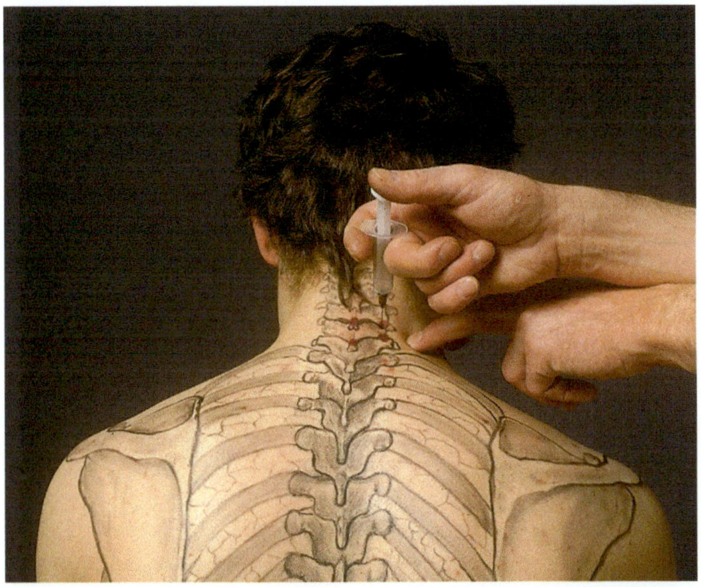

►**Fig. 18.4** Injection to the vertebral joints of the cervical spine.

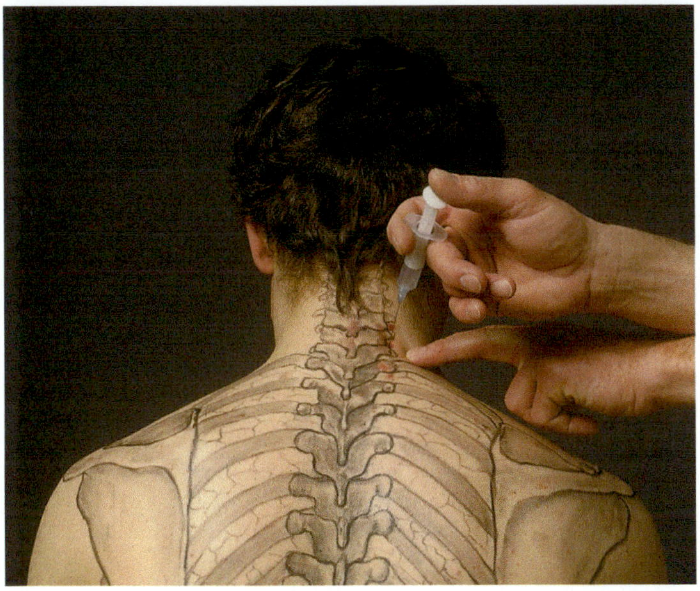

►**Fig. 18.5** Injection to the spinal nerves of the cervical spine.

18.4 Injection to the Thoracic Spine

18.4.1 Indications

The indications given are only a sample of those possible:

- Painful restricted movement of the thoracic spine and ribs after trauma.
- Rib fracture.
- Vertebra fracture.
- Intercostal neuralgia.
- Herpes zoster.
- Myotendinoses.
- Spondylitis
- Reflexive-segmental function impairment in disorders of:
  - The heart (T1–T5).
  - The bronchia and lungs (T1–T4).
  - The pancreas (T6–T10).
  - The liver and the gall bladder (T6–T9).
  - The stomach (T6–T9).
  - The small intestine (T7–L1).
  - The large intestine (T7–L1).
  - The kidneys (T10–L1).
  - The urogenital tract (T10–L2).

The expected success depends, among other things, on the the patient's "interference field situation."

18.4.2 Anatomy and Neurophysiology

The 12 vertebrae of the thoracic spine differ significantly from the other vertebrae in their structure and function. On the one hand, the tip of the spinous process, which is drawn out lengthwise in caudal direction , is at the level of the next lower thoracic vertebra, which should be taken into account in the orientation of the remaining spinal sections and the segmental correlation. On the other hand, the jointed connection to the ribs at the vertebral body and at the transverse process, and the resulting change in the spinal movement, must be particularly taken into account during rotation movements. The segmental division of the nervous system is most clearly delineated in the thoracic region; the course of the ribs is also the "track" of the nerve distribution for both the afferent–efferent somatic as well as the afferent–efferent sympathetic system (► Fig. 18.6, ► Fig. 18.7). This spinal section is clearly useful diagnostically and therapeutically, particularly in allocating the sympathetically innervated organs of the thoracic and abdominal cavities to the corresponding segments of the thoracic spine.

Disorders of internal organs are almost always reflected in impaired functioning of the thoracic spine, whether through pain, muscle tension, position changes in the corresponding section of the thoracic spine, or sensory disturbances in the skin sections associated with the segments. Thus, after resolved or still-present hepatobiliary diseases, for example, the spinous processes of T6–T9 are often sensitive to pressure, the physiological thoracic kyphosis is steeply positioned in this area, and the musculature is tense and sensitive to pressure, with these features more pronounced on the right. On the other hand, irritations of a section of the thoracic spine often simulate diseases of the internal organs, e.g., angina with irritation of the first four thoracic vertebrae when this thoracic portion is overloaded.

In summary, chronic symptoms in the thoracic spine bring to mind both an illness or irritation in the thoracic spine itself and an illness in the internal organ corresponding to the segment, which uses a reflexive pathway to irritate and thus impair the function of this associated thoracic spinal section. The injection of a local anesthetic to the thoracic spine and thoracic structures named above leads to a reduction in the increased afferent nerve impulses related to disease, as well as the somatosensory and, above all, the sympathetic nervous system. After the resulting reduction in pain, muscle tension, and improved movement, circulation is improved via sympatholysis and in the corresponding thoracic segment and via the organ region supplied via the sympathetic reflex arc.

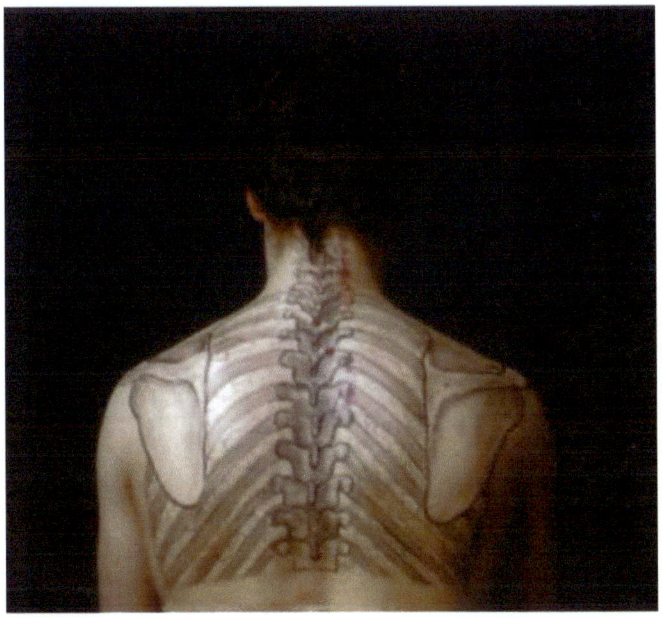

►Fig. 18.6 Injection to the spinous processes, vertebral, and costovertebral joints as well as the spinal nerves of the thoracic spine.

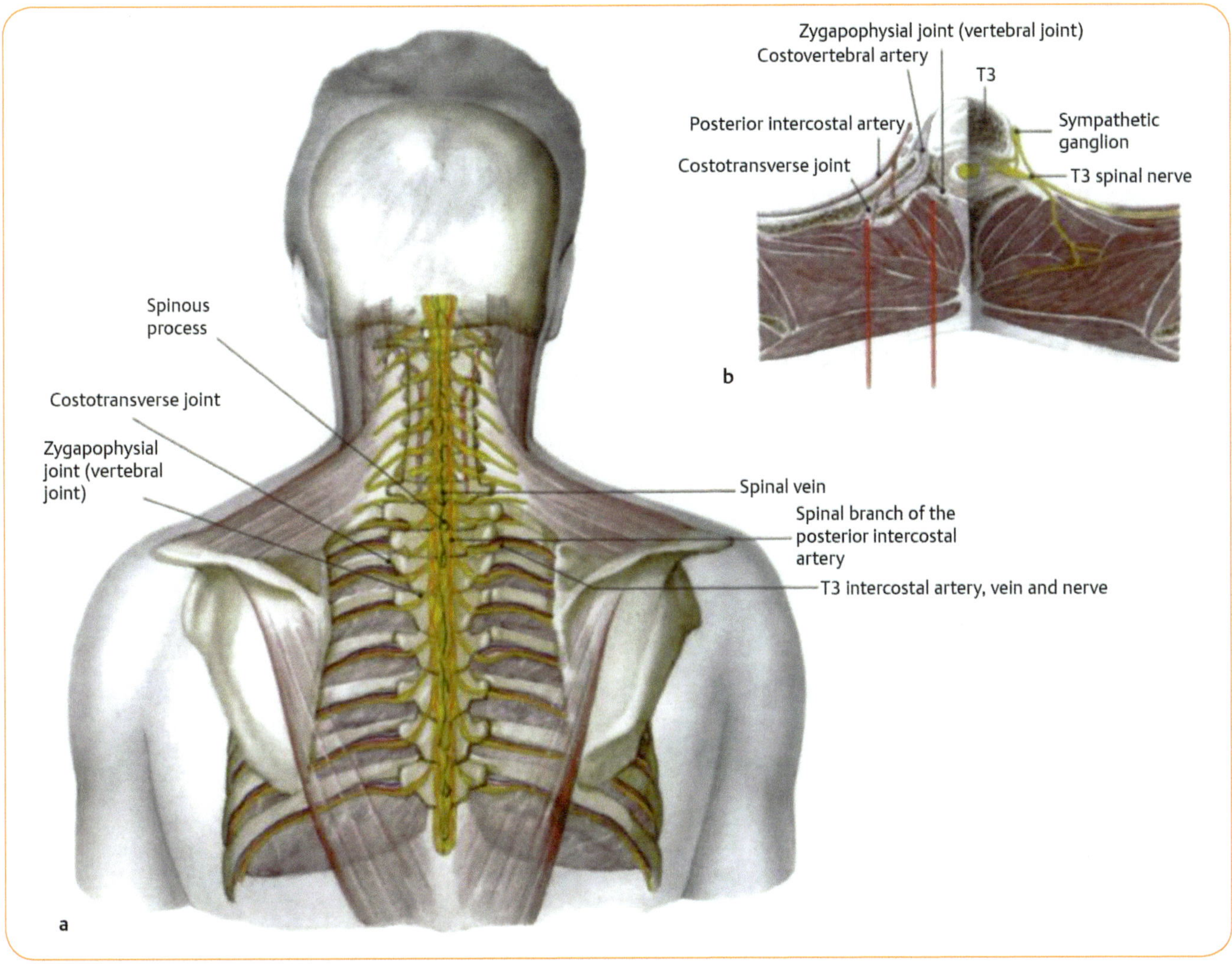

►Fig. 18.7 Topography for injection to the vertebral joints and costovertebral joints of the thoracic spine. **(a)** Topography for injection to the thoracic spine. **(b)** Transverse section for topography of the thoracic spine.

18.4.3 Injection Technique

At the start of the treatment, a wheal series is placed in the diseased thoracic spinal segment via the spinous processes and 3 to 4 cm paravertebral at the same level. The often tense paravertebral musculature is examined for maximum pressure points, and infiltrated with 0.2 to 0.5 mL procaine.

► **Spinous processes**. Bend the patient's body slightly forward and palpate the ends of the spinous processes. The injection is made with a 4-cm needle and the infiltration of 0.5 mL anesthetic, slight withdrawal of the needle, and re-injection at an angle of 45° in cranial direction (► Fig. 18.8). Then infiltration of 1 mL is made at 1.5 cm depth in the supraspinal ligament and the interspinal ligament.

► **Vertebral joints.** Palpation of the spinous processes. The injection point is at the level of the center between the lower spinous process ends and the next highest paramedial spinous process end perpendicular to the skin. The 4-cm-long needle is inserted in sagittal direction until it makes contact with bone at a depth of about 2.5 to 3.5 cm (► Fig. 18.9). Now the needle tip is directly in front of the vertebral joint. After double aspiration and 180° rotation of the needle, 1 mL is infiltrated.

► **Rib–vertebral joints**. Palpation of the spinous processes. The costovertebral joints associated with the thoracic vertebra are approximately at the level of the caudal tip of the next highest spinous process and 3 cm lateral to the spinous process line. The injection is made perpendicular to the vertebral joint—e.g., for the fifth thoracic vertebra it is located at the level of the spinous process end of T4 and 3 cm and lateral to the same (► Fig. 18.10). After about 3 to 3.5 cm depth (not deeper), the bone contact is in the correct needle position. Then, 1 mL is infiltrated after double aspiration and 180° rotation of the needle.

► **Intercostal nerves**. Palpation of the spinous process end. At 3 to 4 cm lateral to this palpable structure, the injection is made perpendicular to the skin with the needle directed slightly in cranial direction (about 5°) (► Fig. 18.11). After about 3 to 3.5 cm depth (in very thin patients, already at 2.5–3 cm depth), the needle makes contact with the rib. The needle tip is retracted and gently lowered; the needle tip may be advanced only 0.5 cm deeper when reinjecting, while the lower edge of the rib should be palpated if possible. Then, after double aspiration, 1 to 2 mL is infiltrated.

18.4.4 Material

Required:

- 5-mL syringe.
- 4 cm long needle.
- Procaine 1%.
- Per injection:
  - To the spinous processes: about 2 mL.
  - To the vertebral joints: about 1 mL.
  - To the rib–vertebral joints: about 1 mL.
  - To the intercostal nerves: about 1–2 mL.

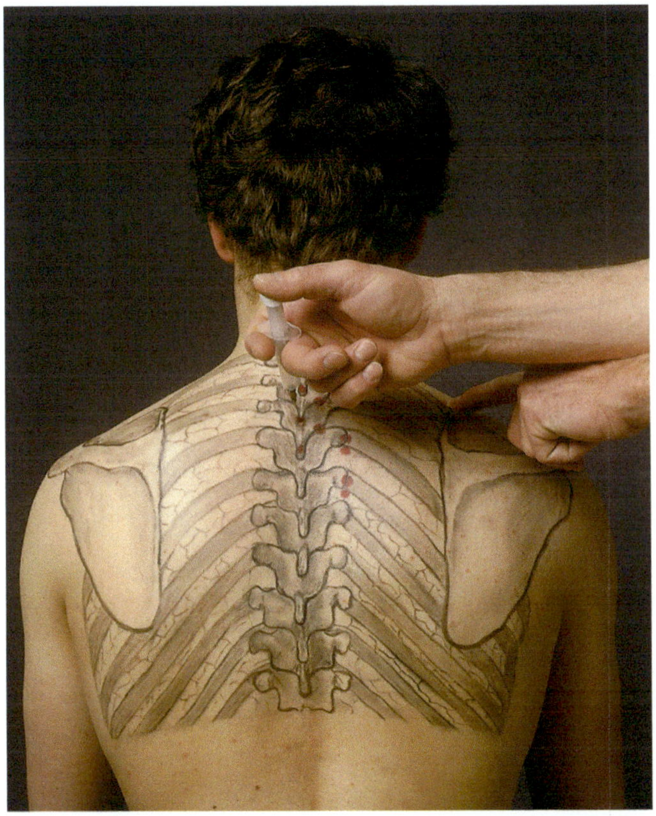

►**Fig. 18.8** Injection to the spinous processes of the thoracic spine.

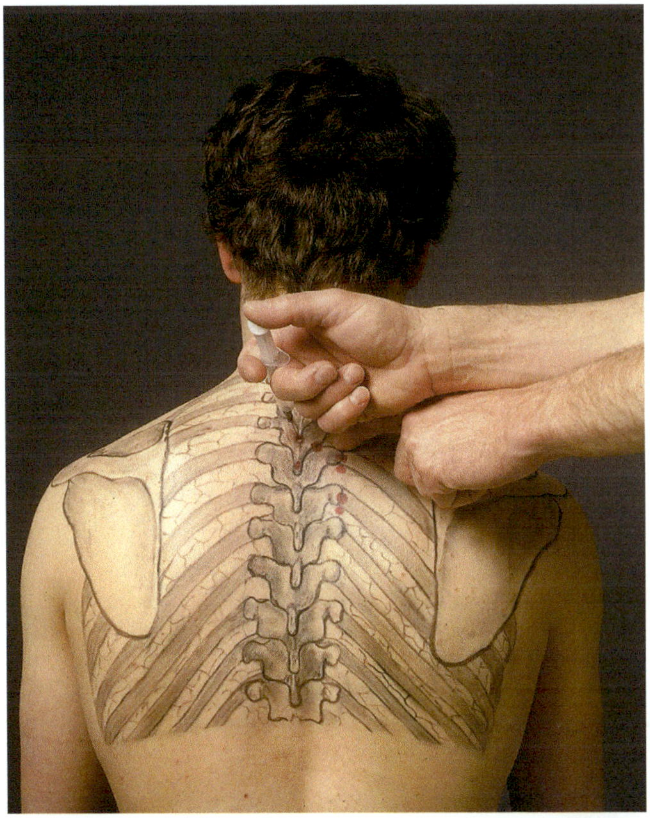

►**Fig. 18.9** Injection to the vertebral joints of the thoracic spine.

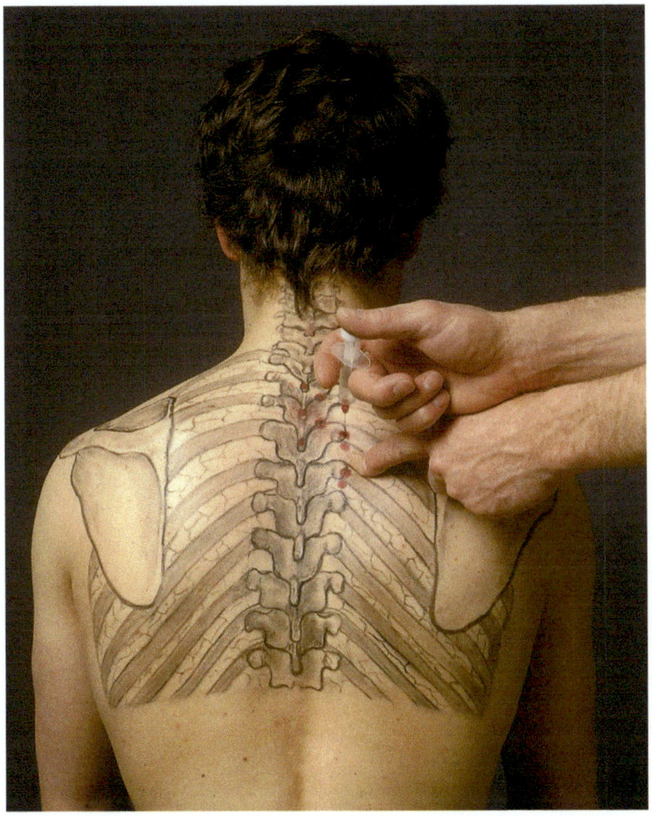

►**Fig. 18.10** Injection to the costovertebral joints.

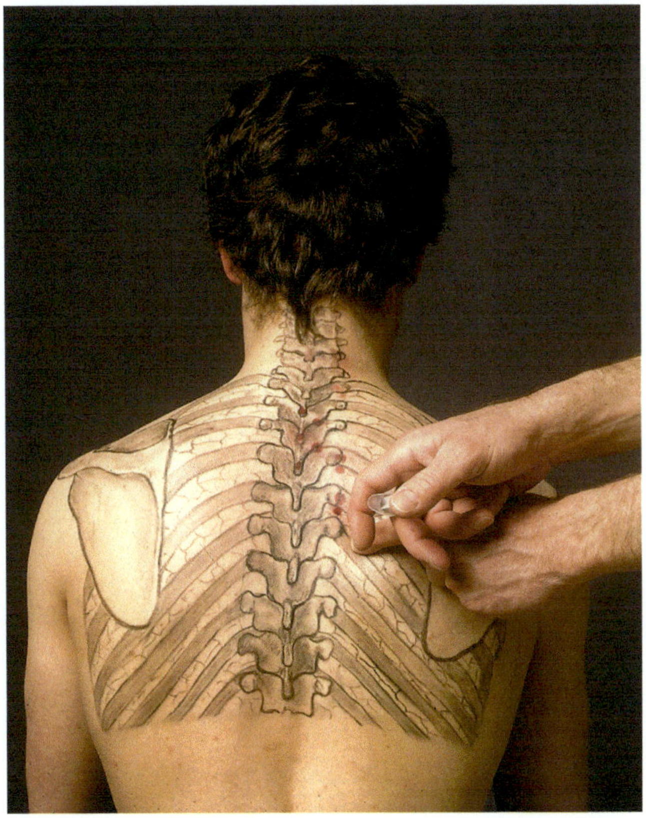

►**Fig. 18.11** Injection to the intercostal nerves and vessels of the thoracic spine.

18.5 Injection to the Lumbar Spine

18.5.1 Indications

The indications given are only a sample of those possible:

- Lower back pain.
- Injuries of the lumbar spine (strains, sprains).
- Overload including "lifting trauma."
- Fractures (old and new, including compression fractures in osteoporosis).
- Scheuermann's disease.
- Degenerative diseases of the lumbar spine.
- Spondylolisthesis.
- Spondylarthrosis.
- Baastrup's disease.
- Spondylodiscitis.
- Myotendinoses.
- Spinal canal stenosis.
- Herniated disk and disk protrusion.
- Root compression syndrome.
- Tumor metastasis pain.

The expected success depends, among other things, on the the patient's "interference field situation."

18.5.2 Anatomy and Neurophysiology

The lumbar spine consists of five vertebrae and is often the site of chronic and acute disorders (▶Fig. 18.12, ▶Fig. 18.13). Generally, there is involvement of all structures that give the lumbar spine its static and dynamic functions, that is, the vertebrae with the intervertebral disks, the vertebral joints, all ligament-capsule structures, the vessels, and the nerves. Due to its topographical position and structure of all spinal sections, the lumbar spine is subject to the strongest stresses, such that this alone can explain the frequency of its disorders. An isolated disorder in one structure is rare, e.g., a single vertebral joint, since the neurophysiological relationships cause a chain reaction with the irritation of one structure affecting others, e.g., vessels, nerves, and muscles.

The clinical result is painful, limited movement of the affected lumbar spine section, with visible and palpable hypertension of the muscles, impaired movement in the form of one or more "fixed" vertebrae, palpable changes in the skin and in the subcutaneous tissue in the form of local edematous swelling (geloses), and local tenderness over the spinous processes, the ligaments, and the muscles, as well as prolonged symptoms in the surroundings, e.g., in the form of pseudoradicular symptoms.

The segmental reaction of the various tissue structures of a lumbar spine section depends on the converging afferent fibers as well as the somatic and sympathetic nervous system via intra- and interneuronal switching and the associated diverging efferent fibers. In summary, the pathological effect consists of a chronically elevated afferent impulse output for all involved nerve structures. In this case the targeted use of the local anesthetic to reduce the afferent impulse output is the neural therapeutic method for restoring physiological balance in the afferent–efferent interconnection and thereby normalizing the spinal function.

The structures mentioned are also injected for the specific purpose of reaching the sympathetic nervous system—i.e., to reach the nerves supplying these structures and interrupt them briefly. With the correct injection technique, and without inducing an interference field, immediate relief of the symptoms can be achieved. The muscles relax, the movement normalizes, the edematous changes in the skin and subcutis are no longer palpable, and there is a slight feeling of warmth in the region as a sign of local sympatholysis.

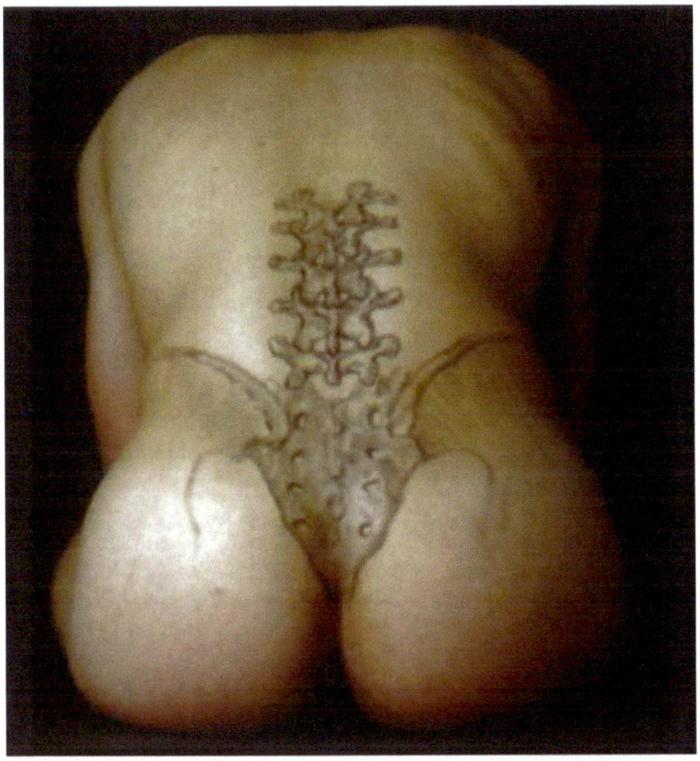

▶ **Fig. 18.12** Osseous topography for injection to the spinous processes and vertebral joints of the lumbar spine.

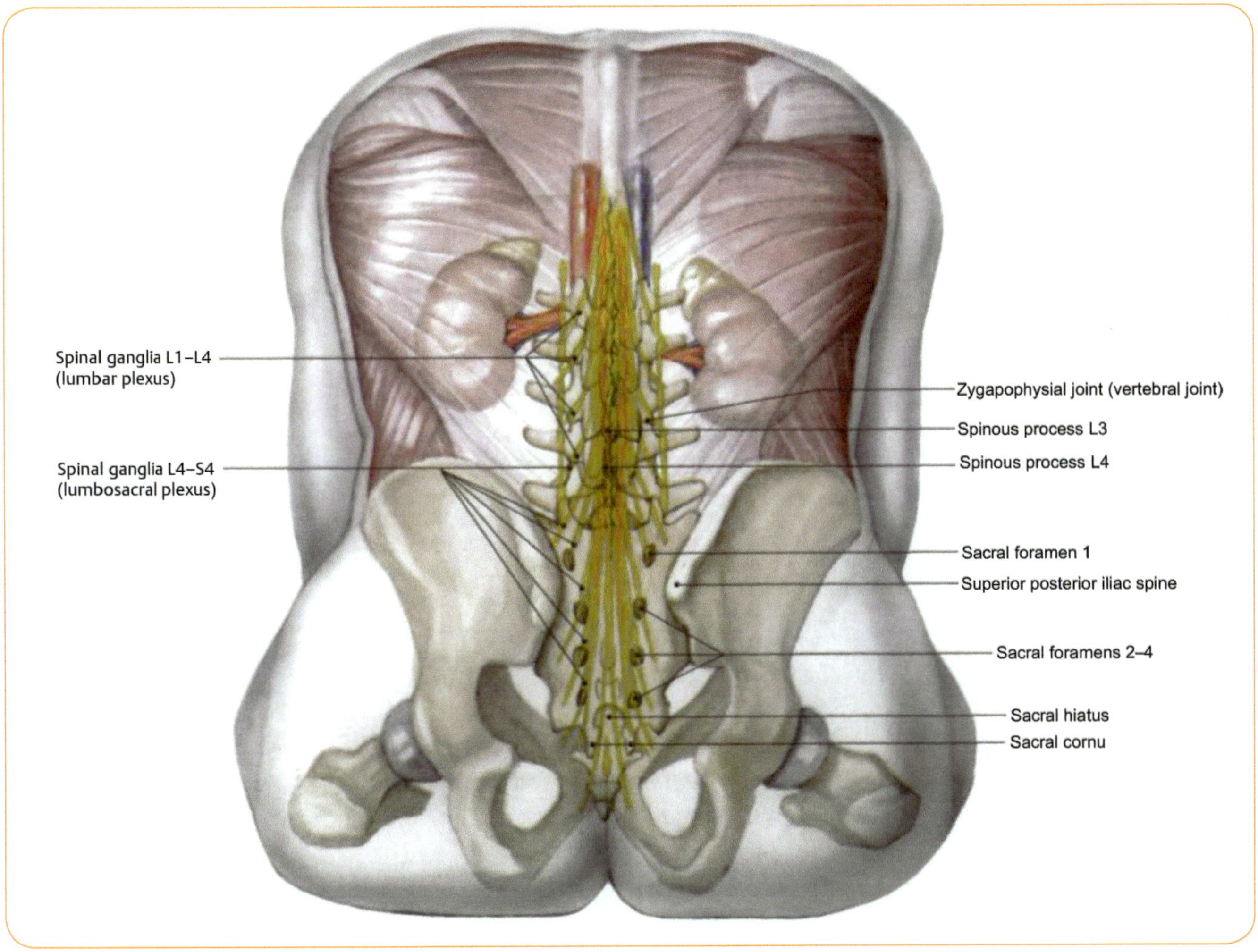

▶ **Fig. 18.13** Topography for injection to the structures of the lumbar spine.

18.5.3 Injection Technique

Primarily, as with treatment of the cervical and thoracic spine, a wheal series is administered as stimulus therapy over the spinous processes of the lumbar spine and at the same level, approximately 3 to 4 cm paravertebral at the level of the diseased segment. In addition, the maximum pressure points, which were detected through palpation of the vertebral musculature, are each infiltrated with 0.5 to 1 mL procaine 1%, as are the frequently palpable subcutaneous geloses.

► **Spinous processes.** Palpation of the pressure-sensitive spinous process. After insertion of a wheal, a needle 2 to 3 cm long is pushed forward until it contacts bone. Inject 0.5 mL, pull back the needle, and infiltrate the supra- and interspinal ligaments running toward the next highest and next lowest spinous process with 0.5 mL by lifting and lowering the needle tip by about 60° (► Fig. 18.14). The injection depth is now about 2 cm.

► **Vertebral Joints.** Palpation of the pressure-sensitive spinous process. The vertebral joints in the area of the lumbar spine are at the level of the spinous process center about 2 to 2.5 cm lateral to the spinous process line at about 4 to 5 cm depth. The 6-cm needle is inserted—with the patient's upper body slightly bent forward—2 cm lateral to the spinous process line and level with the respective center of the spinous process (► Fig. 18.15). With a strictly sagittal puncture direction, contact with the bone must be made after 4 to 5 cm. After two-time negative aspiration with rotation of the needle by 180° in order to exclude intrathecal needle position, 1 mL procaine 1% is infiltrated.

18.5.4 Material

Required:

- Spinous processes:
  - 5-mL syringe.
  - 4 cm long needle.
  - Procaine 1%, 1 mL per injection.
- Vertebral joints:
  - 5-mL syringe.
  - 6 cm long needle.
  - Procaine 1%, 1 mL per injection.

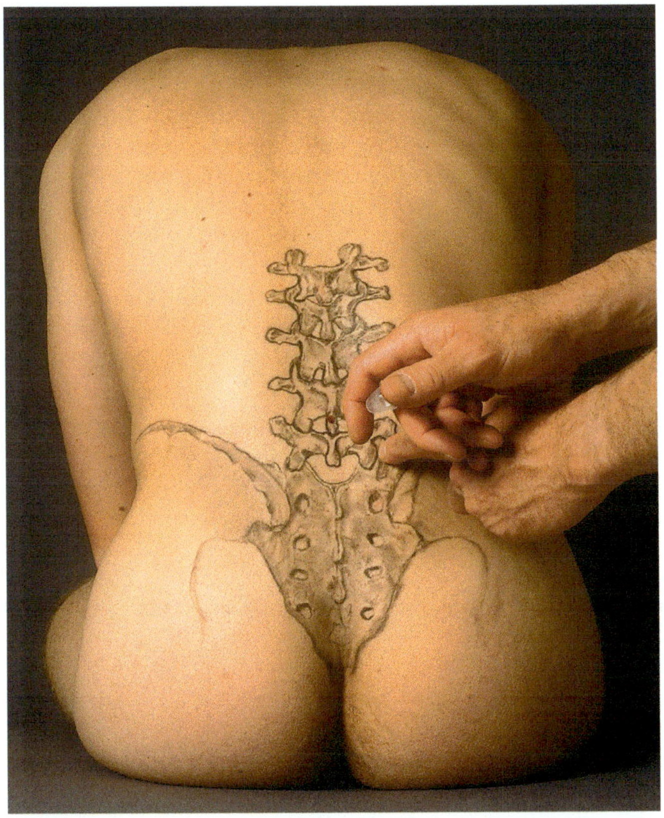

►**Fig. 18.14** Injection to the spinous processes of the lumbar spine.

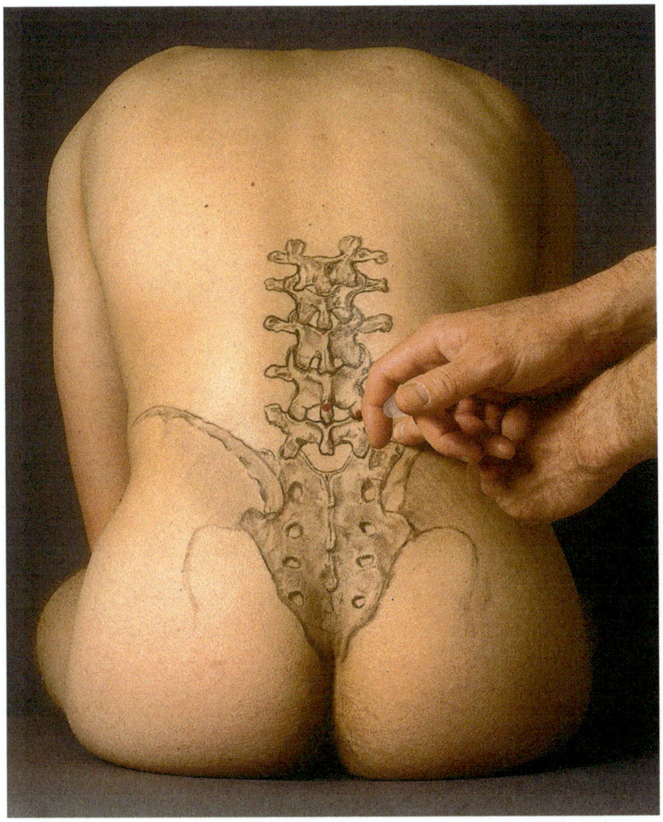

►**Fig. 18.15** Injection to the vertebral joints of the lumbar spine

18.6 Injection to the Spinal Roots L1–S3 (Lumbosacral Plexus)

18.6.1 Introduction

The segmental supply of the lumbar and sacral spine sections and the lower extremity is provided by the spinal nerve system. This includes all the various tissues except for the articular cartilage, which has no nerve structures.

The results of irritation to a spinal nerve are correspondingly found in all tissue parts and can be clinically detected and thus assessed in terms of diagnostics and neural therapy. Depending on the strength of the irritation, simultaneous segment irritation results in variable subjective and objectifiable findings in the area of the lumbar spine, the lower abdomen, the lower extremities, and the gluteal region as well as the small pelvis with its organs. The focus of the following discussion relates to the lumbar spine and lower extremities.

The most common site of spinal nerve irritation can be found at the level of the fifth lumbar vertebra.

Note

The severity of the symptoms and the time of occurrence are important clinical indications for the assessment of spinal nerve irritation, but not for assessing the size of a herniated disc, for example.

Stimulation of the afferent and efferent nerves alone gives rise to the symptoms, so that even a moderate disk protrusion without significant narrowing of the intervertebral foramen can be triggered through stimulation of the sensory and sympathetic nerve fibers of the posterior longitudinal ligament. The irritation potential of the spinal nerve in the area of the intervertebral foramen is diverse, since all afferent and efferent fiber sections in this area—as well as the somatic and sympathetic fibers—are all densely packed next to each other.

This diversity is reflected in the clinical examination, with variable severity of the innervation disturbances. The autochthonous musculature at the level of L5, which receives its motor, sensory, and sympathetic supply via the dorsal branch, is under tension and the skin has impaired sensitivity and moisture as well as palpable edematous swelling. The spinous process of L5 is strongly sensitive to percussion and pressure, as is the palpable supraspinal ligament in the direction of the spinous processes L4 and S1. The gluteal musculature supplied by the superior gluteal nerve (L4–S1) and the inferior gluteal nerve (L5–S2), as well as the tensor fascia latae muscle, which is also supplied via the superior gluteal nerve, shows hypertonic areas, as do the peroneus longus and brevis muscles supplied from the ischiadic nerve (L4–S3) via the common peroneal nerve (L4–S2) and the superficial peroneal nerve, and the anterior tibial muscle, the extensor hallucis longus, and brevis muscles and the extensor digitorum longus and brevis muscles supplied by the deep peroneal nerve. Furthermore, irritation of the ventral branch, which runs afferent sensory fibers next to the efferent motor fibers, causes sensory impairment of the skin in dermatome L5 from the lateral upper thigh and the lateral lower leg, running from the bridge of the foot to the big toe.

Note

The impaired sensitivity of the skin must in no way be continuous as a so-called L5 ligament, but can certainly occur fractionated at various points of the L5 segment, e.g., in the form of a painful big toe or painful outer malleolus.

The sympathetic fiber portion exits the spinal cord with the anterior rootand proceeds via the white ramus communicans to the sympathetic trunk ganglion; from there it extends partially via the gray ramus communicans to the ventral branch of the spinal nerve in the periphery and also connects to the arterial vessels in the form of the periarterial sympathetic network. Stimulation of the sympathetic fiber portion manifests as impaired circulation in the legs. This is often indicated by patients as feelings of cold or early fatigue in the legs.

Up to this point, the stimulation of the spinal nerve L5 has been discussed in terms of fragments. Partial or complete failure shows the partial paralysis of the muscles mentioned as well as full or fractional hypesthesia or anesthesia of the dermatome L5. The failure is possible through mechanical disruption of stimulus conduction as well as through strong reduction of blood supply to the spinal nerve and dorsal root ganglion, due to strong local irritation of the sympathetic nervous system.

From a biomechanical perspective, functional failure in the joints of the lower extremities can be derived from motor dysfunction. Thus, there is the possibility for disease in this area.

Other joint symptoms from irritation of the spinal nerve L5 can be explained through including consideration of the innervation of the joints and the joint capsules. The dorsal capsule section of the hip joint, for example, is partially supplied by spinal nerve L5, via the articular branch and the femoral quadratic muscle branch, or about 60% of the knee joint capsule via the superficial common peroneal nerve (L4–S1) as well as the tibial nerve (L4–S3).

The inner rotation and bending of the knee occurs in part via the semitendinosus and semimembranosus muscles, innervated by the tibial nerve (L4–S3). The hypertension of these muscles (e.g., with L5 irritation including the sympathetic portion) results in varus strain on the knee joint with the long-term consequence of varus gonarthrosis. In neural therapy, causal treatment is carried out in the form of an injection to spinal root L5. This often results in sustained freedom from symptoms, even with advanced varus gonarthrosis detected on X-ray. In this context, with a joint disease in the lower extremities, an irritation of the spinal nerve L5 should always be taken into consideration. The isolated disorder of the spinal nerve L5 was selected as an example to clearly illustrate the neurological relationships contributing to the symptomology of the lumbar spine and lower extremities triggered by this irritation. The same applies to spinal nerves L1–S3.

18.6.2 Injection to the Spinal Roots L1–L4 (Lumbar Plexus)

Indications

The indications given are only a sample of those possible:
- Lower back pain emerging from segments L1–L4.
- Disorders in the adductor muscles of the upper thigh.
- Disorders in the quadriceps musculature.
- Unexplained groin pain.
- Obturator neuralgia.
- Gonarthrosis.
- Neuralgia of the saphenous nerve.

The expected success depends, among other things, on the the patient's "interference field situation."

Anatomy and Neurophysiology

The spinal roots L1–L4 are grouped together because they constitute a functional unit in the diagnosis of diseases of the lower extremities. After exiting the spinal canal, the spinal nerves meet in the lumbar plexus, where they act as peripheral nerves and supply the ventromedial portion of the leg, which leads to "mixing" of the individual spinal nerves (▶Fig. 18.16, ▶Fig. 18.17). This mixture of segmentally articulated spinal nerves to the peripheral nerves (iliohypogastric nerve T12–L1, ilioinguinal nerve T12–L1, genitofemoral nerve L1–L2, lateral femoral cutaneous nerve L2–L3, obturator nerve L2–L4, femoral nerve L2–L4) leads to segmental "mixed innervation" of the muscles, so that failure of one segment causes the failure of various muscle parts, but never a whole muscle. The sensory supply of the leg is analogous to this.

Important to neural therapy is the fact that fiber sections of the sympathetic nervous system run parallel with all spinal nerves and the spinal ganglion is nourished via the vascular system, which in turn is controlled by the sympathetic nervous system.

Injection Technique

▶**Spinal root L1**. The line of the iliac crest is marked as the patient in a sitting position bends forward slightly. The spinous process closest to this line is the spinous process of L4. (The spinous process of L4 is not always on the iliac crest line, but sometimes slightly above it!) Count the spinous processes in cranial direction and the L1 spinous process. With limited experience, it is best to establish all spinous processes through craniocaudal counting and marking. The 8-cm needle is inserted at the level of the lower edge of the spinous process, 3 to 4 cm lateral (depending on the size of the patient). After insertion of a wheal, slightly push the needle forward in a convergent manner. Depending on the size of the patient, there is a flash of pain in segment L1 after a depth of 6 to 7 cm. The patient must be warned in advance about this. Pull back the needle by about 1 to 2 mm and then double aspirate the needle with 180° rotation, to rule out intravascular and intrathecal needle positioning, then infiltrate 2 mL anesthetic. If contact with bone is already made at about 4 cm, the needle position is too far medial and is hitting the vertebra, or it is too far lateral and is hitting the transverse process of L2. If it is not possible to pass the bone by slightly correcting the needle in the lateral or cranial direction, the needle should be completely removed and reinserted after checking the insertion point. Once safely past the bone, without triggering a flash of pain, the spinal nerve can be reached through a larger injection quantity (about 5 mL). If there is CSF in the syringe during aspiration, the needle has been placed intrathecally in a saccular dura protrusion that occasionally occurs in the intervertebral foramen. In this case, the needle is pulled back until there is no more CSF flow, and 2 to 3 mL procaine is infiltrated.

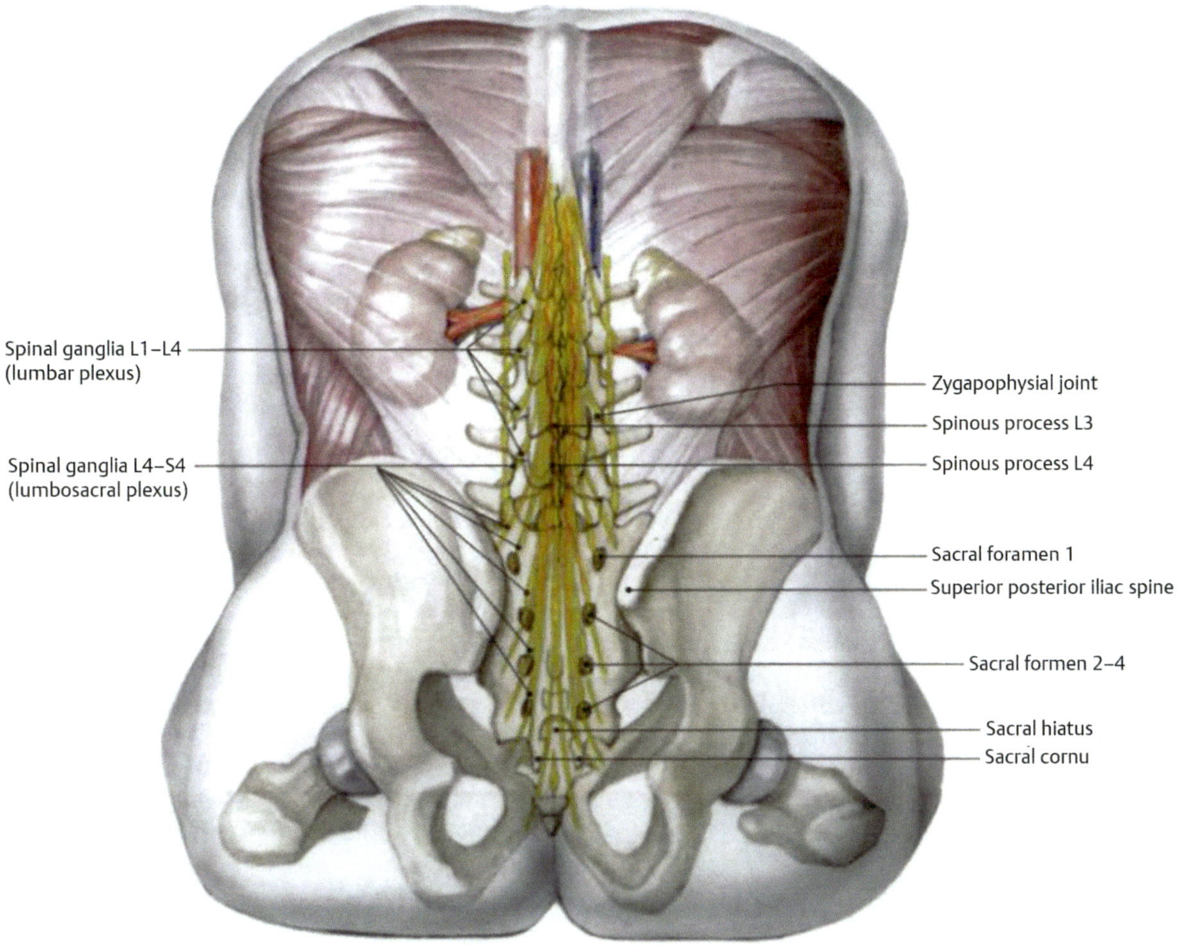

► **Fig. 18.16** Topography for injection to the spinal nerves L1–L4 (lumbar plexus).

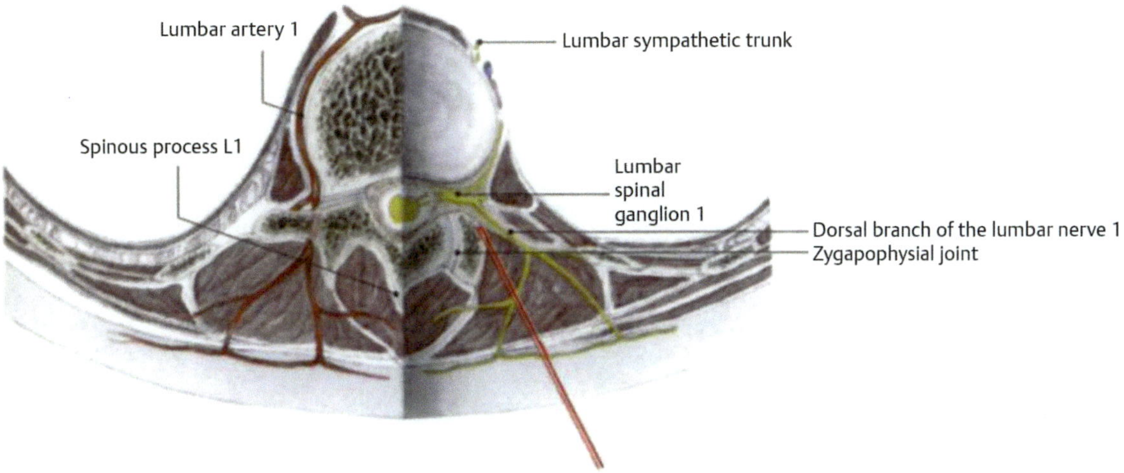

► **Fig. 18.17** Cross-section at the level of L1.

Spinal anesthesia cannot occur in this situation. The correct positioning of the needle should be clinically controlled and documented after a few minutes.

▶**Spinal root L2.** The patient sits slightly bent forward. Mark the iliac crest line and the spinous process of L4, count up to the spinous process of L2 and mark it. When the L2 segment is irritated, the spinous process is sensitive to pressure and percussion. The puncture is made perpendicular to the skin, 3 to 4 cm laterally and at the level of the lower edge of the spinous process. After insertion of a wheal, the needle is pushed forward in sagittal direction until a flash of pain is triggered after reaching 5 to 7 cm depth in segment L2. Retract the cannula by 1 mm and very slowly infiltrate 2 mL procaine. If there is no flash of pain, 5 mL is injected. If the needle was positioned too far laterally, there may be a flash of pain in the next highest segment since this is the path of spinal nerve L1.

▶**Spinal root L3.** The patient sits slightly bent forward for anteflexion of the lumbar spine. Mark the iliac crest line and the spinous process of L4; count up to the spinous process of L3. When segment L3 is irritated, this spinous process is sensitive to pressure. The puncture is made perpendicular to the skin, 3 to 4 cm laterally and at the level of the lower edge of the spinous process (▶Fig. 18.18). After insertion of a wheal, the needle is pushed forward in sagittal direction until a flash of pain is triggered at 5 to 7 cm depth in segment L3. Retract the needle by 1 mm. Double aspirate the needle with 180° rotation to rule out intravascular and intrathecal needle positions and infiltrate 2 mL anesthetic. If there is no flash of pain, 5 mL is injected. After several minutes, check the correct position of the injection and document it.

▶**Spinal root L4.** The patient sits slightly bent forward for anteflexion of the lumbar spine (▶Fig. 18.19, ▶Fig. 18.20). Mark the iliac crest line and the spinous process L4. The puncture with the 8-cm needle is made perpendicular to the skin, 3 to 4 cm laterally and at the level of the lower edge of the spinous process. After insertion of a wheal, the needle is pushed forward, slightly converging in the sagittal direction until a flash of pain is triggered at 5 to 7 cm depth in segment L4. Pull back the needle by 1 mm, aspirate in two levels, and infiltrate 2 mL anesthetic . If a flash of pain is not triggered, infiltrate 5 mL. If the needle was positioned too far laterally, there may be a flash of pain in segment L3.

18.6.3 Material

Required:
- 5-mL syringe.
- 0.6 × 80 mm needle.
- Procaine 1%, 2 to 5 mL per injection.

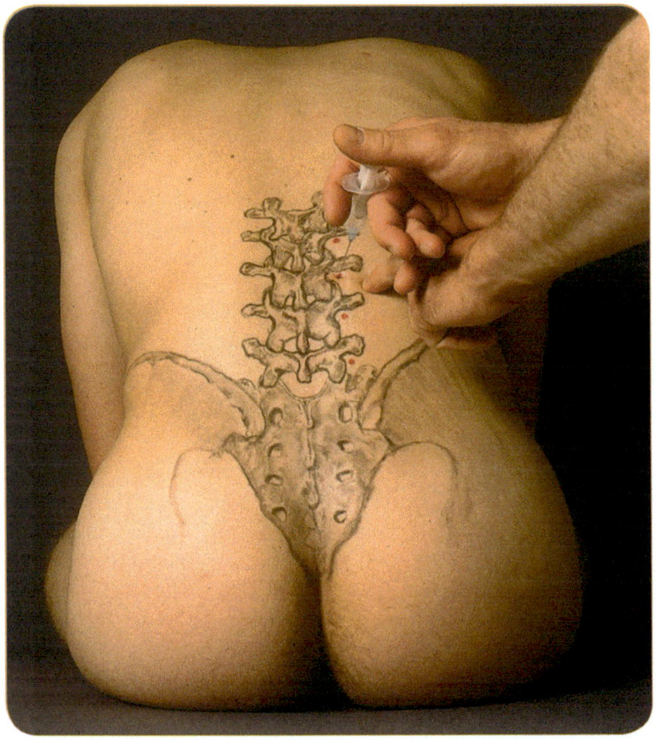

▶ **Fig. 18.18** Injection to the spinal root L3.

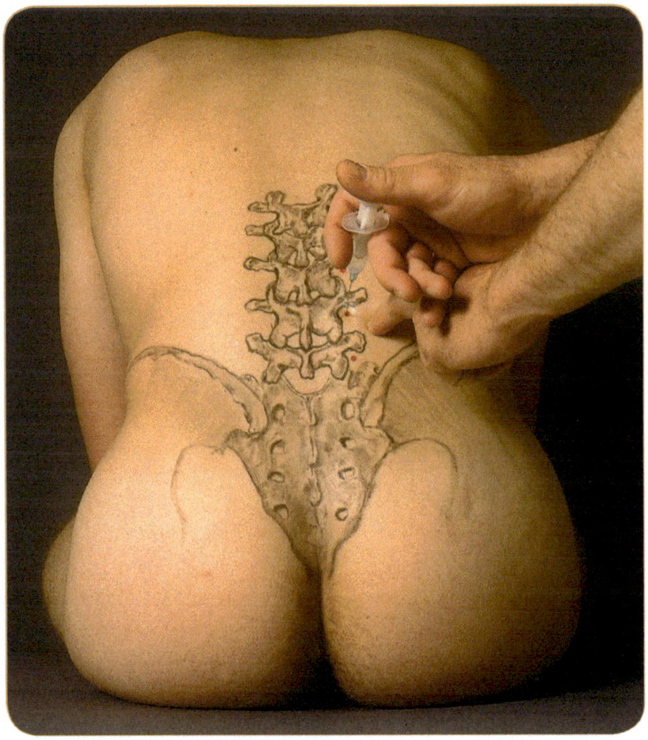

▶ **Fig. 18.19** Injection to the spinal root L4.

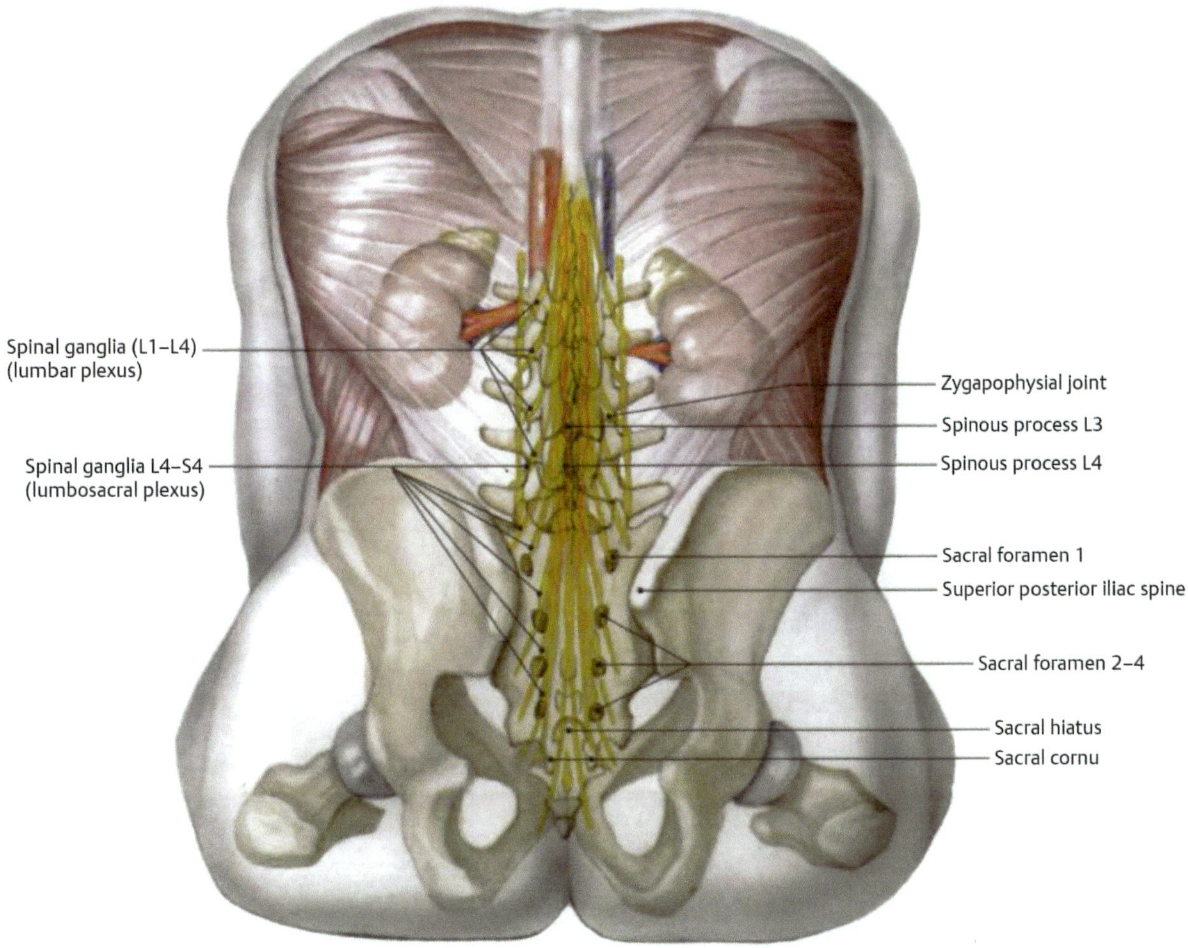

▶ **Fig. 18.20** Topography for injection to spinal roots L1–L4.

18.6.4 Injection to the Spinal Roots L5–S3 (Sacral Plexus)

Indications

The indications given are only a sample of those possible:
- Lower back pain with or without "blockade" of the sacroiliac joints.
- Lumbar sciatica.
- Sciatica.
- Regional pain in the lower extremities in segments L5–S3.
- Impaired muscle function in the gluteal muscles, thigh muscles, lower leg, and foot muscles.
- Old and new peroneal nerve paralysis (L5).
- Disk prolapse L5/S1.
- Varus gonarthrosis (L5).
- Heel spur (S1).
- Achillodynia (S1).
- Patella pain (jumper's knee, retropatellar arthrosis) (S1!).
- "Restless legs" (L5/L4 and S1)
- Coccygodynia.

The expected success depends, among other things, on the the patient's "interference field situation."

Anatomy and Neurophysiology

The sacral plexus consists of the ventral branches of the spinal nerves L5–S3 as well as parts of the ventral branch from L4.

Note

The fact that the structure of the sacral plexus can undergo a caudal or cranial shift by one segment each in about 20% of cases is important for the diagnostics and neural therapeutic treatment.

It is also possible not only that the sacral plexus conducts fiber portions from segment L3, but also that the fiber portion is missing from segment L4. The supply area only includes the flexor side of the lower extremity through the fusion of the ventral branch as well as the dorsal lumbar and sacral region through the dorsal spinal nerve branches not consolidated in a plexus. Thus, stimulation of a spinal nerve causes a clinical response in the region of the lumbar or sacral region as well as the lower extremity.

The most powerful nerve in the human body, the sciatic nerve, originates from the sacral plexus. It contains all afferent and efferent somatic as well as sympathetic fiber portions of a spinal nerve. Another part of the sympathetic system proceeds along the efferent and afferent pathway along with the vessels that supply the lower extremity. An important aspect for everyday clinical practice is that all leg structures—except for the articular cartilage—are innervated, depending on the tissue, by different sections of the somatic nerve system and, in various intensities, by the sympathetic nervous system. Every irritation of a somatic nerve section results in a simultaneous irritation, and vice versa, of the sympathetic nervous system via indirect connections at the spinal level, and all tissue damage (mechanical, thermal, chemical) stimulates the sympathetic nervous system as well as the corresponding somatic system. The sympathetic nervous system, which is so important to neural therapy, is reached by the injection of the local anesthetic in every tissue structure, but more comprehensively with the injection to peripheral nerves and vessels, spinal ganglia, and via the lumbar sympathetic trunk. As opposed to local anesthesia, the simultaneously occurring blockade of somatic nerve portions is secondary for neural therapy. The aim of local and regional sympatholysis is improved microcirculation (affecting the vascular efferent fibers) as well as short-term reduction of the sympathetic afferent fibers—which are increased in the case of illness—with the reflexive effects on the somatic nervous system as well as all remaining tissue structures. This way, the neural therapeutic treatment is carried out via the spinal nerves of the sacral plexus in the case of lumbar spine and sacrum disorders and in disorders of the lower extremity.

Injection Technique

►**Spinal root L5.** With the patient bent slightly forward (►Fig. 18.21, ►Fig. 18.22), identify and mark the spinous process L4 via the iliac crest line. Palpate the spinous process L5 and insert the 8-cm needle 3 to 4 cm laterally, at the

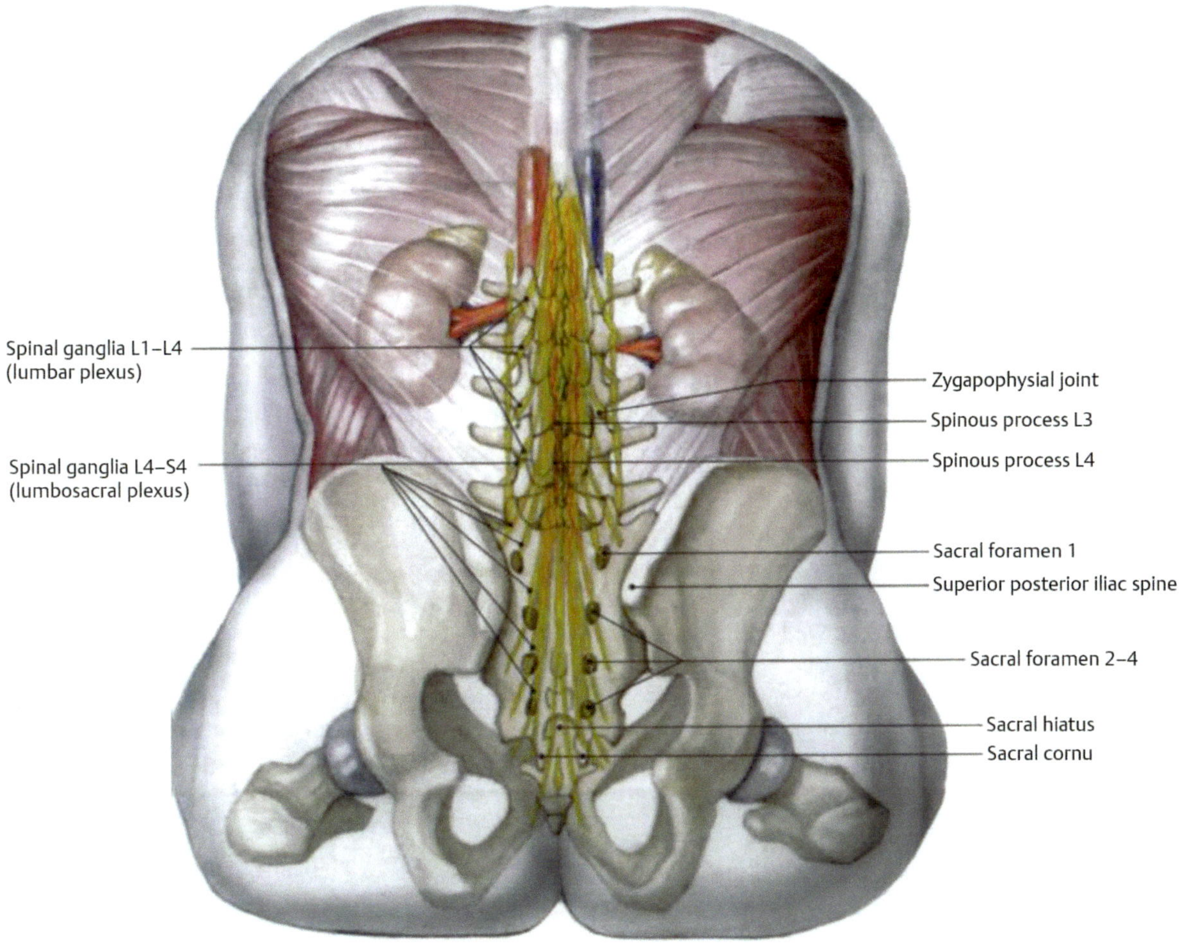

► **Fig. 18.21** Topography of the spinal roots L5–S3.

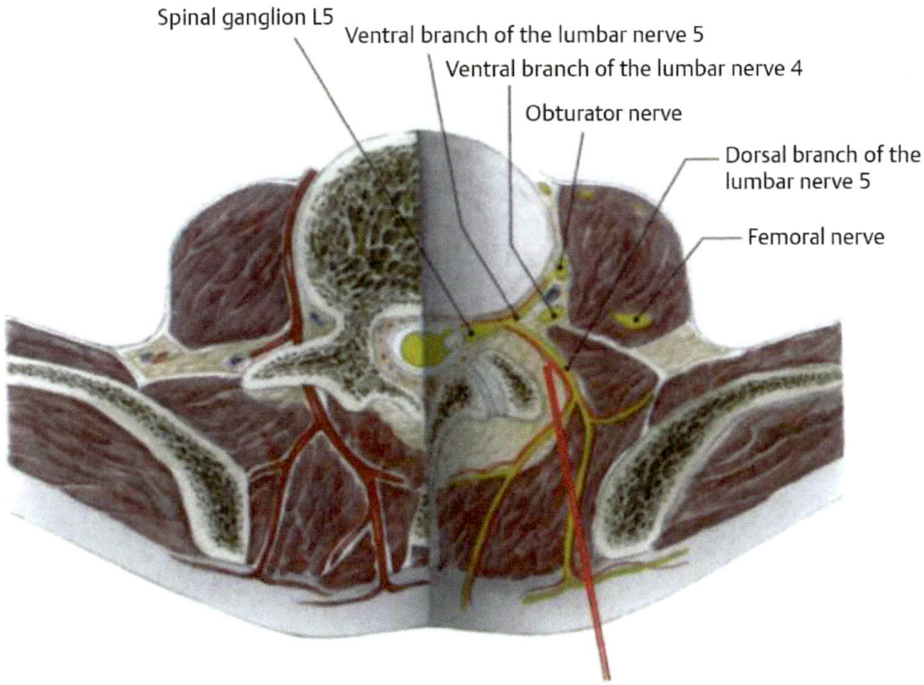

► **Fig. 18.22** Cross-section at the level of spinal root L5.

level of the bottom edge of the spinous process after placing a wheal in the sagittal direction (▶Fig. 18.23, ▶Fig. 18.25). The area of the spinal root L5 is more difficult to reach, since the lateral part of the sacral bone is quite close to the transverse process L5. After 6 to 8 cm, a flash of pain, which indicates the correct needle position, can be triggered in segment L5. After twice- negative aspiration and prior retraction of the needle by 1 mm, infiltrate 2 mL anesthetic after the flash of pain is triggered (infiltrate 5 mL if there is no flash of pain). Because of the proximity of the obturator nerve and the farther lateral femoral nerve along the major psoas muscle, flashes of pain are also possible in segments L2–L4 if the needle is positioned too far in ventral or lateral direction.

▶**Spinal root S1**. Palpation of the superior posterior iliac process. After insertion of a wheal, make the injection at an angle of 45° in caudal direction, two finger-widths above and directly medial to the edge of the palpable iliac crest (▶Fig. 18.24, ▶Fig. 18.25). Pushing the needle forward requires a great deal of sensitivity in order to reach sacral foramen 1. Through 30 to 45° anteflexion positioning of the os sacrum, the first bone contact with the sacral bone can be expected no sooner than 4 to 5 cm depth. The dorsal opening of the foramen is found when the needle can be pushed 0.5 cm deeper (no more). After twice-negative aspiration, slowly infiltrate 2 to 3 mL anesthetic. The flash of pain in segment S1 or a slightly uncomfortable tugging sensation indicates the correct placement of the injection.

▶**Spinal root S2**. Palpate the spinous process S2 and make the injection with the 6-cm needle at this level, 1 cm cranial and almost 2 cm lateral at an angle of about 20° to the skin. The dorsal opening of the foramen S2 is reached at about 2 to 3 cm depth. Push the needle forward by about 0.5 cm and infiltrate 2 to 3 mL anesthetic after twice-negative aspiration. The flash of pain or tugging sensation in segment S2 indicates the correct placement of the injection.

▶**Spinal root S3**. Palpate the spinous process S3 and make the injection with the 6-cm needle at this level, 1 cm cranial and 2 cm lateral perpendicular to the skin and in the sagittal direction. After placement of a wheal, the dorsal opening of the sacral foramen 3, into which the needle is pushed 0.5 cm, is found at 1 to 2 cm depth. After two-time negative aspiration, slowly infiltrate 2 to 3 mL. The flash of pain or pulling sensation in segment S3 indicates the correct placement of the injection.

Material

Required:

- 5-mL syringe.
- 0.6 × 60 to 80 mm needle.
- Procaine 1%, 2 to 5 mL per injection.

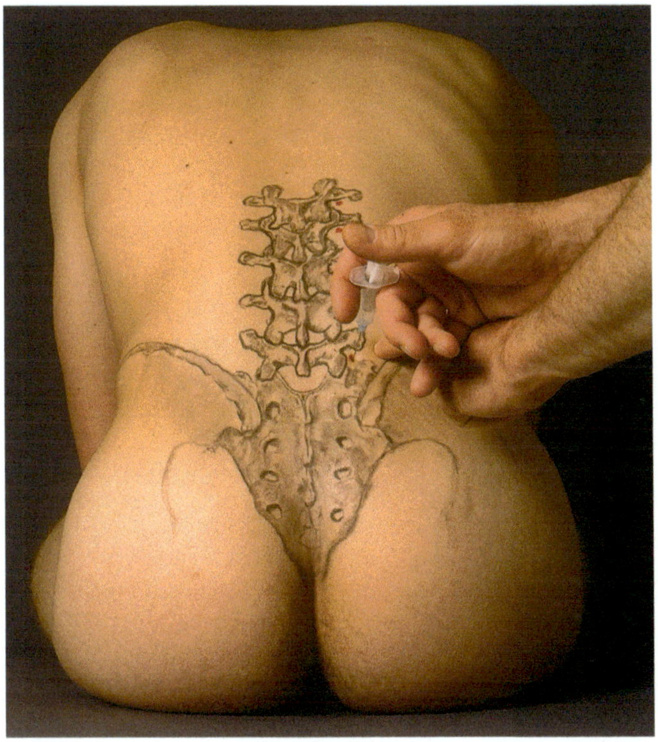

►**Fig. 18.23** Injection to the spinal root L5.

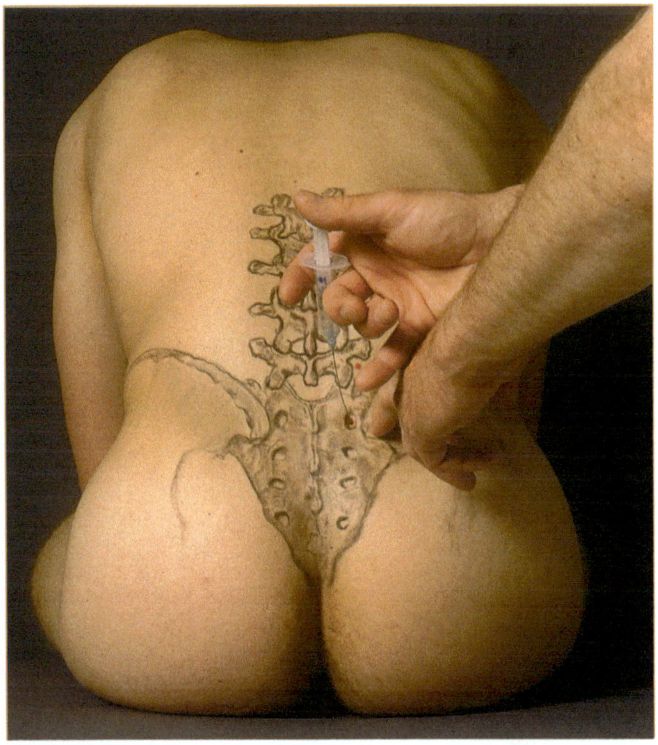

►**Fig. 18.24** Injection to the spinal root S1.

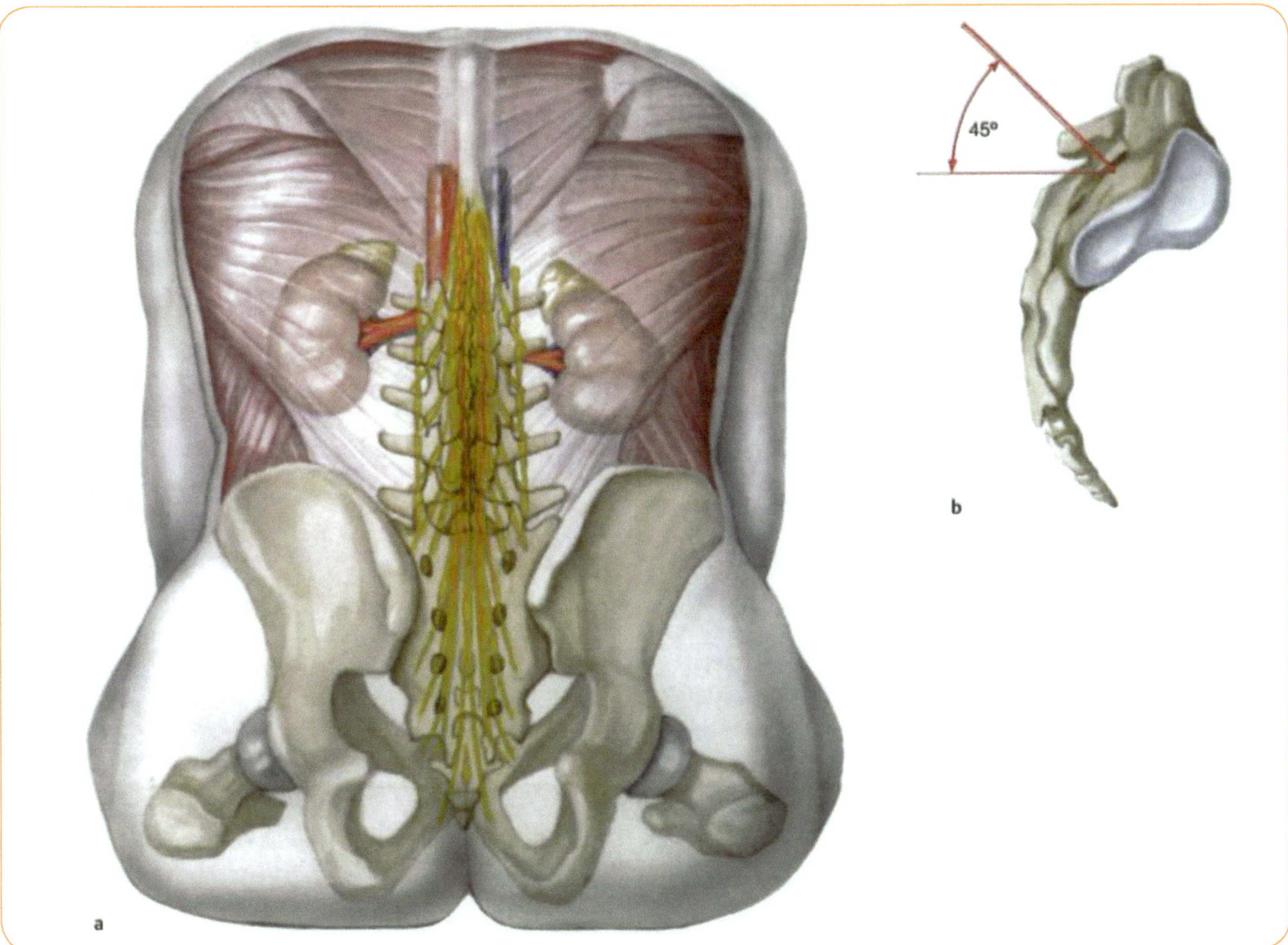

►**Fig. 18.25** Topography for injection to the spinal roots of the lumbar spine and the sacral bone. Note injection angle to sacral foramens 1 to 4. **(a)** Topography for injection to the spinal roots L5–S3. **(b)** Position of the sacral bone when the patient is seated, lateral view of injection in the sacral foramen.

18.7 Injections in the Pelvic Region

18.7.1 Indications

The indications given are only a sample of those possible:
- Acute and chronic lower back pain.
- Pain in the area of the sacral bone, lateral hip region, and symphysis.
- Posttraumatic pelvic pain (particularly after giving birth).
- Ankylosing spondylitis.

The expected success depends, among other things, on the the patient's "interference field situation."

18.7.2 Anatomy and Neurophysiology

The functional three-part pelvis is composed of the left and right os coxa bones and the sacral bone and occupies a special position in neural therapy. As a connection between the spine and the lower extremity, it is subject to various strains resulting from the positioning of the pelvis with regard to the spine and the hip joints. On the one hand, the integral connection of the three bony pelvis sections with each other is made from the very strong ligament structure, the connections to the spine, and to the hip joints. On the other hand, the connection between these bony sections also consists of strong muscle groups which have a significant effect on the position of the pelvis. The key ligamentous structures of the three pelvic sections are the ventral and dorsal sacroiliac ligaments for the iliosacral joint. These are connected with one another via the sacroiliac joint and the symphysis and allow only a slightly springy movement of the bones against each other, (▶Fig. 18.26, ▶Fig. 18.27) and the arcuate pubic ligament for the symphysis, whose bony sections have a springlike connection via a cartilaginous ligament mass—much like an intervertebral disk. The sacrotuberal ligament between the sacral bone and the ischial tuberosity, and the sacrospinal ligament between the sacral bone, coccyx bone, and ischial spine of the ischium complete the ligamentous anatomy. (Another important ligamentous structure worth mentioning here is the connection between the fourth and fifth lumbar transverse process to the dorsal iliac crest in the form of the iliolumbar ligament.)

The nerve supply of the ligamentous structures and the joints of the pelvic ring consists of somatic as well as sympathetic afferent fibers. One part of the sympathetic section always courses together with the somatic afferent fibers, and another part with the vessels supplying the capsule-ligament and is the goal of neural therapeutic treatment. The infiltration of the structures indicated above means, on the one hand, the interruption of the somatic and sympathetic afferent fibers and thus a reduction of the impulse exposure at the segmental-reflexive level of the spine. On the other hand, infiltration with local anesthetic causes peripheral sympatholysis of the perivascular sympathetic nervous system with the positive effect on the supply of the ligament-capsule structures of the pelvic ring. This results in segmental cessation of the pain as well as normalization of the impaired circulation.

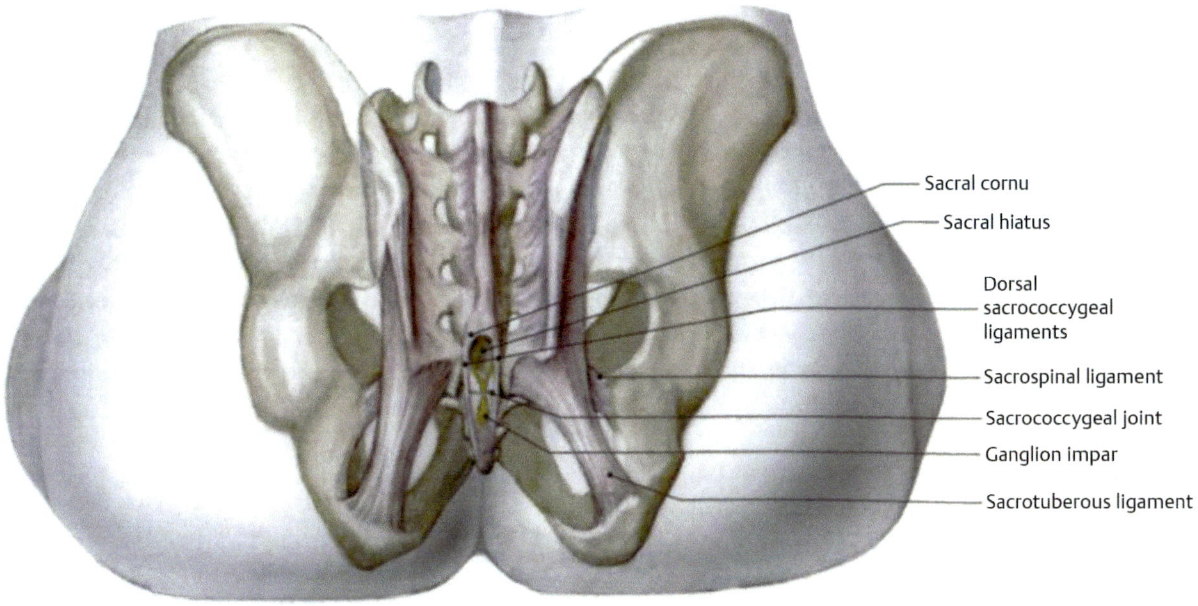

▶ **Fig. 18.26** Dorsal view of pelvis with ligament structures and ganglion impar.

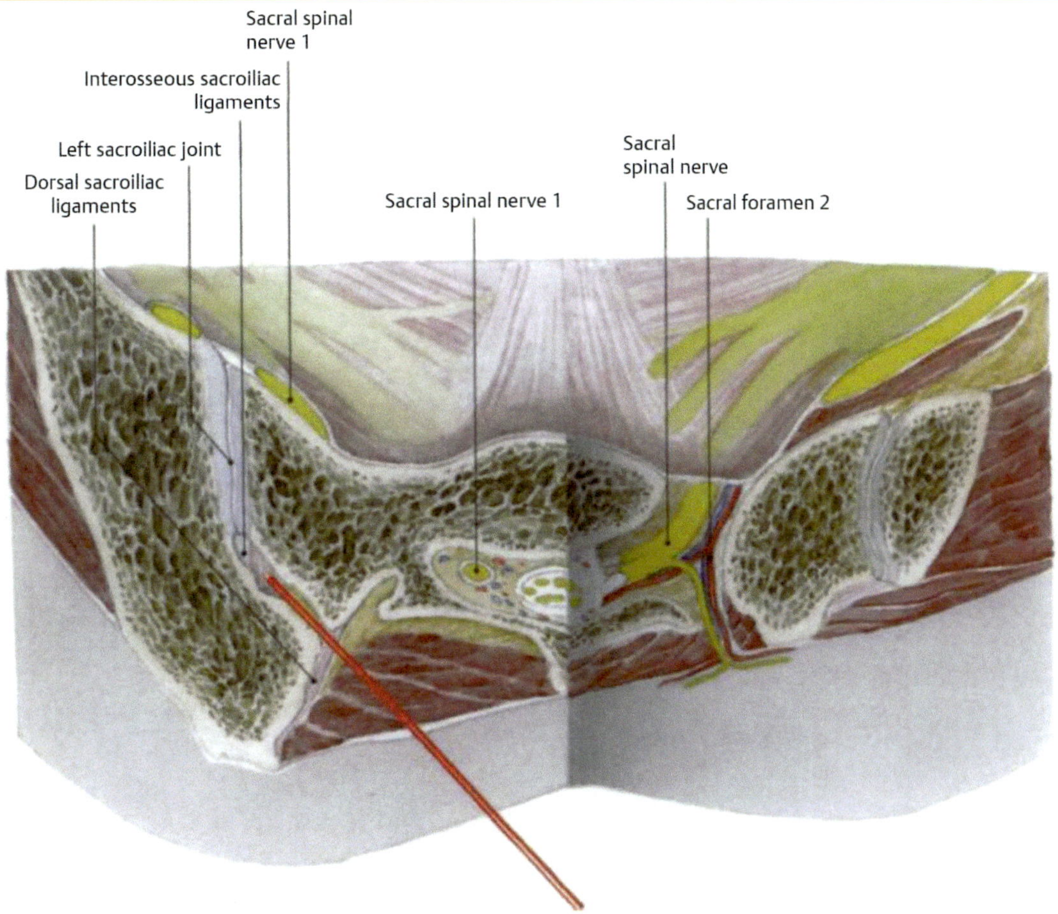

▶ **Fig. 18.27** Topography of the dorsal pelvis in cross-section at the level of sacral foramen 2.

18.7.3 Injection Technique

▶**Sacroiliac joint**. Palpate the superior posterior iliac spine. Aligned with this in caudal and slightly medial direction is the slightly springy portion of the dorsal sacroiliac ligaments. Insert the 6-cm needle perpendicular to the skin at the level of maximum pressure pain. After placement of a wheal, push the needle around the posterior edge of the iliac bone in the lateral direction at an angle of about 40°, until intermediate space between the sacrum and the ilium is reached at about 3 to 5 cm depth. The needle is now in the area of the interosseous sacroiliac ligaments (▶Fig. 18.28). Infiltration of 2 to 3 mL anesthetic is performed.

▶**Iliolumbar ligament**. Palpate the spinous process L4; the spinous processes of L5 are located at the level of its lower edge. The injection is made 4 to 5 cm lateral to the spinous process (▶Fig. 18.29). After insertion of a wheal, the 6-cm needle is pushed forward perpendicular to the skin in the sagittal direction until ligament resistance is felt at 4 to 6 cm depth. Peri- and intratendon injection of 2 to 3 mL is made.

▶**Symphysis** (**not pictured**). Palpate the symphysis. Insert the 6-cm needle in the middle of the symphysis. The superior pubic ligament is reached at 1 to 2 cm depth. Infiltrate 1 mL anesthetic. The caudodorsal arcuate ligament can be reached at about 2 to 3 cm depth with the 6-cm needle, passing by the posterior surface of the symphysis. Infiltrate 1 to 2 mL here as well.

▶**Sacrococcygeal joint**. With the seated patient bent far forward or side-lying with tucked up legs, palpation of the anal cleft of the sacral cornu (▶Fig. 18.26). About 0.5 cm in the caudal direction, insert the 4-cm needle perpendicular to the skin in the midline. After placement of a wheal, infiltrate 1 to 2 mL anesthetic after the needle makes contact with bone at about 0.5 to 1.5 cm depth. The injection should be made without strong resistance. Irritation of the periosteum should be avoided. This injection reaches the joint between the sacrum and the tailbone as well as the dorsal and lateral sacrococcygeal ligaments.

18.7.4 Material

Required:

- 5-mL syringe.
- 4 to 6 cm long needle.
- Procaine 1%, 1 to 3 mL per injection.

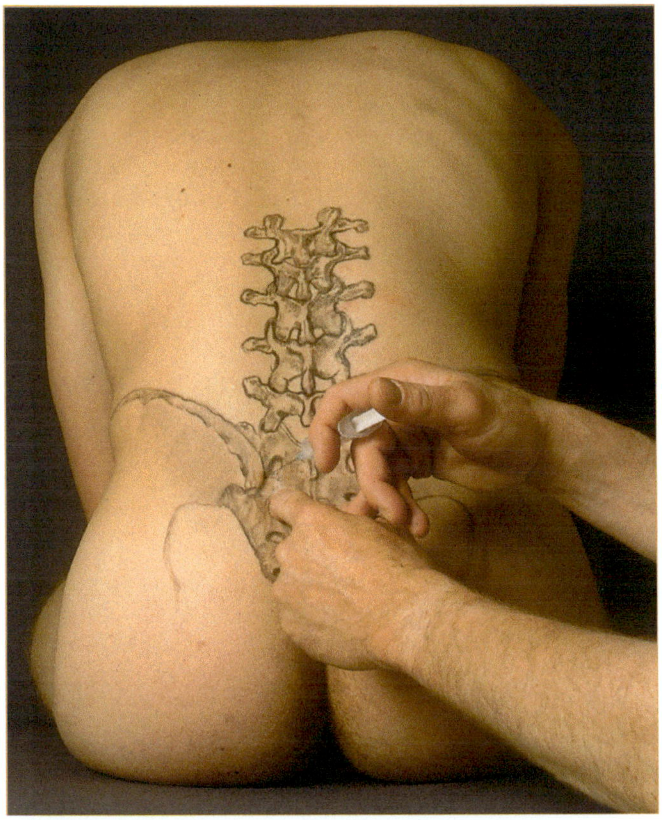

▶ **Fig. 18.28** Injection in the sacroiliac joint gaps and the dorsal and interosseous ligaments.

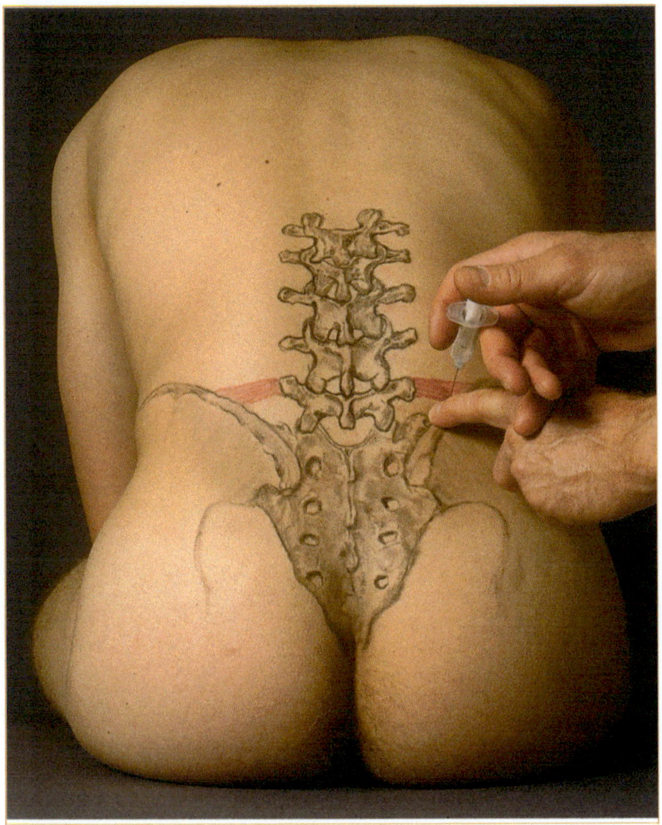

▶ **Fig. 18.29** Injection in the iliolumbar ligament.

18.8 Injection to the Lumbar Sympathetic Trunk

18.8.1 Indications

The indications given are only a sample of those possible:

- Chronic and acute lower back pain.
- Arterial circulation disorders of the pelvis and legs.
- Postoperative lumbar sciatica.
- Postsciatic circulation disorders (dysbasia).
- "Restless legs" investigation.
- Phantom pains.
- Degenerative joint diseases of the lower extremities.
- Venous ulcer.
- Varicosis.
- Thrombosis.
- Thrombophlebitis.
- Postthrombotic syndrome.
- Lymphedema of the lower extremity.
- One-sided spasms of the lower extremity.
- Sudeck's atrophy (CRPS) of the lower extremity.
- Polyneuropathy of the lower extremity with spinal root injections L4–S1.

The expected success depends, among other things, on the the patient's "interference field situation."

18.8.2 Anatomy and Neurophysiology

The lumbar sympathetic trunk has its preganglionic nucleic regions in the lower thoracic and upper lumbar cord of the intermediolateral nucleus. In contrast to the thoracic sympathetic trunk, individuals show substantial differences in the arrangement of the lumbar sympathetic trunk ganglia. Most commonly there are three to four ganglia on the ventrolateral side of the spine, medial to the major psoas muscle.

The sympathetic supply area of the lumbar sympathetic trunk is, on the one hand, efferent as well as afferent supply to the lumbar spine with the associated vessels, capsules, ligaments, muscles, the skin and skin appendages. On the other hand, the supply is to the entire tissue structure of the lower extremity with the exception of the articular cartilage. According to Clara, the lumbar sympathetic trunk is commonly split into multiple stands, whereby the formation of the ganglia and their number appear reduced.[69] There are pronounced right–left connections via the transverse branch. From the upper three lumbar segments, preganglionic fibers as lumbar splanchnic nerves extend to the prevertebral plexus located before the aorta without synapsing in paravertebral ganglia. Thus, judging from the topography of the lumbar sympathetic trunk, the therapeutic use of the sympathetic nervous system in neural therapy is clear; it is particularly useful in improving circulation through sympatholysis.

18.8.3 Injection Technique

With the patient seated and slightly bent forward, find the spinous process of L3. The 8-cm needle is inserted 5 cm (about three finger-widths) lateral to the midline at the level of the middle of the spinous process of L3 (▶Fig. 18.30, ▶Fig. 18.32). Converging about 20° to the midline, the needle is pushed forward after placement of a wheal. Bone contact at about 4 to 5 cm means contact with the transverse process L3, under which the needle should be passed. Depending on the body size, tangential contact with bone is made after 6 to 7 cm (lateral surface of the vertebrae), upon which the needle must be pulled back by about 2 to 3 cm and then tangentially pushed forward by another 3 to 4 cm (▶Fig. 18.31). Now the tip of the needle is at the ventrolateral curvature of the vertebrae. After two aspirations and a negative suction test, slowly infiltrate 3 to 5 mL anesthetic. If blood is aspirated, the needle position must be corrected.

18.8.4 Material

Required:

- 5-mL syringe.
- 8 to 10 cm long needle.
- Procaine 1%, 3 to 5 mL per injection.

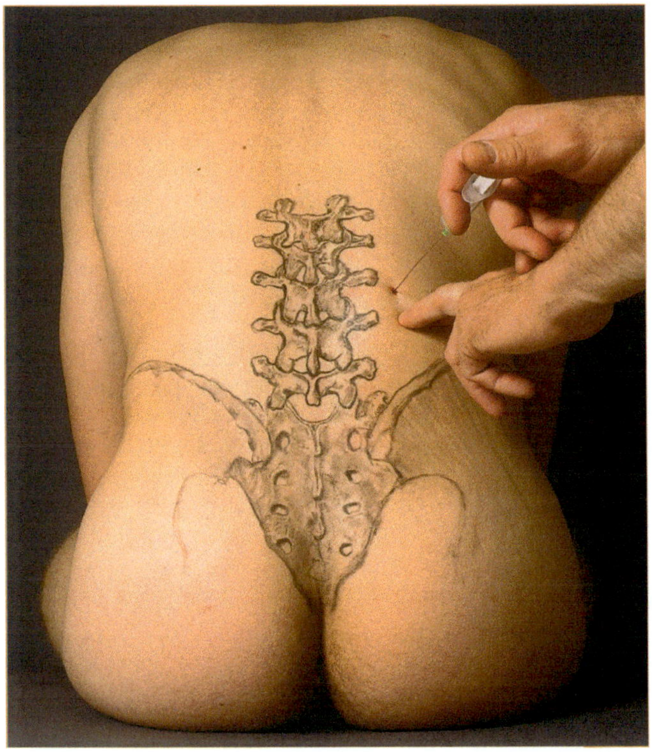

►**Fig. 18.30** Sitting position and puncture point.

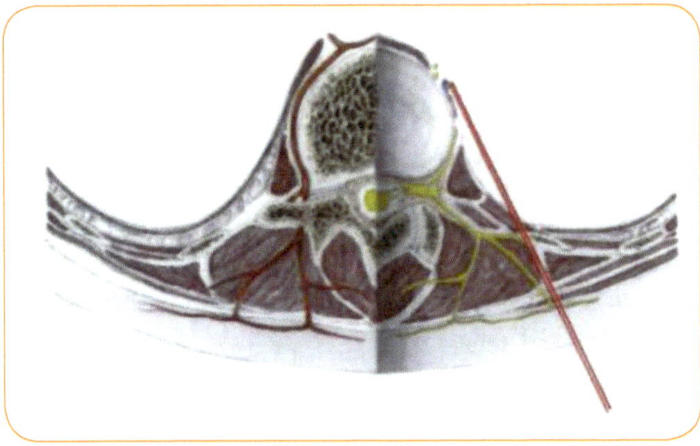

►**Fig. 18.31** Needle position before injection.

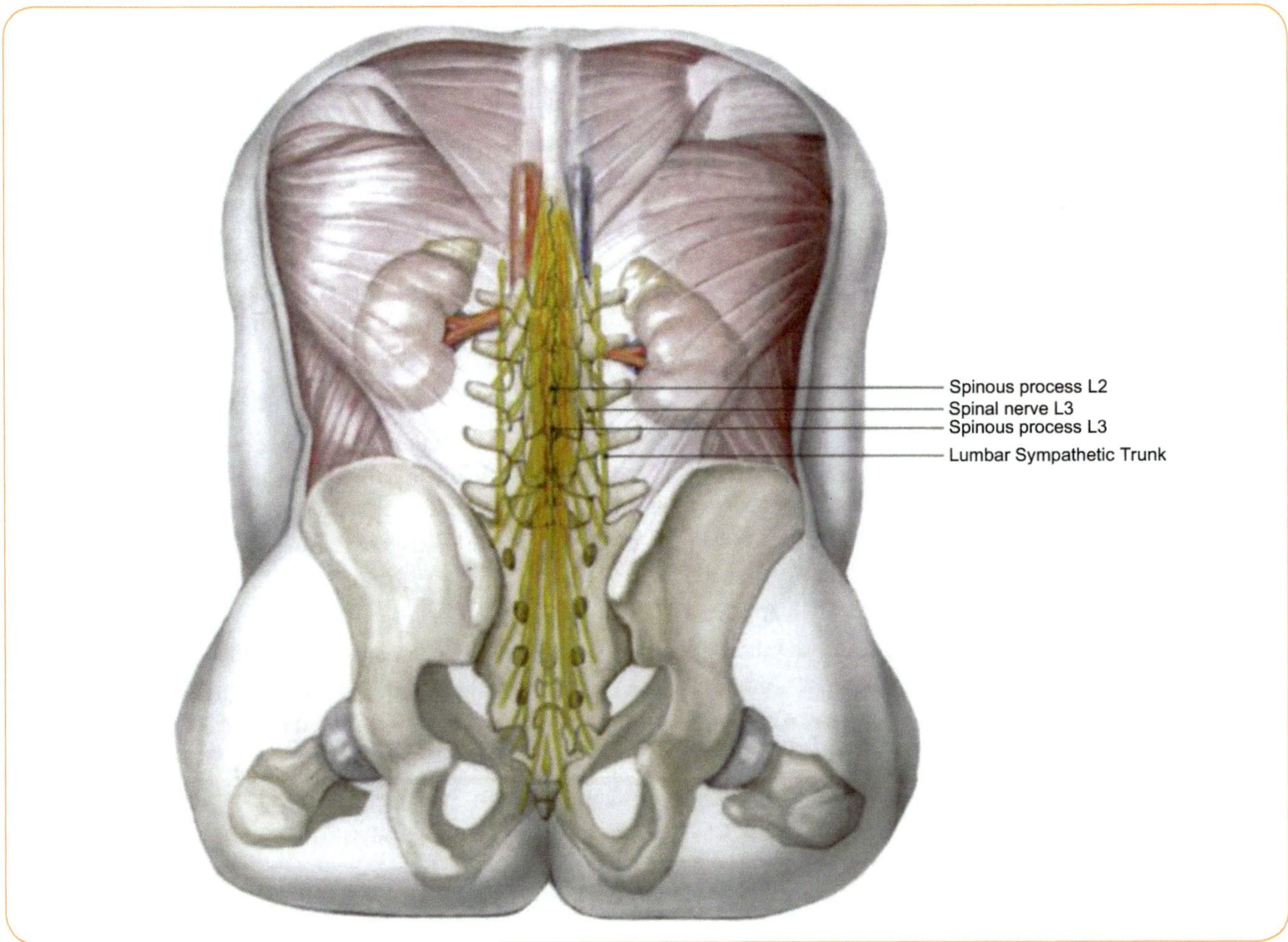

►**Fig. 18.32** Topography for injection to the lumbar sympathetic trunk.

18.9 Injection in the Sacral and Lumbar Epidural Space

18.9.1 Indications

The indications given are only a sample of those possible:

- Chronic lower back pain.
- Chronic sciatica.
- Prostatitis.
- Adnexitis.
- Cystitis.
- Prostate hyperplasia.
- Circulation disorder of the lower extremity.
- Frostbite.
- Venous ulcer.
- Complex regional pain syndrome (CRPS).
- Phantom pain in the lower extremity.
- Chronic osteomyelitis in the area of the pelvis and lower extremity.
- Herpes zoster.
- Thrombophlebitis.
- Postthrombotic syndrome.
- Raynaud's disease.
- Chronic painful conditions after injuries to the lumbar spine and sacral bone.
- Diskitis.
- Pain with metastases in the area of the vertebrae and the spinal canal.

The expected success depends, among other things, on the the patient's "interference field situation."

18.9.2 Anatomy and Neurophysiology

The periosteum of the vertebrae and the vertebral canal space delineated by the dura mater is designated as an epidural or peridural space. This peridural space is filled with connective tissue and fatty tissue, the incoming and outgoing vessels for the cauda equina as well as the dura mater, and the ligament structure within the vertebral canal. Important for neural therapy is the sympathetic innervation of the periosteum of the vertebrae, the dura mater, the vessels in the vertebral canal, and the vasa nervorum which proceeds via a small branch originating via the gray ramus communicans from the dorsal sympathetic root (dorsal artery). The previous presumption that the posterior and anterior root of the spinal cord could be reached in the peridural space was shown to be false since the dura mater, as a coating, reaches up to and including the spinal ganglion and does not start until directly behind the loose connective tissue coating of the spinal nerve.[274] Thus, the local anesthetic reaches initially the spinal nerve, with its fiber portion, distally from the spinal ganglion. The procaine 1% used in neural therapy is not suitable for producing full peridural anesthesia, which is also not the aim. Rather the aim is to reach only the sparsely myelinated autonomic fibers of the sympathetic nervous system in the peridural space. This is also the basis of peridural and epidural infiltration for therapeutic purposes outside of the anesthesia used for operations.

The list of indications for neural therapeutic treatment via the peridural space largely comprises diseases related to regional circulation disorders, i.e., diseases which ultimately correspond to impaired sympathetic nervous system function. Since only the dorsal branch of the sympathetic nervous system is reached with infiltration of the peridural space, sympatholysis of the peridural vessels and improved blood flow to the spinal marrow and the cauda equina are to be expected as well as interruption of the pain-conducting afferent fibers of the dura mater and the periosteum of the vertebrae. The main part of the sympathetic nervous system is initially reached outside of the dura sheath, i.e., outside of the intervertebral foramen.

▸**Sacral epidural space.** For infiltrations to the epidural space (▸Fig. 18.33, ▸Fig. 18.34), it is significant that the spinal ganglia are located within the sacral vertebral canal, whereas in the lumbar spine they are found in the intervertebral foramen. The dural sheath that envelops the cauda equina usually ends at the level of the second sacral vertebra, but may occasionally reach down to the fourth sacral vertebra. The fill volume of the sacral canal is quite variable and is between 12 and 65 mL, which is important for estimating the infusion quantity.[274] Thus, depending on the individual structure of the sacral internal space, an infiltration quantity between 10 and 15 mL is expected with involvement of the lumbar epidural space. If the epidural space must be reached above the level of S1, the injection quantity is increased; 20 mL reaches segment L5, 25 mL is required up to segment T12, and 30 mL reaches approximately the thoracic segments T8–T9. Since procaine 1% or 0.5% (10 mL or more total quantity) is used for infiltration of the epidural space for neural therapeutic purposes, anesthesia and suppression of the motor fiber sections are not expected. In this case, procaine is shown to be particularly useful for selective interruption of the autonomic fibers, especially for outpatient use, since the patient remains able to carry out normal day-to-day activities.

▸**Lumbar epidural space**. The injection in the epidural space (▸Fig. 18.33, ▸Fig. 18.35) bypasses the sacral

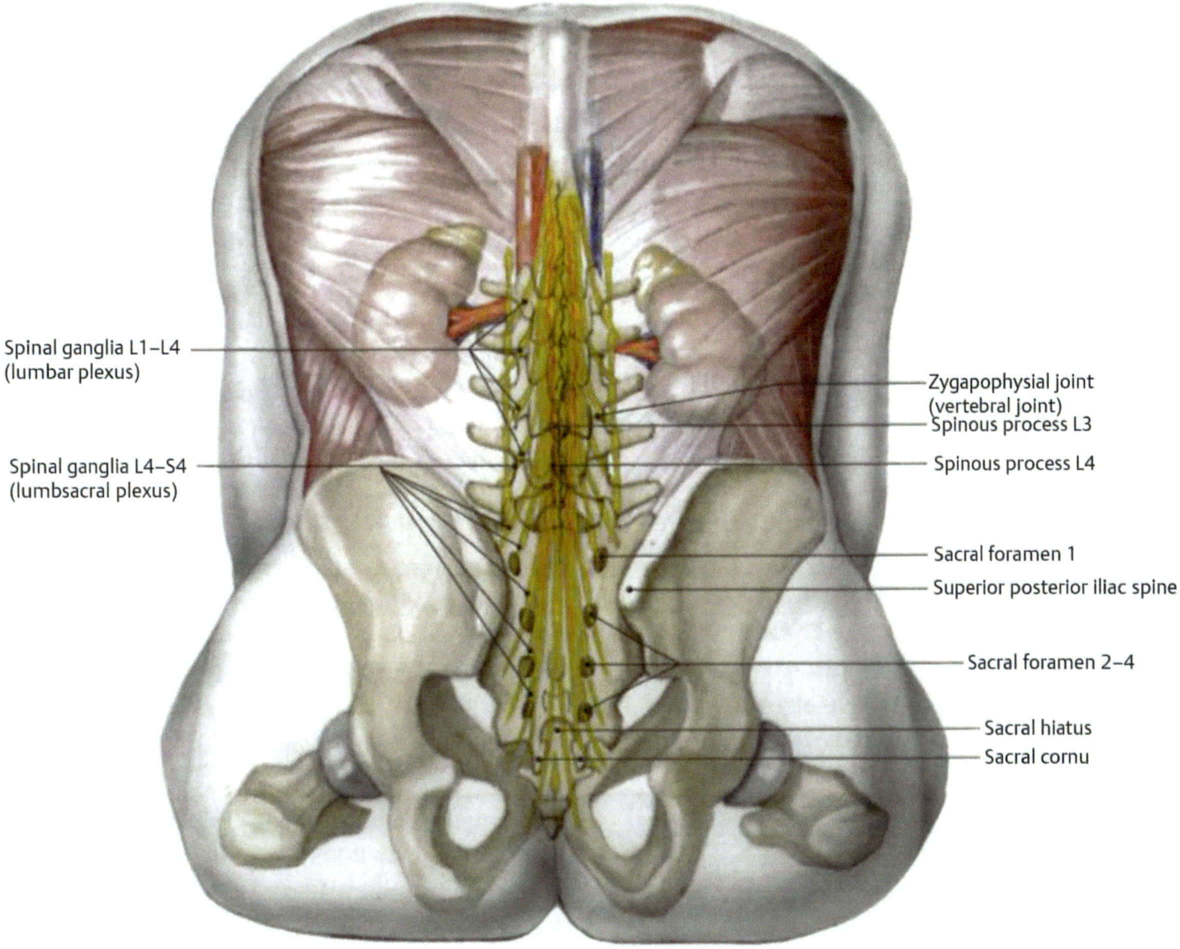

▶**Fig. 18.33** Topography of the lumbar and sacral region.

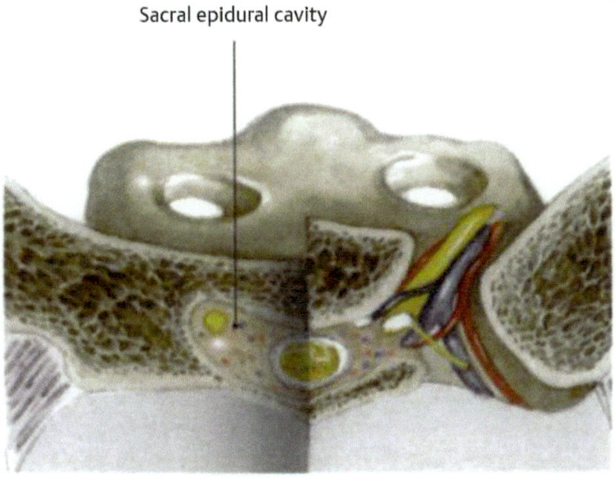

▶**Fig. 18.34** Sacral epidural space.

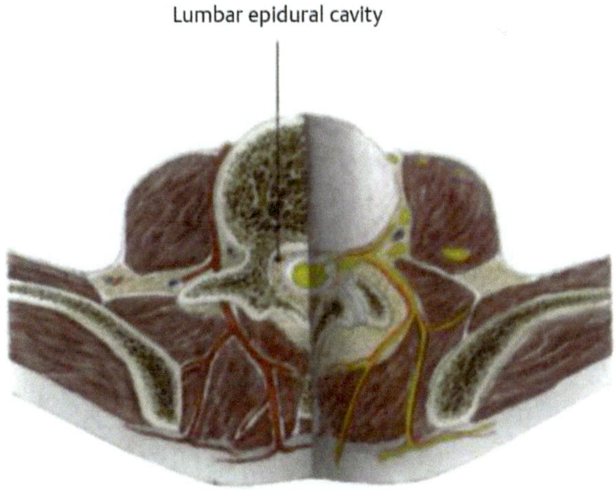

▶**Fig. 18.35** Lumbar epidural space.

epidural space and requires less procaine. Also located here is the anatomical substrate of the sympathetic nervous system, which is used therapeutically in the form of afferent and efferent sympatholysis by way of procaine. On the one hand, this reaches the portion that proceeds with the spinal nerves and, on the other hand, the perivascular portion which controls blood supply, among other things, in the vertebral canal. These anatomical relationships give rise to the indications for lumbar epidural infiltration for disorders of the spine and the surrounding musculature, as well as for disorders of the lower extremity and all of its tissues and functional parts, i.e., bones, joints, ligament-capsule structures, nerves, vessels, and musculature.

Thoracic epidural infiltration provides an excellent opportunity for therapy of diseases and functional disorders of the thorax and abdominal region by utilizing regional-segmental sympatholysis. It has proven effective for the following disorders:

- Lung embolism.
- Intercostal neuralgia.
- Certain forms of pneumonia.
- Diseases of the abdominal organs:
  - Hepatitis (T7–T8).
  - Paralytic ileus (T9–T11).
  - Biliary colic.
  - Renal colic.
  - Spastic constipation.
  - Pancreatitis.
  - Gastric ulcer.

This type of thoracic epidural infiltration is selective sympatholysis of the organs supplied by the sympathetic and parasympathetic nervous systems.

Cave

The injection interrupts the vasomotor function of the abdominal space, so that severe spinal anesthesia with circulatory effects and impaired breathing through motor paralysis of the thoracic musculature is expected with circulatory depression and in the case of accidental intrathecal injection. For this reason, the injection is not suitable for outpatient practices.

The injection to the celiac ganglion (p. 206) is a low-risk and particularly effective therapeutic option for disorders of organs in the abdominal and retro- peritoneal space.

Cervical epidural infiltration is not valuable from a therapeutic perspective since the sympathetic supply of the epidural space, like the connections to the spinal nerves, proceeds via the cervical sympathetic trunk, i.e., it is retrograde from the perspective of the innervation direction. The sympathetic spinal nucleic regions for sympathetic supply of the cervical spine and the neck marrow do not start until segment C8 and reach up to the top five thoracic segments. When treating the cervical spine, the head, the upper extremity, and the thorax including its organs, it is logical to select the ganglia of the cervical sympathetic trunk as the infiltration target, i.e., the stellate ganglion and the superior cervical ganglion.

18.9.3 Injection Technique

▶ **Sacral epidural infiltration (according to Cathelin and Sicard).** The patient is either positioned on the stomach with pelvis raised 20 to 30 cm, or in a side-lying position with tucked up legs, or seated with the upper body bent forward. The seated position shown in ▶ Fig. 18.36 has the advantage of easy orientation to the sacrum for the therapist; it is also c omfortable for the patient. The therapist should select one favored position, since this way the likelihood of an incorrect injection is lowest.

In all cases, the sacral hiatus is identified by palpation of the sacral spinous process line, in order to take into account the frequent anomalies of the sacral hiatus. The normal sacral hiatus is located directly below the spinous process S4 (in about 34% of patients; somewhat deeper in about 19% of patients, and above S4 in about 47% of patients). The second palpable structure is the sacral cornua on both sides, slightly below the spinous process S4. Normally the finger is used to palpate a slightly springy membrane (superficial dorsal sacrococcygeal ligaments) directly below the spinous process S4. After thorough disinfection of the skin, make a sharp medial puncture at the level of the sacral cornu with a 4-cm needle at an angle of about 45° to the skin (▶ Fig. 18.37). After insertion of a wheal, the needle which was previously angled about 30°at the cone is pushed forward through the superficial dorsal sacrococcygeal ligaments. This creates significantly increased resistance which subsides suddenly after 2 to 3 mm, whereby the needle must be directed another 20 to 30° in cranial direction and pushed forward another 1 to 2 cm. After twice-negative aspiration, slowly infiltrate 5 to 30 mL procaine 1%depending on the planned infiltration level:

- 5 mL for S5–S3.
- 10 mL for S5–S2.
- 15 mL for S5–S1.
- 20 mL for S5–L5.
- 25 mL for S5–L1.
- 30 mL for S5–T8/T9.

Cave

Avoid pushing the needle further forward in the sacral canal to prevent injury to the dura mater which generally reaches up to level S2 but can sometimes reach as far as S4.

The injection is performed slowly, whereby the patient can feel a slight sensation of pressure. Place the index finger of your free hand directly above the needle on the sacral hiatus. If the needle is not in the sacral canal, immediately palpate the subcutaneous flowing medication. If blood is aspirated, perform the infiltration again after correcting the needle position and aspirating again. If CSF is aspirated, correct the needle position and perform the injection after negative aspiration. If there is severe pain with the injection and the injection resistance is very high, the needle is in the deep dorsal sacrococcygeal ligament, the extension of the posterior longitudinal ligament. In this case, the needle must be pulled back by about 1 to 2 mm.

Lumbar Epidural Infiltration (According to Dogliotti)

The epidural infiltration in the area of the lumbar spine is indicated for therapeutic purposes if the approach is strictly segmental (e.g., segment L2 or segment L4). The advantage of this peridural infiltration is the ability to work with low amounts of procaine (maximum of 5 mL). A disadvantage is the somewhat more difficult technique, since the peridural space in the lumbar region is only about 1 to 3 mm wide between the yellow ligament and the dura mater.

After marking the spinous process at the planned segmental level (e.g., spinous process L3/L4) and skin disinfection, insert the 6-cm needle somewhat below the lower edge of the upper spinous process perpendicular to the skin and sharply medial. The patient should be in a seated position and bent slightly forward. After insertion of a wheal, slowly push the needle forward with light infiltration.

Note

The attached 5-mL syringe should contain 5 mL saline solution and the opening of the needle should be perpendicular.

Three ligament structures must be penetrated, which is evidenced by increased puncture and injection pressure. First, the thin supraspinal ligament is penetrated; this is followed by the interspinal ligament with only slightly increased injection resistance. The yellow ligament is penetrated last and is characterized by slightly increased puncture resistance and very strong injection resistance. When penetrating the yellow ligament, the needle must be guided with both hands, whereby the free hand is supported on the patient's back and the needle is gripped at the cone.

This ensures that the needle does not enter the spinal canal suddenly through the yellow ligament. The entry of the needle tip is signaled by sudden release of the injection resistance. Since infiltration is done with saline solution, accidental spinal anesthesia is ruled out. After two aspirations with rotation of the needle by 180°, the syringe is changed and filled with procaine 1% this time. Aspirate again at two levels and slowly infiltrate 5 mL anesthetic after a negative suction test.

Note

No pain should occur with the injection.

The anteflexed position of the patient is favorable for the injection to the extent that this slightly translocates the cauda equina and medulla oblongata in the ventral direction and the dorsal epidural space becomes somewhat wider.

18.9.4 Material

Required:

- 5-mL syringe.
- Needle:
  - 0.4 × 40 mm needle for epidural sacral injection.
  - 0.6 × 60 mm needle for lumbar peridural injection.
- Physiological saline solution 5 mL.
- Procaine 1%
  - Sacral: 5 to 25 mL.
  - Lumbar: 5 mL.

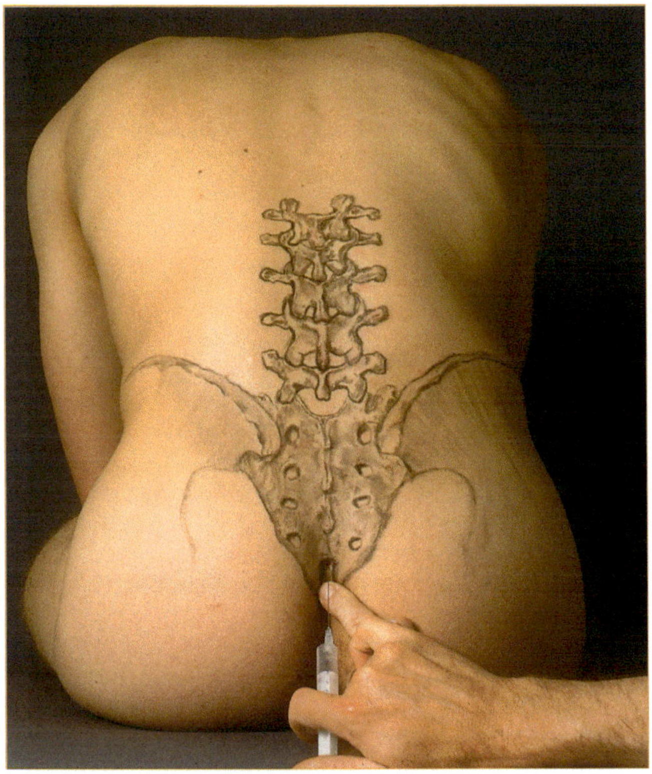

►**Fig. 18.36** Injection in the sacral epidural space.

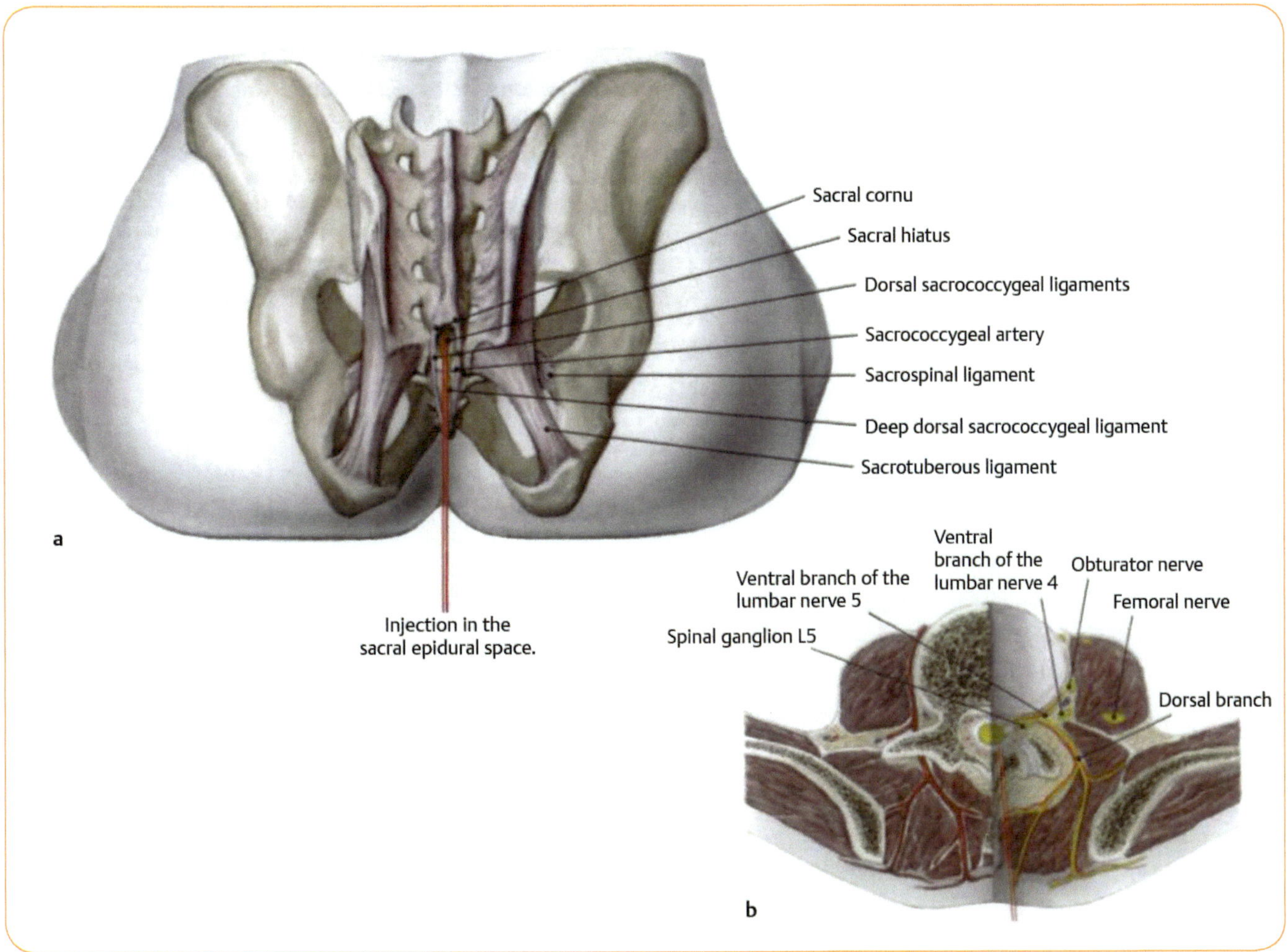

►**Fig. 18.37** Injection in the sacral epidural space. **(a)** Topography for injection in the sacral epidural space. **(b)** Cross-section with epidural needle position at level L2–L3.

19 Abdomen, Retroperitoneum

19.1 Injection to the Renal Hilum and the Renal Plexus

19.1.1 Indications

The indications given are only a sample of those possible:

- Acute and chronic pyelonephritis.
- Nephrolithiasis.
- Renal colic with and without evidence of stones.
- Hydronephrosis.
- Research in kidney function disorders (oliguria, anuria).
- Unexplained flank pain.
- Research in functional disorders of the testes and ovaries.
- Nephrogenic hypertension.
- Research in "essential" hypertension.
- Kidney as an interference field after illness or injury.

The expected success depends, among other things, on the the patient's "interference field situation."

19.1.2 Anatomy and Neurophysiology

The kidneys are positioned bilaterally on both sides of the spine in the retroperitoneal space at the level of the 11th thoracic to the 3rd lumbar vertebrae; the right kidney is positioned about 2 cm further in caudal direction than the left kidney. The renal hilum with its incoming and outgoing vessels and the transition from the renal pelvis to the ureter is normally at the level of the vertebrae L1–L2, i.e., approximately at the level of the spinous process L1, which serves as an important landmark. The sympathetic renal plexus is composed of fiber components from the celiac ganglion, the abdominal aortic plexus, the minor splanchnic nerve, the lowest splanchnic nerve, the lumbar sympathetic ganglion, and the vagus nerve. Running alongside with the renal artery, these nerves supply the renal hilum, renal tissue, kidney cavity system and the ureter. The region of the renal hilum (through which the sympathetic efferent and afferent fibers are easily reached) is the destination of the injection in order to achieve both improved circulation of the kidney as well as reduction of the irritated afferent fibers during illness. At the same time, a therapeutic effect on the testes and ovaries through the testicular plexus or ovarian plexus is possible because this plexus receives a portion of its sympathetic fibers from the renal plexus.

19.1.3 Injection Technique

With the patient seated and bent slightly forward, find the spinous process of L1 (▶Fig. 19.1, ▶Fig. 19.2, ▶Fig. 19.3); three finger-widths in the lateral direction (about 5 cm) make the injection with an 8-cm needle. After placement of a wheal, push the needle forward slightly, whereby the direction of the injection should be about 5° in the medial direction. If bone is contacted at 4 to 5 cm, the needle is too far medial at the spinous process of L2, which the needle should skim past. Depending on the body size, the depth of the injection is between 6 and 8 cm. Proceeding with the infiltration, the medication flows without major plunger pressure after overcoming the muscular resistance of the autochthonous back muscles and the major psoas muscle (only 2 cm thick) as well as the muscle fascia adjacent to the retroperitoneal space. The tip of the needle is now at the level of the renal hilum. After twice-negative aspiration, slowly infiltrate 5 mL anesthetic . The patient may indicate a slight feeling of pressure in the lumbar region. Pain occurs when the fibrous renal capsule is touched by the needle.

19.1.4 Material

Required:

- 5-mL syringe.
- 0.6 × 80 mm needle.
- Procaine 1%, 5 mL per injection.

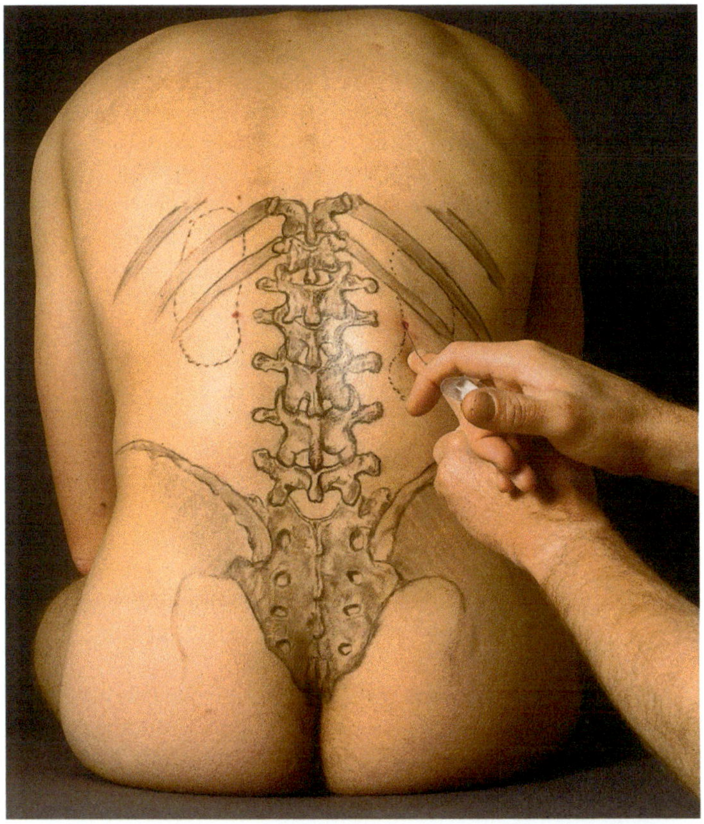

►**Fig. 19.1** Injection to the renal hilum and the renal plexus.

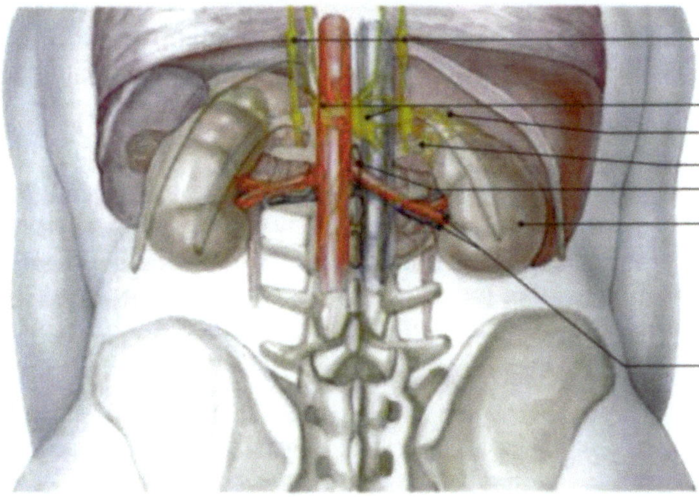

►**Fig. 19.2** Topography for injection to the renal hilum.

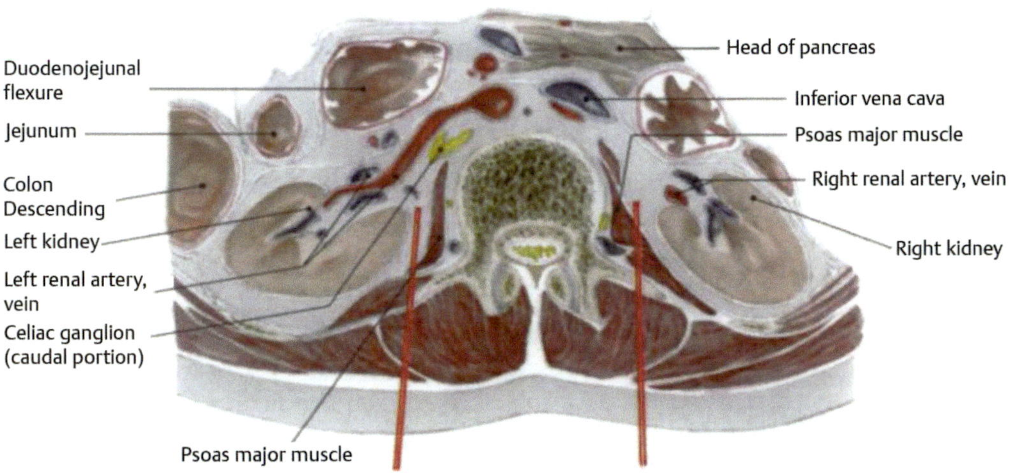

►**Fig. 19.3** Topography for injection to the renal hilum, cross-section at the level of L1–L2.

19.2

Injection to the Celiac Ganglion and the Major and Minor Splanchnic Nerves

19.2.1 Indications

The indications given are only a sample of those possible:

- Chronic digestion disorders (constipation, diarrhea).
- Chronic and acute inflammation of the gastrointestinal tract.
- Ventricular and duodenal ulcers.
- Pyloric spasm.
- Achalasia.
- Reflux esophagitis.
- Gastritis.
- Chronic nausea.
- Pancreatitis.
- Chronic pancreatic insufficiency.
- Hepatitis (toxic, viral).
- Toxic hepatosis.
- Bile secretion disorders.
- Fat metabolism disorders.
- Cholecystitis.
- Cholangitis.
- Gall bladder mucocele.
- Biliary colic.
- Gallstone disease.
- "Postcholecystectomy syndrome."
- Bacterial and viral infections of the gastrointestinal tract.
- Investigations of food intolerance (fat, dairy products, intestinal intoxication, food allergies).
- Crohn's disease (after interference field exploration).
- Ulcerative colitis (after interference field exploration).
- Diverticulitis.
- Diverticulosis.
- Inflammatory and degenerative diseases of the urogenital system.
- Functional disorders of the urogenital system.
- Chronic recurrent vomiting.
- Pre-eclampsia.
- Hepatorenal syndrome.
- Malignant pain of the stomach area.
- Abdominal organs as an interference field during or after illness or injury.

The expected success depends, among other things, on the the patient's "interference field situation."

19.2.2 Anatomy and Neurophysiology

The celiac ganglion is the most powerful network of the autonomic system. It is located on the proximal limb of the abdominal aorta, i.e., on the ventral surface of the aorta, and surrounds it partially on the left and right in a horseshoe shape (► Fig. 19.5). The right portion of the celiac ganglion is partly in contact with the posteromedial wall of the inferior vena cava, so that this ganglion is reached with the injection needle bilaterally from the dorsal direction[274] (modified according to Symington, ► Fig. 19.4, ► Fig. 19.8).

The sympathetic inlets and processes to the celiac ganglion come from T5–T9 (major splanchnic nerve) and T10–T11 (minor splanchnic nerve). The preganglionic efferent fibers are switched partly in the celiac ganglion, partly in the intramural ganglia of the intestine. The sympathetic afferent fibers have the same sequence. They are switched in the spinal ganglia and in the sympathetic trunk ganglia.[69] The splanchnic nerves extend paravertebrally up to the level of the transition of T12/L1, where they radiate into the celiac ganglion after passing through the diaphragm—with the fibers oriented in ventral direction. The first lumbar vertebra is the landmark for the injection to the celiac ganglion and the splanchnic nerves.

The celiac ganglion is not a purely sympathetic ganglion but receives parasympathetic influx particularly from the right vagus nerve, whose celiac branch extends behind the stomach with the left gastric artery on its way to the celiac ganglion and from there with the sympathetic fibers to the pancreas, spleen, liver, small intestine, kidney, and adrenal gland.

Injection of a local anesthetic to the celiac ganglion and the splanchnic nerves results in reduced function of the sympathetic and parasympathetic afferent and efferent fibers. Thus, the broad list of indications is understandable, which concerns the inflammatory, degenerative as well as functional disorders of the organs of the abdomen that can be achieved through suppression of the vasomotor function, as well as disorders of inner and outer secretion, muscle function of the intestine as well as visceral sensitivity. According to clinical experience, the short-term selective interruption of the pathological stimulation of the sympathetic and/or parasympathetic nervous system is sufficient for bringing the body to a state of balanced regional self-regulation.

19.2.3 Injection Technique

With the patient seated and slightly bent forward, palpation of the spinous process of L1 and the 12th rib. Depending on body size make the injection perpendicular to the skin with an 8 to 12 cm needle, one finger-width below the lower edge of the spinous process L1, about 5 cm lateral (three finger-widths) right or left of the medians. After placement of a wheal, push the needle forward slowly with light plunger pressure about 10 to 20° in median direction and about 20° in cranial direction. For relaxation, the patient should breathe normally. The target of the needle tip is the front craniolateral portion of the first lumbar vertebra, which—depending on body size—is reached a depth of between 7 and 9 cm. The distance from the tip of the spinous process to the front edge of the vertebrae is between 7 and 9 cm. Through oblique guidance of the needle, this distance becomes about 0.5 to 1 cm longer. If the needle already makes contact with bone at 4 to 5 cm, the transverse process of L1 has been struck, under which the needle must be inserted. This can result in a flash of pain in segment L1, through irritation of the spinal nerves L1.

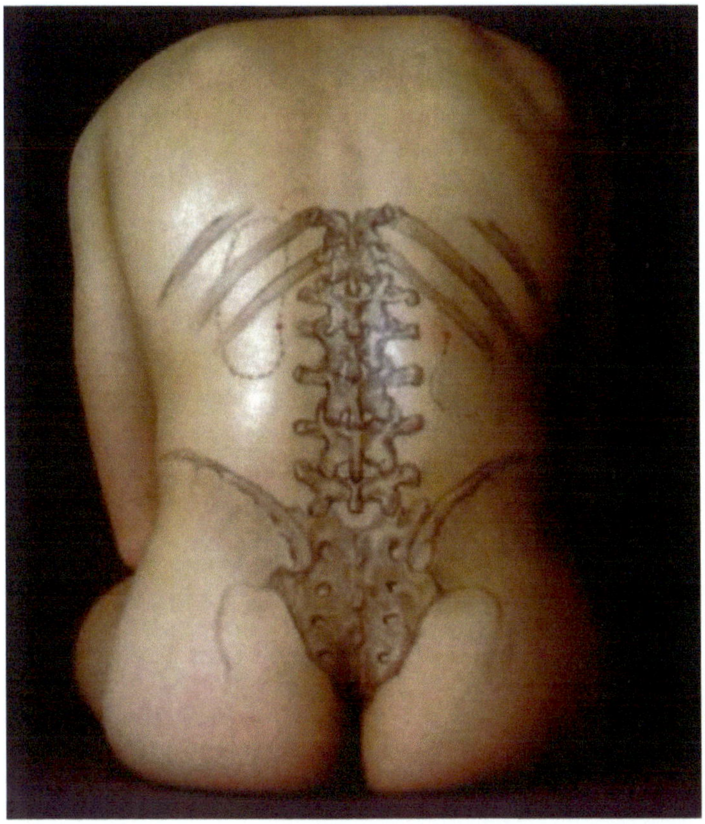

▸**Fig. 19.4** Sitting position for injection to the celiac ganglion and the splanchnic nerves, injection points.

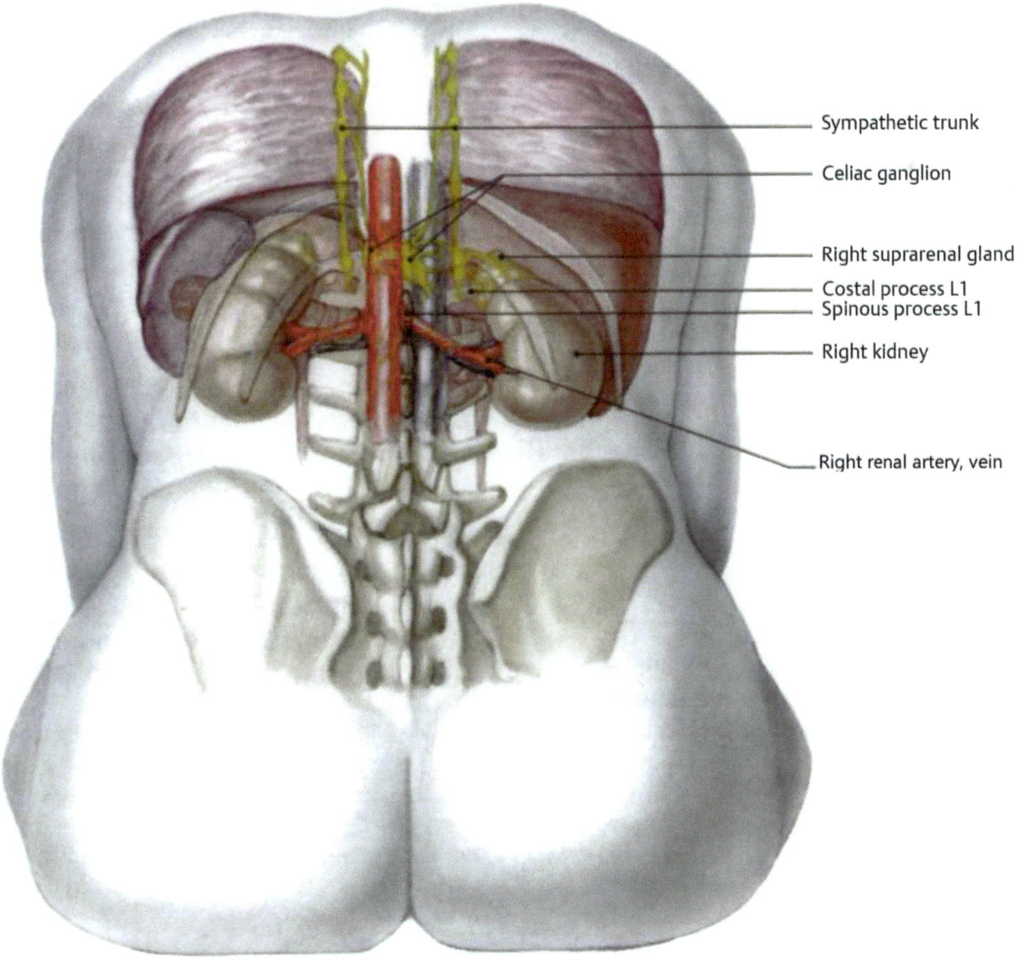

▸**Fig. 19.5** Topography for injection to the celiac ganglion and the splanchnic nerves.

After 6 to 7 cm (after 8–9 cm in larger patients), contact is made with the lateral portion of vertebra L1. After double aspiration with 180° rotation of the needle, 2 to 3 mL anesthetic is infiltrated, since the tip of the needle is near the splanchnic nerves. The medication flows against very slight resistance. Afterward the needle is pulled back about 2 to 3 cm, the convergent direction of the injection is slightly reduced, and then pushed forward again 3 to 4 cm, i.e., 1 cm deeper. Now the needle is directly at the level of the vertebral front edge, on the right behind the inferior vena cava, left dorsolateral to the abdominal aorta. After another double aspiration with 180° rotation of the needle, the medication flows into the retroperitoneum with almost no resistance. An injection quantity of 5 mL is sufficient for partial celiac infiltration. The ganglion itself is about 1 to 2 cm further ventral, anterolateral to the abdominal aorta. Since the celiac ganglion surrounds the aorta in a slight arc form from the ventral direction and the aorta is to the left of the vertebral medians, the distance from the needle tip to the left portion of the celiac ganglion is somewhat shorter than on the other side.

Note

Pain should not occur when advancing the needle nor with infiltration. The patient should only feel slight pressure sensations in the respective flank region or in the course of the autochthonous back musculature.

The vertebra L1, which should be felt with the needle tip, is important for orientation of the needle position, since advancement too far laterally can lead to stabbing of the adrenal gland or kidney, which causes significant pain (► Fig. 19.6, ► Fig. 19.8, ► Fig. 19.9). In this case, the needle must be pulled back and corrected in the medial direction. If the needle is advanced too far, dark blood will appear in the aspiration on the right and light-colored blood in the aspiration on the left, indicating intravenous or intra-arterial needle position, respectively (► Fig. 19.7). After retraction of the needle, infiltration can be performed after negative aspiration. The retroperitoneal hematoma resulting from the puncture hole has no clinical relevance if the coagulation status is normal.

Injury to the lung is not possible if the described technique is complied with.

Practical Advice

The use of imaging procedures is useful only when the anatomical conditions are changed (scoliosis, surgical interventions in the retroperitoneum) or there is insufficient experience with this technique.

The neural therapist's training ensures mastery of this injection without imaging. Reducing the injection risk by using imaging procedures should not be expected, since in addition to the radiation exposure (CT-guided injection), concentrating on a screen or a “transducer” (sonography) is counter to the precise observation of the actual injection procedure on the patient through sensitive handling of the injection tool. Compared to similar injections (spinal root injections, sympathetic trunk injections, renal plexus injections), injection to the celiac ganglion/splanchnic nerves involves an injection procedure in which the needle must be advanced only 1 to 2 cm further in the ventral direction.

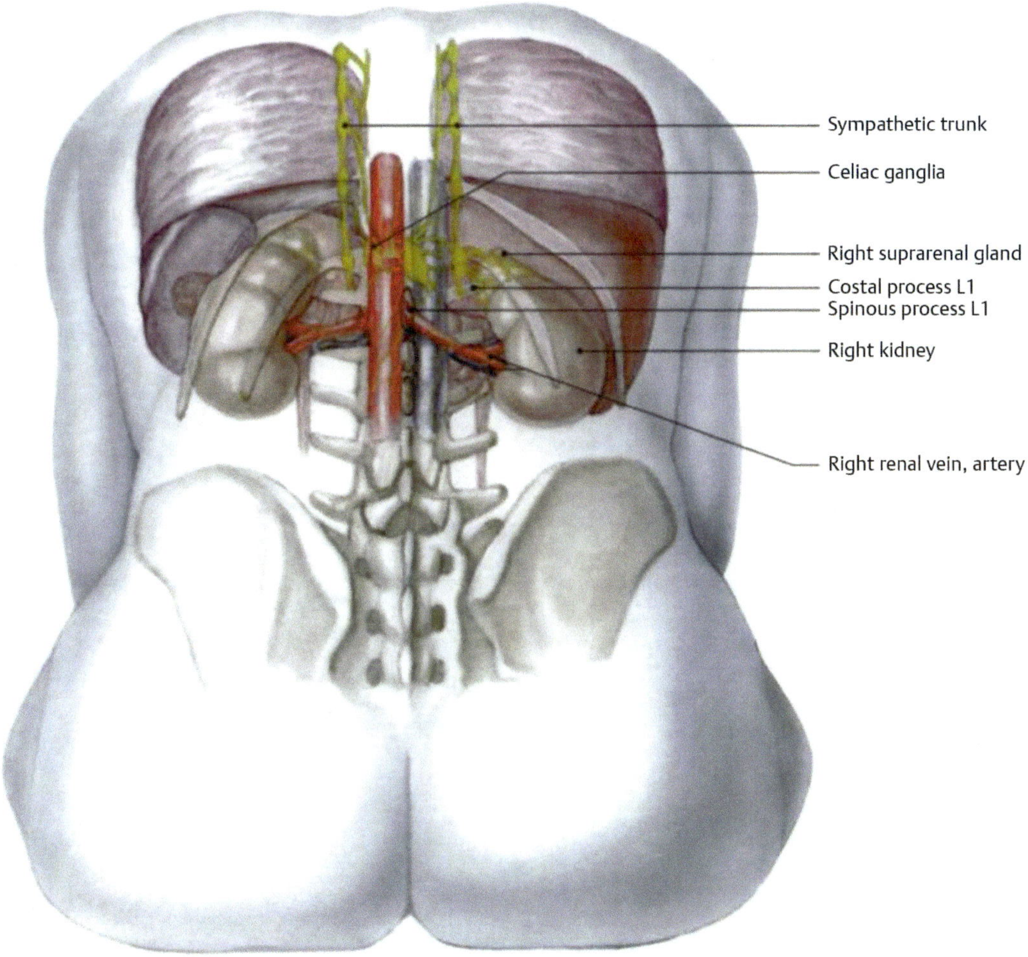

▶ **Fig. 19.6** Topography for injection to the celiac ganglion and the splanchnic nerves.

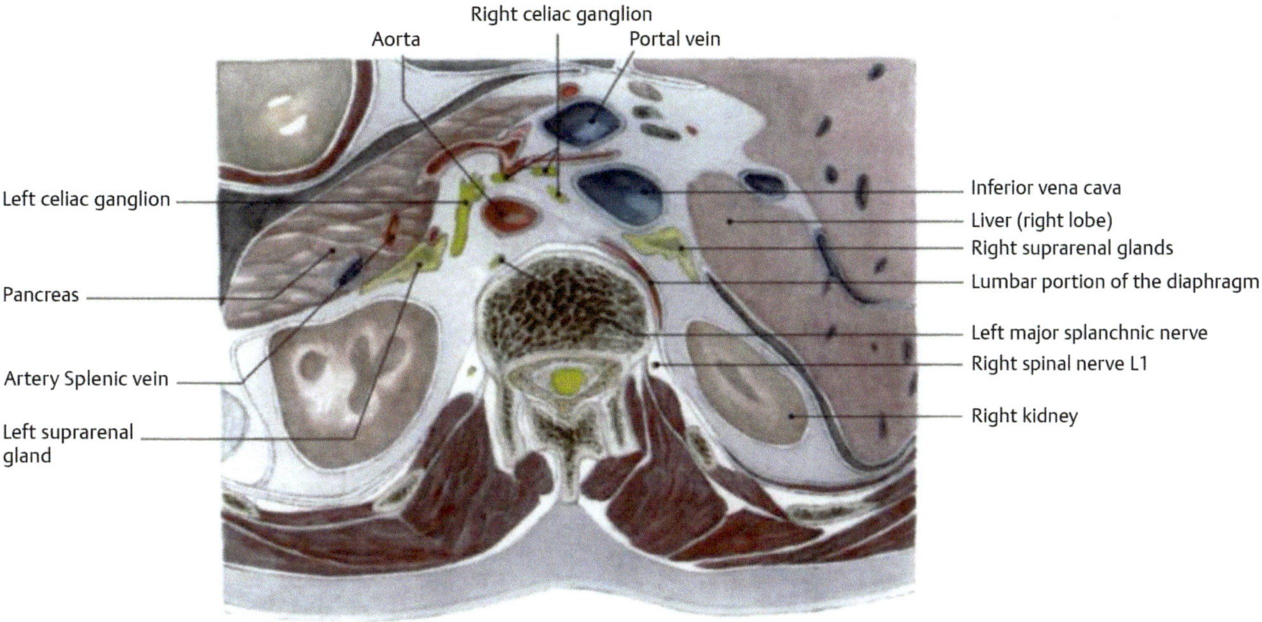

▶ **Fig. 19.7** Topography for injection to the celiac ganglion and the splanchnic nerves, transverse section at the level of the upper edge of L1.

If the symptomology remains unaffected by the first injection, the injection to the celiac ganglion should be repeated one to two times using double the injection amount (10 mL procaine) in order to ensure that the ganglion is reached.

19.2.4 Material

Required:

- 10-mL syringe.
- 0.6/0.8 × 80 to 100 mm needle.
- Procaine 1%, 5 to 10 mL per injection.

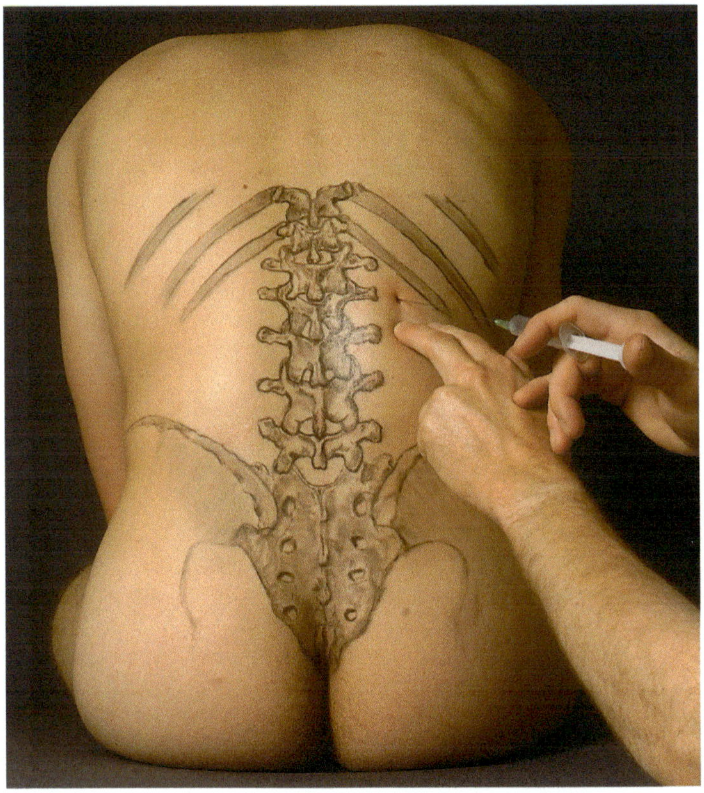

►**Fig. 19.8** Injection to the right celiac ganglion, needle guidance (modified according to Symington), insertion point.

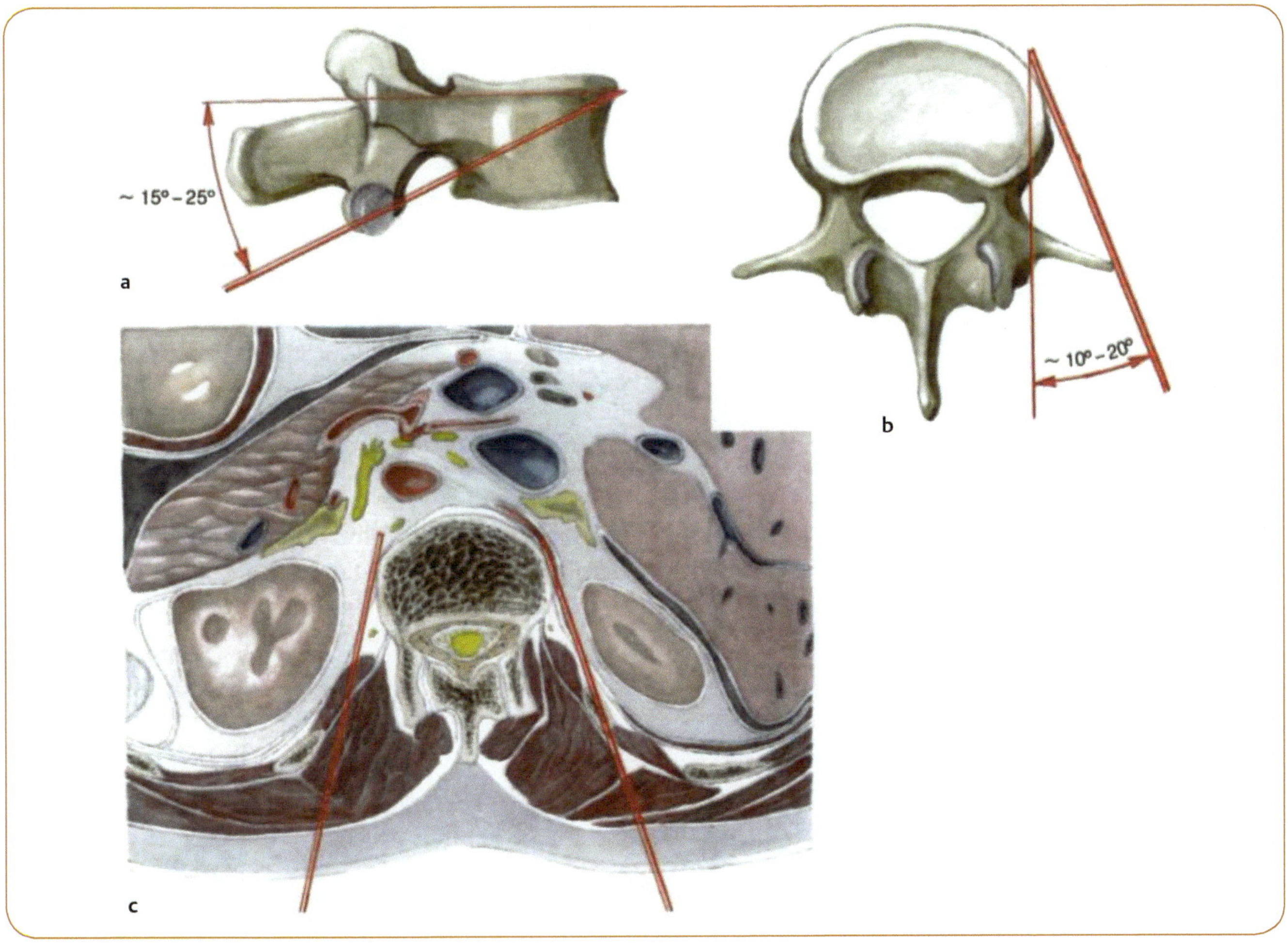

►**Fig. 19.9** Needle guidance. **(a)** Side view. **(b)** Sagittal view. **(c)** Needle position for injection to the right and left celiac ganglion. Horizontal section for upper third of L1 vertebra.

19.3 Injection to the Branches of the Inferior Hypogastric Plexus (Pelvic Plexus)

19.3.1 Indications

The indications given are only a sample of those possible:

- Amenorrhea.
- Dysmenorrhea.
- Fertility disorders.
- Chronic pelvic pain.
- Endometritis and parametritis.
- Acute and chronic adnexitis.
- Sexual dysfunction.
- Impaired genital function.
- Vaginal discharge.
- Menopausal symptoms (mood swings up to and including depression, adynamia, sleep disorders, "hot flashes").
- Cystitis (acute-chronic, bacterial, nonspecific).
- Bladder function disorders (dysuria, incontinence, voiding disorder).
- Organs of the small pelvis as an interference field (e.g., after giving birth, after operations, after inflammations).

The expected success depends, among other things, on the the patient's "interference field situation."

19.3.2 Anatomy and Neurophysiology

The autonomic innervation of the small pelvis and its organs is, on the one hand, sympathetic via the portion of the superior hypogastric plexus advancing with the aorta, which receives its fibers from the lumbar sympathetic nucleic regions (► Fig. 19.10, ► Fig. 19.11); on the other hand, it is from the pelvic paravertebral ganglia medial to the pelvic sacral foramen. The sympathetic nucleic regions are in the lower thoracic spinal cord and extend up to segment L2/L3. In addition to the supply via the sympathetic nervous system—similar to the sympathetic and parasympathetic composition of the celiac ganglion—the parasympathetic portion is additionally activated via the pelvic splanchnic nerves, whose nucleic regions are in the sacral spinal cord between S2 and S4. The "main gathering point" of these sympathetic–parasympathetic nerves is called the "inferior hypogastric plexus" or "pelvic plexus" and innervates the organs in the pelvis and the external genitalia. From this inferior hypogastric plexus, the following other plexuses emerge:

- Inferior and medial rectal plexuses to supply the rectum.
- Prostatic plexus for the prostate.
- Differential plexus, which proceeds with the vas deferens and supplies this and the epididymis as well as the seminal vesicles.
- The uterovaginal plexus (Frankenhäuser), which corresponds to the deferential plexus but has a considerably greater supply of ganglia cells; it is responsible for the innervation of the uterus and the vagina, and part of the tubes and the ovaries.
- Vesical plexus for supplying the bladder and the bladder voiding function (parasympathetic portion of sphincter relaxation and contraction of the bladder muscles), as well as the cavernous nerves of the penis and clitoris for activation of the cavernous bodies.

Through the pronounced vascular supply of the organs in the small pelvis, the vessel-bound afferent and efferent conducting sympathetic nervous system is also noteworthy. It is responsible for the circulation of these organs and is targeted by the neural therapeutic injections.

Local anesthetic injection in the branches of the inferior hypogastric plexus or pelvic plexus causes partial disruption of the pathological efferent and afferent fibers of both the sympathetic and the parasympathetic nervous systems, resulting in normalization of organ dysfunction.

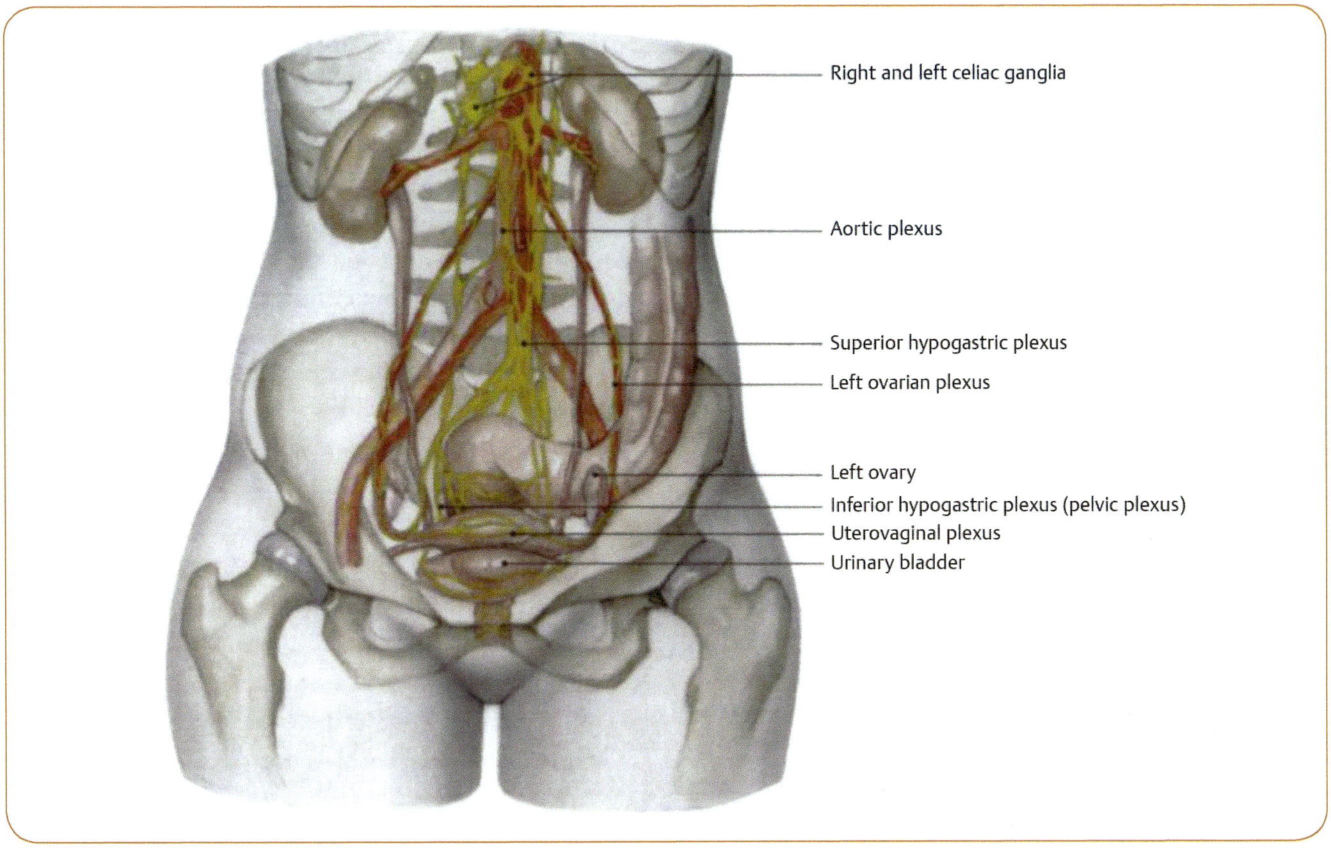

►**Fig. 19.10** Topography of the female urogenital tract.

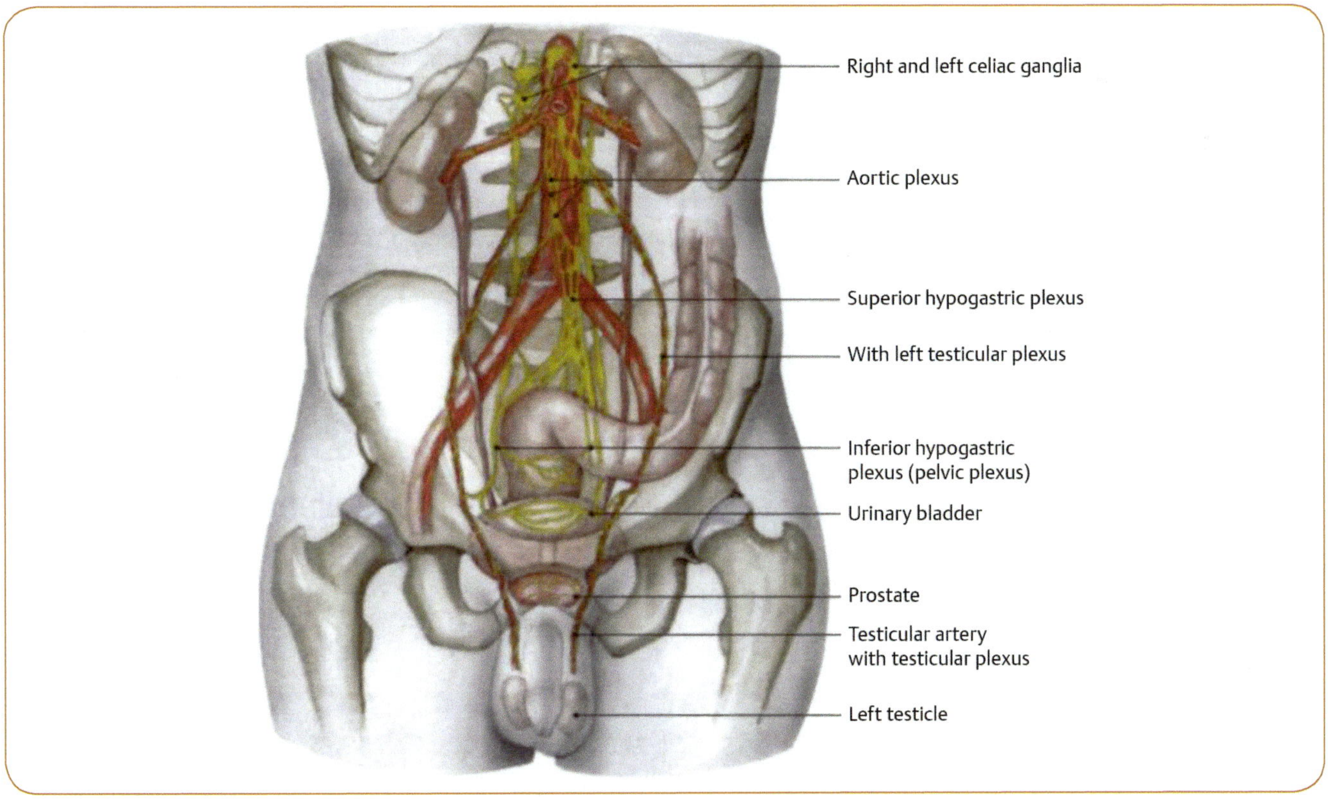

►**Fig. 19.11** Topography of the male urogenital tract.

19.3.3 Injection Technique

Injection to the Branches of the Uterovaginal Plexus

▶ **Suprapubic access.** Palpation of the symphysis and the right and left pubic tubercle into which the inguinal ligament is inserted. About a finger-width cranially at the level of the pubic tubercle with deep pressing of the abdominal wall by 3 to 4 cm, a 4 to 8 cm needle (depending on the strength of the abdominal wall) is inserted perpendicular to the skin. The bladder must be empty.

> **Cave**
>
> **The injection must not be made further laterally due to the risk of injuring the inferior epigastric artery.**

Cranially to the pubic bone transitioning to the symphysis, after insertion of a wheal the needle is advanced by about 30 to 40° in caudal direction and about 10°convergent, if possible without making contact with bone (▶Fig. 19.12, ▶Fig. 19.13). With light pressure on the plunger, the needle is inserted 4 to 8 cm deep depending on anatomical conditions until the patient indicates slight dysesthesia in the area of the urethra, the bladder, and the vagina. Double aspiration with 180°rotation of the needle is performed in order to rule out intravascular or intravesicular needle placement. After negative aspiration, 3 to 5 mL procaine 1% is infiltrated and the needle is removed. If blood is aspirated, the needle position should be corrected and infiltration can be repeated after negative aspiration. If urine is aspirated, the needle and syringe should be removed and the injection repeated with a new syringe, whereby the needle should be slightly (less than 5° convergent) pointed in the median direction.

19.3.4 Complications

Accidental puncture of the bladder is clinically insignificant. Puncture of a vein, or more rarely, puncture of an artery causes a hematoma in the uterovaginal space, possibly resulting in a feeling of moderate pressure in the bladder for several days. A strong feeling of pressure or dysuria persisting for several days without a hematoma is the so-called **reaction phenomenon** and almost always indicates an interference field disorder of the small pelvis, and so the appropriate diagnostics (p. 81) should be performed.

With intact anatomy, intraperitoneal needle positioning with the above injection technique is precluded

> **Cave**
>
> **Puncturing too far in the cranial direction can injure the branch of the superficial epigastric artery, resulting in a painful abdominal wall hematoma. A needle positioned too far laterally (lateral to the pubic tubercle) can injure the inferior epigastric artery causing a preperitoneal hematoma which may require surgical removal.**

With normal coagulation status, injury to the inferior or superior epigastric vein does not cause any relevant hematoma formation.

Transvaginal access to the branches of the uterovaginal plexus will not be described. It requires special instruments as well as a "gynecological" examination chair since the procedure must be performed in the lithotomy position. The injection corresponds to paracervical blockade and is familiar to doctors trained in gynecology.

19.3.5 Material

Required:

- 5-mL syringe.
- 0.4–0.6 × 40–80 mm needle.
- Procaine 1%, 5 mL per injection.

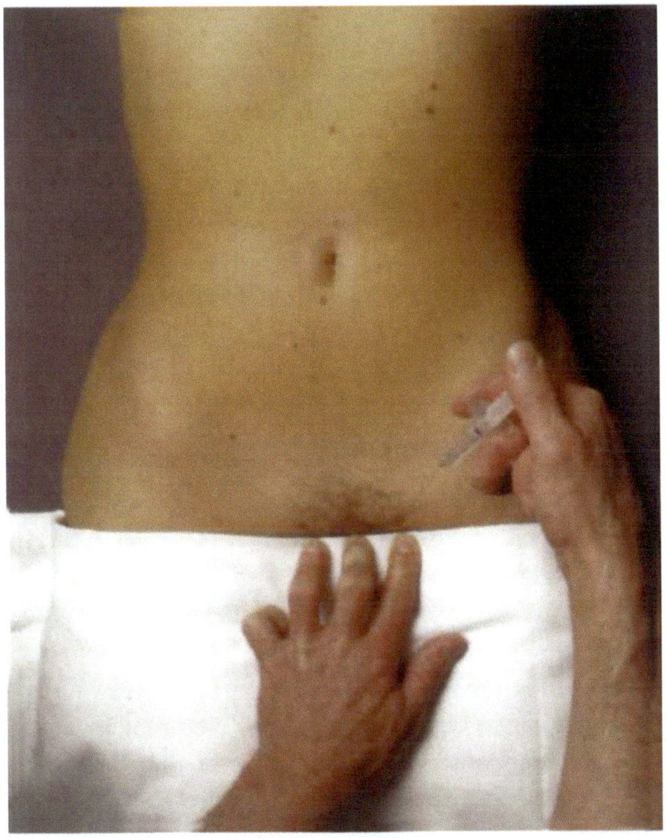

► **Fig. 19.12** Injection to the branches of the uterovaginal plexus in the uterovaginal space.

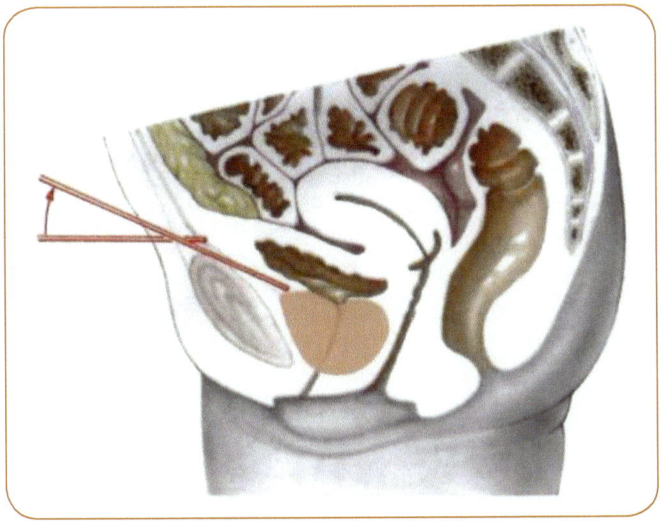

► **Fig. 19.13** Injection to the branches of the uterovaginal plexus at the level of the uterovaginal space.

19.4 Injection to the Branches of the Prostatic Plexus, in the Prostate

19.4.1 Indications

The indications given are only a sample of those possible:

- Acute and chronic prostatitis and cystitis.
- Urination disorders.
- Prostate hyperplasia with and without urination disorders.
- Dysuria after surgical interventions (catheters, cystoscopy, transurethral resection).
- Erectile dysfunction.
- Prostate and bladder as interference fields after illness.

The expected success depends, among other things, on the the patient's "interference field situation."

19.4.2 Anatomy and Neurophysiology

The neuroanatomic and neurophysiological relationships of the male pelvis correspond to those of the female pelvis (p. 240).

19.4.3 Injection Technique

► **Suprapubic/perineal access.** Palpation of the symphysis and the right and left pubic tubercle. The insertion point for the 6 to 8 cm needle is just one finger-width above the pubic tubercle. After insertion of a wheal, the injection is performed perpendicular to the skin. With light pressure on the plunger, the needle is placed above the pubic bone, with the abdominal wall pressed inward 3 to 4 cm, and then advanced past the pubic bone 30 to 40° in caudal direction and 10° convergent (► Fig. 19.14) until the patient indicates a slight burning pain in the glans. Now the needle is positioned directly at the prostate (► Fig. 19.15). After double negative aspiration with rotation of the needle by 180°, 3 to 5 mL procaine 1% is infiltrated. If the needle is advanced about 1 cm further in the same position, the prostate will be punctured. This is indicated by significantly increased plunger resistance and increased pulling in the glans. In case of infiltration in the prostate, the injection quantity should be about 1 to 2 mL.

Note

This injection should be performed slowly, otherwise increased pain can occur during the injection procedure.

In perineal injection, the 8-cm needle is inserted 2 cm anterior to the anal ring and just over 1 cm lateral to the raphe. Beforehand, the prostate is digitally palpable transanally. The injection is made along with transanal finger-palpation of the prostate. The slight injection pain in the glans with perforation of the prostate capsule and further advancement of the needle by 1 cm in the prostate parenchyma demonstrates the correct needle position. Then 2 to 3 mL procaine is slowly infiltrated; another 2 mL is injected periprostatic and the needle is removed.

19.4.4 Complications

If the aspiration draws blood, the needle must be pulled back slightly before an injection is performed after a repeated negative aspiration. The aspiration of urine indicates accidental bladder puncture. In this case the syringe and needle are removed and the injection is repeated with a new instrument.

In the case of pronounced venous vascular supply of the connective tissue surrounding the prostate, the formation of a hematoma is certainly common, but clinically insignificant. A slight feeling of pressure in the bladder region can be caused by such a hematoma.

If the injection is made into the prostate, the patient should be informed about possible resulting slight bleeding from the urethra or bloody ejaculate. These events have no therapeutic consequences.

19.4.5 Material

Required:

- 5-mL syringe.
- 0.6 × 80 mm needle.
- Procaine 1%, 2 to 5 mL per injection.

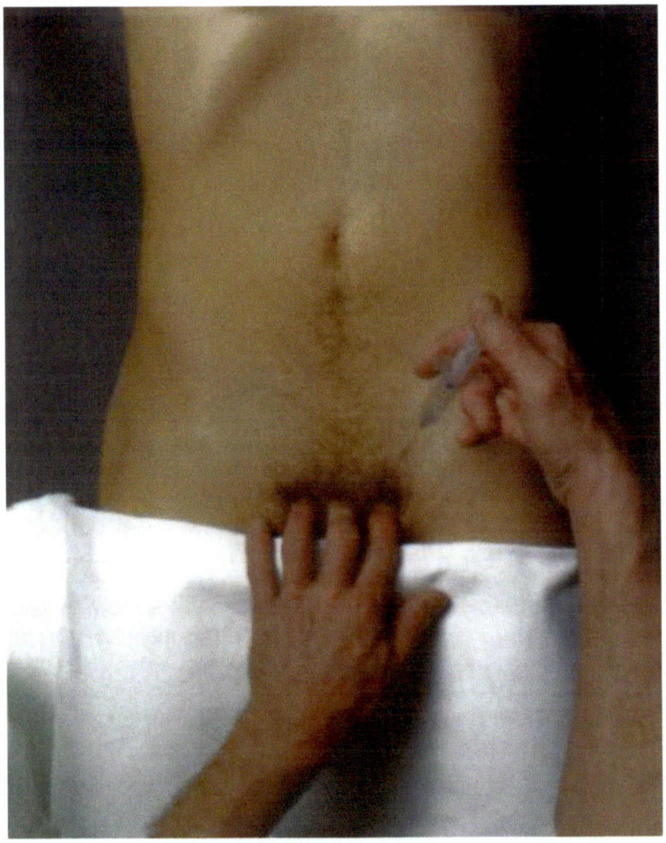

►**Fig. 19.14** Suprapubic injection to the prostatic plexus, in the prostate.

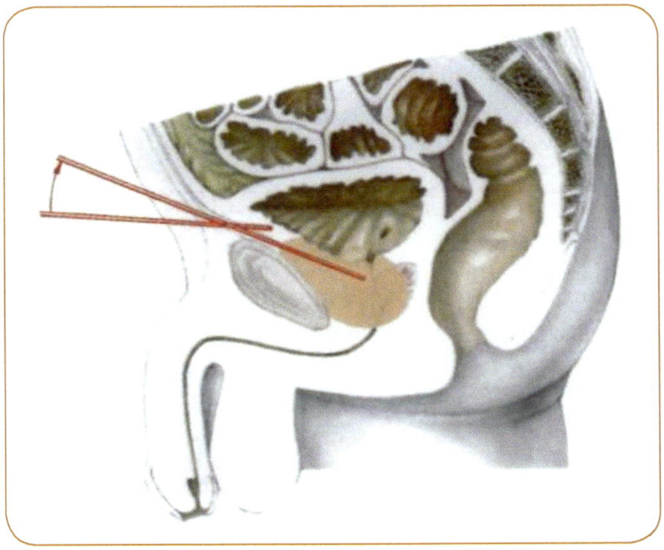

►**Fig. 19.15** Needle position for injection to the prostatic plexus, in the prostate.

20 Joints

20.1 Injection to the Shoulder Joint and Shoulder Girdle

20.1.1 Indications

The indications given are only a sample of those possible:

- New and old injuries to the shoulder joint (without indication for surgery).
- Acute (nonbacterial) and chronic inflammation of the shoulder joint.
- Degenerative diseases.
- Posttraumatic (and postoperative) pain in the shoulder girdle.
- Inflammatory and degenerative diseases of the capsular ligament apparatus (rotator cuff), the tendons, and bursae.
- The shoulder joint as an interference field after illness or injury.

The expected success depends, among other things, on the patient's "interference field situation" and the stimulation status of the spinal nerves supplying the shoulder joint.

20.1.2 Anatomy and Neurophysiology

The shoulder joint is a ball joint with the greatest range of motion of all the joints. This is ensured by a relatively small, shallow articular cavity relative to the humeral head. This creates the necessity for good muscular guidance and a strong joint capsule. Due to the comprehensive change in position of the joint socket, which is made possible by the synchronous sliding motion of the shoulder blade, the total range of motion of the shoulder joint is "well-buffered" and significantly expanded at the same time. Functionally, the joints of the collarbone between the sternum and shoulder blade are part of the shoulder joint. The collarbone, which acts counter to the musculature as a "tie rod," ensures stabilization of the shoulder joint to the trunk.

The vascular supply of the shoulder joint proceeds from the anterior and posterior circumflex humeral arteries (▸ Fig. 20.1, ▸ Fig. 20.2). With the vessels, the perivascular sympathetic nervous system conducts to all shoulder joint structures supplied by the arterial system, except the joint cartilage. The sensory innervation of the shoulder joint is very complex and originates from the articular branch of the axillary nerve (C5/C6), the musculocutaneous nerve (C5–C7), the subscapular nerve (C4–C6), and the suprascapular nerve (C5/C6). With these somatosensory nerves, sympathetic fibers also conduct to the sensory-supplied tissue structures. The supply to the shoulder via the sympathetic nervous system is afferent, in addition to the somatosensory supply, and efferent for managing the perfusion of the joint structures. The nucleic regions of the sympathetic efferent fibers are in segments C8 and T5 and are partially switched to the second neuron in the stellate ganglion. The sympathetic afferent fibers proceed partially with the somatosensory nerves up to the spinal ganglia of segments C5–T5 and are switched here. In part, they proceed with the vessels to the sympathetic trunk ganglia T1–T5 and to the stellate ganglion. Thus, the locations of the neural therapeutic injections are derived from the topography of the sympathetic nervous system.

20.1.3 Injection Technique

Before starting the injection to more deeply positioned structures of the shoulder joint and shoulder girdle, a wheal should be inserted in the area of the shoulder (dermatome C4 and C5) as well as subtle trigger point infiltration of the musculature responsible for moving the shoulder joint and shoulder blade!

▸ **Subacromial space.** With the patient's arm hanging down, palpation of the dorsal edge of the acromion. The insertion point for the 6-cm needle is one transverse finger medial to the lateral margin of the acromion and just over one transverse finger in the caudal direction. The needle is advanced 3 to 4 cm in strictly sagittal direction through the deltoid muscle, then directed slightly obliquely (about 5°) cranial. If there is early contact with bone, this means the head of the humerus has been reached. The needle must then be slightly retracted and directed further in cranial direction. After aspiration, inject 3 to 5 mL procaine. This injection reaches the subacromial bursa, the pericapsular fatty tissue, the cranial capsule portions, and the tendon of the supraspinatus muscle, which should be infiltrated directly in case of stimulation.

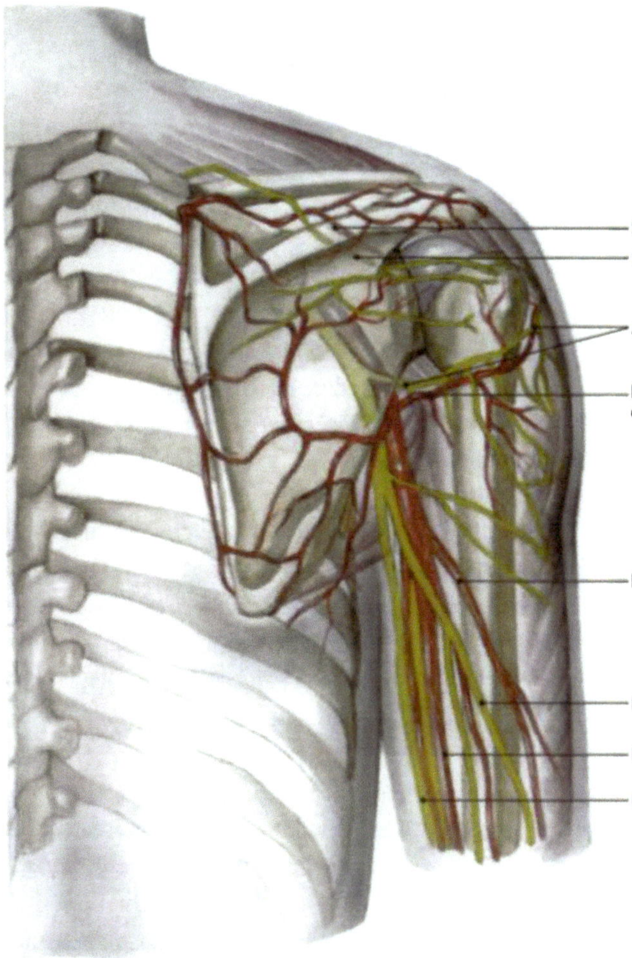

► **Fig. 20.1** Topography of the nerves and arteries of the right shoulder, dorsal view.

► **Muscle attachment of the infraspinatus muscle and teres minor muscle.** Palpation of the dorsal edge of the acromion at the transition to the lateral edge. The insertion point is 2.5 finger-widths perpendicular, caudal to this transition. The 4-cm needle makes contact with bone at about 2.5 to 3.5 cm depth. It is located in the area of the infraspinatus muscle tendon as well as the dorsal joint capsule at the level of the greater tubercle. After aspiration, infiltrate 2 to 3 mL procaine.

► **Axillary nerve and posterior humeral circumflex artery.** With the patient's upper arm hanging down, the insertion point is three to four transverse finger-widths below the acromion and one to two transverse finger-widths medial to the lateral acromion tip. The needle is advanced 3.5 to 4.5 cm in sagittal direction. Now the tip of the needle is in the immediate vicinity of the axillary nerve and the posterior humeral circumflex artery, which proceed at the level of the surgical neck of the humerus. After aspiration, infiltrate 2 to 3 mL procaine. A sensation of warmth in the shoulder as well as abductor weakness indicates the correct position of the needle.

► **Ventral shoulder joint capsule, tendon of the subscapular muscle, biceps tendon (intertubercular groove).** Palpation of the lateral margin of the acromion and its front edge. The insertion point for the 4-cm needle is in the perpendicular passage of the acromioclavicular joint, three transverse finger-widths below the acromion. With a strictly sagittal insertion position, the tendon of the subscapular muscle as well as the ventral joint capsule portion of the shoulder joint is reached. If there is contact with bone, the needle must be retracted 2 to 3 mm before 1 to 2 mL procaine is infiltrated after aspiration. A slightly lateral insertion direction (about 10°) reaches the lesser tubercle, the root of the subscapular muscle. Here, 1 mL procaine is infiltrated. About 1 cm further lateral is the intertubercular groove, in which the biceps tendon glides. Here again, 1 mL procaine is injected.

► **Axillary artery.** With the patient in a prone position with 90° abducted shoulder joint, palpate the clearly pulsating axillary artery in the cranial ventral region of the armpit. The patient should turn slightly to the side on which the injection will be performed, in order to relax the pectoral muscle behind which the artery proceeds. The palpating finger remains on the pulsating artery. The 4-cm needle is inserted directly above the palpating finger and, after insertion of a wheal, the needle is slowly pushed forward in cranial direction. The axillary artery is reached at 2 to 3 cm depth, which is proximal to the branches of the humeral circumflex artery. In the case of arterial puncture, intra-arterial injection of 1 to 2 mL procaine is performed. If the puncture is not successful, 3 to 4 mL is infiltrated perivascular in order to reach the sympathetic nervous system associated with the vessels.

Cave

There may be irritation of the radial or ulnar bundle which the patient indicates as a slight flash of pain in the course of the radial nerve or ulnar nerve. In these cases, the needle should be retracted slightly. Pain should not occur with this injection.

A sensation of warmth in the arm is clinical evidence of the correct injection. This injection also reaches the articular branch of the subscapular nerve, the musculocutaneous nerve, and the axillary nerve.

► **Suprascapular nerve.** Palpate the coracoid process. The 4-cm needle is inserted one transverse finger-width in the medial direction at the same level. At a depth of 2 to 3.5 cm, the needle is located at the base of the coracoid process, in the immediate vicinity of the scapular notch. The patient indicates a moderate pulling sensation in the ventral shoulder region. After aspiration, infiltrate 1 to 3 mL procaine.

► **Acromioclavicular joint.** The acromioclavicular joint is easily visible two transverse finger-widths medial to the lateral acromion edge. By way of the acromioclavicular ligament, the joint space with an articular disk can be palpated as a small trough. Another two transverse finger-widths medial, the ligaments (coracoclavicular ligaments)—which is often injured in shoulder compression—holds the clavicles between the coracoid and the clavicle, similar to the transverse ligament of the knee joint with its joint area at the coracoid. The 2-cm needle is inserted cranially above the joint space so that it is located only slightly below the skin in the ligaments. Infiltrate 0.5 to 1 mL procaine.

► **Sternoclavicular joint.** The sternoclavicular joint is clearly visible one finger-width lateral to the jugular. The head of the clavicular joint is supported by the sternal joint area and is held by the interclavicular ligament, costoclavicular ligament, and the joint capsule and is buffered by an articular disk. The 2-cm needle is inserted at the lower joint margin after insertion of a wheal. After retraction of the needle, the pericapsular infiltration of 0.5 to 1 mL procaine in craniomedial direction (not intracapsular or intra-articular) is completed through injection of 1 mL to the ligament between the medial clavicle and the first rib at a depth of about 1 cm.

► **Shoulder joint.** The injection to the shoulder joint is most successful from the dorsal direction. The insertion point is a finger-width below the dorsal acromion edge and two finger-widths medial to lateral margin of the acromion. After insertion of a wheal, at a depth of 1.5 to 3.5 cm the 4-cm needle reaches the deltoid muscle and the infraspinatus muscle through the capsule in the inner joint space. 2 to 3 mL procaine is infiltrated.

20.1.4 Material

Required:

- 5-mL syringe.
- 0.4 to 0.6 × 4 × 6 cm needle.
- 2 to 5 mL procaine 1%.

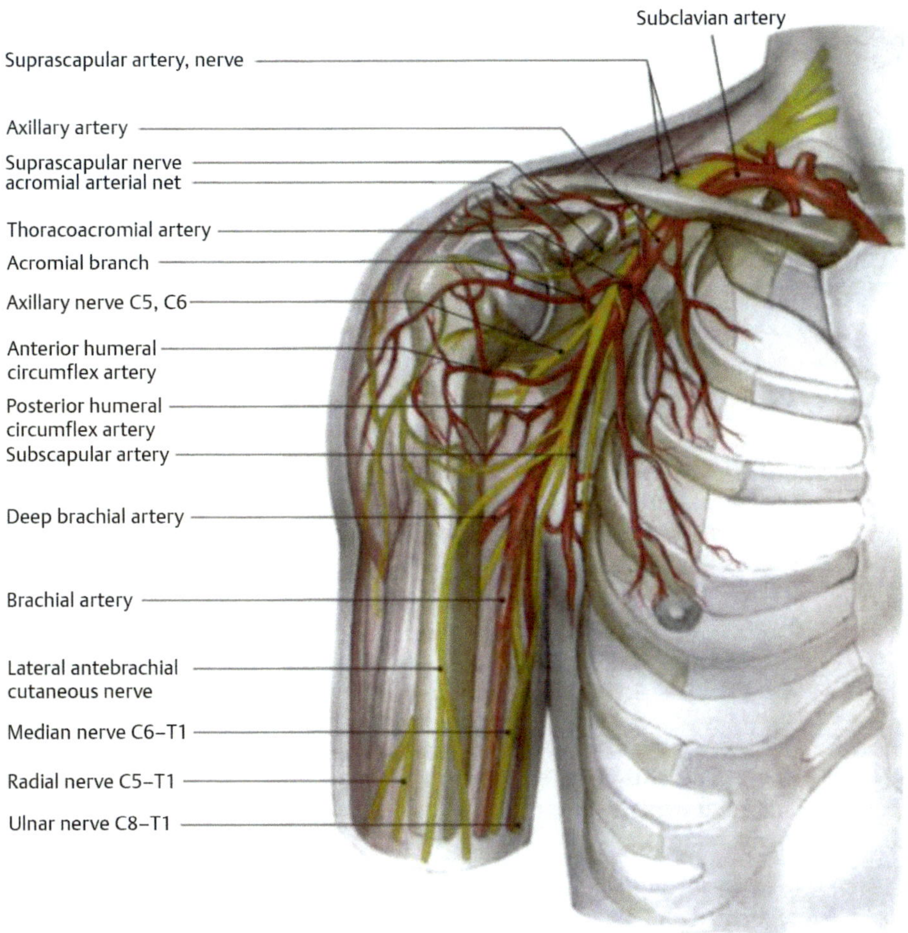

► **Fig. 20.2** Topography of the shoulder girdle with nerves and arteries, ventral view.

20.2 Injection to the Elbow Joint

20.2.1 Indications

The indications given are only a sample of those possible:

- Old and new injuries to the elbow joint (without indication for surgery).
- Acute and chronic inflammation (nonbacterial).
- Epicondylitis.
- Insertion tendinopathy.
- Degenerative diseases of the elbow joint.
- Cubital tunnel syndrome.
- Elbow as an interference field after illness or injury.

The expected success depends, among other things, on the the patient's "interference field situation."

20.2.2 Anatomy and Neurophysiology

The elbow joint is formed from three bones which form the connection between the upper and lower arm. The humeroulnar joint is the main part of the joint, while the humeroradial joint is an accompanying joint that enables axial turning movements of the lower arm against the upper arm. Both joints are connected with each other in the inner space of the joint. The easily palpable bone structures are the olecranon, the ulnar epicondyle, and the radial head.

The blood supply and thus the sympathetic innervation of the joint as well as the capsule proceeds via an arterial network (rete cubiti) from the ulnar collateral and radial arteries, the regressive recurrent radial and ulnar arteries, and the interosseous recurrent artery (▶Fig. 20.3). The sensory supply of the joint proceeds via the articular branches of the radial and ulnar nerves on the extensor side, on the flexor side via the articular branches of the median nerve on the ulnar side, and on the articular branch of the radial nerve on the radial flexor side. Parts of the sympathetic nervous system responsible for joint and capsule supply also course with these somatosensory nerves.

20.2.3 Injection Technique

Note

Before starting the injection to the elbow joint, muscular trigger points of the lower arm extensor and flexor musculature must be ruled out and, if necessary, infiltrated.

▶**Ulnar and radial humeral epicondyle.** Both epicondyles are easily palpable under the skin. Attached to these are the collateral ligaments of the elbow joint and the main portion of the extensors radially and, for the ulna, the main portion of the flexors of the lower arm, hand, and fingers. The 2-cm needle is inserted directly above the epicondyle and infiltration of 1 mL procaine to the epicondyle is conducted without bone contact.

▶**Radial collateral ligament and the humeroradial joint.** Palpation of the radial epicondyle. With the elbow slightly bent, the insertion point is about 0.5 cm distal to the epicondyle in the center between the palpable radial head and the epicondyle. Puncture in the collateral ligament is only required with isolated pressure pain and should proceed very slowly with pressure on the syringe plunger. The 2-cm needle can be advanced peritendinously with infiltration of 0.5 to 1 mL procaine 1 cm above the humeroradial joint on the flexor side.

▶**Ulnar collateral ligament and the humeroulnar joint.** Palpation of the ulnar epicondyle; the insertion point for the 2-cm needle is about 0.5 cm distal to the epicondyle. After insertion of a wheal, the infiltrating needle should be advanced 1 to 1.5 cm very slowly through the roots of the flexors inserted at the epicondyle. The needle is now in a periarticular position and 1 to 2 mL procaine is infiltrated after aspiration.

▶**Brachial artery.** The brachial artery is recognizable by its clear pulsation in the distal third of the upper arm on the inner side. The 2-cm needle is inserted between two palpating fingers slightly tensioning and holding the artery. After insertion of a wheal, 1 to 2 mL procaine can be infiltrated subcutaneously. The same technique is used for intra-arterial injection. The intravascular position is ascertained via aspiration; 2 mL procaine is injected.

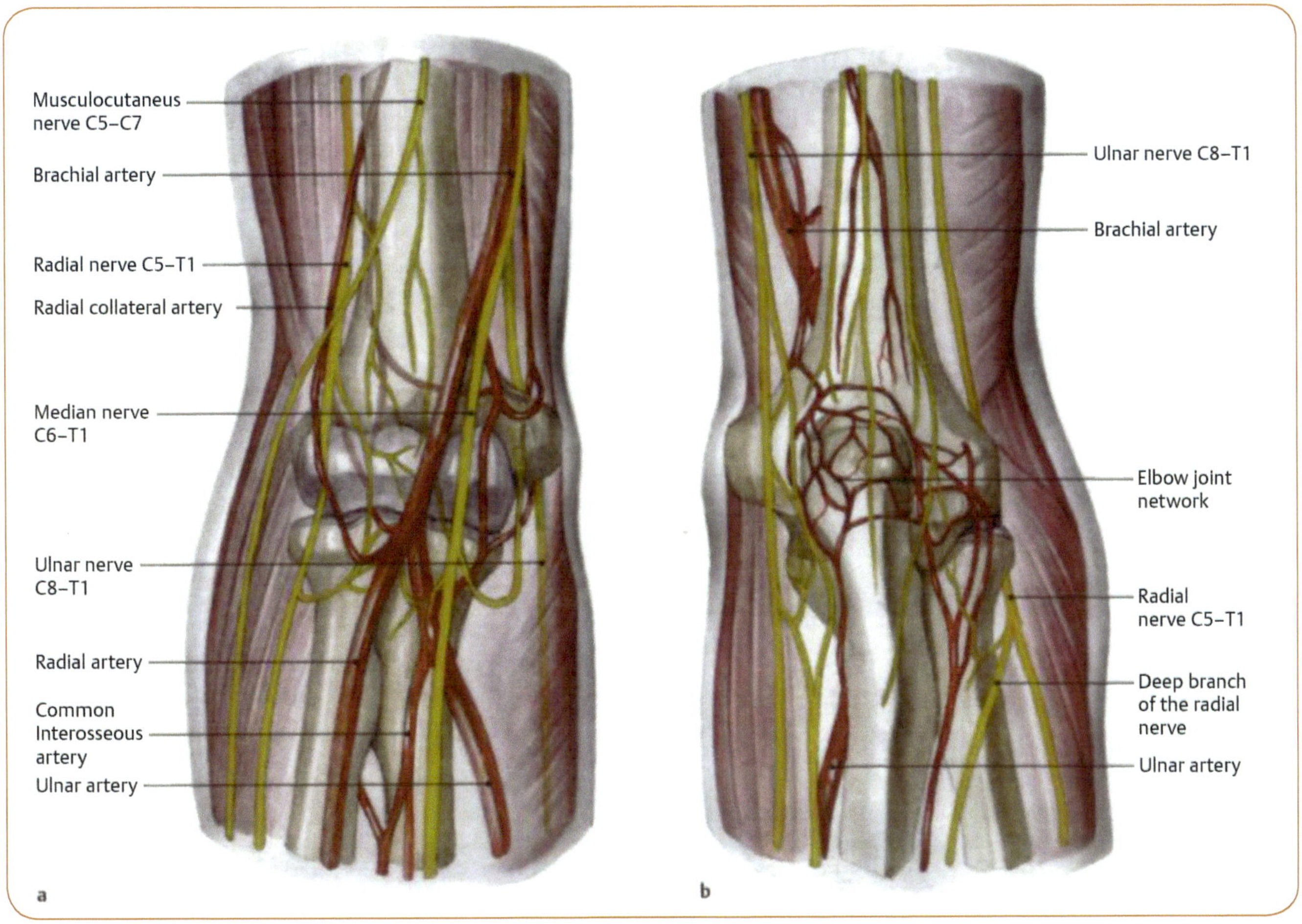

▶ **Fig. 20.3** Topography of the elbow joint with arteries and nerves. **(a)** Ventral view. **(b)** Dorsal view.

▶ **Ulnar nerve in the ulnar nerve groove.** Palpation of the ulnar epicondyle and the ulnar nerve groove. The insertion point for the 2-cm needle is directly in front of the tendinous arch of the flexor carpi ulnaris, under which the ulnar nerve extends. Slow perineural infiltration of 0.5 to 1 mL procaine, which simultaneously reaches the superior collateral ulnar artery belonging to the elbow joint artery network.

▶ **Elbow joint.** Under strict aseptic conditions, and with the elbow bent 90°, the 4-cm needle is inserted two transverse finger-widths above the olecranon tip. After insertion of a wheal, the needle is advanced 2 to 3 cm through the enthesis of the brachial triceps muscle, with the tip slightly in the caudal direction, until contact is made with bone. Now the needle tip is in the olecranon fossa, which is connected with the joint space via the synovial recess. Here, 2 to 3 mL of procaine is instilled after aspiration.

20.2.4 Material

Required:

- 5-mL syringe.
- 0.4 × 4 cm needle.
- 1 to 3 mL procaine 1%.

20.3 Injection to the Wrist and to the Finger Joints

20.3.1 Indications

The indications given are only a sample of those possible:

- New and old injuries of the wrist, carpus, metacarpus, and phalangeal joints in the absence of indication for surgery.
- Specific and nonspecific inflammatory and degenerative diseases of the wrist, carpus, and finger joints.
- Diseases and injuries of the capsular ligament system in the absence of indication for surgery.
- Dupuytren's contracture.
- Tendovaginitis.
- Tendinitis (e.g., trigger finger).
- Carpal tunnel syndrome.
- Wrist and finger joints as an interference field after illness or injury.

The expected success depends, among other things, on the the patient's "interference field situation."

20.3.2 Anatomy and Neurophysiology

The wrist is the movable joint between the forearm and hand. The actual pure wrist movements take place between the distal radius, the scaphoid bone (navicular bone), and the lunate bone. The articulated connection between the proximal and distal ends of the ulna and the radius to each other and the sole joint formation between the ulna and proximal humerus and the radius and distal carpus enable the pronation and supination of the forearm and therefore the hand. These movements are functionally on a par with the pure wrist movement.

The arterial blood supply to the wrist, its stabilizing and moving units, proceeds via the radial artery and ulnar artery (▶Fig. 20.4, ▶Fig. 20.5). The arterial supply of the hand and fingers takes place via the same arteries that form an extensive collateral circulation in the palm of the hand through the superficial and deep palmar arches. With these arteries, the perivascular sympathetic nervous system activates up to the terminal vascular capillary and controls the circulation of all tissue components.

The somatic innervation of the wrist and the hand is ensured by the ulnar nerve, medial nerve and the radial nerve. These nerves also activate efferent and afferent portions of the sympathetic nervous system, responsible for the function of the skin glands (sebum, sweat), arrector pill muscles, and for protopathic sensitivity. The nucleic regions of the efferent fibers are between C8 and T6 and are partially switched to the second neuron in the stellate ganglion. To provide a therapeutic effect on the different tissue components of the wrist, hand, and fingers, the injection of a local anesthetic is not only sensible for the "diseased" or "injured" structure, but also for the vessels, peripheral nerves, and stellate ganglion.

20.3.3 Injection Technique

Note

Before injections to the wrist, the carpus, the metacarpus, or fingers, muscular trigger points of the forearm muscles must be excluded and, if necessary, infiltrated!

▶**Wrist and distal radioulnar joint.** Palpation of the distal radius on the extensor side; the puncture site for the 2-cm needle is somewhat radial of the center line and thus radial to the extensor compartment. After insertion of a wheal, the tip of the first vertically inserted needle is pointed slighted radially and inclined 1 cm and lightly advanced backward by hand under the thumb extensors. Now the needle tip is above the dorsal wrist capsule and 1 mL procaine can be infiltrated. The needle is retracted into the subcutaneous space and re-advanced slightly obliquely to the ulnar side under the extensors of the fingers. At 1 cm depth, the needle tip is in front of the distal radioulnar joint and here 1 mL procaine is also infiltrated.

▶**Finger joints.** Palpation of the finger joint to be injected. With the 2-cm needle, 0.5 mL procaine is infiltrated subcutaneously radial and ulnar at the level of the joint gap in the area of the collateral ligament structure. Through tangential advancement of the needle toward the extensor side and flexor side, each re-infiltration of 0.5 mL procaine reaches the dorsal and ventral neurovascular bundles, and hence the accompanying sympathetic nervous system.

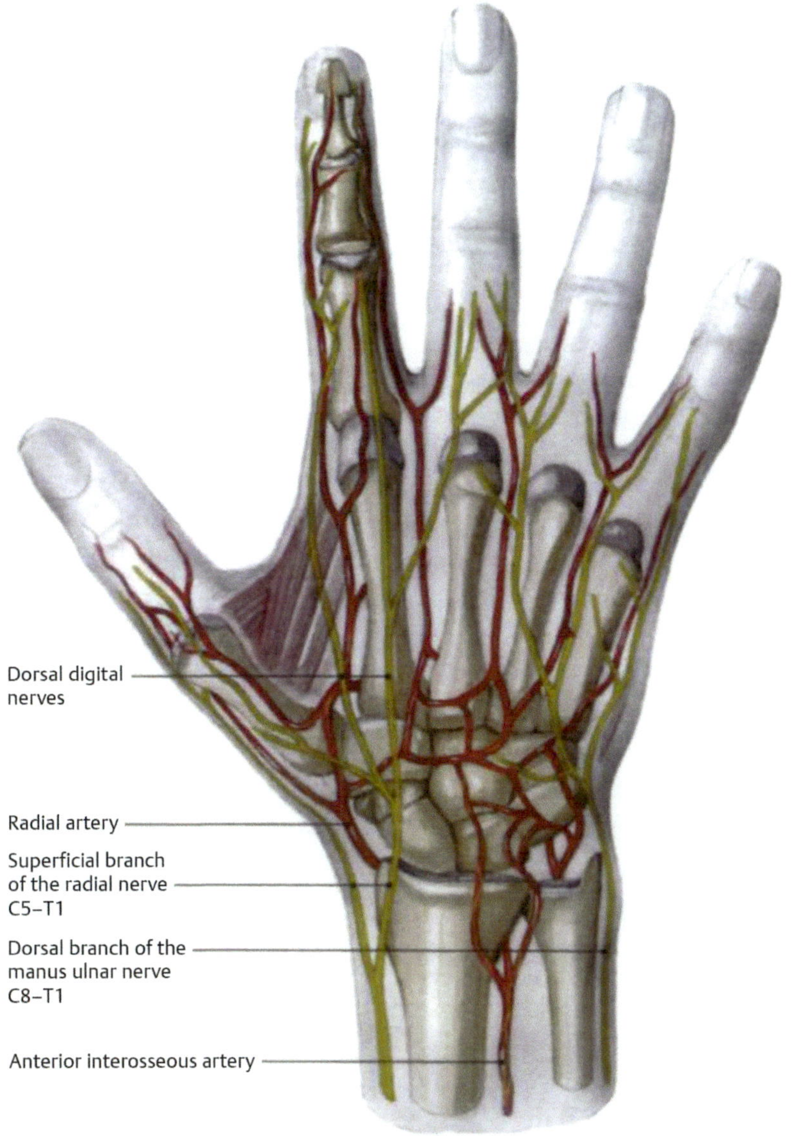

▸**Fig. 20.4** Topography of the hand with arteries and nerves, dorsal view.

▸**Wrist joint.** The transverse dorsal edge of the distal radius is palpated under strict aseptic conditions. The 2-cm needle is inserted vertically through a narrow gap between the thumb extensors and the extensors of the fingers. At a depth of 0.5 to 1 cm, the needle is already in the wrist joint and 2 mL of procaine is instilled after aspiration. The drug then flows into the joint without much resistance.

▸**Radial artery.** Palpation of the radial artery on the flexor side over the distal radius end. When the lower arm is tensioned, the pulsation of the radial artery is often easily visible. The injection with the 2-cm needle is made between two fingers palpating the arteries and by slightly spreading the fingers. At 0.5 cm deep, the radial artery is flooded with 1 mL procaine to reach the perivascular sympathetic nerve plexus. The puncturing of the artery is performed with the same technique, whereby the aspiration informs the intravascular needle position. Then 1 mL procaine is administered intra-arterially after which the puncture site is lightly compressed.

▸**Ulnar artery.** Palpation of the pisiform volar ulnar bone. The pulsating ulnar artery is palpated radially between 0.5 to 1 cm. At a depth of 0.5 to 1 cm, the 2-cm-long needle reaches the arteries and their sympathetic perivasal nexus. Infiltrate 0.5 to 1 mL procaine. Since the ulnar artery is very thin, the puncture is difficult.

▸**Ulnar nerve.** Immediately dorsolateral to the palpable ulnar artery, the peripheral ulnar nerve runs parallel and can be reached with the same injection technique for injection to the ulnar artery; a slight "electrification" of the fifth and fourth finger shows the correct needle position.

▸**Median nerve.** Palpation of the palmaris longus tendon, being the most prominent of the flexor tendons, can be easily determined near the wrist. Immediately radially, adjacent to the tendon, a 2-cm needle is inserted perpendicular to the skin; this may lead to a burst of pain toward the palm, indicating that the superficial extending branch was irritated (palmar branch of the median nerves). Occasionally, there is even a slight sparklike feeling in the area of the ulnar nerve due to an arc forming between a nerve branch of the median nerve and the ulnar nerve (communicating branch of median nerve with ulnar nerve). The cannula, pointing slightly to the palm of the hand, is advanced up to about 1 to 1.5 cm depth between the tendon of the palmaris longus and the tendon of the flexor carpi radialis muscle until a sparklike pain in the palm of the hand and in the third and fourth fingers indicates irritation of the median nerve. Retraction of the cannula by 1 mm and very slow infiltration of 0.5 mL procaine.

Note

No pain should occur during the injection procedure!

The drug is distributed under the flexor retinaculum.

This injection is particularly suitable as a conservative form of treatment for carpal tunnel syndrome. When performed at intervals of 3 to 4 days, and later at longer intervals, surgical treatment in which the full width of the flexor retinaculum is split can often be avoided. The conservative "decompression" of the ulnar nerve by procaine is made possible by the anti-edematous effect of the drug with simultaneous improvement in the microcirculation of the tendon sheaths of the flexor tendons running under the flexor retinaculum.

20.3.4 Material

Required:

- 5-mL syringe.
- 0.4 × 2 cm needle.
- 1 to 2 mL procaine 1%.

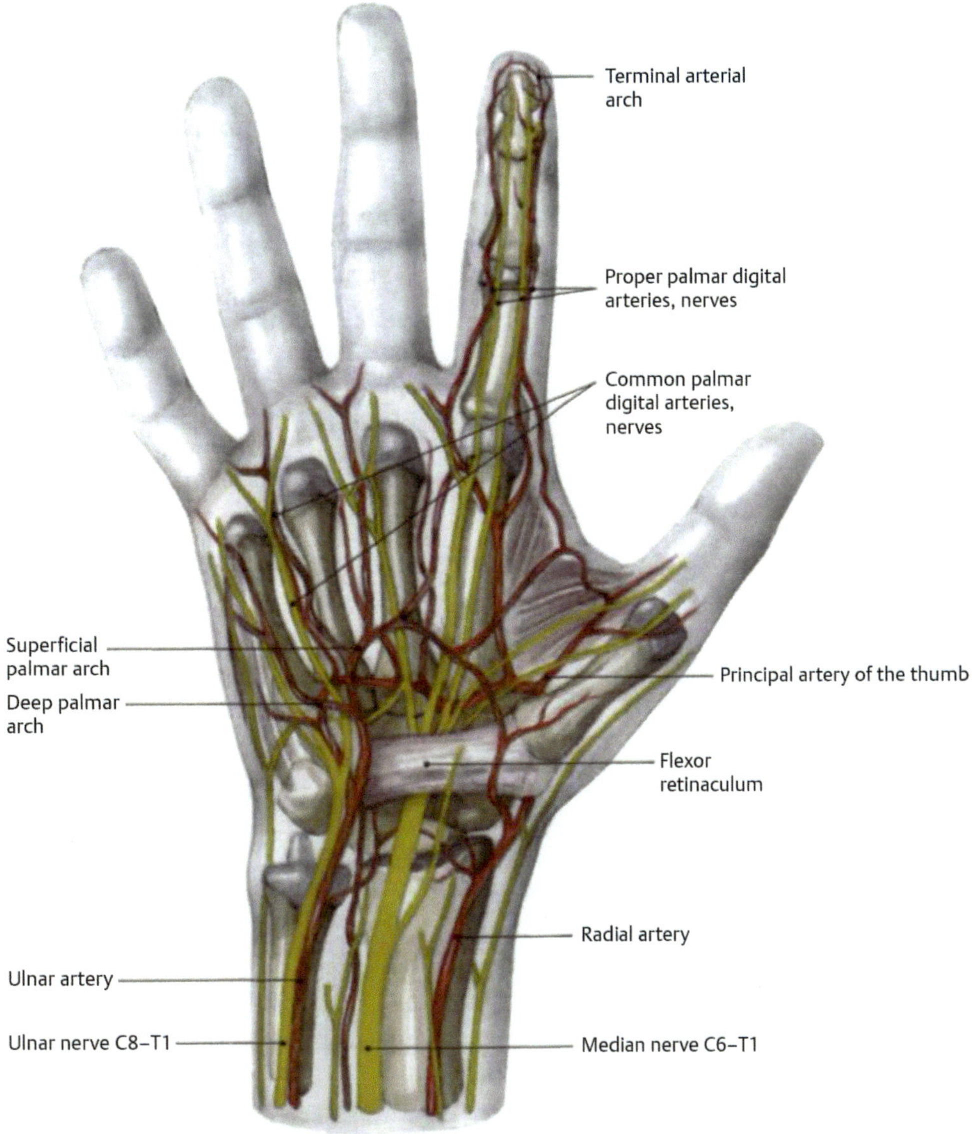

► **Fig. 20.5** Topography of the hand with arteries and nerves, palmar view.

20.4 Injection to the Hip Joint

20.4.1 Indications

The indications given are only a sample of those possible:

- New and old injuries to the hip joint (without indication for surgery) and inflammatory disorders of the hip joint.
- Research in hip dysplasia.
- Snapping hip.
- Root tendinopathy of the muscles responsible for movement of the hip joint.
- Hip joint as an interference field after injury or illness.

The expected success depends, among other things, on the patient's "interference field situation" and the stimulation status of the spinal nerves supplying the hip joint.

20.4.2 Anatomy and Neurophysiology

The hip joint is the articulation between the pelvis and thigh in the form of a ball joint, with a corresponding wide range of motion. The three ligaments combined in the capsular ligament structure—the iliofemoral, pubofemoral, and ischiofemoral ligaments secure the femoral head to avoid luxation in the acetabulum at the topmost level of the range of motion. Two clinical features should be highlighted. Of all the joints, the hip joint has the highest rate of malformations (dysplasia) and the highest rate of degenerative changes that can lead to clinical symptomology. The severe mechanical stress and easily irritable arterial vasculature may also play an essential role.

The arterial supply of the hip joint basically proceeds via the medial and lateral circumflex arteries starting from the femoral artery. The arterial vessels supplying the portion of the head near the socket, the inferior and superior nutrient branches of the head, have the longest distance to travel. Immediately in this portion of the femoral head, X-ray images show the "degeneration zone" in the form of "cysts" in hip osteoarthritis or, in acute cases of interrupted nutrition, necrosis of the femoral head, which is primarily due to the spastic or embolic occlusion of these vessels. The arterial supply via the femoral head ligament is often no longer present in adults.

The perivascular plexus of the sympathetic nervous system extends along with the arteries supplying the hip joint. It controls the vessel width and thus the nutrient supply of the joint, the capsule ligament apparatus, the synovium and thus indirectly also the articular cartilage.

The somatic nerves (afferent) are supplied by the obturator nerve (▶Fig. 20.6, ▶Fig. 20.7), the accessory obturator nerve, and the femoral nerve; the dorsal joint region receives its sensory supply from the articular branch of the quadratis femoris muscle which originates from the sacral plexus. Thus the joints are supplied from spinal segments L2–S3. These somatic afferent nerves extend along with the efferent sympathetic fibers that control the function of the synovium as well the afferent fibers responsible for protopathic conduction of pain.

Neural therapeutic treatment of the hip is performed with the application of a local anesthetic directly to the "diseased" tissue structure that is supplied by the sympathetic nervous system, as well as on spinal nerves and arterial vessels that control the nutrition of the joint and its other structures via the accompanying sympathetic fibers.

20.4.3 Injection Technique

▶**Hip joint.** Palpation of the greater trochanter. Nearly one finger-width above the trochanter, insert the 8-cm needle vertically and insert it deeply after placement of a wheal. The needle must be pushed through the gluteus maximus muscle, the gluteus medius muscle, and gluteus minimus muscle to finally arrive at the transition from the femoral neck to the femoral head of the joint capsule. Located here are also the branches of the medial and lateral femoral circumflex arteries radiating to the femoral head, which are responsible for the nutrition of the capsule and bone and the synovium and are accompanied by the perivascular sympathetic nervous system. After aspiration, infiltrate 3 to 5 mL procaine.

▶**Sacral plexus at the level of the greater sciatic foramen.** With the patient in sitting position, palpate the posterior superior iliac spine; three finger-widths perpendicular from this point in the lateral direction is the insertion point for the 8 to 10 cm needle, which is pushed forward in sagittal direction after placement of a wheal. Beyond a depth of 6 to 9 cm, there is a flash of pain (which the patient should be prewarned about) in the leg and buttocks, which indicates the correct position of the needle. Pull the needle back by about 1 to 2 mm and slowly infiltrate 1 to 2 mL procaine.

The patient must be informed that he or she will be unsteady in standing and walking during the active time of the local anesthetic and will not be "street worthy" during this period. A clear feeling of warmth in the leg indicates the correct injection.

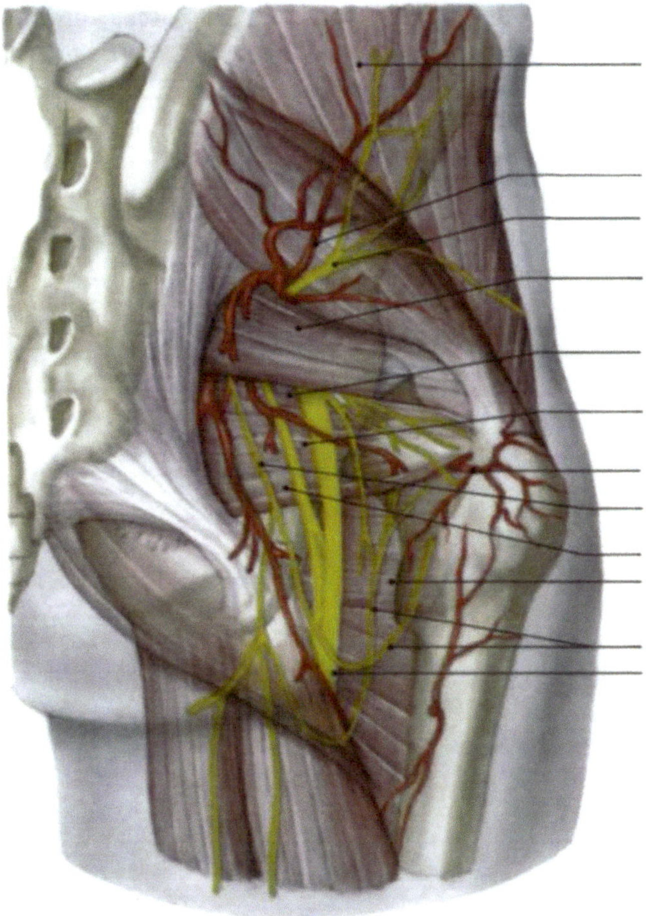

▶ **Fig. 20.6** Topography of the hip joint with arteries and nerves, dorsal view.

▶ **Femoral artery.** Below the inguinal ligament, about two finger-widths lateral to the pubic tubercle, palpate the pulsation of the femoral artery. Insert the 4-cm needle perpendicular between two of the fingers palpating the artery. The ongoing aspiration indicates the intravascular position of the needle, whereby the blood flows into the syringe in a lightly pulsating manner. At a normal $p0_2$, the blood is light red and can be easily differentiated from the venous blood. A dose of 2 to 3 mL procaine is injected. While pulling back the needle, infiltrate 1 to 2 mL procaine perivascularly in order to reach the sympathetic nerve plexus extending along with the femoral artery.

▶ **Femoral nerve.** The femoral nerve courses along the iliopsoas muscle about one to two finger-widths lateral to the pulsating femoral artery. The femoral nerve supplies the thigh extensors, the skin and the ventral parts of the hip joint. The injection is made with the 4-cm needle below the inguinal ligament after insertion of a wheal. In the immediate vicinity of the needle tip at a 2.5 to 3.5 cm depth, there is a slight flash of pain in the side of the thigh extensor. Pull back the needle by 1 mm and infiltrate 1 to 2 mL procaine perineurally. A feeling of warmth in the side of the thigh extensor indicates the correct position of the injection.

▶ **Lateral femoral cutaneous nerve.** Palpation of the anterior superior iliac spine and the lateral root of the inguinal ligament. The puncture with the 4-cm needle is carried out by inserting a wheal perpendicular to the skin just a finger-width medial to the spine. At a depth of 3 to 4 cm, there may be a flash of pain in the groin and the lateral proximal thigh. Infiltrate 2 to 3 mL procaine. A slight feeling of warmth as well as numbness over the lateral thigh region indicates the correct injection.

▶**Obturator nerve**. Palpation of the pubic tubercle. Insert the 8-cm needle just lateral to the tubercle, one finger-width below. After insertion of a wheal, turn the needle tip about 10° lateral and push it forward. At a depth of 6 to 8 cm, the needle is in the area of obturator nerve at the level of the obturator foramen under the pubic bone. A flash of pain in groin and in the mediodorsal region of the knee joint indicates the correct position of the needle. Pull back the needle by 1 mm and infiltrate 1 to 2 mL procaine. If there is no flash of pain in the area indicated above, infiltrate 5 mL procaine.

▶**Articulatio coxae.** Under aseptic conditions, palpate the greater trochanter. Somewhat ventral to the middle, insert the 12-cm needle just 1 cm above the trochanter, perpendicular to the skin, in a precisely lateral direction. After passage through the gluteal muscles the needle reaches the cranial joint capsule. This produces a moderate pain in the hip region. After infiltration of 1 mL procaine and a short wait, push the needle forward slowly with light pressure on the plunger. The capsular tissue can hardly be infiltrated due to its coarse structure. With sudden release of the infiltration pressure, the tip of the needle is intra-articular. The aspiration results in an amber-colored aspirate in the presence of joint effusion. Instill 3 mL procaine. The depth of the insertion varies widely and depends on the specified soft-tissue ratios and the position of the femoral neck.

20.4.4 Material

Required:

- 5-mL syringe.
- 0.4 to 0.6–0.8 × 8 to 12 cm long needle.
- 1 to 5 mL procaine 1%.

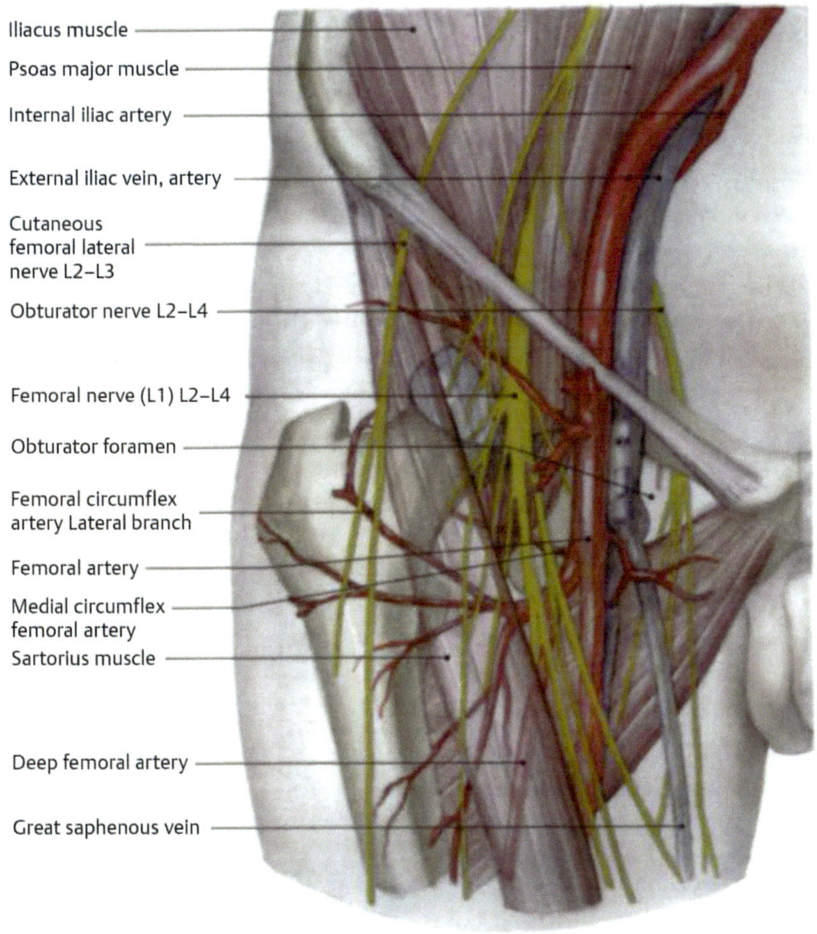

► **Fig. 20.7** Topography of the hip joint with arteries and nerves, ventral view.

20.5 Injection to the Knee Joint

20.5.1 Indications

The indications given are only a sample of those possible:

- New and old injuries to the hip joint and the patella (without indication for surgery).
- Degenerative and abacterial inflammatory diseases of the knee joint and the patella.
- Knee joint as an interference field after injury or illness.

The expected success depends, among other things, on the patient's "interference field situation" and the stimulation status of the spinal nerves supplying the knee joint.

20.5.2 Anatomy and Neurophysiology

The knee joint is the largest joint in the human body. Mobility at all levels is framed by the capsular ligament structure. The bone structure, as present in its most pronounced form in the ball joint, is reduced to the dimensions of the slightly trough-shaped tibia. Malfunction of the muscles that move and stabilize the knee can cause improper loading of the medial and lateral compartments, which has clinical relevance. Varus or valgus stress loading can occur in the knee joint with hypertension of a muscle group, which eventually leads to damage to the medial or lateral knee joint component and the capsular ligament structure.

The blood is supplied to the knee joint and the patella via an arterial plexus (articular rete, patellar rete), whose basic design is similar to the plexus for the ulnar joint. Numerous collaterals ensure "circulatory security," which persists even with different levels of tension in the soft tissues during movement and loading of the joint, and is accompanied by corresponding compression of the arteries. With this arterial plexus, the sympathetic nervous system extends up to the terminal vessels and controls the blood flow to the knee and its capsular ligament structures up to the synovial membrane.

The sensory supply of the knee joint and its capsular ligaments proceeds in the dorsal direction via the articular branches of the obturator nerve, tibial nerve, and common peroneal nerve (▶Fig. 20.8). On the extensor side, the nerve supply proceeds via the articular branches from the branches of the femoral nerve to the vastus lateralis muscle, vastus intermedius muscle, and vastus medialis muscle as well as from the saphenous nerve (▶Fig. 20.9). These somatic nerves also carry sympathetic fibers that are responsible for protopathic sensitivity.

The injection of a local anesthetic directly into or on the knee joint with its stabilizing or moving structures as well as to the relevant vessels and nerves always reaches the corresponding sympathetic nerve portions that control the nutrient supply and thus the tissue function.

20.5.3 Injection Technique

Note

Before injections to the knee, muscular trigger points of the upper and lower leg muscles must be excluded and, if necessary, infiltrated!

▶**Popliteal artery.** With the patient lying on his or her side and the knee bent about 10°, palpate the popliteal artery in the popliteal center at the level of the joint gap. Insert the 6-cm needle somewhat medial to the midline. After insertion of a wheal, push the laterally pointing needle tip forward slightly until it reaches the immediate vicinity of the vascular nerve bundle at 3 to 4 cm depth (popliteal artery, popliteal vein, tibial nerve). After aspiration, infiltrate 2 to 3 mL procaine. In case of a flash, retract the needle 1 to 2 mm.

Note

If a flash of pain is triggered in the calf and the sole of the foot, this means the needle position was too far lateral.

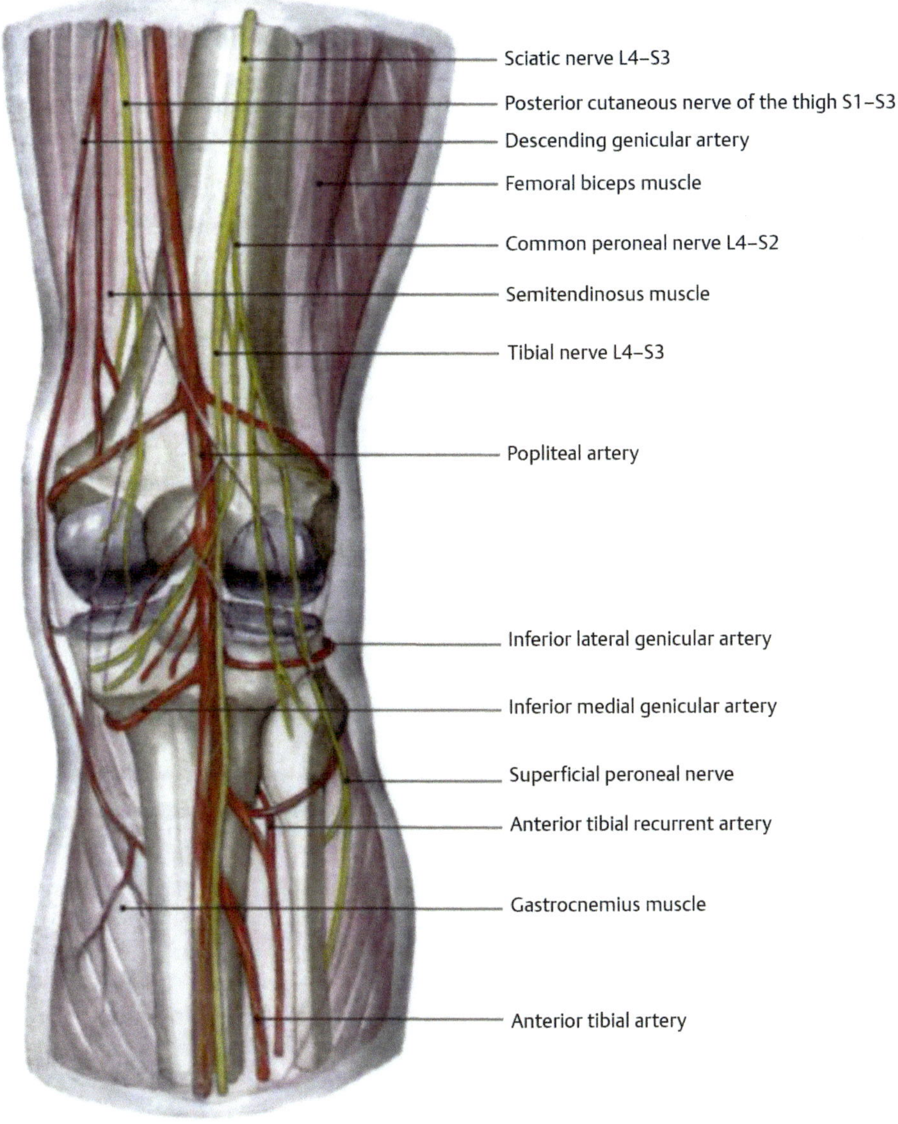

►**Fig. 20.8** Topography of the knee joint with arteries and nerves, dorsal view.

►**Cruciate ligaments (intra-articular injection!).** Under strict aseptic conditions, insert the 6-cm needle perpendicularly, one-half finger-width medial to the pulsating popliteal artery. The patient should be side-lying with knees slightly bent (about 5°). At 4 to 5 cm depth, the needle tip is already in the joint at the level of the posterior cruciate ligament. The joint capsule is thin in the dorsal direction and offers no resistance to the needle. The femoral attachment of the anterior cruciate ligament is also in close proximity to the rear inner surface of the lateral femoral condyle. After aspiration, inject 2 to 3 mL procaine.

►**Collateral ligaments.** Palpate the lateral femoral epicondyle; one finger-width above the joint space there is a firmer, lighter projection indicating the femoral attachment of the lateral ligament. Insert the 2 cm needle perpendicular to the skin. After insertion of a wheal, infiltrate 0.5 mL procaine subcutaneously. The injection to the fibular root of the lateral ligament is done in the same way after palpating the proximal fibula head. The same procedure is used for the medial collateral ligament, whereby the distal root of the ligament is just one finger-width below the joint gap at the head of the tibia. The collateral ligament roots are very often remarkably tender in knee disorders and therefore easy to locate.

►**Patellar insertions of the extensor mechanism and the tibial tuberosity.** Palpate the upper edge of the patella upper edge (base patella) where the major portion of the quadriceps tendon is inserted. Insert the 1 to 2 cm needle just above the bone edge perpendicular to the skin; after insertion of a wheal, subcutaneously infiltrate 0.5 mL procaine, 0.2 mL in the tendon. Use the same procedure at the bony root of the patellar ligament of the patella and the tibial tuberosity. Infiltrate the quadriceps tendon as well as the patellar ligament using the same technique after checking for localized (pinhead sized) pain points.

►**Superficial peroneal nerve.** Palpate the head of the fibula. Just about one finger-width below the top, the superficial peroneal nerve proceeds from the oblique craniodorsal direction to the caudolateral direction. The nerve, which extends along the bone, is easily palpable subcutaneously against the bone. This is also the location at which the nerve can be damaged from external pressure (cast, position, contusion, sprain). The 2-cm needle is positioned perpendicularly over the nerve before insertion. After placing a wheal, perform subcutaneous perineural infiltration of 0.5 mL procaine.

►**Tibiofibular joint.** Palpate the head of the fibula from the ventrolateral direction. A trough to the tibial plateau indicates the puncture point of the 2-cm needle. After placing a wheal, push the needle forward at an angle of 45° to the palpated trough. At 1 to 1.5 cm depth, the needle is in front of the anterior ligament of the head of the fibula. Now proceed with periligamental and intraligamental infiltration of 1 mL procaine.

►**Knee joint.** Under strict aseptic conditions, the knee joint is placed on a roll at an approximate angle of 25°. Palpate the lateral cranial edge of the patella. One finger-width above the patella and one finger-width lateral from the patella, insert the 4-cm needle from the lateral direction. After placing a wheal push the needle forward in medial direction, whereby the needle can be lightly lowered to the thigh extensor side. After penetrating the lateral patellar retinaculum, the needle "falls" into the upper lateral recess. After aspiration, which may contain effusion from the joint instill 3 to 5 mL procaine into the knee joint.

20.5.4 Material

Required:

- 5-mL syringe.
- 0.4 to 0.6 × 4 to 6 cm needle.
- 1 to 5 mL procaine 1%.

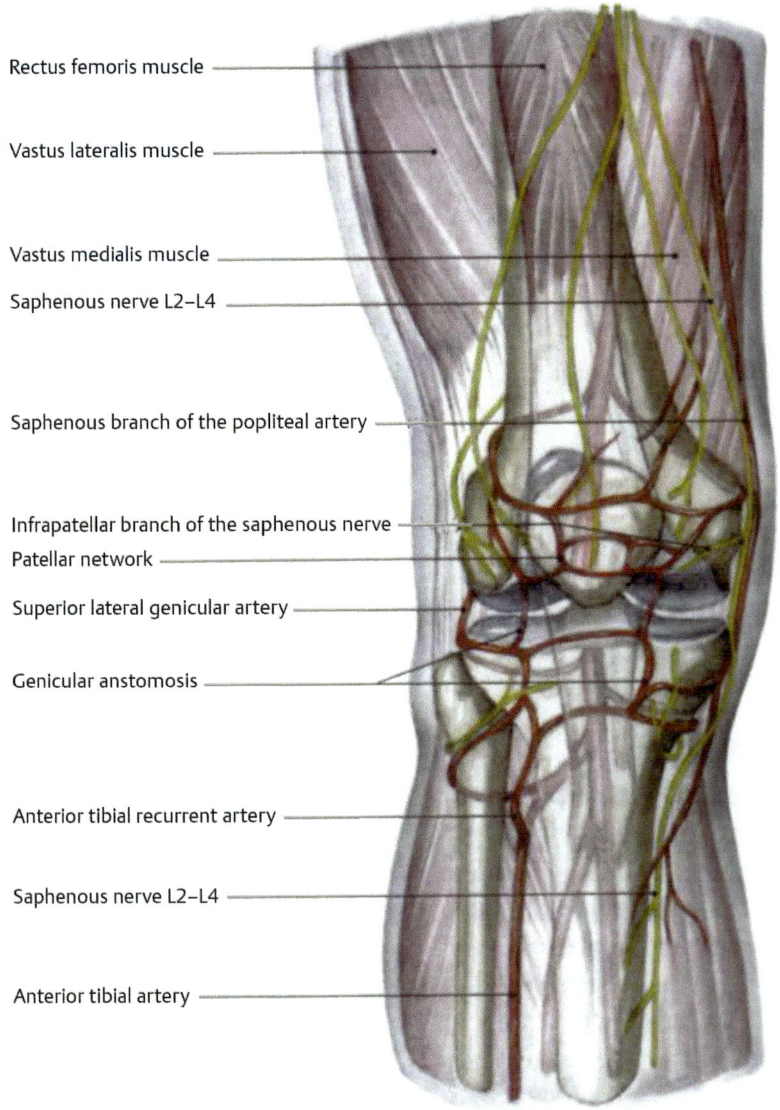

▸ **Fig. 20.9** Topography of the knee joint with arteries and nerves, anterior view.

20.6 Injection to the Upper and Lower Ankle Joints, the Tarsal/Metatarsal Joints, and the Toe Joints

20.6.1 Indications

The indications given are only a sample of those possible:

- New and old injuries to the ankle, foot, and toe joints (without indication for surgery).
- Degenerative and inflammatory diseases of the joints, the capsular ligament structure, and the structures responsible for moving the joints.
- The foot as an interference field after injury or illness.

The expected success depends, among other things, on the patient's "interference field situation" and the stimulation status of the spinal nerves supplying the ankle, the tarsus, the midfoot, and the toes.

20.6.2 Anatomy and Neurophysiology

The upper ankle joint, formed by the tibia, fibula and talus, which is controlled by the ankle mortise in its range of motion, enables dorsal and plantar movement; the lower ankle between the talus and calcaneus enables pronation and supination. Despite solid bone structure, the joint motion of the ankle joint is dependent on stable ligaments for resilient fixation of the ankle mortise. This ligamentous structure (deltoid ligament, anterior and posterior talofibular ligaments, anterior and posterior calcaneofibular ligaments, anterior and posterior tibiofibular ligaments) is often involved in injuries to the foot.

The tarsal bones form the minimally movable bony transition to the metatarsal bones; this in turn forms the connection to the toes, which—thanks to their good mobility—have an important function in the rolling gait and the imprint of the foot. As with the anatomical structure of the hand, there are numerous bursae and tendon sheaths, which significantly influence the mobility of the foot and the stasis of the foot skeleton. Thus, weaknesses of the lower leg muscles and short foot muscles have a decisive influence on the shape of the foot skeleton.

The arterial blood flow begins with the anterior and superior tibial arteries as well as the peroneal arteries and continues down to the paired arteries on the extensor and flexor sides of the toes via an arterial plexus of both malleoli and the calcaneus and the tarsal and metatarsal regions over multiple collaterals (▶Fig. 20.10). Following these arteries, the sympathetic nervous system—as a perivascular plexus—extends to the terminal vessels and thereby controls the supply of all tissue components. A disorder of the sympathetic nervous system function causes a disturbance of the supply of the tissue with subsequent disturbance of the functions of the corresponding tissue.

The sensory supply of the ankle originates from the tibial, saphenous, and deep peroneal nerves and from the sural nerve; the sensory innervation of the joints of the tarsus, the metatarsus and the toes originates from the tibial nerve, the superficial nerve, and deep peroneal nerve. Sympathetic fibers for protopathic sensitivity course with these somatic sensory nerves. The local anesthetic used for therapy reaches the sympathetic nervous system through injection to each structure of the ankle and the joints of the tarsus, the metatarsus, and the toe joints as well as via injection to the vessels, spinal nerves, and the lumbar sympathetic trunk.

20.6.3 Injection Technique

▶**Sural nerve.** The entry point of the 2-cm needle is a good four finger-widths above the lateral malleolus tip and one finger-width dorsal to the palpable rear edge of the fibula. After insertion of a wheal, push the needle forward about 1 to 1.5 cm.

Note

In the case of direct needle contact with the sural nerve, there will be a flash of pain all the way to the small toes.

Retract the needle by 2 mm and infiltrate 0.2 to 0.5 mL procaine. If there is no flash of pain, infiltrate 2 mL.

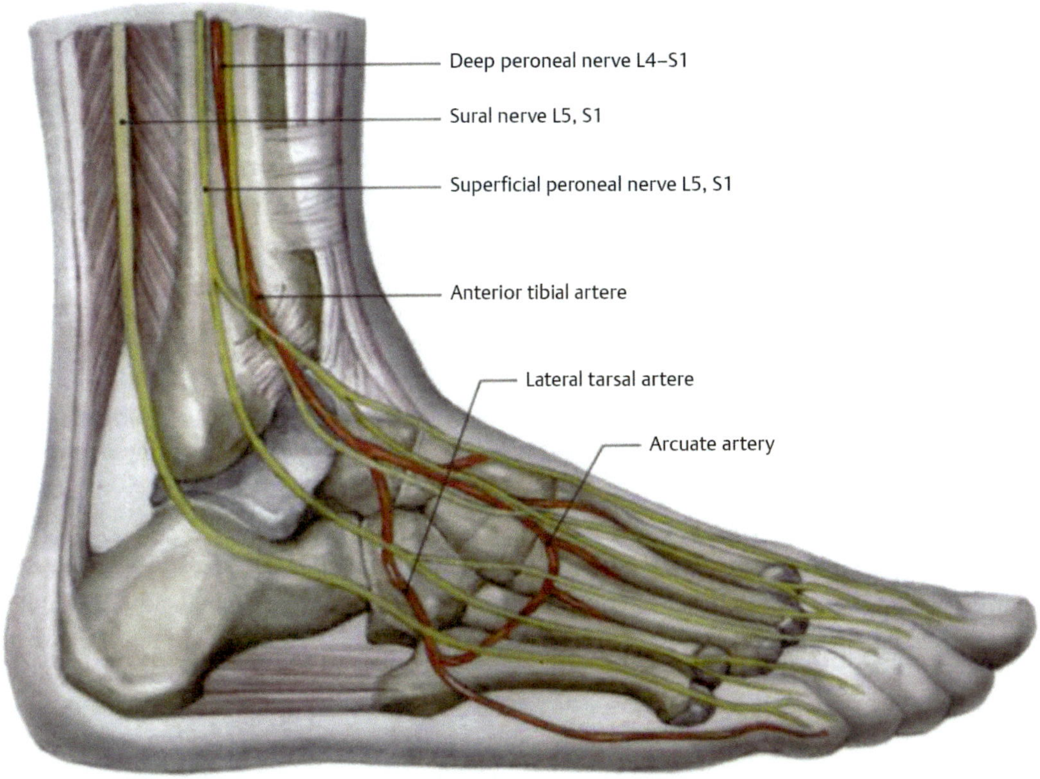

▸**Fig. 20.10** Topography of the foot with arteries and nerves, fibular view.

▶ **Superficial peroneal nerve.** Palpate the distal fibula. The anterior edge of the ankle is the site of the superficial peroneal nerve, which is easily palpable by sliding the finger under in ventral and dorsal direction. Make the insertion with the 2-cm needle directly next to the palpating finger. Perform perineural infiltration of 0.5 to 1 mL procaine.

▶ **Anterior and posterior tibiofibular ligament and the upper ankle joint.** The anterior tibiofibular ligament is palpable one finger-width above the lateral malleolus tip and extends from the ventral fibula obliquely upward to the tibia. The rough ligament, approximately 1.5 to 2 cm wide, is easily palpable in a plantar-flexed and pronated foot. Insert the 2-cm needle directly above the ligament and subcutaneously infiltrate 0.5 to 1 mL procaine. From the same puncture with the tip pointed in the ventral direction, push the needle a further 1.5 cm under the palpable extensor tendon. Here 1 to 2 mL procaine is deposited in the anterior joint capsule.

▶ **Lateral capsular ligament structure of the upper and lower ankle.** The puncture point of the 2 cm long needle is one finger-width below the lateral malleolus tip center. After insertion of a wheal, guide the needle in the dorsal and then in ventral direction while subcutaneously injecting 1 to 2 mL procaine. From the same initial position, push the needle forward (strongly in the lateral direction) to a depth of 1 to 2 cm at the front edge of the easily palpable calcaneofibular ligament until contact with bone; there, after retracting the needle by 1 to 2 mm, inject again 1 to 2 mL procaine to the lateral capsular ligament of the lower ankle joint.

▶ **Dorsalis pedis artery.** The dorsalis pedis artery (▶ Fig. 20.11) is subcutaneously palpable on the midline of the back of the foot, one to two finger-widths distal to the ventral ankle crease. Insert the 2-cm needle in front of the palpating finger. Perform subcutaneous perivascular infiltration of 0.5 to 1 mL procaine.

▶ **Toe joints.** Presentation of the toe joints through passive movements. The tibial and fibular injection is made with the 2-cm needle directly at the level of the collateral ligament structure. An amount of 0.5 mL procaine is used per injection.

▶ **Vascular nerve bundle of the toes (Oberst's anesthesia).** In the tibial and fibular directions at the base of the toes, at the level of the basic group, insert the 2-cm needle on the extensor side perpendicular to the toes. After subcutaneous infiltration of 0.5 mL procaine, push the needle forward to the flexor side of the toe and infiltrate 0.5 mL procaine there also.

▶ **Saphenous nerve.** One finger-width above the angle between the inner front edge of the malleolus and the distal tibia, the great saphenous vein courses with the saphenous nerve (▶ Fig. 20.11) and is easily palpable there. Insert the 2-cm needle in front of the palpating finger and perform perineural infiltration of 0.5 to 1 mL procaine.

▶ **Posterior tibial artery and tibial nerve.** The tibial artery is visible and palpable at the rear edge of the medial malleolus. Guiding with the fingers, insert the 2-cm needle. Perform perivascular infiltration of 1 mL procaine at a depth of approximately 0.5 cm. The tibial nerve extends a few millimeters dorsal to the artery and can also be reached there through the same injection with the same technique.

▶ **Ligament structure of the inner malleolus and the subtalar artery.** Insert the 2-cm needle one finger-width below the tip of the inner malleolus. At a depth of about 0.5 cm, 1 to 1.5 mL procaine is infiltrated to the deltoid ligament in ventral and dorsal directions.

The medial capsular ligament structure is located scarcely two finger-widths below the tip of the inner malleolus. The 2-cm needle is inserted here. At a depth of about 1.5 cm, perform pericapsular injection of 1 mL procaine each in the ventral and dorsal direction by turning the needle.

20.6.4 Material

Required:

- 5-mL syringe.
- 0.4 × 2 cm needle.
- 0.5 to 2 mL procaine 1%.

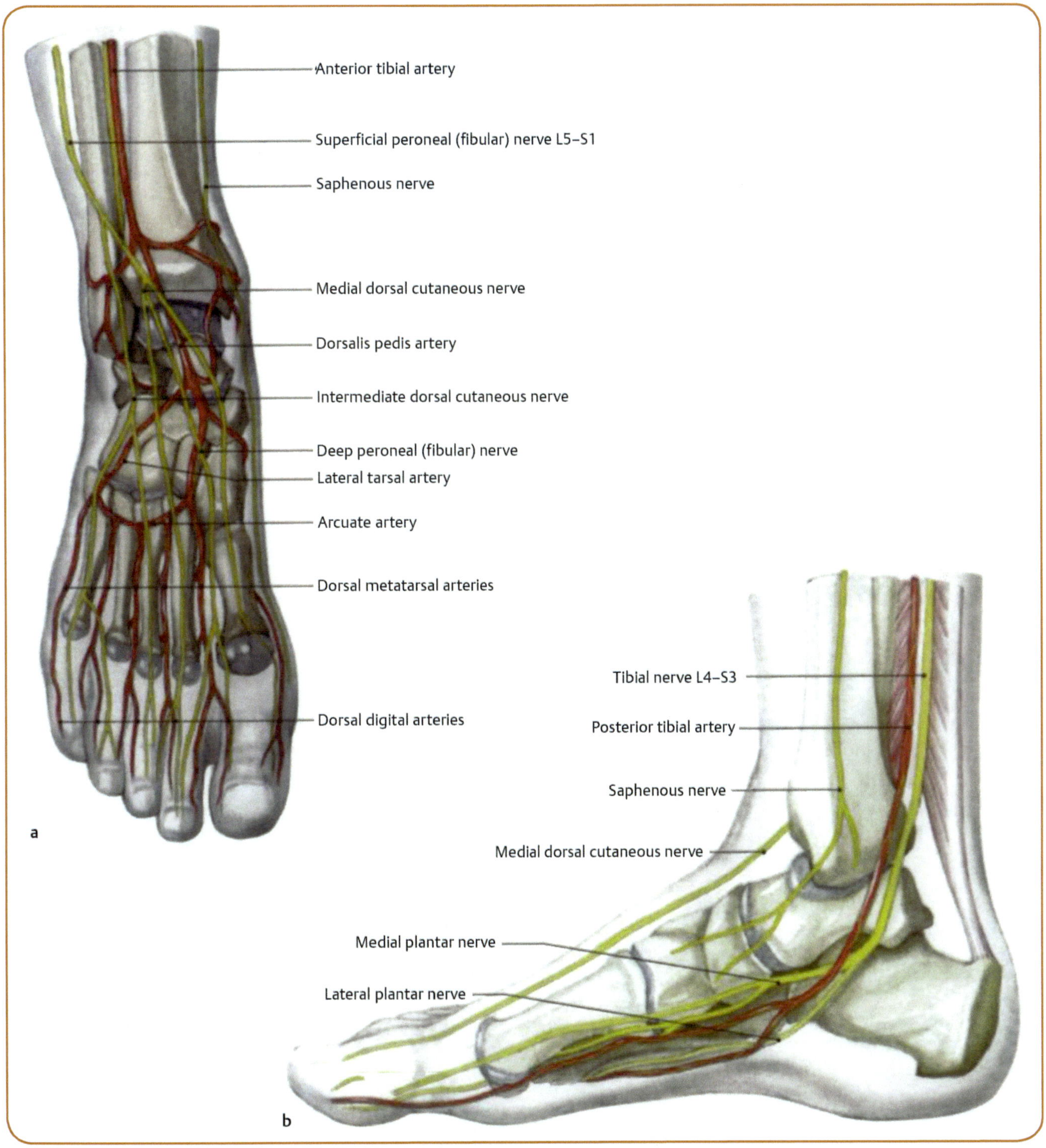

▶ **Fig. 20.11** Topography of the foot with arteries and nerves. **(a)** Ventral view. **(b)** Medial view.

Part 4
Indications and Therapy

21 Indications and Therapy

21.1 Introduction

The sympathetic nervous system is ubiquitously distributed in the body; virtually no disease progresses without its involvement. Furthermore, the sympathetic nervous system provides the opportunity for regulatory influence through neural therapy, and in particular the possibilities for the use of neural therapy according to Huneke are very extensive. The method is applicable in almost all medical fields, thus appealing to both the general practitioner and the specialist physician.

In general, the range of indications includes all illnesses that are associated with acute or chronic stimulus and functional impairment of the sympathetic nervous system and thus leads to **impaired microcirculation**. This includes degenerative and inflammatory diseases of the tissues, whereby nonspecific infections can be reached just as well as bacterial or viral infections. Parasitic diseases are excluded, however. All types of functional disorders of the musculoskeletal system, especially organ dysfunction, are included in the catalog of indications, as well as immunological (e.g., allergies) diseases. Neural therapy is only an adjuvant measure for tumors, but it can have a positive influence on some tumor pain. If we focus on symptoms, it is most frequently the pain that can be very successfully treated using neural therapy, in particular by means of interference field therapy.

Limitations to the indications are found in psychosomatic symptoms, in which the primary cause of the disease is likely a situation of mental conflict. Since the transitions and the real causal relationships for a psychosomatic disease are not always clear, a treatment trial in cases of doubt is indicated, since all too often the psychosomatic illness is revealed as somatopsychic by way of neural therapy.

Note

Excluded from the indications for neural therapy are disorders requiring surgical operations, psychosis, neurosis, and genetic defect diseases. Illness-related or medicinally induced coagulation disorders are among the relative contraindications.

The cooperation of the patient is of crucial importance for the success of the therapy. Since neural therapy according to Huneke is an injection treatment, each treatment is associated with pain—albeit reasonable—that must be tolerated by the patient. The fear of injections can impair detailed communication between the doctor and patient. If it is not possible to cure the patient of this "fear of needles" within the first or second treatment, the treatment should be discontinued even if there is an indication for neural therapy.

The treatment of children requires special empathy on the part of the therapist, a very "delicate" touch, and the trusting consent of the accompanying parents. The tolerance of most children should not lead one to overlook any child who is affected too strongly by the injection treatment. The symptomology and the treatment method of neural therapy should always be weighed against one another. For interference field conditions, and therefore the medically necessary suppression of the interference field, injections cannot be avoided for a curative approach.

Principally, we should aim to carry out neural therapy as monotherapy in order to ensure clear monitoring of success; this is certainly possible for numerous diseases. For patients with multiple morbidity whose existing medication cannot be changed, this success monitoring is sometimes more difficult, since some medications restrict the regulatory ability of the body.

Note

Corticosteroids, cytotoxic drugs, psychotropic substances, and numerous antibiotic therapies are able to impede or eliminate the self-regulation made possible by neural therapy, so that neural therapeutic success is difficult to achieve or even not possible to identify.

Thus, depending on the medical condition, it is necessary to weigh whether these products can be discontinued or "tapered off" and gradually reduced over a long time in parallel with the neural therapeutic treatment.

Neural therapy can also be carried out as adjuvant therapy. On the one hand, this is possible in combination with other therapy methods—even regulatory medicine procedures such as homeopathy and acupuncture—whereby the interference field therapy surely dominates from the perspective of neural therapeutic treatment.

On the other hand, neural therapy is also possible for use in **acute disorders** that endanger the life of the patient. For example, in:

- Lung embolism.
- Heart attack.
- Cerebral attack.
- Kidney failure.
- Cardiac insufficiency.
- Infectious diseases, e.g., bacterial or viral pneumonia, typhus, cholera, and dysentery.

In these situations, too little use is made of the opportunity to improve or eliminate the illness-related impaired performance of the sympathetic nervous system and to shorten the duration of the illness via improved tissue perfusion by normalizing sympathetic activity.

The following representation of diagnoses and pathologies that can be treated with neural therapy is certainly incomplete. However, this last chapter is the necessary framework in which the neural therapeutic mindset and therapeutic strategy are presented comprehensively, so that it becomes possible to incorporate unlisted diseases in your own list of indications. Many diagnoses are only oriented toward symptoms and pathogenetic aspects, and the actual etiology is unclear; in contrast, the neural therapy concept includes the crucial element of the search for etiology through **relational diagnostics**. If the context of a disease is not found, there is no therapeutic effect from neural therapy. This situation becomes especially clear in the diagnosis and treatment of pain disorders in which the painful structure can be detected but not the causality chain that led to this disorder. These cases are often clarified through segment diagnostics (p. 53) and interference field diagnostics (p. 81).

The diagnoses are not performed individually with subsequent therapy, but are consolidated according to body region since the therapeutic intervention for each disease (even the same diagnoses) must be individually adapted to the relationships of the patient's illnesses. The therapeutic guideline consists of only the basic approach to perform a segment treatment first or, in case of a lack of success, conduct interference field exploration and interference field therapy of the corresponding symptomology.

In summary, for all listed disorders, the impaired perfusion and microcirculation, which are induced by the sympathetic nervous system and determine the pathogenetic sequence, have an effect on the tissue involved in the disorder and form the decisive component of a symptomology from which the indication for neural therapy must originate. Only after successful completion of the treatment is the etiological relationship of the symptomology clarified at the same time.

22 Head

22.1 Headache

22.1.1 Diagnoses

The following headache diagnoses are the most commonly occurring forms (over 90%):

- **Tension headaches, episodic, chronic:**
  - No clearly defined periods.
  - No typical characteristics of attack.
  - Frequent daily headaches.
  - In 60% of patients: predominately bilateral, more frequently frontotemporal, less frequently occipital.
  - More common in women than in men.
  - Sometimes associated with tension of the cervical spine and facial muscles.
  - Overlap of symptoms with migraine and vascular headaches; spasm of the vessels of the head, neck, or facial muscles is suspected.[117,121,219,242,305]
- **Migraine:**
  - Paroxysmal frontotemporal headache.
  - One-sided and bilateral over 4 to 72 hours.
  - One to four times a month.
  - More common in women than in men.
  - Nausea.
  - Vomiting.
  - Sensitive to light and noise.
  - Various triggers (stress, distress, cycle, contraceptives, diet).
  - Concomitant symptoms: aura, e.g., scintillating scotoma.
  - Special forms of migraine:
    - Ophthalmoplegic migraine.
    - Retinal migraine.
    - Basilar migraine.
    - Hemiplegic migraine.
    - Dysphrenic migraine.
  - Among other things, migraine is characterized by an initial vasospasm with subsequent vasodilation advancing from the occipital to the frontal direction; this shows the initial involvement of the sympathetic and parasympathetic nervous system in the pathogenesis of migraine.[13,79,98,352,357,389]
- **Vascular headache:**
  - No firmly defined periods.
  - Unilateral, bilateral, and also occurring in a diffuse ring form around the head.
  - Can be triggered by specific noxa (sodium glutamate, nitrite, cold, nicotine, alcohol, sleep deprivation).
  - Autonomic symptoms (induced by the sympathetic/parasympathetic nervous system).[336,483,505]:
    - Hyperhidrosis.
    - Tachycardia.
    - Acrocyanosis.
    - Dizziness.
    - Hypotension.
    - Accompanied by vasodilation and increase in capillary permeability with edema.
- **Cluster headaches**[6,95,165,319,366,398]:
  - Migraine-related form of headache.
  - Strictly one-sided.
  - Episodes localized around one eye.
  - Ipsilateral rhinorrhea.
  - Lacrimation.
  - Eye redness (incomplete Horner's syndrome).
  - Hypoxia of the pterygopalatine ganglion, connections via parasympathetic vasodilators to the brain vessels.
  - Duration of the episodes: 15 minutes to 2 hours, sometimes multiple times a day.
  - More frequent at night than during the day.
  - Men more frequently affected more than women.
  - Months-long intervals with no symptoms.
- **Posttraumatic headache:**
  - Initial occurrence after skull/brain injury or operation.
  - No uniform symptomatology.
  - Sometimes regional or diffuse.
  - Sometimes progressing with other, nonpainful symptoms:
    - Difficulty concentrating.
    - Rapid fatigability.
    - Learning difficulties.
    - Dizziness.
    - Irritability.
    - Depression.
  - Associated with impaired brain circulation in accordance with a slowdown in microcirculation induced by sympathetic nervous system.

The remaining, rarer forms of headache generally can be treated like forms of headache that only partially fulfill the criteria for the respective headache definition in accordance with the International Headache Society guidelines.

22.1.2 Therapy

The **neural therapeutic** treatment of all forms of headache is focused on the treatment of perfusion and impaired microcirculation of the nociceptive nerve structure, which is known as the pathophysiological correlate for the various forms of headache. The perfusion-impaired structure determines the clinical symptomology and thus the diagnosis. The effects of the pathologically stimulated sympathetic nervous system on the spinal nerves C2 and C3 supplying the trigeminal nerve, glossopharyngeal nerve, facial nerve, and the skull, or the vasa ganglionares of the trigeminal ganglion, the pterygopalatine ganglion, and the otic ganglion—and the resulting hypoxia with increased irritability—are also seen in the various symptomologies. The hypoxia-related change to the neurotransmitter profile and the release of pain-generating neuropeptides from the corresponding cell structures are a direct result of the chronic stimulation of the sympathetic nervous system in a chronic painful illness. The overall clinical appearance, such as edema, redness, swelling, and impaired muscular function, including pain, can be thoroughly explained by the distribution systematics and function of the sympathetic nervous system. The sympathetic nervous system is distributed via the vessels as well as the cranial/spinal nerves supplying the brain and skull. This distribution pattern clarifies such things as the pathogenesis of migraine and its special forms, tension headaches and cluster headaches, and the neural therapeutic intervention to its logical result.

Mumenthaler and Mattle noted the following in their textbook[362]: "Head pain and facial pain can be either symptomatic, i.e. the expression of a specific cranial structure disorder, or it is much more likely a result of vasomotor or neural regulation disorders."

Furthermore, it should be noted that in the development of the headache, the responsiveness of the sympathetic nervous system supplying the vessels can vary individually. With the principal therapy concept of normalization of microcirculation, neural therapy demonstrates some parallels to classic medicinal treatment which also seeks—through a different pathway—to remedy the vascular-related pain symptomology with corresponding medications. However, the advantage of neural therapy lies in the fact that it can selectively and lastingly interrupt the regional disruption of the sympathetic nervous system, without the side effects of a general medicinal therapy. Thus, in contrast to traditional treatment, it is possible to relieve the headache disorder by way of autoregulative mechanisms (perfusion control).

Neural therapeutic treatment of headache varies from patient to patient, even with the same diagnosis. The therapy in the segment consists of subgaleatic injections, infiltrations of scars or impact sites including contrecoup, injections to the temporal artery, maxillary artery, facial artery, and the nerve exit points of the trigeminal nerve and the neurovascular bundle of the major and minor occipital nerves. The skull and facial pressure points personally indicated by the patient must always be infiltrated as well, along with the pressure-sensitive points found during palpation. In the case of predominantly occipital symptoms, the cervical spine must be involved in the diagnosis and treatment. In the case of one-sided headache on the ipsilateral side, intravenous injection of 1 mL of procaine into the cubital vein is obligatory. If unsuccessful, injections to the stellate ganglion or superior cervical ganglion are indicated. In the case of diffuse headache, these injections are performed alternately right and left, and primarily ipsilaterally for one-sided headache symptoms.

The injections for segmental treatment of headache described so far are not all applied in each session. The injections are based on the exam findings and the subject ive information from patients, which needs to be re-evaluated at each new treatment. If one or a maximum of two segmental treatments do not result in a change in the headache or even cause temporary worsening, segmental therapy is no longer indicated and interference field diagnostics should be performed after taking the history (p. 81).

Therapy monitoring is simple for chronic long-term headache or even for acute headache, since improvement in the symptoms occurs shortly after treatment (a few minutes up to 24 hours). With interval-type headache or episodic headache, the monitoring of success is more difficult since only prolonged absence of these headaches indicates the correctness of the treatment.

According to neural therapy experience, every chronic headache disorder can also be induced by an interference field, whereby the induction of the interference field is often varied.

For the following headaches, the presence of an interference field is much more common than for posttraumatic headache:

- Cluster headache.
- All forms of migraine.
- Tension headache.
- Vascular headache.

If the migraine is cyclical, occurs for the first time after pregnancy, with menstruation or menopause, or after curettage, cesarean section, or uterus extirpation, neural therapeutic interference field diagnostics should be performed by way of injection to the branches of the uterovaginal plexus. If the migraine is absent afterward or if it is changed in severity and frequency, the same injection should be continued until the patient is permanently asymptomatic; additional stabilization of the therapeutic result is achieved through parallel injections in both thyroid lobes as well as intravenous injection.

If the headache is triggered by alcohol, certain foods, or medications, abstention from the corresponding triggers must be taken into account along with an interference field situation in the abdominal organs, most commonly originating from the liver. In this case, injections are made to the right celiac ganglion and the Vogler pressure point on the right costal margin, coupled with the preperitoneal and intraperitoneal injection into the middle of the upper abdomen and—in the case of pressure sensitivity—to the right supraorbital neurovascular bundle as well. If the migraine, tension headache, cluster headache, or other headache that cannot be added to these traditional diagnoses is caused by cold drinks, eating ice cream, or drinking highly concentrated alcoholic beverages, the interference field can be assumed—with a high level of certainty—to be located in the oral cavity and the throat, i.e., in the area of the teeth or tonsils. Stimulation from cold or other stimuli from concentrated alcohol on the tonsils or an infected tooth is the trigger for the headache disorder.

Note

No matter the type of headache, it is crucial to explore the medical history of the affected patient. It should be noted that it is not the specific diagnosis of a headache that determines the therapeutic pathway, but the associated conditions under which the headache occurs.

In headache diagnostics, the international headache classification refers to these relationships, though not in a comprehensive manner. Thus, headache is observed in internal medicine, ophthalmic, or otorhinolaryngologic diseases as well as the multiple autonomic “concomitant symptoms” that provide the decisive indication for the etiology of the headache disorder from a neural therapeutic perspective. Thus, the neural therapeutic application of local anesthetics seems logical with the goal of interrupting the pathological stimulation of the sympathetic nervous system, the normalization of the microcirculation, and the termination of the chronic irritation from afferent pain fibers, including autonomic concomitant symptoms.

Similarly, we should evaluate treatment regimens in which stimulators are implanted, for example, in order to interrupt such disorders as cluster headache or migraine. The nonphysiological (“therapeutic”) electrical stimulation leads to regional “sympatholysis,” i.e., a comparable effect to local anesthetic sympatholysis, and therefore to interruption of the pain process induced by the sympathetic nervous system. This neural therapeutic process is comparable to a nervous “desensitization,” since after successful ending of the therapy the former triggering noxa loses its triggering function, much like an allergen which no longer triggers an allergic reaction after desensitization.

The neuraltherapeutic treatment pathway which targets normalization of the impaired vascular function including microcirculation is less specific than the pathway of classical headache therapy in which the definition of the headache type determines the essentially standardized symptom-oriented treatment approach.

Practical Advice

In every case, diagnostics by a specialist are necessary before neural therapeutic treatment, to ensure that conditions such as vascular anomalies, tumors, or subarachnoid bleeding which require surgery are not overlooked.

The specialist assessment of the headache patient should be available before the start of neural therapy and, in cases of doubt, should be repeated if diagnostic uncertainties remain. The ophthalmologist, otorhinolaryngologist, orthopaedist, internist, and dentist should be involved in the diagnostics if applicable, in order to objectivize or rule out the findings that trigger the headache.

The considerable number of patients with headache whose diseases cannot be categorized into classical diagnoses or demonstrate mixed symptomology with proportions of different types of headache can benefit from neural therapy.

Especially in these patients, precise examination and documentation of the headache symptoms are important so that changes attributable to neural therapy are not overlooked. Multiple interference fields can be responsible for headache symptomology, which means that sustained freedom from symptoms can only be achieved by taking into account all interference fields at the same time. On the one hand, individual symptoms of the headache disorder can be relieved through segmental treatment, while others can only be relieved via one or more interference fields, so that a combined segmental–interference field therapy becomes necessary.

With subtle diagnostics and follow-up monitoring, neural therapeutic treatment of headache is successful in most cases. Sustained freedom from symptoms should be considered as therapy success, but from a neural therapeutic standpoint this is only possible by interrupting the pathological causes. Therefore, the exact diagnosis, e.g., of migraine, is only possible after successful completion of treatment and might involve the following: migraine with aura, caused by a tooth infection or dysfunction of the internal genitalia.

22.2 Neuralgias

22.2.1 Diagnoses

The term “neuralgia” is an etiological description of various pain conditions in which the distribution of pain corresponds to the sensory supply area of a peripheral nerve, a nerve plexus, a nerve root, or a ganglion. Often, there are no or only slightly obvious neurological pathologies, since the lesion of the nerve involved is very slight. The characteristic feature is the sudden, short-term shooting pain **from the central region to the peripheral** (i.e., against the actual afferent pain conduction) occurring in most cases in the supply area of the involved nerves.

However, a deeper, duller, constant pain is also possible. Known causes of neuralgia of the cranial nerves supplying the head and oropharynx are local viral, bacterial, or nonspecific inflammation of the nerves or their supplied tissues; however, the etiology remains unclear in many cases. From a neural therapeutic perspective, the sympathetic nervous system–induced neuronal perfusion with hypoxia via the vasa nervorum or vasa ganglionares is definitely able to explain pathological stimulation of the affected cranial or spinal nerves as the etiological cause. What remains unclear is the spread of the pain usually described by patients as antidromic, i.e., proceeding centrally from the neuron axonal direction toward the periphery in the opposite direction, which is typical of neuralgia pain.

▸**Trigeminal neuralgia**. Sudden, shooting, violent pain in the course of the peripheral branches of the trigeminal nerve, mostly involving the second and/or third branch, rarely the first and second branch or all three branches, and only in exceptional cases the first branch alone. In most cases, there are specific trigger mechanisms; neurobehavioral pathologies are often lacking. It occurs more frequently after the age of 50 years, and is more common in women than in men. In addition to the violent, shooting pain, slight pressure pain may be present as a subjective finding. In terms of etiology, degenerative inflammatory changes in the trigeminal ganglion (degeneration through impaired microcirculation) and compressions from vascular abnormalities or tumors are known causes.

▶ **Raeder's syndrome (very rare)**. Neuralgia of the supraorr bital nerve. Clinically, there are flashes of pain in the supply area of the nerve as well as simultaneous incomplete Horner's syndrome without enophthalmus. In terms of etiology, there is an irritation of the ophthalmic nerve as well as the parallel running sympathetic fibers from the internal carotid plexus, induced by inflammatory (ethmoid sinusitis, frontal sinusitis), tumorous, or traumatic lesions.

▶ **Charlin's syndrome (nasociliary neuralgia)**. Clinically, there are short-term, violent attacks of pain in the corner of the eye, the eyeball, and the bridge of the nose with unilateral rhinitis, severe rhinorrhea, conjunctivitis, lacrimation, and sweat on the ipsilateral portion of the forehead. The etiology is supposedly an inflammation-related irritation of nasociliary nerve and the ciliary ganglion (ethmoid sinusitis, frontal sinusitis).

▶ **Sluder's neuralgia (neuralgia of the pterygopalatine ganglion)**. Clinically, there is 10-minute to 2-hour, persisting, one-sided pain in the area of the orbits, the base of the nose, and the upper jaw, from the throat to the soft palate, and fits of sneezing. Soyka sees similarities with cluster headache (p. 244).[466]

In terms of etiology, irritation of the pterygopalatinum ganglion associated with inflammatory diseases of the paranasal sinuses is assumed.

▶ **Neuralgia of the auriculotemporal nerve (rare)**. The clinical symptomology includes paroxysmal, burning pain in the area supplied by the auriculotemporal nerve, as well as redness and hyperhidrosis. It occurs by way of irritation of the auriculotemporal nerve (third trigeminal branch) as well as the parallel running sympathetic fiber portions. The etiology is predominantly a disease in the parotid gland, the lower jaw (teeth), and the mandibular angle (inflammation, tumor, postoperative state, lymph nodes, abscesses).

▶ **Neuralgia of the intermediate nerve (Hunt's neuralgia, very rare)**. The clinical symptoms consist of shooting, acute pain, initially for a few seconds, later for minutes or even hours, in the external auditory meatus, to the mastoid, neck, upper jaw, and palate, sometimes associated with facial palsy. Known causes are viral (herpes zoster) infections of the geniculate ganglion as well as inflammatory disorders of the inner ear, the middle ear, and the petrous bone region.

▶ **Neuralgia of the glossopharyngeal nerve (rare)**. Clinically, there is a strictly one-sided flash of shooting pain in the throat, base of the tongue, the tonsil region, and the soft palate, sometimes with radiation into the ear, and from the ascending mandibular branch to the teeth. Prodromes are dry mouth, viscous saliva, and abnormal taste sensations as signs of regionally increased stimulus of the sympathetic nervous system. Pain-free intervals often supersede painful phases. The most common causes are inflammatory disorders of the tonsils or scarlike changes after tonsillectomy. The trigger zone is located there.

▶ **Neuralgia of the superior laryngeal nerve**. The symptomology consists of strictly one-sided sharp pain lasting a few seconds to minutes at the level of the lateral larynx, radiating to the lower jaw, ear, and sometimes to the shoulder. Numerous daily attacks give way to long pain-free intervals. Trigger points can be found at the passage of the nerve between the lateral hyoid branch and larynx into the thyrohyoid membrane. The attack can be triggered by neck rotation, yawning, coughing, swallowing, or speaking. In terms of etiology, inflammatory diseases of the larynx come into question.

▶ **Neuralgia of the major occipital nerve (very rare)**. The pain symptomology of occipital neuralgia consists of episodic, shooting, sharp pain in the occipital region. Sometimes, multiple attacks occur in sequence with lon ger pain-free intervals. Triggers are slight stimuli in the cutaneous supply area (crests, pressure) as well as cervi cal movements or digital pressure on the occipital nerve exit point. Possible causes are inflammatory irritations in the area of the occipital nerve exit point at the level of the muscle fascia or other proximal stimuli of the dorsal branch up to and including spinal ganglion C2.

22.2.2 Therapy

Neuralgia in the head region, as presented according to the classification of the International Headache Society, provides the framework for a wealth of painful head disorders whose prominent pathological basis is the primarily fulgurant antidromic pain propagation in the area of the respective cranial nerves and the first three cervical spinal nerves. The decisive criterion for the therapy is the hypoxia-induced involvement of the sympathetic nervous system, which—from a neural therapeutic perspective—has the leading role in the etiology of neuralgia. Thus, from clinical observation, the perfusion-increasing effect of the procaine injection has a therapeutically lasting effect both directly in the affected nerves as well as the corresponding sympathetic ganglia if the pathological sympathetic nervous system stimulus originates from the area supplied by the cranial or spinal nerves.

The flash of shooting pain, present in essentially all neuralgias of the head, which is characteristic of neuralgia, represents only part of the possible stimulus conditions for the corresponding nerves when the indicated symptomology is closely observed. Only the maximum stimulation of the nerve, which causes shooting pain from the slightest additional stimulus, is taken into account. The less severe pain conditions—whether wavelike or persistent—that can occur in the supplied area of the above-named cranial and spinal nerves, are caused only by a weaker pathological stimulus of the sympathetic nervous system which controls the perfusion.

Note

In neural diagnostics and therapy, the intensity of the pain is of minor importance; only the fact is important that nerve irritation is involved.

Finding the primary cause of a neuralgia is of particular relevance if the neuralgia is in the area supplied by the corresponding nerves (teeth, gingiva, oral mucosa, facial skin, tonsils) or if it is external in the form of an interference field (e.g., in the supplied area of the vagal nerve via the link to the spinal nucleic regions of the trigeminal nerve). Symptomatic treatment of neuralgia is not possible with neural therapy: the therapy is only successful if the cause of the irritation, i.e., the stimulus itself, is found.

▸**Trigeminal neuralgia**. With neuralgia of the cranial nerves, the full supply area from which the neuralgia is originating should be diagnostically explored first and foremost. With trigeminal neuralgia, the dominant involvement of the second and third branches is already an indication that suggests the teeth as a possible cause, because the teeth are supplied by the second and third trigeminal branch and the sympathetic nervous system. This means neural therapeutic testing of teeth. The infection diagnostics of the dental and maxillofacial region in accordance with the generally customary vitality test and an X-ray diagnosis are insufficient because the various "subclinical" inflammatory changes cannot be detected in full. Exactly these inflammatory changes of the tooth, the periodontium, and the jawbone as well as persistant osteitis after tooth extraction, dental residues, or foreign objects represent the stimulus that can exist locally without any symptoms, but can lead to chronic irritation of the trigeminal nerve via the sympathetic nervous system and its strongest form of stimulus in clinically impressive trigeminal neuralgia.

If these pathological relationships are taken as a basis, the diagnostic classification of trigeminal neuralgia is more comprehensive. When neuralgia is classified in terms of neural therapy, all gradations of the trigeminal nerve irritation are simultaneously detected and treated in the same way. Thus, a part of the therapy involves the subtle restoration of the dental and maxillofacial region in accordance with the diagnosis stated above and repeated injection to the existing scars (empty maxillary regions).

If there is a chronic inflammation of the paranasal sinuses, which are also supplied by the trigeminal nerve, the injections take place at the nerve exit points (supraorbital nerve, supratrochlear nerve, infraorbital nerve) or more central to the pterygopalatine ganglion and the maxillary artery. In the case of simultaneous tooth infection, this must be eliminated first, since this is the only way inflammation of the paranasal sinuses can be normalized sustainably. Scars in the supplied area of the trigeminal nerve must always be infiltrated, since an irritation of the trigeminal nerve originating from these scars is quite possible (ephapses, chronic inflammatory changes in the scar).

Note

The trigeminal neuralgia can subside only when all causes of the trigeminal stimulus induced by the sympathetic nervous system are eliminated.

Since there is no uniform cause of trigeminal neuralgia, the goal of neural therapy must be subtle reduction in the peripheral sympathetic stimulus. If the vascular supply of the gasserian trigeminal ganglion is considered in terms of hypoxia-induced neuralgia, analogous pathophysiological possibilities are the result. The arterial supply and thus the connection to the sympathetic nervous system come from the internal carotid artery immediately after its entry in the inner skull. The sympathetic supply proceeds via the superior cervical ganglion and the cervical sympathetic trunk, whereby the efferent nucleic areas are in the region C8–T5/T6. In this way, all chronic stimuli in this area of influence from the sympathetic nervous system are theoretically able to induce and maintain a trigeminal neuralgia via the sympathetic conduction arc.

The normal function of the trigeminal nerve is bound to normal delivery of blood, which in turn is dependent on the function of the sympathetic nervous system. Based on the clinical symptoms of trigeminal neuralgia, which is tantamount to a seizure disorder, sympathetic nervous system–induced neuronal hypoxia is quite conceivable as a principal cause. In connection with the multiple stimulus possibilities from the peripheral supply area of the trigeminal nerve and the parallel stimulation of the sympathetic nervous system and the resulting disruption of blood flow to the nerve itself, trigeminal neuralgia is also quite explicable in all of its nuances. As a therapeutic consequence, this results in repeated injection to the affected trigeminal branch, including the vascular bundle or at a higher level to the **stellate ganglion**, on the side of the trigeminal neuralgia.

In case of additional or isolated interference field exposure, interference field exploration is necessary. Again, promising procedures are primarily the testing of the teeth, the tonsils or tonsillectomy scars, the paranasal sinuses, and the middle ear or the further exploration of the interference field in accordance with the medical history and examination findings.

▸**Neuralgia of the pterygopalatine ganglion**. With chronically inflammatory, generally asymptomatic disorders of the teeth, the paranasal sinuses, and the tonsils, interference fields surely represent the most common causes of neuralgia of the facial skull owing to their mutual sympathetic supply via the superior cervical ganglion; thus injections are performed on the suspicious teeth, the paranasal sinuses, and the tonsils. In the case of clinical, X-ray, or neural therapeutic evidence of a tooth lesion, restoration generally should not be avoided. The same approach applies to cluster headache.

▸**Neuralgia of the intermediate nerve**. This neuralgia primarily involves an asymptomatic disease of the middle and inner ear, hence the treatment is performed via injections to the mastoid and to the superior cervical ganglion. If this local treatment fails, an interference field induced via the teeth, paranasal sinuses, or tonsils should be considered. Scars in the area of the ear after operations or even scars from earrings should also be infiltrated in every case.

▸**Neuralgia of the glossopharyngeal nerve**. In terms of neural therapy, this disorder is generally easily influenced via repeated injection to the tonsils or tonsillectomy scars. Impacted wisdom teeth must be included in the therapy, or removed if necessary. A more proximal affecting step is the injection to the superior cervical/stellate ganglion, in which the glossopharyngeal nerve is also included. If local treatment fails, interference field diagnostics (p. 81) should be added, starting with the tooth/jaw region, the paranasal sinuses, and the middle ear.

▶**Neuralgia of the superior laryngeal nerve**. The therapy consists of repeated injection to these nerves, and to the superior cervical ganglion if unsuccessful. If this neuralgia still cannot be affected, interference field diagnostics should be performed with a focus on the tonsils, the teeth, and the paranasal sinuses.

▶**Occipital nerve neuralgia**. This disorder is often induced by an interference field, so that direct injection to the nerves has a low chance of long-term success. Nevertheless, it should be performed as a first treatment step.

Note

The most common interference field localizations are in the tooth/jaw region as well as the paranasal sinuses, i.e., the area supplied by the trigeminal nerve.

The neurological connection between the major occipi tal nerve (C2) and the trigeminal nerve is via the spinal nucleic regions of the trigeminal nerve, which extend up to cervical segment C2/C3 and have a synaptic connec tion with these. The neural therapeutic treatment proceeds via injection to the teeth, to the nerve exit points of the trigeminal nerve, or to the pterygopalatine gan glion. Other common interference field locations are the palatine tonsils and the pharyngeal tonsils. Scars of the scalp and the facial skeleton must be infiltrated in any case.

Last but not least, the connection of the spinal nucleic regions of the trigeminal nerve with the afferent fibers of the vagal nerve and thus also with the first three cervical spinal segments is a prerequisite for interference field disorders in the trigeminal supply area. Therefore, segmental therapy in the area supplied by the vagal nerve (thoracic and abdominal organs) is the logical choice for "interference field treatment" of occipital neuralgia.

22.3 Illnesses and Injuries of the Brain

22.3.1 Diagnoses

- Circulation disorders (cerebral sclerosis, cognitive disorders, apoplectic stroke, postapoplectic symptoms).
- Encephalitis, encephalomeningitis, meningitis (bacterial, viral).
- Symptoms following resolved inflammation.
- Research on multiple sclerosis, Parkinson's disease, amyotrophic lateral sclerosis.
- Head injuries with brain involvement (skull/brain trauma I–IV).
- Posttraumatic and postoperative brain function disorders.

22.3.2 Therapy

The goal is to normalize the disturbed circulatory conditions as quickly as possible via regional repeated sympatholysis. This general concept in neural therapy allows for treatment of **cerebral insult** based on vascular spasm, bacterial or viral-induced **inflammatory circulation disorders**, and circulation disorders following **skull/brain trauma** or surgery.

Note

The earlier the therapy is initiated, the greater the likelihood of preventing permanent brain damage. Already established tissue necroses can no longer be resolved.

The injections to be performed are reciprocal injection to the stellate ganglion or—evenly more effectively—to the superior cervical ganglion. The actuality of the symptomology determines the frequency of the injections. Initially, injections are performed once a day to multiple times daily and the reaction is awaited in the short term. Owing to ease of control, procaine is preferred over other local anesthetics.

In the case of **cerebral stroke**, injections should be performed chiefly on the side of the brain damage, i.e., contralateral to the peripheral paralysis. For inflammatory disorders of the brain and the cerebral membranes, injections are performed with a minimal interval of 1 hour to the right and left of the named ganglia; in the case of **brain/skull trauma**, **insolation**, or even circulation disorders after surgery to the skull, the stellate ganglion or the superior cervical ganglion is infiltrated alternately on the left and right with an injection interval of at least 1 hour. For skull/brain traumas, possible impact sites and contrecoup should also be treated with procaine infiltrations. Level I and II skull/brain traumas can sometimes be normalized very quickly through infiltration of the injury sites and multiple subgaleatic injections, so that no additional treatment is necessary.

Overall, the neural therapeutic measures in the mentioned acute illnesses are successful as very useful adjuvant treatment with the aim of improving the tissue perfusion.

The effect of an antibiotic treatment in the case of **bacterial encephalitis** or **meningitis** is significantly improved since the medication can become more effective via sympatholysis at the perfusion-impaired inflammation site. The same is true for circulation disorders of the brain in the case of cerebral sclerosis or following brain trauma, since the oxygen supply to the tissue, among other things, should be normalized quickly when the vascular spasm is reduced.

The therapy for **chronic circulation disorders** of the brain, for cerebral sclerosis, and for the aftermath of a stroke, a trauma or inflammatory illness, is performed in the same way but with lengthier treatment intervals (about 1 week). The following symptoms are easily influenced by injections below the scalp in the area of the cranial sutures, to the temporal and facial arteries, and to the occipital nerves in the case of tenderness on palpation.

- Sleep disorders.

- Concentration difficulties.
- Drive disorders.
- Seizure disorders.
- Impaired cognitive function, motor function, and sensitivity.
- Headache.
- Dizziness.
- Depression.

Scars following trauma or operations, even old impact sites, personal pressure points, or pressure tenderness noticed upon palpation should also be infiltrated.

Patients often report significant improvement in the symptoms already after the first treatment. If there is no change in the pain symptoms, an attempt should be made via injection to the cervical sympathetic trunk ganglia at weekly intervals alternating right and left. If there is still no success after one or two attempts, exploration of an interference field is useful in any case. Furthermore, therapeutic treatment of **early dementia** through complex interference field therapy (interference fields: intestine, teeth, paranasal sinuses, internal genitalia, pharyngeal tonsils) and segmental therapy of the skull is promising. The intravenous injection of 1 mL procaine as a bolus concludes each treatment.

The treatment of **multiple sclerosis**, whether the cerebral or spinal, is limited to adjuvant measures for various motor or sensory innervation disorders, which can be partially improved.

Thus, injections to the sympathetic cervical trunk are occasionally able to relieve an existing spasm. Subgaleal injections can certainly improve the patient's general well-being, and peridural infiltrations can improve the function of the bladder or intestine. Furthermore, consistent interference field therapy (e.g., intestine, teeth, sinuses) performed according to anamnestic data and neural therapeutic experience is valuable.

Note

Normalization of multiple sclerosis symptomology should not be expected in any case. But the progression of the illness can be mitigated or interrupted. These limited therapeutic options should be explained to the patient in detail to avoid unrealistic expectations.

Amyotrophic lateral sclerosis (ALS) is treated from a similar perpective as multiple sclerosis. In this case, interference field exploration is always the dominant approach (teeth, paranasal sinuses, tonsils, abdominal organs), whereby particular attention should be given to **inflammatory** changes of the teeth and paranasal sinuses. Surgical correction is always necessary in the case of bacterial tooth lesions. Segmental treatment of the skull (trigger points, scars, personal pain points) as well as overriding injection to the cervical sympathetic trunk and the superior cervical ganglion (both sides alternately) enhances the neural therapeutic process. Fast progression of the illness can be interrupted. Physical therapy on a neurophysiological basis is required. The earliest possible start of treatment is paramount.

In the case of **Parkinson's disease** (morbus Parkinson, postencephalitic, posttraumatic), injections to the vertebral artery and the stellate ganglion are therapeutic options. An attempt should be made to influence impaired dopamine synthesis through sympatholysis of the obligate degenerative modified substantia nigra supplied by the auxiliary branches of the vertebral arteries. The three main symptoms of stiffness, tremor, and akinesia as signs of impaired dopamine levels can be somewhat improved, whereby the medicinal substitution can even be reduced occasionally. In addition, especially with concurrent cognitive deficits, depression, and impaired consciousness—e.g., after encephalitis, craniocerebral trauma, surgery, or as part of cerebral sclerosis—injection at the superior cervical ganglion and the internal carotid artery has proven successful, since a portion of the arterial supply takes place via anastomoses between the internal carotid artery and the circle of Willis. In any case, subtle interference field therapy must be included in the treatment since—as with all chronic illnesses—Parkinson's symptomology can indeed be induced by an interference field.

22.4 Eye Disorders

22.4.1 Diagnoses

Neural therapeutic treatment is primarily performed to improve the microcirculation of the diseased or injured tissue via the sympathetic nervous system in order to initiate the healing process and regeneration:

- Blepharitis.
- Hordeolum.
- Chalazion (hailstone).
- Dacryocystitis.
- Dacryoadenitis.
- Unspecific conjunctivitis.
- Shingles.
- Keratitis.
- Iridocyclitis.
- Choroiditis.
- Chorioretinitis.
- Diabetic retinopathy.
- Arterial and venous occlusions.
- Degenerative retinal diseases.
- Macular degeneration.
- Neuritis of the optical nerve.
- Glaucoma.
- Eye injuries not requiring surgery (e.g., contusion, superficial injuries to the cornea).

22.4.2 Therapy

Depending on the location of the finding, circulation disorder can be reached through direct injection in the tissue, i.e., for disorders of the eyelid, the tear glands, and the tear duct system as well as through injection to the peripheral nerves, vessels, and ganglia, when the eye itself is affected.

Practical Advice

Depending on the severity of the symptomology, injec tions to the supraorbital and infratrochlear nerves and the instillation of procaine (without any additives) in the conjunctival sac are indicated. This way, disorders at the surface layers can be reached (eyelid, tear and sebum glands, cornea, and retina).

In addition to the sympatholytic effect of the local anesthetic, procaine also demonstrates its vasodilatory properties and capillary sealing and general cell membrane stabilization. Injection to the ciliary ganglion or, even better, retrobulbar infiltration is the more invasive measure, as not only the parasympathetic ganglion but also the sympathetic fiber portions of the eye can be reached, resulting in increased overall tissue perfusion of all tissue components, which is impaired in the case of inflammatory and degenerative diseases as well as in eye injuries.

Injection to the pterygopalatine ganglion is also well suited for the treatment of eye disorders, because from here the orbital branches supply the tear ducts and the optical sheath. The third invasive injection available for eye disorders is injection to the superior cervical ganglion or to the stellate ganglion, which improves tissue perfusion of the ipsilateral half of the head. This is important because not only the eye but also other tissue components (e.g., teeth, tonsils, paranasal sinuses) are reached which can affect an eye disorder by way of an interference field during illness. Under no circumstances, however, should this injection replace the interference field treatment that is required for chronic or chronically recurring eye disorders. Interference field diagnostics (p. 81) and therapy (p. 82) involve injection in or to the interference field, or via sympathetic inflow and discharge (peripheral nerves, arteries, ganglia) if the interference field cannot be reached directly.

Note

In case of diagnostic uncertainty, specialist medical diagnostics should be used to maximum advantage, also in regard to the objectification of treatment outcomes.

The following allocates the most important injections to the corresponding diseases. The following disorders are treated by injecting a few increments of procaine in the inflamed eyelid tissue and to the supraorbital and infraorbital nerves:

- Blepharitis.
- Hordeolum.
- Chalazion.
- Dacryocystitis.
- Dacryoadenitis.

Adding one to two drops of procaine 1% several times daily into the conjunctival sac is also very useful for treating pain. Already after the first treatment, there is generally a significant improvement in the inflamed tissue, so that a maximum of two to three treatments are required until the end of the therapy. Injections to the lymphatic drainage of the facial skull in the mandibular angle are also helpful. If there is no significant improvement after the first treatment, injection to the ipsilateral stellate ganglion or the superior cervical ganglion is indicated.

Neural therapeutic treatment of the following illnesses involves injection to the ciliary ganglion and the pterygopalatine ganglion:

- Iritis.
- Iridocyclitis.
- Chorioretinitis.
- Cataract.
- Diabetic retinopathy.
- Arterial or venous occlusion.
- Degenerative retinal diseases.
- Macular degeneration.
- Neuritis of the optical nerve.
- Glaucoma.
- Eye injuries not requiring surgery.

If there is no significant improvement after the second treatment, additional injection to the stellate ganglion or the superior cervical ganglion on the side of the disorder is indicated.

In the case of **chronic forms of illness**, an interference field origin should always be considered, whereby chiefly the teeth, the paranasal sinuses, and the tonsils come into question. It is important to note that for the treatment of inflammatory, especially bacterial and viral, illnesses procaine is superior to all other local anesthetics due to its pharmacological properties.

22.5 Disorders of the Nose and Paranasal Sinuses

22.5.1 Diagnoses

Neural therapeutic treatment is primarily performed to improve the microcirculation of the diseased or injured tissue via the sympathetic nervous system in order to initiate the healing process and regeneration:

- Acute/chronic sinusitis.
- Subbronchial syndrome.
- Pollinosis.
- Allergic diathesis.
- Angioedema.
- Ozena.
- Chronic recurrent rhinitis.
- Nonmechanically induced nasal congestion.

22.5.2 Therapy

Disorders of the paranasal sinuses, and to a lesser extent the nose, and the resulting consequences are given special consideration in neural therapy. This applies particularly to the different pathologies that originate from the paranasal sinuses and can affect the entire body. In addition to the local pain symptoms that occur most clearly in acute sinusitis, a wealth of chronic local ailments indicates evidence of sinus disorder. These include:

- Alternating or permanent disorders of nasal breathing.
- Expectoration from the nasopharyngeal space in the morning.
- Nasal speech.
- Repeated feeling of temporal pressure (sphenoid sinus):
  - Behind the eyes (ethmoid sinus).
  - Over the forehead (frontal sinus).
  - Over the maxillary sinuses.
- Different unilateral or bilateral edema of the eyelids.
- Disturbed sense of smell.

From a neural therapeutic perspective, bronchopulmonary complaints such as **chronic dry cough**, recurring **bronchitis** up to **spastic bronchitis** and **bronchial asthma**, pain, or even tension in the occipital region and around the upper cervical spine are evidence of frequently chronic, somewhat asymptomatic sinusitis. Allergic disorders, such as **pollinosis**, allergies against different substances, or even **angioedema**, are often based on a chronic disorder of the sinuses, so that their neural therapeutic treatment leads to stopping the allergic reaction despite constant exposure to allergens.

The suggestion of paranasal sinus treatment as causal therapy against a definite allergy presents an approach that differs from traditional allergy treatment, since the autonomic supply of the paranasal sinuses, and the microcirculation and the function of the mucosa are normalized. Of course, other interference fields can initiate an allergic illness, just as the paranasal sinuses are often an interference field for nonallergic chronic illnesses. Precisely because of this duality, it should be mentioned once again that the paranasal sinuses should always be part of the exploration in interference field diagnostics (p. 81), even without symptoms or indications in the medical history.

The following injections are for neural therapeutic treatment of the paranasal sinuses or the illnesses stemming from these (interference field) as well as diseases of the nose:

- Injection to the nerve exit points of the first and second trigeminal branch (supraorbital nerve, infratrochlear nerve, nasal branch, external nasal branch of the nasociliary nerve).
- Alternatively, injection to the pterygopalatine ganglion on both sides and to the maxillary artery, particularly in the case of acute sinusitis with pain, fever, and effusion.
- Injection to the superior cervical ganglion or even the stellate ganglion, if the prior injections resulted in inadequate success.
- Intravenous injection of 1 mL procaine in the cubital vein.
- Additional subcutaneous injection in the mandibular angle at the level of lymphatic drainage of the facial skull and the paranasal sinuses.
- Nasal spray procaine 1% without additives, or cotton carriers soaked in procaine in the upper nasal cavity. If local treatment fails, when performing interference field exploration the primary focus should be on tooth diseases as well as disorders originating from the tonsils. Scars on the skin of the face or head, as well as in the neck area (e.g., boil scars), must also be infiltrated. Special attention should be given to chronic or resolved diseases of the gastrointestinal tract, which remarkably often are the basis for chronic disorders of the paranasal sinuses.

22.6 Disorders of the Ear and Vestibular Organ

22.6.1 Diagnoses

Neural therapeutic treatment is primarily performed to improve the microcirculation of the diseased or injured tissue via the sympathetic nervous system in order to initiate the healing process and regeneration:

- Acute/chronic otitis media.
- Otitis externa.
- Unclear otalgia.
- Tinnitus.
- Hypoacusis and hyperacusis.
- Sudden hearing loss.
- Vertigo.
- Sea and motion sickness.
- Meniere's disease.

22.6.2 Therapy

Neural therapeutic treatment for disorders of the ear and the vestibular organ is based on those in which the impairment has a primary or secondary relationship to impaired microcirculation, whether as part of degeneration, inflammation, or overuse. The illness to be treated and the corresponding symptomology are the clinical result of the respective functionally impaired section of the ear or vestibular organ. If the circulation ratios are to be normalized, the location of the corresponding injection is always linked to vascular nerve bundles which are—independently of the diagnosis—carriers of the sympathetic innervation supplying the ear. These are for:

- The outer ear:
  - Superficial temporal artery.
  - Maxillary artery.
  - Occipital artery.
- The inner ear:
  - Labyrinthine artery and basilar artery from the vertebral arteries.
- The middle ear:
  - Anterior and posterior inferior superficial tympanic arteries, medial meningeal, ascending pharyngeal, maxillary, and stylomastoid arteries—all from the external carotid artery.

Since the vessels extending to the middle and inner ear cannot be reached directly, the injections take place more peripherally, i.e., to the vertebral artery and external carotid artery or to the stellate ganglion and superior cervical ganglion.

Injections near the ear for neural therapeutic treatment of the middle and inner ear are made to the mastoid, whereby the mastoid branch of the occipital artery and the posterior auricular artery are reached. For disorders of the outer ear, an additional injection should be made to the superficial temporal artery as well as direct infiltration in the pathologically modified tissue. Scars of the pinna (e.g., **freezing, burns, earring scars**) as well as tender points in the region of the mastoid and temporal bone should be infiltrated with a smal volume of procaine. For inflammatory illnesses, subcutaneous injection in the mandibular angle supports improved lymph drainage.

Practical Advice

If there are scars on the tympanic membrane after inflammation or injury or if signs of acute inflammation are found, a few drops of procaine on the eardrum are helpful.

A significantly more invasive approach, which should not be used as a first therapeutic step, is injection to the stellate ganglion or—even better—to the superior cervical ganglion on the side of the illness, and alternately left and right in the case of bilateral illness. Exceptions are **sudden hearing loss** and **Meniere's disease** in which the injection to the stellate ganglion must always be performed in addition to local treatment. In every case, even with acute onset of illness, an interference field should be considered because there could have been an interference field related to the inner ear or vestibular organ that existed before the acute onset of illness.

In **pediatric otitis media**, sole injection to the mastoid is often amazingly successful, so that the clinical symptomology and the local findings subside after a short time, provided that the injection is performed within the first 24 hours after the start of the illness if possible, and if otitis was not previously treated several times with antibiotics. In these cases, the injection should be repeated at daily intervals until the inflammation subsides. In the case of **otalgias** during a cold with involvement of the paranasal sinuses or tonsils, local treatment via the mastoid generally is not sufficient. In this case, infiltrations in the area of the mandibular angle performed two to three times a day are more successful.

Tinnitus and hypoacusis or hyperacusis, as they occur after infectious illnesses, should be subjected to neural therapeutic treatment as early as possible. Injections to the stellate ganglion are indicated in addition to injections to the mastoid, to the lymphatic drainage in the mandibular angle, and to the otic ganglion. If there is no improvement after the first two to three treatments, subtle interference field exploration should be performed. Here, the wisdom teeth and tonsils should be mentioned as possible interference fields first and foremost. Particularly when treating tinnitus, early neural therapeutic treatment is clearly more successful; however, in isolated cases normalization of the findings is possible even when the tinnitus started in the distant past.

The treatment of **otogenic dizziness** is local via injection to the mastoid or to the stellate ganglion if local treatment fails.

Note

In the medical history provided by patients, it is important to ascertain the conditions under which the otogenic dizziness occurred.

If there is known **seasickness or motion sickness**, injection to the mastoid on both sides as well as injection in the thyroid immediately before the start of the trip can prevent the sometimes unpleasant symptoms.

22.7 Disorders of the Mouth and Throat

22.7.1 Tonsils and Pharynx

Diagnoses

Neural therapeutic treatment is primarily performed to improve the microcirculation of the diseased or injured tissue via the sympathetic nervous system in order to initiate the healing process and regeneration:

- Acute and chronic tonsillitis.
- Pharyngitis.
- "Lateral funiculus angina," particularly after tonsillectomy.
- Mononucleosis (Pfeiffer's glandular fever).
- Chronic recurrent eustachian catarrh.
- Unexplained dysphagia.
- Recurring infections of the nose and throat region.
- Tonsil hyperplasia.

Therapy

Disorders of the **lymphatic pharyngeal ring**, particularly the inflammations with very few symptoms, have special significance in neural therapy, because the tonsils not only may cause infectious or toxic diseases at entirely different locations (e.g., heart, kidneys, joints), but also can cause a wide variety of noninfectious diseases much more commonly via the autonomic nervous system, especially the sympathetic nervous system.

Note

Remarkably often, the tonsils take on the function of an interference field, which is referenced in a vast number of case reports. The same applies to scars that arise after tonsillectomy.

A possible cause is the topographical proximity to the cervical sympathetic trunk.

Acute tonsillitis is treated by repeated infiltration in the area of the lymphatic drainage in the jaw angle through multiple subcutaneous injections. The inflammation subsides quickly with daily repetition over the course of 2 to 3 days. **Diphtheria** and **scarlatina** should be treated primarily with antibiotics while continuing injections in the area of the lymphatic drainage. In all cases, after 2 to 3 weeks, injection to the tonsils several times in weekly intervals is indicated. As in chronic tonsillitis, slight irritation is to be expected after the first injection to the tonsils. This subsides after a few hours, or after 1 to 2 days at the latest. Injection to the tonsils should be repeated in weekly intervals until no more irritation occurs in the throat.

In the case of **recurring tonsillitis**, **recurring eustachian catarrh**, or **tendency to infection** of the nose/throat area, with recurring **pharyngitis** or lateral funiculus angina after tonsillectomy, repeated injection to the tonsils or in the tonsillectomy scars results in normalization of the inflammations if there are no further chronic inflammations, particularly in the teeth and the maxillodental region.

Note

In each treatment of the tonsils, it is important that the pharyngeal tonsils are not forgotten, otherwise "treatment failures" occur more frequently.

Practical Advice

A special case is morning irritation of the tonsils which subsides over the course of the day and recurs the next morning. This is generally the result of an interference field causing stress on the intestine. Therefore, the treatment is performed via segmental therapy of the intestine. Injection to the tonsils is unsuccessful.

Very rarely, after treatment, a **peritonsillar** abscess can occur which is not of iatrogenic origin but is identified as the exacerbation of an existing chronic bacterial inflammation. In this case, immediate specialist medical support with antibiotic therapy and, if necessary, surgery should be initiated. The healing of the wound is accelerated by daily flushing of the wound region with procaine multiple times and, after healing of the wound, repeated infiltration with procaine; this treatment applies to all wounds with bacterial inflammation. In addition to the accelerated healing, rapid pain relief or even pain-free status can be achieved. It must be emphasized again that only the ester-structured procaine can be used to infiltrate infected wounds since amide-structured local anesthetics cause local vasoconstriction at the injection site and thus worsen the tissue perfusion and increase the inflammation, possibly leading to phlegmonous proliferation.

A further possibility for neural therapeutic treatment of acute tonsillitis is injection to the stellate ganglion or superior cervical ganglion, alternately left and right at daily intervals. Rapid improvement of the local inflammation as well as concomitant symptoms such as fever, pain, and general malaise is often observed even after the first injection.

Due to the high success rate for neural therapeutic treatment of chronic or chronic recurring tonsillitis, tonsillectomy should only be indicated after the failure of this conservative treatment option. It is important to note that, like chronic sinusitis, subtle dental diagnostics and, if necessary, dental restoration must be taken into consideration before each tonsillectomy. Since the tonsils very often take on an interference field function, injection to the tonsils or tonsillectomy scars is part of every interference field exploration in connection with other diseases, even if the history or the local findings do not indicate a prior illness of the tonsils.

In turn, **pharyngitis** in the **acute form** is treated through repeated injection at daily intervals to the lymphatic drainage area in the jaw angle. For the **chronic recurring form**, injections to the tonsils as well as subtle interference field exploration are promising (especially frequently: intestine, sinuses, teeth). **Chronic eustachian catarrh** is treated in the same way, since in many cases a chronic inflammatory disorder of the lymphatic pharyngeal ring or chronic paranasal sinus inflammation is present. In these cases, the injection is made to the nerve exit points of the trigeminal nerve or to the pterygopalatine ganglion on both sides.

Swallowing difficulties that occur after recurrent tonsillitis or after tonsillectomy are generally successfully treated by injection to the tonsils or infiltration of the tonsillectomy scars.

For **hyperplasia** of the tonsils, especially in childhood, peritonsillar infiltration over several weeks at 2- to 3-week intervals as well as in the area of the lymphatic drainage in the jaw angle is promising. Often, there is symptom-free chronic otitis or paranasal sinus inflammation, so injection to the sinuses or to the pterygopalatine ganglion and mastoid is indicated. In small children, injection to the maxillary sinuses on the fold of the upper teeth and upper lip is sufficient.

22.7.2 Salivary Glands, Oral, and Pharyngeal Mucosa

Diagnoses

Neural therapeutic treatment is primarily performed to improve the microcirculation of the diseased or injured tissue via the sympathetic nervous system in order to initiate the healing process and regeneration:

- Chronic and acute sialadenitis.
- Epidemic parotitis.
- Unspecific parotitis.
- Unexplained pain in the salivary glands.
- Herpes simplex.
- Infection of the oral mucosa (gingivostomatitis, canker sores).

Therapy

Inflammatory disorders of the salivary glands are treated by infiltration of the inflamed gland with procaine. This leads to rapid reduction in the inflammation and the subjective pain symptoms.

This is demonstrated very impressively in **epidemic parotitis** as well as in **unspecific parotitis**. In this case, two to three treatments on consecutive days are usually sufficient. For **stone diseases** of the salivary glands, the same injection treatment should be carried out before surgical stone removal or removal of the entire salivary gland, since this neural therapeutic form of treatment often leads to freedom from symptoms.

Inflammatory disorders of the oral mucosa, often of **viral origin**, are successfully treated through direct infiltration with procaine. In addition to fast pain relief, the wound healing process is significantly shortened. It is striking that in chronic recurrent **herpes simplex diseases** of the oral mucosa and lips, the herpes infection no longer occurs at the "old location" after two or three procaine infiltrations, and often subsides entirely. If the corresponding skin or mucosal zone is infiltrated early enough—at the start of the infection, which manifests for the patient in familiar itching—there is often no more blister formation or development of a skin or mucosa defect.

22.7.3 Teeth, Periodontal Apparatus, and Gums

Diagnoses

Neural therapeutic treatment is primarily performed to improve the microcirculation of the diseased or injured tissue via the sympathetic nervous system in order to initiate the healing process and regeneration:

- Difficult teething.
- Unexplained tooth pain.
- Periodontitis.
- Paradontosis.
- Unexplained pain after dental treatment or tooth extraction.
- Wound treatment after tooth extraction.
- Gingivitis.

Therapy

The treatment of dental disease through neural therapy is essentially limited to diseases that do not require a dental surgery or jaw surgery. These are mainly unexplained symptoms associated with discomfort or pain without radiographic–pathologic findings or impaired vitality from a traditional perspective. With **unexplained tooth pain** in individual teeth, whether already treated by a dentist or not, repeated injection to the tooth and, in particular, intraligamental injection is successful. Of these, "bridge abutments" are affected in the same way as teeth with unremarkable exam and X-ray findings. The sometimes persisting symptoms following **crowns**, **fillings**, or **root canals** can often be eliminated through neural therapy. **Painful tooth eruption** with inflammatory response of the gums is made sustainably pain-free after one treatment through infiltration of the gums and careful paradental injection. Teeth that serve as support pillars of a partial denture can easily be treated in the same way.

Wounds following tooth extraction heal more quickly through repeated infiltration, such that antibiotic therapy is not needed. Sustained freedom from pain is often achieved after the first treatment. The vasoconstrictors often still used as an additive to local anesthetic during dental extractions are more likely to disturb the wound healing process, because the trophism of the infiltrated tissue deteriorates significantly. This effect is successfully eliminated with procaine. Discomfort after wound healing in the former parodontium or toothless branches of the jaw can be safely treated by repeated procaine infiltrations if there is no osteitis of the jawbone that cannot be reached by procaine, in which case, surgical removal of the osteitis is indicated.

Widespread **parodontosis** and chronic recurring **periodontitis** are resolved through repeated procaine infiltrations. Intraligamental injection of affected teeth with the carpule syringe reaches not only the periodontal gums, but also the proximal alveolar region which is also affected. Pain and bleeding gums usually subside after the first two to three treatments. This treatment should be performed in a repeated series of six to seven infiltrations two to three times a year in order to interrupt the oft-associated horizontal bone degradation. Neural therapeutic treatment of periodontal disease through infiltration of the gums and the periodontium involves repeated infiltration until sustained normalization of the blood flow which is disrupted in chronic inflammation. With profound bone involvement, restoration through oral surgery is inevitable, followed by neural therapeutic "follow-up treatment" for nonirritated wound healing.

The possibility of observing the normalization of inflammatory tissue components under treatment with procaine reaffirms its valuable properties.

Note

Interference field induction is quite possible with periodontal disease, whereby the tonsils, sinuses, the intestines, and the gynecological and andrological space represent the most frequent sites.

Gingivitis, above all the chronically recurring form, responds to repeated procaine infiltration or just as well to daily flushing with procaine 1%. The associated **gum pockets** become smaller, and the gums lose their erythematous, slightly glassy structure. With crowned teeth, there is regularly an inflammation of the gum surrounding the tooth, whereby an inflammatory exudate is often expressed or flushed out during the infiltration between the tooth and gum. Thus, the local osteitis is eliminated and bone loss does not occur.

Like the teeth, the periodontal apparatus, gums, and jawbone are interference fields for other illnesses remarkably often. If the tooth or multiple teeth are clearly identified as an **interference field**, treatment should be based on neural therapy before tooth removal, in order to rule out the possibility that an interference field originating from the teeth can also be eliminated without tooth extraction. However, if the symptomology always improves for only a short time (a few days), tooth extraction and curettage of the alveoli cannot be avoided.

23 Neck

23.1 Disorders and Dysfunctions of the Thyroid

23.1.1 Diagnoses

Neural therapeutic treatment is primarily performed to improve the microcirculation of the diseased or injured tissue via the sympathetic nervous system in order to initiate the healing process and regeneration:

- Goiter.
- Hyper/hypothyroidism.
- Grave's disease.
- Thyroiditis.
- Vegetative dystonia.
- Sleep disorders.
- Hyperhidrosis.
- Impaired concentration.
- Hyper/hypomenorrhea.
- Dysmenorrhea.
- Recurring miscarriage.
- Imminent abortion.
- Globus sensation.
- Depression.
- Anxiety disorders.
- Exhaustion.
- Change of life (male, female).

23.1.2 Therapy

Diseases of the thyroid and the different symptomologies originating from its functioning are viewed more comprehensively, but also less specifically, in neural therapy than in traditional assessment of this organ. Neural therapy addresses not only the hyperactivity and underactivity confirmed by laboratory chemistry, but also numerous other diseases and symptoms that can be attributed to a functional disorder of this organ without changes shown by chemical analysis. Many diseases also demonstrate psychological involvement in addition to the somatic symptoms.

Pure hyper- or hypothyroidism with or without organ enlargement and euthyroid goiter are treated by repeated weekly infiltration of both thyroid lobes, whereby short-term laboratory tests and especially the associated clinical symptoms indicate normalization of the organ's function. If there is no improvement within 2 to 3 weeks, interference field exploration must be initiated immediately, whereby the teeth as well as the internal genitalia most commonly come into question. **Autonomic adenoma** as well as the severely enlarged thyroid with compression symptoms of the trachea must be treated surgically.

Thyroiditis is almost always induced by an interference field (teeth, tonsils, sinuses), so that interference field diagnostics should be started as a priority (p. 81). Here, too, the subjective impression of the patient and checking laboratory parameters for monitoring results is required. If the interference field is found, there is a noticeable improvement in the concomitant symptoms (normalization of the sleep disorder, discontinuation of the sweating/freezing, elimination of internal unrest) and simultaneous gradual normalization of the lab values.

Functional disorders of the organ without findings detectable clinically or through lab chemistry general ly indicate symptomologies much like those occurring in objectifiable thyroid hyperfunction and underfunction in various combinations. From a traditional standpoint, however, a functional disorder of the thyroid is not attributed to the lack of these objective findings. This includes **disorders in the menstrual cycle**, **the course of pregnancy**, and **menopause** with its many symptoms. Treatment of the thyroid as well as the gynecological or andrological area results in normalization of the symptomology after just a few treatments carried out at weekly intervals. In the same way, the following symptoms can be eliminated through just a few repeated infiltrations of both thyroid lobes.

- Sleep disorders.
- Vegetative dystonia.
- Exhaustion.
- Impaired concentration.
- General hyperexcitability.
- Depression.
- Anxiety disorders.
- Fever in stress situations.
- Other symptoms occurring under stress or distress.
- Globus sensation.
- Hyperhidrosis.

Unexplained disorders such as listlessness, rapid fatigue, restlessness, "nervousness," irritability—in short, disorders within the context of normal exposure—almost always improve through repeated thyroid treatments performed at weekly intervals. It is regularly observed that patients with more agitated symptoms describe an economization of their daily routine already after the first treatment. Sometimes, these patients experienced so-called compulsive crying after the first treatment. The repeated injection into the thyroid gland for the treatment of supposed psychosomatic diseases often eliminates this after only a few sessions.

Note

A "true" psychosomatic illness cannot be affected by neural therapy.

Additional neural therapeutic treatment of thyroid disorders via the stellate ganglion is only necessary when pure organ infiltration does not result in sustained improvement and if interference field therapy was also unsuccessful.

23.2 Disorders and Dysfunctions of the Larynx

23.2.1 Diagnoses

Neural therapeutic treatment is primarily performed to improve the microcirculation of the diseased or injured tissue via the sympathetic nervous system in order to initiate the healing process and regeneration:

- Acute and chronic laryngitis.
- Neuritis of the superior laryngeal nerve.
- Chronic hoarseness.
- Chronic dry cough.
- Sensation of a lump.

23.2.2 Therapy

Diseases not requiring surgery and functional disorders of the larynx and its supplying nerves are treated with repeated injection to the superior laryngeal nerve and the vessels extending along with it. **Laryngitis**, in its acute form with impaired respiration and pain, improves significantly after a few repeated injections to the vascular nerve bundle. Inhalation of procaine 1% through a cold atomizer supports this treatment. Chronic laryngitis is just as treatable if an interference field induction (paranasal sinuses, tonsils) is not present.

Chronic hoarseness, which sometimes appears after a viral infection of the upper airway, as well as **chronic dry cough** and the sensation of a lump or foreign body are eliminated after two to three treatments.

Note

If there is diagnostic uncertainty, chronic hoarseness must always be examined by a specialist to rule out a tumor.

After exclusion of a tumor and unsuccessful local treatment, chronic **dry cough** should bring to mind a primary illness of the paranasal sinuses in accordance with a sinubronchial syndrome, and less commonly chronic tonsillitis in accordance with an interference field disorder.

One special feature is **hoarseness** and **weak speech** from disruption of the recurrent laryngeal nerve function. This disorder is most commonly seen after thyroid surgeries. The inadvertent severing of the nerve is certainly a rare cause of "recurrent nerve paralysis." The vocal cord function can generally be normalized through repeated weekly infiltration of the cicatricial thyroid remnant and its surroundings. Interference field exploration (teeth) should be initiated if local treatment fails. This would not be possible in the case of a severed nerve.

24 Thorax

24.1 Disorders of the Bronchia and Lungs

24.1.1 Diagnoses

Neural therapeutic treatment is primarily performed to improve the microcirculation of the diseased or injured tissue via the sympathetic nervous system in order to initiate the healing process and regeneration:

- Acute and chronic bronchitis.
- Bronchial asthma.
- Pneumonia (bacterial, viral).
- Interstitial pneumonia.
- Pneumonitis (e.g., through radiation).
- Lung emphysema.
- Silicosis.
- Lung fibrosis.
- Pleuritis.
- Lung contusion.
- Lung embolism.
- Rib fracture.
- Intercostal neuralgia.

24.1.2 Therapy

Bronchial and lung disorders as well as injuries to the thorax are treated according to the neural therapeutic treatment regimen—depending on the severity and duration of the symptomology—via the reflexive pathway or via regional sympatholysis through injection to the stellate ganglion or through the interference field. The easiest method is segmental treatment of T1–T4, a wheal series on both sides paravertebral to the thoracic spine and parasternal, and additional intravenous injection to the cubital vein. Scars in the area of the thorax as well as trigger points of the thoracic musculature must always be infiltrated as well. This treatment is particularly suitable for chronic illnesses such as **chronic bronchitis**, **lung emphysema**, **lung fibrosis**, **silicosis**, **pneumonitis**, and **pleuritis**. With insufficient success, reciprocal infiltration of the stellate ganglion is indicated and should be carried out at 1-week intervals. If there is no significant improvement after one to two treatments, interference field exploration is indicated.

Acute bronchitis is initially treated with a wheal series in the thoracic spine and parasternal as well as with trigger point infiltrations of the thorax and sternum. Under this treatment, directly after therapy there is longer sustained subjective and objective improvement in respiration, relieving expectoration in the case of dry concomitant cough, and a reduction in chronic or severe bronchial secretion. In the case of insufficient effect, the stellate ganglion should be injected alternately on the left and right. Generally, two to three treatments are sufficient for eliminating the symptoms.

Along with a thoracic wheal series and trigger point infiltration, **pneumonia** is most quickly treated by way of reciprocal stellate infiltration, regardless of the pathogen, since sympatholysis leads to a significant improvement in the impaired microcirculation related to the infection. The effect of the antibiotic treatment necessary in the case of a bacterial pneumonia is greatly enhanced and the treatment time is significantly shorter.

Practical Advice

Initial stellate injection along with "blind" antibiotic therapy is the optimal treatment approach since evidence of the pathogen—which is important for targeted antibiotic therapy in bacterial pneumonia—is not confirmed for 2 to 3 days or even later. Short-term X-ray follow-ups document well the normalization of the lung findings.

Both **viral** and **interstitial pneumonia** should be treated in the same way through reciprocal stellate infiltration at daily intervals. Atypical pneumonia caused by viruses or mycoplasma pneumoniae often do not show the initial severe symptomology typical of bacterial pneumonia. Sputum testing can provide a rough orientation in the clinical assessment:

- Putrid, possibly bloody sputum indicates aerobic, bacterial pneumonia.
- Malodorous, purulent sputum indicates anaerobic infection with, e.g., bacteroides or peptostreptococci. Nonpurulent sputum is a sign of viral or mycoplasma pneumonia.

Concomitant symptoms of pleuritis can be significantly improved and often eliminated through wheals over the painful thoracic region as well as injections to the intercostal nerves in the same region.

As a polyetiological disease, **bronchial asthma** is rarely affected by local treatment of the thoracic space, but primarily via interference field therapy. The interference fields are most commonly found in the dental and maxillofacial region, in the paranasal sinuses, the tonsils, in the ears, in internal genitals, and in scars. In the short term, the asthma attack can be improved through stellate infiltration. The hyperresponsiveness of the bronchial system, which manifests itself in the form of bronchial obstruction and a thick mucus production, is an expression of an excessive, regional activity of the sympathetic nervous system (primary microcirculatory disturbance of the bronchial system) which requires normalization. Medical history detailing the circumstances under which the asthma started or is triggered can be very helpful (allergen induction, after trauma, after infection, after pregnancy).

Note

An existing medication, particularly steroids, should never be discontinued. The medications should be reduced slowly, depending on the course of the neural therapy.

The asthmatic patient's own familiar medication for asthma attack must be considered in each case. If interference field exploration fails, twice-weekly reciprocal injection to the superior cervical ganglion should be attempted.

Taking into account the autonomic, sometimes deleterious concomitant symptoms, **lung embolism** can be treated with reciprocal stellate ganglion infiltration at intervals of 30 minutes, whereby circulation is stabilized. The fact that a "derailment" of the sympathetic and parasympathetic functions is likely involved, triggered by a sudden shift in the pulmonary circulation, is evidenced by patients whose lung tissue was surgically removed (segment resection, pneumonectomy) without resulting in heart/circulatory decompensation. If indicated, the aim should be immediate thrombolytic therapy to dissolve the embolus.

Closed **injuries to the lungs not requiring surgery**, e.g., **contusion** with or without rib fracture, should also be treated with stellate infiltration in order to achieve improved perfusion through sympatholysis. At the same time, the injured areas of the thoracic wall are treated with wheals and through infiltration of the intercostal musculature. **Rib fractures**, which generally mean significantly impaired respiration, become painless or less painful long past the anesthesia time after infiltration with 1 to 2 mL procaine. The examiner's palpating finger is the best diagnostic method for injection, e.g., in comparison to X-ray diagnostics.

If there is no interference field, **intercostal neuralgia** is safely treated by injection to the corresponding intercostal nerves. In case of zoster neuralgia in the area of the ribcage, the infiltration treatment should be performed as soon as possible and initially carried out daily, possibly with simultaneous stellate ganglion infiltration to the affected side, since this is the safest way to restore the patient's condition. As a reminder, persistent symptoms after zoster neuralgia are often improved by simultaneous segmental and interference field therapy. Basically, it is much easier to abate fresh symptoms of zoster neuralgia than old postzoster pain symptoms.

24.2 Disorders of the Heart and the Mediastinal Space

24.2.1 Diagnoses

Neural therapeutic treatment is primarily performed to improve the microcirculation of the diseased or injured tissue via the sympathetic nervous system in order to initiate the healing process and regeneration:

- Coronary heart disease with and without pectoral angina.
- Heart rhythm disorders.
- Cardiac insufficiency.
- Endo/myocarditis.
- Functional heart disorders.

24.2.2 Therapy

Neural therapeutic treatment of heart disease is carried out, on the one hand, as an adjuvant measure with existing traditional medication in order to improve persistent symptoms and often to conserve medications as well. On the other hand, it is an option as monotherapy in illnesses that do not require immediate acute cardiological care.

Cave

Acute heart disorders, particularly those with manifest or imminent decompensation, are excluded from neural therapy.

The treatment itself proceeds via the sympathetic nervous system on the reflexive pathway of the heart segment from C8–T5, through stellate ganglion infiltration or interference field therapy. By improving the heart muscle circulation in the area of the arterioles and the capillary system, the basic goal of the treatment is to have a therapeutic effect on degenerative and inflammatory diseases of the heart muscle and its nervous conduction.

Coronary heart disease with and without **pectoral angina** can be improved through repeated insertion of precordial and thoracic wheals in segments T1–T5 on the left. Often isolated, subcutaneous, very pressure-sensitive points in the medioclavicular line are one to two finger-widths below the parasternal clavicle in the first to fifth intercostal space as well as immediately precordial. Frequently, patients will indicate these points or other points that lead to relief of the heart symptoms when massaged. This is infiltrated along with paravertebral pressure points in the autochthonous musculature or pressure-sensitive spinous processes of thoracic segments T1–T5. Scars in these segments must always be infiltrated. If there is no longer-lasting significant improvement in the symptoms after the first treatment, injection to the left stellate ganglion is indicated. If there is no change in the coronary symptomology after the first or second repetition, interference field exploration should be ruled out in which the teeth[173] and tonsils play a major role. For each treatment, 1 mL procaine is injected in the cubital vein.

Heart rhythm disorders without signs of decompensation can normalize through intravenous cubital injection of 1 mL procaine as well as additional precordial wheals and infiltrations to the pressure pain points in the thoracic segment T1–T5 on the left. Alternating left and right stellate ganglion infiltration at intervals of several days is indicated in the case of inadequate success, whereby another one to two injections should result in normalization of the rhythm disorders that can be further stabilized with repeated injections. Often, rhythmization comes only after interference field exploration, in this case particularly in the area of the teeth[173] (wisdom teeth). Indeterminate **tachyarrhythmia** or **tachycardia** can often be eliminated in neural therapy by way of additional injection in the thyroid, whereby manifest hyperthyroid is generally not present.

Endocarditis, with its common complication of valve insufficiency or stenosis, can be treated with adjuvant neural therapy. Antibiotic treatment of bacterial endocarditis, low-dose long-term aspirin therapy, and valve correction requiring surgery cannot be replaced. Subjective alleviation of pain in the segment is achieved through wheal insertion and infiltration of trigger points. If the result is inadequate, alternating stellate ganglion infiltration is indicated. The focus of the therapy, however, is primarily in the neural therapeutic suppression of the interference field and surgical removal of bacterial lesions, whether through tonsillectomy or oral surgical removal of bacterially contaminated teeth or the jawbone. Since endocarditis essentially has a "rheumatic" background and the bacterial colonization of the heart valves is an additional destructive component in the metastatic pathway via the vessels, interference field exploration and therapy should be carried out thoroughly and swiftly to minimize the pathological cardiac valve changes. The aim is to eliminate the nonspecific rheumatic inflammation through segmental therapy and interference field therapy.

The procedure for **myocarditis** is the same as the procedure for endocarditis. The adjuvant neural therapeutic treatment of this illness induced by viruses or bacteria aims to improve myocardial microcirculation via the reflexive pathway through the heart segment and by way of bilateral alternating injection to the stellate ganglion, thereby eliminating the inflammation process in the heart muscle more quickly. If segmental therapy fails, interference field therapy, also taking into account special consideration of the teeth, tonsils, and paranasal sinuses, should be immediately initiated in order to inhibit all dystrophic interference field effects induced by the sympathetic nervous system. Initially, the treatments should be performed two to three times a week. The use of interference field therapy and segmental treatment should be alternated.

Neural therapeutic treatment of **cardiac insufficiency** is limited if the heart musculature shows severe degenerative changes. Precise diagnostics of the heart/circulatory system and the lungs must always be performed before attempting neural therapeutic treatment. Repeated segmental therapy of the heart and lungs should have an influence on the microcirculation of the diseased organ via the perfusion-improving effect of the neural therapy, thereby improving function. However, this is to be expected only to the extent that the tissue-damaged organ still has available "regeneration reserve."

Interference field therapy based on the medical history, alternating with comprehensive segmental therapy, has the greatest chance of success. Infected teeth, the tonsils, and paranasal sinuses as well as the intestine are the most common interference fields.

After previous interventions on the heart (ablations, stent implantations, or bypass/valve surgeries), after heart attacks or resolved inflammations, patients also report improved mood and alertness, reduced tightness of the chest, easier respiration, and, as a result, better performance.

Cave

A heart attack requires immediate intensive care.

After the heart attack, there are neural therapeutic treatment options for heart rhythm disorders, remaining heart symptoms, and impaired performance and impaired mental health common to heart disease. Subtle interference field therapy is also indicated for heart attack patients since chronic inflammations of the tooth/jaw region (particularly wisdom teeth), the paranasal sinuses, and the intestine are often present. Comprehensive studies show a significantly more frequent incidence of infarction with preexisting tooth lesions.[173]

24.3 Mammary Gland Disorders

24.3.1 Diagnoses

Neural therapeutic treatment is primarily performed to improve the microcirculation of the diseased or injured tissue via the sympathetic nervous system in order to initiate the healing process and regeneration:

- Mastitis.
- Mastodynia.
- Reclus' disease.

24.3.2 Therapy

Mastitis is treated with the insertion of wheals over the inflamed mammary gland section and infiltration of the inflamed mammary gland tissue as well as ipsilateral stellate ganglion infiltration. At the same time, subcutaneous infiltration should be performed in the area of the axillary lymph nodes to improve lymph drainage. With daily treatment, significant improvement is seen as early as 1 to 2 days, allowing the treatment intervals to be extended. Antibiotic therapy is unnecessary as a rule.

As with all local infections, only procaine 1% should be used as a neural therapeutic agent since the tissue trophism is improved with procaine but worsened with amide-structured local anesthetics.

Degenerative diseases of the mammary gland, such as Reclus' disease or functional painful disorders such as **mastodynia** are improved by local treatment of the mammary gland itself (wheals, infiltration of painful or hardened tissue areas) as well as by injection to the branches of the uterovaginal plexus and infiltration of the thyroid. The treatment intervals should take place weekly until the symptoms subside.

With an existing allergy to procaine, which is very rare, another product must be used, e.g., lidocaine.

25 Abdomen, Small Pelvis, and Retroperitoneum

25.1 Stomach Disorders

25.1.1 Diagnoses

Neural therapeutic treatment is primarily performed to improve the microcirculation of the diseased or injured tissue via the sympathetic nervous system in order to initiate the healing process and regeneration:

- Gastritis (acute, chronic).
- Gastric ulcer.
- Hyper-/hypoacidity.
- Pyloric spasm.
- Bacterial inflammation of the mucous membranes of the stomach.
- Dumping syndrome (postgastrectomy syndrome).
- Functional stomach disorders.

25.1.2 Therapy

The inflammatory and functional disorders of the stomach are well suited for neural therapy as adjuvant or monotherapy. In case of diagnostic uncertainty, gastroscopy must always be performed first. The function and circulation of the mucosa are particularly linked to unimpaired autonomic innervation, so that a regional therapeutic effect on the autonomic nervous system is apparent. Pure segmental therapy is available and is the first therapeutic step for the illnesses mentioned. The following are simple injections that often show an immediate effect for minor manifestations of the diseases: wheals in segment T6–T9, left paravertebral injections in any tense muscle extensions, infiltration of the left Vogler's pressure point at the front costal arch at the level of the mammary line (T8), pre- and intraperitoneal injection three finger-widths below the xiphoid tip, and the infiltration of pressure-sensitive points of the abdominal wall in the left upper abdomen. With several repetitions, at 1- to 2-day intervals for an acute case and weekly intervals for a chronic illness, symptom-free status and normal function can be achieved after three to four treatments.

If there is no significant improvement in the symptoms after the first or second treatment, injection to the left celiac ganglion is indicated. This injection is also primarily indicated for the mentioned diseases with increasing symptoms, particularly in the case of acute diseases. With chronic symptomologies that show no significant improvement after the first or second injection, interference field diagnostics (p. 81) should be performed. For **stomach problems**, **gastritis**, or **ulcers** that occur **under the effect of stress**, repeated injection in the thyroid should be performed along with the local treatment of the stomach. With recurrent epigastric pain without pathological changes in the gastric mucosa, there can be chronic relapsing, oligosymptomatic appendicitis, such that the required therapy consists of wheals in the right lower abdomen in segments T10–T12 and a preperitoneal injection in the area of the McBurney point or injection into the right celiac ganglion.

In neural therapy, infected teeth and paranasal sinuses are often interference fields for stomach disorders. The infiltration of scars, particularly in the stomach wall, is just as important for interference field diagnostics as the infiltration of the navel.

Acute hyperacidity with and without esophageal reflux is often helped immediately by oral administration of 5 mL procaine two to three times every hour and can even be sustained with 2 to 3 days of repetition.

25.2 Disorders of the Small and Large Intestine

25.2.1 Diagnoses

Neural therapeutic treatment is primarily performed to improve the microcirculation of the diseased or injured tissue via the sympathetic nervous system in order to initiate the healing process and regeneration:

- Duodenitis.
- Duodenal ulcers.
- Terminal ileitis.
- Ulcerative colitis.
- Chronic appendicitis.
- Viral infection of the intestine.
- Chronic constipation.
- Diarrhea.
- Paralytic ileus.
- Irritable colon.
- Meteorism.
- Spastic functional disorders of the intestine.
- Diverticulitis.
- Abdominal angina.
- Anal fissure.
- Increased sphincter tone.
- Hemorrhoids.

Adjuvant therapy for:

- Dysbioses.
- Fungal diseases.
- Typhus.
- Dysentery.
- Salmonellosis.

Investigation of:

- Mesenteric infarction.
- Inoperable mesenteric thrombosis.
- Tumor pain in inoperable tumors.

25.2.2 Therapy

The intestinal tract has a mucosal surface of approximately 400 m². The innervation is autonomic in principle, modulated via the vagus nerve and the sympathetic nervous system via the spinal sympathetic portion from sacral segments S2–S4. The sympathetically and parasympathetically controlled capillary system and the submucosal immune system are further basic anatomical entities that, from a neural perspective alone, have multiple segmental as well as centralized and thus far-ranging cross-segmental effects on the whole body. In pathological processes of the intestine, corresponding multiple reactions that affect the entire body (interference field effect) occur via the afferent fibers. The direct afferent process of the vagus nerve from the intestine to the brain stem and the resulting pathological effects of a chronic intestinal disorder on central neurohumoral processes suggest which effects are possible from the intestine to the overall organism. This explains the high "interference field effect" of the intestine in many inflammatory-degenerative (i.e. arthritis) as well as psychological illnesses (i.e. depression). Toxic stress to the liver in the case of intestinal disorders (leaky gut?) is quite possible, even if laboratory chemical findings cannot be determined, for example, although autonomic innervation of the liver is involved.

In the treatment of intestinal diseases with neural therapy, the autonomic reflexive pathway is selected for the reduction of pathological impulse inputs via the sympathetic and parasympathetic afferent fibers (cutivisceral, splanchnic nerves, celiac ganglion), just as the same injections are intended to improve microcirculation of the intestine via the efferent pathway.

In minor cases, treatment of intestinal diseases can be attempted via the segmental-reflexive pathway of spinal segments T10–L3 and S2–S4, whereby the cutivisceral pathway is taken into account through wheals as well as trigger-point infiltrations of the abdominal wall up to the peritoneum and paravertebral muscular tension between T10 and L3. The diseases listed above are additionally treated through injection to the splanchnic nerves and the celiac plexus. For acute illnesses, these injections are performed two to three times at daily intervals if a surgical procedure is ruled out, and in weekly intervals for chronic illnesses. Continuation of the infiltrations is determined from the result of the first or second treatment. If the symptomology does not change after the second segmental therapy, interference field diagnostics should be added (p. 81). This particularly applies to **chronic appendicitis**, **terminal ileitis**, and **ulcerative colitis**, in which the interference field is often in the dental and maxillofacial region and the paranasal sinuses.

Note

Acute appendicitis is excluded from neural therapy.

For **irritable bowel syndrome**, subtle segmental treatment of the intestine usually results in a significant improvement in symptoms. In particular, locating the trigger points of the abdominal walls, which are almost always to be found, **all scars**, and epidural sacral infiltration with 10 mL procaine, can improve the prolific symptoms. The interference fields are found remarkably often in the teeth and paranasal sinuses. Long-term treatment is crucial, initially at weekly intervals, then increasingly longer intervals every 3 to 4 weeks. Particular attention should be paid to triggering causes (e.g., nutrition) since irritable bowel syndrome is often a multifactorial disease, of which only the symptoms caused by autonomic factors can be addressed with neural therapy.

Segmental therapy of the intestine, including daily injection to the celiac ganglion on both sides for **acute bacterial infections of the intestine** including **diverticulitis**, results in better tissue perfusion of the intestinal mucosa via sympatholysis, so that regeneration and the antibiotic effect improves at the inflammation site and symptoms and clinical findings are normalized within a few days.

Repeated infiltration of the celiac ganglion on the right and left in the case of **inoperable tumors** as well as possible intra-abdominal injection of 5 mL procaine in the area of worst pain is a successful pain treatment to the extent that strong analgesics and spasmolytics can be reduced and neither paralytic symptoms nor tenesmuses occur, if no tumor-related obstructions are present. These are not amenable to neural therapy.

Disorders of the rectum can be treated very successfully by way of neural therapy. For example:

- Anal fissure.
- Anal pruritus.
- Increased sphincter tone.
- Hemorrhoids with pain during defecation.

In this case, direct infiltration of the fissures, the anal mucosa, the external sphincter, and the visible hemorrhoids with procaine 1% is usually successful after only one to two treatments. A reduction of hemorrhoids is quite possible; however, surgical removal is necessary for severe cases.

25.3 Disorders of the Liver and Bile Ducts

25.3.1 Diagnoses

Neural therapeutic treatment is primarily performed to improve the microcirculation of the diseased or injured tissue via the sympathetic nervous system in order to initiate the healing process and regeneration:

- Acute hepatitis (nonspecific and viral).
- Chronic persistent hepatitis.
- Hepatosis (after infection, after toxic contamination).
- Liver function disorders with impaired digestion.
- Hepatorenal syndrome.
- Postcholecystectomy syndrome.
- Cholangitis.
- Cholecystitis.
- Biliary colic (with and without evidence of stones).

25.3.2 Therapy

The segmental-reflexive treatment of liver and biliary diseases consists of insertion of a wheal series paravertebral and at the level of the right upper abdomen at the corresponding spinal segments T8–T11, the infiltration of muscular tensions in the right paravertebral region at the same level, and injection at the Vogler's pressure point on the right costal arch (T8) and possibly to the right supraorbital nerve in the case of pressure sensitivity. This segmental therapy is suitable for chronic disorders of the liver and bile ducts. For acute illnesses and in case of indeterminate success with segmental therapy, injection to the right celiac ganglion is promising. This injection is indicated in numerous different diseases since it improves the circulation in the liver and bile ducts and relaxes the muscles of the bile ducts and gall bladder. This not only normalizes organ-related disorders, but also the intestinal function disorders caused by these diseased organs, such as:

- Diarrhea.
- Constipation.
- Nausea.
- Loss of appetite.
- Tympanites.
- Intolerance to various foods.

As with all organ-related **viral infections**, injection to the corresponding sympathetic ganglia triggers accelerated healing of the infection. This also applies to **acute hepatitis**, regardless of the virus type. Injection to the celiac plexus and the splanchnic nerves not only improves the subjective symptoms, but also accelerates the normalization of transaminases. A significant improvement should occur after no more than two to three injections at daily intervals, so that individual treatment intervals can be extended.

With **chronic persistent hepatitis** as well as **autoimmune hepatitis**, suspicion of a focal disease needing ugent attention is engendered if the first two to three celiac infiltrations do not result in subjective and objective improvement. In this case, subtle interference field diagnostics should be initiated.

Hepatosis as a result of toxic damage (alcohol, drugs, occupational exposure, food) can be treated with neural therapy through weekly repeated right and left celiac infiltrations to the extent that the quite different pathologies of the abdomen (dyspepsia, recurrent nausea, anorexia, food intolerance, meteorism, headaches) can be eliminated. Interruption of the toxin load is necessary in any case. The normalization of occasionally elevated transaminases points to the positive influence of liver cell perfusion through improved microcirculation.

The neural therapeutic treatment of **postcholecystectomy syndrome**, which is based on the fact that similar symptoms persist before and after a cholecystectomy, takes place by way of interference field therapy in most cases. The symptoms are not to be interpreted as adhesion symptoms but as a **reaction phenomenon** from the perspective of neural therapy. In any case, infiltration of the cholecystectomy scar to the peritoneum and repeated injection to the right celiac ganglion should be considered. If there is a temporary worsening or no reaction after the first treatment, interference field induction is almost guaranteed.

Cholangitis and **cholecystitis** are treated through injection to the right celiac ganglion. Subjective symptoms and inflammatory parameters disappear after the first two to three treatment sessions, which should take place at daily intervals.

Note

Gall bladder empyema is excluded from neural therapy and should be treated immediately by surgery.

Surgery is necessary for **cholecystolithiasis**. Biliary colics without detected stones can be diminished through the spasmolytic effect of celiac filtration without further therapy. In the case of closure of the cystic duct or the common bile duct with formation of jaundice, expulsion of the stone can be expected with small concretions through bilateral celiac infiltration. Sonography of the bile ducts with evidence of stones should determine the decision for either surgery or neural therapy.

25.4 Disorders of the Pancreas

25.4.1 Diagnoses

Neural therapeutic treatment is primarily performed to improve the microcirculation of the diseased or injured tissue via the sympathetic nervous system in order to initiate the healing process and regeneration:

- Pancreatitis (acute, chronic).
- Pancreatic insufficiency.

25.4.2 Therapy

The injection of the left celiac ganglion is probably the most effective treatment for **acute** and **chronic recurring pancreatitis**. The often considerable symptoms subside and laboratory findings normalize in a remarkably short time. A significant decrease in mortality of acute pancreatitis and a decrease in complicated disease progression are seen with this treatment.[119] The injection is given daily (twice daily in the case of severe progression). As the subjective and objective symptoms decrease, the injection intervals can be extended if deemed appropriate.

Note

Before neural therapeutic treatment, a tumor of the pancreas must always be excluded!

Chronic pancreatitis is treated on the segmental-reflexive pathway via the thoracic segment T8 on the left through paravertebral wheals, injection to the pressure-sensitive spinous process, and injection into existing trigger points—especially in segment T8. After the palpation findings, there are mainly isolated pressure-sensitive points in the mid and upper abdomen which are also infiltrated up to the peritoneum, as well as the Vogler's pressure point at the left costal arch, which is usually very painful when pressed. If unsuccessful, injection to the left celiac ganglion is an option. A focal disease should always be considered in the case of chronic pancreatitis, thus interference field diagnostics (p. 81) should be initiated after two to three unsuccessful injections to the left celiac ganglion. In addition to the teeth and sinuses, being frequent localizations for interference fields, foci in the liver should be considered and occasionally also an interference field disease originating from the parotid gland after mumps.

Chronic excretory pancreatic insufficiency with its effect on digestion is also treated by injection to the left celiac ganglion. The aim is to improve the secretion capacity of the still-functional tissue through improved microcirculation of the pancreas. In case of insufficient success, a combined disorder of liver and pancreas function should be considered, i.e., the right celiac ganglion should also be infiltrated. Since an interference field may be present, as with all chronic illnesses, interference field diagnostics is indicated if there is no effect on the pancreatic insufficiency.

25.5 Disorders of the Kidneys and Efferent Urinary Tracts

25.5.1 Diagnoses

Neural therapeutic treatment is primarily performed to improve the microcirculation of the diseased or injured tissue via the sympathetic nervous system in order to initiate the healing process and regeneration:

- Pyelonephritis.
- Cystitis.
- Nephrolithiasis.
- Nephrosis (after infection or toxic exposure).
- Nephritis.
- Renal colic.
- Investigation of renal insufficiency.
- Persistent functional symptoms after kidney operations.
- Functional stress incontinence.
- Prostate hyperplasia.

25.5.2 Therapy

Treatment of **kidney disorders** via the segmental-reflexive pathway proceeds via spinal segments T10–LI and additionally via segments S2–S4 for bladder disorders and diseases of the internal genitals. Again, the simple neural therapeutic approach is through paravertebral wheals in these segments, injections to spinous processes with pressure pain, into muscular trigger points found mainly in the flank region, and possibly into the scars present there. The intravenous injection concludes each treatment. Interference field diagnostics (p. 81) should be performed if there is no improvement after the first two treatments or if there is rapid deterioration. Injections to the renal plexus should be done on both sides if the symptoms do not fully subside.

The same injection is indicated for **acute pyelonephritis**, whose antibiotic treatment is supported by improved kidney circulation via regional sympatholysis. This injection significantly shortens the course of the illness and the pain usually subsides immediately after the first injection, even without antibiotics.

In **nephritis**, which occurs as interstitial inflammation of the kidneys after bacterial and viral infections or may be drug induced, injection to the renal plexus is useful not only for treating pain, but also particularly as a targeted "anti-inflammatory" measure by way of improved microcirculation of the renal parenchyma. The intravenous injection strengthens this anti-inflammatory effect. It is important for the neural therapy to address the primary location of the disease, i.e., prior location of the infection, and to perform interference field therapy as well. Essentially, the tonsils, sinuses, teeth, and the intestine play an important role here.

Note

Tonsillectomy followed by neural therapeutic follow-up treatment of the tonsillectomy scars may be required in the case of nephritis, as well as precise restoration of the teeth.

In **glomerulopathies** (acute/chronic nephritis, progressive nephritis, minimally persistent urine abnormality, nephrotic syndrome), the glomeruli (podocytes) are essentially affected. Comorbidities include bacterial infections, gold treatments, mercury, vaccines, or malignant tumors. Systemic diseases such as lupus, polyarteritis nodosa, scleroderma, Wegener's granulomatosis, and glomerulopathies (in diabetes mellitus) are also observed. There are various distinct inflammatory degenerative changes that lead, depending on the course of the disease, to correspondingly faster or slower loss of kidney function. The primary goal of neural therapy is to use sympathicolysis to improve microcirculation of the kidney tissue and interrupt the pathological process, and to improve the elimination capacity with the still-viable tissue. Comprehensive interference field therapy over several weeks at intervals of 1 to 2 weeks is required, alternating with segmental therapy including injection to the renal plexus. Timely lab test follow-ups should be ordered to document the course of the therapy.

Again, **kidney stone disorders** are treated via the segmental-reflexive pathway and through injection to the renal plexus in order to improve organ perfusion. **Colicky pain**, with and without evidence of stones, subsides quickly after repeated daily injection to the renal plexus.

Note

Stones that cannot pass through the urethra because of their size must be removed surgically or via lithotripsy.

Injection to the renal plexus is also indicated for **ureter stones**, whereby the colicky pain is eliminated and expulsion of the stone is made possible through relaxation of the ureter.

Neural therapeutic treatment of **acute cystitis** involves prevesical infiltrations to the branches of the vesical plexus as well as infiltration of 3 to 5 mL procaine 1% in the bladder. This not only leads to fast improvement of the dysuria symptoms, but also reduces bacteria physiologically through improved mucosal circulation. Repeated injection in a daily pattern can thus reduce the bacterial count to normal values after two to three treatments, often without antibiotics. Urinalysis after completion of treatment is mandatory for follow-up monitoring.

Dysuric pain without bacteriuria should be treated in the same way. The same technique can also be used successfully to treat **urge incontinence** as well as the incontinence that primarily occurs in women after giving birth, after gynecological procedures, or in association with a descending uterus. Successful treatment can often eliminate the need for corrective surgery of the bladder, the pelvis, or the genitals. In this context, prevesical infiltration should extend to the branches of the uterovaginal plexus. Surgical scars from gynecological procedures must always be infiltrated. If segmental therapy fails, interference field exploration represents an additional therapy option (incisors).

Analogously to micturition disorders in women, in men these are often associated with **prostate hyperplasia**. Prevesical infiltration to—or even more effectively—in the prostate is performed in this case. Not only does this result in improved incontinence and dysuria, but also the residual urine volume is reduced and the closure pressure of the sphincter system is improved.

Along with injection in both thyroid lobes, neural therapeutic treatment of **bladder function disorders** is a successful nondrug method that should be attempted before any surgical procedure. If there is insufficient success, weekly repeated epidural sacral infiltration should be carried out as well.

25.6 Disorders of the Female Internal Genitals

25.6.1 Diagnoses

Neural therapeutic treatment is primarily performed to improve the microcirculation of the diseased or injured tissue via the sympathetic nervous system in order to initiate the healing process and regeneration:

- Cycle disorders.
- Dysmenorrhea.
- Amenorrhea.
- Fertility disorders.
- Recurring miscarriage.
- Spastic parametropathy.
- Sexual dysfunction.
- Vaginal discharge.
- Menopausal symptoms (hot flashes, insomnia, adynamia, depression).
- Parametritis.
- Endometritis.
- Adnexitis.

25.6.2 Therapy

Segmental-reflexive treatment of diseases and disorders of the female genitals is possible via spinal segments T12–L3 (sympathetic nervous system) and sacral segments S2–S4 (parasympathetic nervous system). The spinous processes S2–S4 are often very sensitive to pressure only in the sacral bone area; furthermore, as displaceable subcutaneous tumors, geloses indicate a reflexive perfusion disorder of the subcutis. This reflexive treatment approach is reflected in wheals in these segments, the infiltration of geloses, injection to pressure-sensitive spinous processes, and in tensed muscle portions. It should be used as the first treatment step for functional disorders as well as chronic courses of illness. For nonlasting success, epidural sacral infiltration (10 mL) is an effective injection that can be administered with simultaneous injection of the celiac ganglion in the case of acute inflammation.

The direct neural therapeutic treatment approach involves the infiltration of the local anesthetic immediately near the organ via the branches of the uterovaginal plexus from the inferior hypogastric plexus. Scars in the segmental area of the outer and inner genitals (scars from herniotomy, appendectomy, Pfannenstiel incisions, or episiotomy) must always be infiltrated. If the indirect reflexive or direct treatment fails, interference field therapy should be the next step. Remarkably, the wisdom teeth region (even without tooth germ) and the incisors of the upper jaw are the most common locations for interference fields.

When treating **cycle disorders,fertility disorders**, **sexual dysfunction**, **spastic parametropathy**, **recurring miscarriage**, and symptoms of **menopause** injection to the thyroid lobe as well as intravenous injection should be carried out in addition to the segmental-reflexive or direct injections described above which affect the genitals.

Practical Advice

Note that if a patient is medicated with psychotropic drugs for depression associated with menopause, neural therapeutic treatment is not as successful as it would be without antidepressants. In these cases, attempts should be made to achieve a better therapeutic result by slow reduction of the medication while continuing the neural therapeutic treatment at 1- or 2-week intervals. Without antidepressants, the menopausal symptoms can be treat ed at weekly intervals and monthly thereafter. Successful treatment of the menopausal symptoms can be success fully concluded after 3 to 4 months.

For acute parametritis, endometritis, and adnexitis, the reflexive treatment approach is less successful than injection to the branches of the uterovaginal plexus, infiltration of the sacral epidural space, and injection to the celiac ganglion. The aim of treatment is improved tissue perfusion through sympatholysis, leading to a therapeutically effective influence on the inflammation and allowing it to subside. Existing foci, e.g., in the dental and maxillofacial region, the tonsils, or sinuses, should be treated with neural therapy or surgery in the context of interference field therapy if the local inflammation in the genital region does not subside after two to three treatments with the indicated injections.

25.7 Disorders of the Male Internal and External Genitals

25.7.1 Diagnoses

Neural therapeutic treatment is primarily performed to improve the microcirculation of the diseased or injured tissue via the sympathetic nervous system in order to initiate the healing process and regeneration:

- Prostate hyperplasia with and without urination disorders.
- Nonspecific prostatitis.
- Adjuvant measures for bacterial prostatitis.
- Functional disorders of the genitals.
- Male menopause.
- Epididymitis.
- Orchitis.

25.7.2 Therapy

Injection to and in the prostate is first-line therapy for neural therapeutic treatment of urination disorders in men due to **prostate hyperplasia** and **nonspecific prostatitis** as well as adjuvant measures for **bacterial prostatitis.** Daily injections are performed for acute illnesses and weekly injections for chronic illnesses. Additional injections in the thyroid improve the therapeutic result for urination disorders due to prostate hyperplasia as well as for male menopause. In case of insufficient success, infiltration of the sacral epidural space (10 mL) and injection to the celiac ganglion should be considered as an alternative or combination option. Scars in the area responsible for male genitalia and supplied by spinal segments T12–T13 (herniotomy, appendectomy, circumcision or sterilization scars) as well as spinal segments S2–S4 should always be infiltrated. The most common locations for interference fields are found in the teeth and paranasal sinuses.

Orchitis and **epididymitis** are generally successfully treated with neural therapy, except for cases where the cause is an interference field. Even with the most delicate needle, the injection is painful. But patients are happy to take their chances since a successful result can be expected immediately. In orchitis, injection to the easily palpable and highly pressure-sensitive spermatic cord is the first therapeutic step, followed by injection into and to the testicles which are significantly painful when touched.

Note

The differential diagnosis of testicular torsion is important as it requires immediate surgical treatment.

The severe pain of orchitis and inflammatory swelling usually disappear continuously after the first treatment, so that repetition of the injection is rarely needed.

The treatment approach is the same for **epididymitis,** whereby the spermatic cord and the easily palpable and highly pressure-sensitive epididymis are infiltrated. The immediate pain relief and fast abatement of symptoms "compensate" the patient for this painful treatment.

26 Spine and Pelvis

26.1 Degenerative and Inflammatory Diseases, Injuries

26.1.1 Diagnoses

Neural therapeutic treatment is primarily performed to improve the microcirculation of the diseased or injured tissue via the sympathetic nervous system in order to initiate the healing process and regeneration:

- Osteochondrosis.
- Spondylarthrosis.
- Degenerative disk development with protrusion/ prolapse.
- Spinal canal stenosis.
- Lumbago.
- Lumbar sciatica.
- Ankylosing spondylitis.
- Coccygodynia.
- Spinal cord injuries.
- Postspinal headache.

26.1.2 Therapy

The neural therapeutic treatment of chronic degenerative diseases of the spine begins with a series of wheal injections paravertebral to the area of the painful spinal segment. Weekly repeated injections to pressure-sensitive spinous processes in strained muscle sections, and to irritated vertebral joints and their capsular system, may further help to resolve the quite varied symptomology. A subtle clinical examination helps to identify the structure most clearly affected. Repeated injection to two or three vertebral joints can often stop lumbago, for example.

Note

The degree of degenerative changes in no way limits the possible therapeutic success.

The statement often expressed after radiographic findings that “nothing more can be done” with regard to these severe changes is factually incorrect. While the degenerative deformities cannot be normalized, the pain can almost always be improved by interrupting the inflammatory degenerative process and the associated disrupted function. Peridural infiltration in the lumbar and sacral spine section and injection to the paravertebral sympathetic trunk are also very helpful. Local sympatholysis to improve persistently impaired tissue perfusion at the site of the degeneration and the interruption or reduction of pain with its reflexive negative effect on the vasomotor system is the therapeutic mainstay of treatment with local anesthetics.

The **narrowing of the spinal canal** or **intervertebral foramen** through a **prolapse**, protrusion of the intervertebral disk, or **osteophytes** is neither absolutely connected with pain nor with a neurological disorder in the corresponding spinal segment. Impaired microcirculation of the dorsal root ganglion and vertebral joints, resulting in local inflammation by way of pathological sympathetic nervous system stimulation, is the basis of pain, sensory disturbances, or impaired motor function. The duration and extent of the neurological finding is decisive for a possible surgical procedure.

Note

Acute disk herniation with motor and sensory deficits as well as bladder and bowel evacuation disorders must be treated promptly with neurosurgery.

Discrete neurological disorders of varying intensity can often be completely eliminated by repeated injections to the affected spinal ganglia and the lumbar sympathetic chain, and by infiltration of the epidural space in the area of the herniated disk, such that there is no need for a surgical procedure.

A remarkable number of chronic degenerative **diseases of the spine** originate from an interference field disorder, especially in young patients. The teeth, tonsils, sinuses, internal genitals, bowel, and scars represent the primary contingent of interference field localizations; therefore interference field diagnostics (p. 81) are promising, especially in the case of a temporary worsening of spinal pain after localized treatment. After the completion of interference field therapy, any “residual symptoms” can usually be completely resolved through segmental therapy. In scoliosis as well, the neural therapeutic treatment in both the segment and via the interference field is quite promising since interference fields, according to therapeutic experience, very often demonstrate their impact as a recurrence in already damaged organs or tissues.

Lumbago, as a collective term for pain in the lumbar spine and the adjacent tissue components, is a “collective diagnosis” for acute and chronic cases with the primary symptom of lumbosacral pain of various origins. These include:

- Irritation of the spinal joints through malposition or stress.
- Irritation of the sacroiliac joints.
- Stress on the associated strong ligament system.
- Tension in the psoas muscles and the paravertebral musculature.
- Irritation of the ligaments of the vertebral joints, the anterior and posterior longitudinal ligament, and the flavum ligament.

In addition to the lumbago symptoms, in **lumbar sciatica** there is also irritation of spinal nerves in the area of segments L4–S3. Thus, depending on neurological findings, an additional intervertebral injection must be made into the affected spinal nerves at the level of the intervertebral foramen. Occasionally, sole injection to the spinal nerves is sufficient for resolving the symptoms immediately. If local infiltration of the above structures does not significantly help to improve the pain and the resulting dysfunction after the first two treatments, an interference field origin is usually the cause, which must be determined through neural therapy. Again, the teeth, tonsils, sinuses, internal genitalia in the small pelvis, and scars are the dominant locations for an interference field.

Ankylosing spondylitis is primarily viewed as interference field–induced, so that interference field exploration should take place early on before significant loss of function of the spine and partly also of the large joints (hip, shoulder joint, knee joint). If the interference field is found (scars, teeth, tonsils, internal genitalia), which is reflected in reduced pain and improved range of motion, more functional improvements are possible through segmental treatment, as long as bony stiffening of the vertebrae has not occurred over the anterior and posterior longitudinal ligaments.

Coccygodynia is caused by irritation of the ligaments between the sacrum and coccyx or improper stress on the joint. Bruises, sprains, or birth trauma usually trigger this sometimes very painful medical condition. If local infiltration of the ligaments, taking into account the ganglion impar, provides no significant improvement in symptoms after the first or second treatment, an interference field induction is often present, which is found especially in the minor pelvis in the form of impaired internal genitalia.

Injuries of the spine and sacroiliac joints from excessive stress (e.g., lifting injury, carrying of heavy loads), from **distortion** (whiplash), and from **contusion**, **sprain**, and **compression** with structural injury to the vertebrae (transverse process tear, vertebral body compression factor) are easily accessible for neural therapy through local infiltration of the structures involved. Injury-induced hemorrhages or edema are absorbed much faster, and pain is greatly reduced or eliminated. Unstable vertebral fractures with dislocation can generally only be stabilized through surgery. If there is a compression fracture of the vertebral body, the injection to the vertebral body and the sympathetic trunk and the spinal nerves at the same level, with clinically detectable irritation, leads to clear persistent pain reduction—even in the presence of osteoporosis with continuity of the vertebral canal. Furthermore, bone fractures heal more quickly through interruption of the injury-induced irritation of the sympathetic nervous system, which always means a deterioration of tissue perfusion. Thus, the desired functional treatment is possible early on and certainly shortens the normally lengthy downtime. It is important to note that chronic symptomatology often appears, for example, in the form of lumbar sciatica involving the L5 segment, which can only be resolved via injection to an old vertebral fracture elsewhere, e.g., an old compression fracture of the 11th thoracic vertebra.

The fact that an **acute spinal injury** such as **whiplash** can be subject to an interference field effect and is therefore inaccessible to local treatment is shown again and again in practice. It is regularly apparent that local treatment is more likely to result in worsening of the symptoms. The cause then often lies in an interference field in the tonsils, teeth, or sinuses, which existed before the accident and gained clinical relevance by the acute spinal injury as a "second strike". In this situation, the injury is treatable only via the interference field.

The **postspinal headache** that may occur after spinal anesthesia or spinal fluid collection can generally be relieved neurotherapeutically after the first or second injection to the occipital nerves as well as through subgaleal injections. If the patient does not remain asymptomatic, peridural procaine infiltration should take place in the area of the dural puncture site.

Note

The "blood seal" recommended in anesthesiology, which is a mixture of intravenously drawn blood and a local anesthetic for "bonding" the puncture hole of the dura, is more elaborate and riskier than neural therapeutic treatment.

27 Extremities and Joints

27.1 Degenerative Disorders, Inflammations, and Injuries

27.1.1 Diagnoses

Neural therapeutic treatment is primarily performed to improve the microcirculation of the diseased or injured tissue via the sympathetic nervous system in order to initiate the healing process and regeneration:

- Chronic degenerative joint disorders.
- Nonspecific inflammatory joint disorders.
- Polyarthritis.
- Insertion tendinopathy.
- Bursitis.
- Tendinitis.
- Tendovaginitis.
- Carpal tunnel syndrome.
- Cubital tunnel syndrome.
- Tarsal tunnel syndrome.
- Dupuytren's contracture.
- Injuries of the extremities and joints.

27.1.2 Therapy

There are numerous neural therapeutic options available for treating joint disorders. Local treatment consists of the insertion of wheals at the level of the intra-articular space, infiltration of the generally pressure-sensitive ligaments, injection to the joint capsule, and the infiltration of painful pressure points in the immediate joint area. Scars near the joints are always infiltrated as well. As further segmental therapy, injections can be made to and in the supplying vessels (e.g., femoral artery, axillary artery) as well as those peripheral nerves responsible for supplying the joints (e.g., axillary nerve for the shoulder, femoral and ischiadic nerves for the hip joint). For toe and finger joints, the injection takes place in the neurovascular bundle at the level of the proximal phalanx. If there is no significant improvement in the symptoms after the first treatment, injection to the sympathetic trunk is indicated. Injection to the stellate ganglion is suitable for the upper extremities, while injection to the lumbar sympathetic trunk at the level of L3 is suitable for the lower extremities.

The differentiated assessment of the joint with special emphasis on **pain localization** and **pain radiation** as well as consideration of the innervation of the corresponding joint-moving muscles often provides important indications as to whether the disease is primarily a disease of the joints or, for example, a primary irritation in the spine or an irritation of adjacent joints. Medially focused knee joint pain (even with existing varus gonarthrosis) is frequently eliminated through injection to the bilaterally identical spinal root L5, less frequently at L3–L4. Hip joint pain is eliminated through injection to spinal roots L5 or S1 for dorsal pain symptoms and to spinal roots L3 or L4 for ventral symptoms. The variety of patella symptoms, "heel spurs," and nocturnal leg cramps or "achillodynia" frequently have an irritation of the bilaterally identical spinal root S1 in common. Similarly, the isolated pain of the metatarsophalangeal joint can be solely due to the irritation of the bilaterally identical spinal root L5 or L4, whereby radiology can detect degenerative changes of the metatarsophalangeal joint as well as completely normal X-ray findings.

Note

In diseases of the joints, examination of the corresponding spinal segment is always required in addition to examination of the joint, even if the patient subjectively indicates no spinal pain.

From a neural therapeutic perspective, intra-articular injections are only very rarely necessary and useful, as the nerves and vessels responsible for the perfusion and microcirculation of the joints and capsular ligament apparatus are located outside of the joints. Exceptions are found in posttraumatic joint degeneration and inflammation following intra-articular injections.

The accompanying examination of adjacent joints is very important for diagnosing a joint disorder. Thus, knee-joint pain can originate entirely from coxarthrosis which remains clinically asymptomatic, just as hip problems can arise from irritation or arthritis of the bilaterally identical sacroiliac joint.

Furthermore, much of the pain felt in the shoulder joint originates from the acromioclavicular joint, so that sole treatment of this joint eliminates the shoulder joint problems. If there is no differentiating inclusion of the spine and adjacent joints in the joint examination, there is a risk of misdiagnosis and corresponding maltreatment.[56]

In the case of **chronic degenerative joint disorders**, if there is no improvement or even temporary deterioration after the first or second local treatment, a focal illness should be considered and interference field exploration should be carried out. Especially in young patients with degenerative joint disorders, an interference field disorder is often seen. The majority of interference fields are found in the maxillodental region, in the tonsils, the paranasal sinuses, the intestine, and the liver as well as in scars.

The majority of **nonspecific inflammatory joint disorders** are due to foci; therefore, interference field diagnostics (p. 81) are a priority. This is especially true for monarthritis and rheumatoid arthritis. The neural therapeutic treatment of these consists of subtle interference field exploration and interference field removal if necessary, particularly in the dental and maxillofacial region, the sinuses, the intestine, and the liver. Initial neural therapeutic removal of the infection is especially important in rheumatoid arthritis, on the one hand, in order to forestall rapidly progressive and irreversible joint destruction and, on the other hand, to avoid the oft-used drug therapy with cortisone or cytostatic agents.

Practical Advice

Patients taking medication such as cortisone or cytostatic agents that affect the basic regulatory system are significantly less responsive to neural therapy than patients without corresponding medication. The dosage must be very carefully reduced with simultaneous neural therapeutic treatment performed at intervals of 1 to 2 weeks. Reducing the cortisone or cytostatic medication requires an overlapping treatment with NSAIDs, which has a lower negative impact on the base regulation system. In some cases, a drug-free, solely neural therapeutic treatment of the illness can be achieved, with complete disappearance of pain and the biochemical signs of inflammation.

Far more often, additional treatment with nonsteroidal anti-inflammatory drugs (NSAIDs) is given alongside the neural therapy, although in lower doses. In these cases, progression, albeit very slow, of the inflammatory joint changes can be expected. As experience shows, in the juvenile form of rheumatoid arthritis, the prospect of success at the end of the neural therapeutic treatment is significantly greater. Low-pain or pain-free joints are of primary importance for patients undergoing conservative treatment. The medical assessment of the symptomology of each affected joint should always incorporate the surgical treatment options, be it synovectomy, arthrodesis, or—in the large joints (hip, knee, shoulder, elbow joint)—prosthetic replacement with corresponding joint destruction. Local joint treatment for rheumatoid arthritis has no prospect of success in the acute stage. However, when the inflammation has subsided, persistent joint pain can frequently be improved for a longer time with local treatment.

Insertion tendinopathy (e.g., "tennis elbow" [lateral epicondylitis]), **tendinosis, tendovaginitis**, or **bursitis** can be treated by neural therapeutic local infiltration of the pathologically altered tissue. Contact of the needle with bone should be avoided as much as possible in epicondylitis, since temporary severe pain is to be expected. Subcutaneous infiltration over the bone and subsequent distribution of the procaine through light massage is the more gentle approach. In the examination of the cervical spine, there is often distinct paravertebral tenderness at the level of C6 (radial epicondylitis) or C8 (ulnar epicondylitis). In these cases, the epicondylitis can be ended with a few infiltrations of the corresponding spinal root, carried out at weekly intervals. Simultaneous injections of the cervical sympathetic chain or the stellate ganglion are indicated in the case of insufficient success. If there is no significant improvement of the epicondylitis symptomology after the first or second treatment, an interference field induction is virtually certain, often starting from the teeth, the middle ear, sinuses, tonsils, or the intestines and the liver.

Before every surgical intervention, **tendinitis** should be treated through local infiltration of procaine 1 to 2 times a week into the easily palpable inflammatory swelling of the tendon. In general, the reduction of the inflammatory tendon swelling is usually so advanced after the second and third treatments that the **trigger finger** phenomenon is no longer present. With a little patience, the tendon can be completely normalized.

Dupuytren's contracture is also well suited to neural therapy. Weekly direct infiltration of the scarred contracting portions of the palmar or plantar aponeurosis results in a significant reduction in scar tension and improves the stretchability of the affected fingers or toes after only a few treatments. If the flexion contracture is not too far advanced and consistent neural therapeutic treatment is carried out, a surgical procedure is usually avoidable.

For **carpal tunnel syndrome** (CTS), **ulnar nerve entrapment** (URS), and **tarsal tunnel syndrome** (TTS), perineural infiltrations at weekly intervals often improve the symptoms after only two to three treatments, to the extent that a surgical procedure becomes unnecessary. In these diseases, the corresponding spinal segment should be examined in each case, since irritations of the corresponding segments are frequently responsible (median nerve: C7–T1, ulnar nerve: C8–T1, tibial nerve: L4, S3). If there is no improvement of symptoms after the first local treatment, injection to the corresponding spinal nerves in the region of the spine segment is indicated. If this injection also does not lead to significant improvement, an interference field induction may very well be present, so that interference field diagnostics must be carried out.

Joint injuries, if there is no indication for surgery, are responsive to neural therapy through direct infiltration of the traumatized structure. These include:

- Distortions.
- Strains.
- Contusions.
- Bruises.
- Misuse and overloads.

In particular, the ligaments and the joint capsule are almost always remarkably pressure-sensitive clinically and are infiltrated with a small quantity of procaine, as are **bruises** or **hematomas**. This way, the healing process is significantly shortened and pain is eliminated after the second or third treatment, which should initially take place at daily intervals. Immobilization is often not necessary. With local treatment, **muscle injuries** particularly also **torn muscle fibers** usually become pain-free after the first treatment, as do **tendon segment ruptures** not requiring surgery. In these cases, the injury should be protected for 4 weeks. The treatments are carried out initially at daily intervals three to four times, then at increasingly long intervals. Older injuries are treated at longer intervals (1–2 times per week); they also show a significant reduction in pain after the first treatment. Additional injection to the associated sympathetic trunk supports this process.

Prior to the injury of a joint, if there are disorders in the relevant spinal nerve segment, e.g., in the form of a root irritation of spinal root L5 in the case of an ankle sprain, sole treatment of the ankle injury often does not lead to complete freedom from symptoms, but only additional injection to the spinal root L5. If the L5 symptomatology is induced by an interference field, e.g., an impacted wisdom tooth, it must be infiltrated or even possibly removed to gain freedom from symptoms.

With repeated local procaine infiltrations, **fractures** heal significantly faster than without this treatment. This observation was already made over 60 years ago, but is still not part of routine treatment in traumatology.[302] Regardless of whether a bone fracture is to be treated surgically, or if it has to be fixed by external splinting or not, the pain after two to three infiltrations is almost always reduced to the extent that mobilization is much easier and the development of pseudarthrosis or reflex sympathetic dystrophy and their incidence is significantly reduced.

Note

The sooner the neural therapeutic treatment of fractures is initiated, the lower the therapeutic effort and greater likelihood of fast healing of the broken bone.

Fatigue fractures ("march fractures") or **overload fissures** ("dancer's leg," cortical avulsion of the tibia cortex in dancers and athletes) should be treated in the same way, whereby irritation of the spinal segments should always be taken into account. In the case of overload pain in the bones and joints, there are often preexisting spinal symptoms in the corresponding segment or an interference field situation which must be elicited through detailed interference field diagnostics. For all injuries discussed here, injection to the corresponding sympathetic trunk also promotes healing.

Pseudarthrosis should be infiltrated two times a week to exploit the conservative treatment option of neural therapy before the surgical option. If surgical treatment has already been performed, local procaine infiltration accelerates osseous development and reduces the risk of recurrence. Here too, the associated sympathetic trunk should be infiltrated and the blood circulation in the area of pseudarthrosis should be improved by repeated periarterial and intra-arterial injections in the relevant arteries.

For unspecific as well as bacterial **osteitis**, local procaine infiltration and the injection of the supplying vessels and the corresponding sympathetic trunk are very helpful—not only because of the rapid decrease in pain. Normalization of the microcirculation, which is impaired in any inflammation, illustrates the basic concept of neural therapy and is the body's own prerequisite for complete healing. The surgical procedure in the form of detailed debridement targets the same process. Therefore, enteral or parenteral antibiotic therapy alone is often unsuccessful because the necessary antibiotic concentration "on-site" is not sufficient because of the impaired microcirculation. Surgical debridement along with topical application of bone cement, for example, which was mixed with an effective antibiotic according to an antibiogram, is an effective surgical procedure for treating **osteomyelitis**. In these cases, neural therapy as an adjuvant measure can certainly improve the local circulation disorder through weekly repeated local infiltrations, injections to the sympathetic trunk, and injections to and in the afferent arterial vessels.

28 Nerves

28.1 Disorders of the Peripheral Nerves and Cranial Nerves

28.1.1 Diagnoses

Neural therapeutic treatment is primarily performed to improve the microcirculation of the diseased or injured tissue via the sympathetic nervous system in order to initiate the healing process and regeneration:

- Neuritis.
- Neuralgia.
- Investigation of peripheral, posttraumatic paresis.
- Phantom pains.
- Investigation of polyneuropathy.

28.1.2 Therapy

Neuritis is treated by direct injection of procaine to the affected nerve at the level of the spinal ganglion and to the affected nerve branch for cranial nerves. Scars in the corresponding segment should be infiltrated in each case. Very often the cause is a focal illness that causes the inflammatory nerve disease, such that the inflammation can only subside through suppression of the interference field. Injections to the sympathetic trunk at the same segment level and to the corresponding ganglia and vessels for the optic nerve and trigeminal nerve of the cranium are also indicated in order to reach all possible portions of the sympathetic nervous system.

Neuralgia should be treated in the same way, whereby interference field exploration once again represents the primary task. Zoster neuralgia should be treated as early as possible through specific infiltration of the corresponding spinal ganglia, paying special attention in chronic cases to the localization of the diseased segment. In the corresponding supply area, very often there is a preexisting or lapsed organ disease whose neural therapeutic treatment finally enables the neuralgia to subside (herpes zoster in the liver segment after hepatitis or in hepatosis, in the region of the trigeminal branch in tooth infections, in the course of a spinal nerve in degenerative disk disease).

Note

According to the classical view in neurology, paresis of the peripheral nerves following trauma or inflammation is usually considered an untreatable final state of nerve damage. However, a neural therapeutic attempt is highly appropriate.

This is done by local infiltration at the former site of injury and by injection to the corresponding paravertebral sympathetic ganglia, the spinal nerve exits in the spine, and in scars in the area supplied by the nerve. If the individual axons are not severed by the trauma, functional regeneration is definitely possible. The function of the peripheral nervous system is linked to intact microcirculation controlled by the sympathetic nervous system. The fact that the peripheral nervous system including ganglia is supplied by an extensive capillary network, demonstrates the importance of the microcirculation for sufficient neuronal metabolism. Interference fields can also hinder the regeneration of a nerve lesion as a "first strike." In private practice, two complete peroneal pareses that existed for years were sustainably eliminated in one case by infiltrating an epigastric midline incision scar, and in the other case by injection at the branches of the uterovaginal plexus. Although the number of possible successes in the treatment of injuries to the peripheral nervous system is small, a treatment attempt is always carried out since the findings cannot be worsened.

In contrast, **pain** occurring after peripheral nerve lesions is almost always eliminated with the help of neural therapy through the treatments described above. This is especially true for **phantom pain**, which may be partially caused by shorted afferent–efferent ephapses formation in the area of the nerve injury, and in the stimulation of the nerve stumps by nonspecific inflammation in the scar area or stress, for example, from prostheses. The contralateral pain treatment recommended by Gross for phantom pain, which is very often successful, goes back to the form of acupuncture treatment that was used before neural therapy.[197]

Practical Advice

The treatment option for phantom pain is based on the fact that trigger points on the healthy limb can often be found by palpation, and are mirrored almost exact ly in the area of the primary injury to the amputated limb. As an example, there is violent pressure pain (not spontaneous pain) in the healthy left lower leg in the same region where a bullet went through the right lower leg, which subsequently led to the amputation. If these trigger points on the left leg are infiltrated, the phantom pain of the right lower leg can almost always be relieved and ultimately eliminated with correspondingly repeated treatment.

Polyneuropathies are divided in terms of their etiological aspects:

- According to genetic causes in the case of metabolism disorders and deficiency disorders.
- According to infections in the case of arteriopathies (connective tissue disease, among others) and toxic exposure (heavy metals, among others).
- As an autoimmune illness.

The neural therapeutic treatment of polyneuropathy is carried out only from the standpoint of a neuronal and general microcirculation disorder resulting in inflammatory degeneration of the peripheral nerves. This pathogenetic relationship is responsive to neural therapy in that the therapy can improve the microcirculation.

The disease generally starts peripherally in the extremities, affects multiple spinal nerves, usually occurs bilaterally, and is characterized by a primary lack of sensation and loss of epicritical sensitivity advancing slowly from the periphery to the center. The disorders can be contained and slowly improved through injections to corresponding spinal ganglia, the lumbar and cervical trunk, and epidural and, above all, intrathecal injections at L1–L2 (0.5% procaine, 2–3 mL).

Note

With intrathecal application of procaine 1% solution, motor deficits and inability to walk should be expected for 60 to 90 minutes!

To prevent postspinal headache, additional injection to the occipital nerves has proven effective. Especially the pain, which is especially prominent in some cases, is easily influenced.

The treatment is to be carried out in the long term. Initial weekly dose intervals can be extended to 2- to 4-week intervals depending on the degree of improvement. Greater success is achieved by alternating interference field exploration with the segmental therapy described above. The slow improvement—which varies from person to person—determines the treatment intervals and the alternation of interference field and segmental therapy. After previous comprehensive specialist medical diagnostics, and depending on the breakdown of the results, an additional substitution therapy for deficiency disorders, a detoxification, or an improvement in the metabolic state (e.g., diabetes mellitus) is required in every case.

29 Vessels

29.1 Disorders of the Arterial Vessels

29.1.1 Diagnoses

Neural therapeutic treatment is primarily performed to improve the microcirculation of the diseased or injured tissue via the sympathetic nervous system in order to initiate the healing process and regeneration:

- Arterial occlusive disease.
- Temporal arteritis.
- Raynaud's disease.
- Frostbite.

29.1.2 Therapy

Arterial occlusive disease of the extremities, **particularly the lower extremities**, should be treated with neural therapy if there is no indication for surgery, if stent insertion is not possible, or if both have already occurred. As always, the aim of neural therapy is to improve the circulatory conditions, in particular the microcirculation of the affected tissue. This is possible, albeit in a limited sense, even with advanced sclerotic changes in the vessels. Exact documentation (e.g., walking distance, ischemic pain during exercise) is essential for the treatment intervals.

Weekly injections to the lumbar sympathetic trunk on both sides at the level of L3 are among the standard injections. Intra-arterial (5 mL procaine 1%) and periarterial injections in and to the femoral artery also help improve tissue perfusion. Subtle palpation over the course of the vessels can detect painful pressure points, particularly in the calf muscle, that must also be infiltrated.

At the first signs of **gangrene**, for example, of the toes, repeated daily infiltration of the neurovascular bundle and the transition zone to the vitality-disturbed tissue with procaine is also indicated. Interference field exploration performed in parallel provides the opportunity to further improve the circulation conditions. Since each arterial plaque formation starts with an intimal inflammation, the interference field diagnostics (p. 81) should particularly focus on chronic inflammation of the tooth/jaw region, the paranasal sinuses, and the intestine, which should be treated accordingly with neural therapy. Bacterial foci of the teeth and jaw must be surgically removed.

For **Raynaud's disease**, repeated injection to the four neurovascular bundles of the affected toes and fingers is very often sufficient to sustainably relieve the recurrent spasticity of the vessels. In case of insufficient success, injection to the axillary artery or femoral artery as well as to the responsible sympathetic trunk is indicated. Interference field exploration is the last option.

Frostbite at the extremities, especially the toes and fingers, can be effectively treated immediately and with regard to the long-term consequences by infiltration of the neurovascular bundle and direct infiltration of the affected tissue with procaine. Repeated injection to the responsible sympathetic trunk increases the perfusion-strengthening effect.[57]

29.2 Disorders of the Venous Vessels

29.2.1 Diagnoses

Neural therapeutic treatment is primarily performed to improve the microcirculation of the diseased or injured tissue via the sympathetic nervous system in order to initiate the healing process and regeneration:

- Phlebitis.
- Thrombophlebitis.
- Postthrombotic syndrome.
- Varicose symptom complex.
- Leg ulcers.

29.2.2 Therapy

Through perivascular and intravascular infiltration of 1 to 2 mL procaine, **phlebitis** is rendered painless already after the first treatment. The inflammation is largely eliminated after another two to three treatments. The same treatment is indicated for superficial **thrombophlebitis**. Even in phlebitis which can occur after infusion therapy or accidental paravascular injected drugs, immediate procaine infiltration is superior to all other treatments.

The possible complications of a bacterial infection or tissue necrosis do not occur through local sympatholysis. Pre-existing trophic disorders are normalized significantly faster. In the case of extensive edema, additional subcutaneous infiltration in the area of the regional lymph nodes is very helpful, as is injection to the responsible sympathetic trunk.

Neural therapeutic treatment of **postthrombotic syndrome** of the lower extremities is performed at weekly intervals through repeated injection to the lumbar sympathetic trunk at L3 and extensive infiltration (5 mL) below the inguinal ligament. In addition to the subjective pain symptoms that generally subside completely, there is almost always a reduction in leg swelling and an improvement in the walking distance. If the therapy described does not result in success after the second or third treatment, the cause may be a lesion, so interference field exploration should be carried out.

The **varicose symptom complex** is responsive to neural therapy to the extent that pain symptoms over the varicose convoluted tubule as well as inflammatory indurations are generally significantly reduced or completely eliminated after one to two repeated treatments with perivenous procaine infiltration in the vascular lacuna.

Note

Varicose crossectomy or endovenous sclerotherapy cannot be avoided in the long term despite successful neural therapy.

Leg ulcers, which are often accompanied by varicose veins, are healed significantly faster through local infiltration of the rough margin wall, the ulcer bed, and injection to the supplying arteries and possibly to the lumbar sympathetic trunk at L3, than through the typical local treatments with ointment. Neural therapy should not be expected to bring about a change in the varicose vessels. Along with wound cleansing, and for improved epithelization, procaine-soaked mull patches are an option. These must be changed two to three times daily. This often results in rapid cleansing of the generally putrid wound bed, which is evident from the improved microcirculation and the improved local resistance to infection.

30 Lymphatic System

30.1 Disorders of the Lymphatic Channels and Lymph Nodes

30.1.1 Diagnoses

Neural therapeutic treatment is primarily performed to improve the microcirculation of the diseased or injured tissue via the sympathetic nervous system in order to initiate the healing process and regeneration:

- Lymphangitis.
- Lymphadenitis.
- Lymphedema.
- Angioedema.

30.1.2 Therapy

The neural therapeutic treatment of **lymphangitis** consists initially of repeated daily intracutaneous and subcutaneous infiltration of the affected tissue section, in particular a possible existing skin lesion. This can be as small as an insect bite, which develops into an areal inflammation of the regional lymphatic vessels. After the first treatment there is often already a cessation of pain as well as lightening of the stripelike reddening of the cutis in the affected section of skin. When there is simultaneous involvement of the lymph nodes (**lymphadenitis**), these are usually spontaneously painful or painful on pressure and enlarged. Local infiltration of these lymph node sites and direct lymph node infiltration allows the pain as well as the swelling to subside quickly after a few treatments without further therapy. Additional injection to the associated sympathetic trunk supports this "anti-inflammatory" effect.

Lymphedema after an injury of any kind should be treated just as quickly by local treatment as described above. Older scars, especially in the lymph node sites (e.g., herniotomy scars, abscess scars of the axilla and the groin, scars after lymphadenectomy) should also be infiltrated. In case of insufficient success, injection to the responsible sympathetic trunk is indicated. This is especially true for lymphedema occurring after lymphadenectomy (e.g., from breast cancer) or after radiation therapy of regional lymph sites in tumor diseases. For nonspecific lymphedema, which can affect all parts of the body without the existence of any injury or primary disease of the lymphatic system (excluding malignancy), interference field diagnostics (p. 81) should be carried out in the event of unsuccessful local treatment.

After one to two daily treatments without further treatment, **angioedema**, which is characterized as a variably severe edematous swelling of the face in allergic diseases, is often eliminated by injection to the nerve exit points of the trigeminal nerve or by injection to the pterygopalatine ganglion with additional stellate infiltration.

31 Skin

31.1 Disorders and Injuries of the Skin and Its Appendages

31.1.1 Diagnoses

Neural therapeutic treatment is primarily performed to improve the microcirculation of the diseased or injured tissue via the sympathetic nervous system in order to initiate the healing process and regeneration:

- Eczema.
- Seborrhea.
- Acne.
- Rosacea.
- Pruritus.
- Neurodermatitis.
- Psoriasis.
- Lupus erythematosus.
- Scleroderma.
- Alopecia.
- Boils.
- Carbuncles.
- Paronychia.
- Ingrown nails.
- Panaritium.
- Erysipelas.
- Herpes simplex.
- Infected and noninfected wounds.
- Ulcerations.
- Burns.
- Acid or alkali injuries.
- Keloids.

31.1.2 Therapy

The neural therapeutic treatment of eczematous skin diseases usually requires subtle interference field exploration. The attempt at local infiltration treatment of diseased skin sections is warranted, but should only be continued through long-term weekly treatments if the first treatment already leads to subjective and objective improvement. Occasionally, infiltration of the skin area on which the eczema began is sufficient. The most common interference field localization is found in the area of the intestine and the liver, the teeth, the paranasal sinuses, the tonsils, and in scars (navel). Rosacea and eczema of the hands, fingers, soles, and toes often originate from the interference fields of the intestine, liver, and sinuses. This connection results in treatment in the form of injection to the celiac ganglion on both sides, the navel and scars of the abdomen, and injections to the nerve exit points of the trigeminal nerve and the pterygopalatine ganglion on both sides.

Neurodermatitis in infants and small children is often induced solely by the interference field of the navel. In adults, eczema more commonly depends on two or more interference fields (e.g., colon, sinuses, tonsils, teeth, scars), such that multiple interference fields must be infiltrated simultaneously. For food intolerance, a change in diet is necessary.

Seborrhea, **acne**, **pruritus**, **psoriasis**, **lupus erythematosus**,**scleroderma**, and **alopecia** are partially responsive to neural therapy alone or in combination with other available methods, whereby the neural therapeutic treatment focus clearly lies in interference field therapy. Despite the expected limited success rate for response to neural therapy alone, the diseases mentioned repeatedly show the importance of eliminating the interference field, without which other regulation medical therapies remain ineffective.

The **furuncle**, a liquefying bacterial infection of a hair follicle and its surroundings, can be healed quickly by infiltration with procaine after a few daily treatments, whereby an existing abscess is not a limitation for neural therapy.

Practical Advice

In addition to infiltration, a procaine-soaked mull dressing as a moist wrap changed two to three times a day supports elimination of the furuncle or spontaneous perforation of an abscess. It is important that only procaine—as an ester-structured neural therapeutic agent—is used, since amide-structured local anesthetics (e.g., lidocaine) lead to slight vasospasm at the injection site and impaired tissue perfusion. Therefore, these local anesthetics are contraindicated.

The **carbuncle**, a collection of closely spaced furuncles, is treated in the same way through local infiltration with procaine, a repeatedly moistened procaine wrap, and possibly through additional injection to the corresponding sympathetic trunk. Thus, the significantly traumatizing surgical treatment of excision and open wound treatment is usually not necessary.

Paronychia, **ingrown nails**, and **panaritium** heal after two to three local infiltrations daily with procaine and the infiltration of the neurovascular bundle at the proximal phalanx, hence surgical treatment can be omitted. Here too, the addition of consistently moist procaine wraps that are changed several times a day relieve pain and promote healing.

Erysipelas, a streptococcal skin infection usually from a small break in the skin, can be healed after a few daily treatments through multiple intradermal procaine infiltrations without further antibiotics, whereby the portal of entry, which can be a small skin defect or a larger wound, must be infiltrated thoroughly with procaine. A wrap with procaine-soaked dressing and a moisture-retaining seal speeds up the healing process.

Herpes simplex disease of the skin and mucous membranes should be treated with neural therapy as soon as it is safely possible. In the early stage, when there is no blister formation, the pain can be immediately and sustainably relieved with proper, strict intradermal infiltration that must include the entire infected skin area. In most cases the herpes infection does not recur at this site as is otherwise typical for herpes. If the disease is already in the blister stage, treatment at daily intervals should be repeated two to three times.

Neural therapeutic treatment of **noninfected wounds** that require no primary treatment with surgery (e.g., excision, suture) and the treatment of **infected wounds** involves repeated local infiltration and a moist procaine wrap. This leads to accelerated wound healing and to simultaneously reduced infection of wounds. In any case, this treatment results in fast relief of the wound pain. Fresh wounds that are primarily considered to be infected—such as bite wounds, lacerations or punctures by nails, as well as injuries with objects contaminated with bacteria—usually heal rapidly without complications.

When undergoing the same procedure, **chronic ulcerations** of the skin show the same rapid healing tendency. For chronic ulcers of the lower leg, injection to the sympathetic trunk should be carried out, as with tenderness in the lumbar segment corresponding to the ulcer area. Perivascular injection to the respective arterial vessels should be included in the treatment.

First and second degree burns (including sunburn!) with skin defects and nonirritated, accelerated healing tendency are immediately relieved with moist procaine wraps (procaine-soaked mull dressings) that are changed three to four times a day. The treatment should be concluded after 1 to 2 days.

Acid or alkali injuries should be thoroughly rinsed with water as soon as possible and then covered with procaine-soaked dressings which must be changed in hourly intervals initially.

Note

Acid or alkali injuries cause direct damage to the skin, and also a massive stimulation of the sympathetic nervous system, which leads to substantial, progressive vasospasm of the tissue, extending to tissue necrosis.

In addition to the local treatment with procaine-soaked mull dressings, early infiltration of the skin may be indicated for the treatment of pain, and to improve tissue perfusion and minimize tissue damage as much as possible.

Injuries to the skin from **bites** or **stings** by insects, snakes or spiders can be successfully treated through early thorough infiltration of the injury site, and by intravenous procaine administration, insofar as the allergic or toxic reactions are absent locally or systemically. The experimentally reproducible absence of anaphylactic reactions with repeated injection of endotoxins, the Sanarelli–Shwartzman phenomenon (p. 63), in which procaine was infiltrated at the site of the endotoxin injection, proves the dominant role of the sympathetic nervous system in the symptomatology of anaphylaxis.[461] Thus, it is understandable that a disease which is immunological at first glance can be treated via the sympathetic nervous system by using a local anesthetic.

Keloids after injuries can largely be normalized through neural therapy with repeated procaine infiltration. After the first two to three treatments at weekly intervals, there is already a blanching effect on bulbous, often distorted scars. Occasionally, a parallel interference field exploration is necessary if the region has already been stressed due an interference field prior to emergence of the scar. The age of the keloid is not relevant to the neural therapeutic treatment.

32 Tumors

32.1 Malignant Diseases

Note

Malignant tumors must not be treated with neural therapy, even if procaine shows a limited antitumor effect in vitro.[492,493]

Basal cell carcinomas are an exception. In this case, according to my own experience, repeated direct infiltration (once a week) of the basal cell carcinoma is worth a try, whereby the procaine must reach the "healthy" skin beyond the edge of the tumor. In case of visible reduction in tumor size after two to three treatments, the infiltrations are continued until the tumor has completely regressed. Especially with basal cell carcinomas of the facial skin, after consultation with the patient this treatment can be attempted "under visual control," since surgical extraction is considerably more extensive. In each case, detailed documentation of the decrease in basal cell carcinoma and the medical monitoring should be pursued in the interests of the patient.

However, for inoperable tumors, accompanying pain or discomfort can often be improved. Therefore repeated injections to the tumor tissue, insofar as this can be reached, are successful for pain reduction and decreasing the inflammatory tissue reaction in the immediate vicinity of the tumor, as well as reducing the need for pain medications. Additional injections, which can even be performed daily depending on the pain evaluation, are injections to the stellate ganglion for tumors of the head, neck, chest and the upper extremities, as well as repeated injection to the celiac ganglion on both sides for tumorous diseases of the abdominal space. For inoperable tumors localized in the small pelvis, repeated epidural sacral infiltration with procaine should be attempted for pain reduction.

Cytostatic therapy, which frequently has a significant negative impact on patients' general well-being, has fewer side effects when neural therapy is performed at the same time. Daily repeated intravenous procaine injections and repeated injections to the celiac ganglion on both sides improve symptoms such as nausea, loss of appetite, or fatigue. **Radiation therapy** is tolerated better with simultaneous targeted infiltration of the irradiated tissue two to three times a week and through intravenous treatment.

33 Summary

"*The wise use of the autonomic system will someday make up the majority of the medical arts.*" This quote by Karl Ewald Hering (1834–1918), director of the Leipzig Institute of Physiology, drew attention early on to the possibility of diagnostic/therapeutic utility of the autonomic nervous system. Today, the search is primarily for drug-based solutions directed toward the pathological function of the sympathetic nervous system which is causally involved in a pathophysiological process (inflammation, degeneration, allergy, pain), whether as sympathicolytic or receptor-based therapy regimen. This approach is problematic because of the expected side effects from the nonpathologically irritated—and thus uninvolved—sympathetic nervous system. In contrast, the selective treatment of the sympathetic nervous system by way of neural therapy has proved successful for decades in humans, since this "wise use" can be realized without the related side effects.

Knowledge of the physiological functions of the autonomic nervous system as well as its characteristics and its pathophysiology provides a considerable expansion of present-day therapeutic possibilities, in particular for the treatment of chronic diseases. The possibilities for using neural therapy to treat disease have certainly not been exhausted, and the method's mode of action and variability of the therapeutic tactic allow the list of indications to be further expanded.

Through selective use of the autonomic nervous system for diagnostic and therapeutic purposes and taking into account the autoregulation mechanisms, neural therapy works on the pathogenesis of an illness via the regulatory function of the autonomic nervous system having an **impaired information** condition and resulting **impaired regulation**, i.e., before the therapy processes. Therefore the approach is based on the pathogenetic status of the **functional impairments** and **structural impairments**.

Relational diagnostics, which are necessary in neural therapy, mean that the causal relationships of an illness must be found. Otherwise, the treatment will fail. The **etiology** of a disease only becomes clear during the diagnostic and therapeutic interventions, so that a clear diagnosis in the strict sense is only possible at this stage.

In each patient, similar diseases have a remarkably different causality chain, particularly in the **presence** of **neuromodulatory effective interference fields**. This should also explain why, with the same symptomologies, the therapeutic course is generally so variable with regard to scope of the interventions and the time spent. However, with this there is the possibility of ending the course of chronic diseases and shortening the course of acute illnesses. This represents an expansion of the therapy options, particularly in comparison with primarily symptomatic therapy regimens .

Part 5
Appendix

34 Literature

[1] Adamec RE, Stark-Adamec C, Saint-Hilaire JM, Livingston KE. Basic science and clinical aspects of procaine HCl as a limbic system excitant. Prog Neuropsychopharmacol Biol Psychiatry . 1985; 9(2):109–119

[2] Ader H. 10 Jahre neuraltherpeutische Ambulanz an der Universitätskinderklinik Wien. In: Dosch P, Hrsg. Neuraltherapie nach Huneke - Freudenstädter Vorträge. Band 7. Heidelberg: Haug; 1981

[3] Adler E. Störfeld und Herd im Trigeminusbereich. 6. Aufl. Bissenhofen: Sieber; 2013

[4] Agassandian K, Fazan VP, Adanina V, Talman WT. Direct projections from the cardiovascular nucleus tractus solitarii to pontine preganglionic parasympathetic neurons: a link to cerebrovascular regulation. J Comp Neurol. 2002; 452(3):242–254

[5] Ajijola OA, Shivkumar K. Neural remodeling and myocardial infarction: the stellate ganglion as a double agent. J Am Coll Cardiol. 2012; 59(10):962–964

[6] Albertyn J, Barry R, Odendaal CL. Cluster headache and the sympathetic nerve. Headache. 2004; 44(2):183–185

[7] Aldrete JA, Johnson DA. Evaluation of intracutaneous testing for investigation of allergy to local anesthetic agents. Anesth Analg. 1970; 49(1):173–183

[8] Althoff H. Therapie mit Novokain. In: Kilian H, Hrsg. Lokalanästhesie und Lokalanästhetika. 2. Aufl. Stuttgart: Thieme; 1973

[9] Anderson RU, Sawyer T, Wise D, Morey A, Nathanson BH. Painful myofascial trigger points and pain sites in men with chronic prostatitis/ chronic pelvic pain syndrome. J Urol. 2009; 182(6):2753–2758

[10] Anselmino KJ. Neue Wege der Eklampsie- und Präeklampsiebehandlung: Die Blockade des Nierenbereichs und des Ganglion stellatum. Schweiz Med Wochenschr. 1959; 52:1373

[11] Ashina S, Bendtsen L, Ashina M. Pathophysiology of tension-type headache. Curr Pain Headache Rep. 2005; 9(6):415–422

[12] Ashkenazi A, Blumenfeld A, Napchan U, et al; Interventional Procedures Special Interest Section of the American. Peripheral nerve blocks and trigger point injections in headache management - a systematic review and suggestions for future research. Headache. 2010; 50(6):943–952

[13] Avnon Y, Nitzan M, Sprecher E, Rogowski Z, Yarnitsky D. Autonomic asymmetry in migraine: augmented parasympathetic activation in left unilateral migraineurs. Brain. 2004; 127(Pt 9):2099–2108

[14] Bahekar AA, Singh S, Saha S, Molnar J, Arora R. The prevalence and incidence of coronary heart disease is significantly increased in periodontitis: a meta-analysis. Am Heart J. 2007; 154(5):830–837

[15] Barbagli P, Bollettin R. Therapy of articular and periarticular pain with local anesthetics (neural therapy of Huneke). Long and short term results [in Italian] Minerva Anestesiol. 1998; 64(1–2):35–43

[16] Baron R, Binder A, Ulrich W, Maier C. Komplexe regionale Schmerzsyndrome. Sympathische Reflexdystrophie und Kausalgie. Schmerz. 2003; 17(3):213–226

[17] Baron R, Jänig W. Schmerzsyndrome mit kausaler Beteiligung des Sympathikus. Anaesthesist. 1998; 47(1):4–23

[18] Baron R, Jänig W. Sympathetically maintained pain. In: Bountra C, Munglani R, Schmidt WK, eds. Pain. New York, NY: Marcel Dekker; 2003:309–320

[19] Baron R, Schattschneider J, Binder A, Siebrecht D, Wasner G. Relation between sympathetic vasoconstrictor activity and pain and hyperalgesia in complex regional pain syndromes: a case-control study. Lancet. 2002; 359(9318):1655–1660

[20] Barop H. Neuraltherapie nach Huneke als adjuvante und alternative Behandlung in der Knochen- und Gelenkchirurgie. In: Dosch P, Hrsg. Neuraltherapie nach Huneke - Freudenstädter Vorträge. Band 13. Heidelberg: Haug; 1988

[21] Barop H. Gutachten über Procain zur Anwendung in der Neuraltherapie nach Huneke. Gutachten, eingereicht dem Bundesgesundheitsamt Berlin als Beitrag für die Erstellung der Procain-Monografie. Berlin; 1991

[22] Barop H. Klinische Studie über den Wirksamkeitsnachweis der Neuraltherapie nach Huneke (basierend auf Praxis-Dokumentation H. Barop). Erfahrungsheilkunde. 1991; 40(3):158–161

[23] Barop H. Neuraltherapie nach Huneke aus der Sicht der Relationspathologie Rickers. In: Dosch P, Hrsg. Aktuelle Beiträge zur Neuraltherapie nach Huneke. Band 15. Heidelberg: Haug; 1994

[24] Barop H. Lehrbuch und Atlas Neuraltherapie nach Huneke. Stuttgart: Hippokrates; 1996

[25] Inauen W. Akute Pankreatitis: Konservative Therapie. Ther Umsch. 1996; 53(5):342–345

[26] Bayer L. Über eine Möglichkeit therapeutischer Beeinflussung akuter Magengeschwüre. Dtsch Med Wochenschr. 1936; 62:636

[27] Becke H. Die Neuraltherapie und ihre Einsatzmöglichkeiten in der medizinischen Grundbetreuung - dargestellt an der Behandlung des lumbosakralen Schmerzes und der Migräne[Dissertation (Habilitationsschrift)]. Berlin: Akademie fürärztliche Fortbildung; 1991

[28] Becke M. Procain und die Diskussion um die Allergie. Ärztez Naturheilverf. 1996; 37:908–912

[29] Becke H. Neuraltherapie bei Kreuzschmerz und Migräne. 2. Aufl. Stuttgart: Hippokrates; 2000

[30] Becke H, Gerlich B. Neuraltherapeutische Behandlungsergebnisse der Migräne. Ärztez Naturheilverf. 1991; 32(9):716–720

[31] Becker A. Die kombinierte Störfeld-Segmentbehandlung in der Neuraltherapie nach Huneke. Erfahrungsheilkunde. 1978; 1:12–15

[32] Bellinger DL, Millar BA, Perez S, et al. Sympathetic modulation of immunity: relevance to disease. Cell Immunol. 2008; 252(1–2):27–56

[33] Bergouignan H, Benoit P, Boussagol P, Brun G. Neuralgic syndrome of dental origin simulating an essential facial neuralgia [in French] Rev Odontostomatol Midi Fr. 1969; 27(2):124–125

[34] Bergsmann O. Herdwirkung in der Pulmologie. Therapiewoche. 1965; 15:1284–1287

[35] Bergsmann O. Neuraltherapie und ihr Anschluss bei Erkrankungen der Lunge. Phys Med Rehabil. 1979; 11:233–237

[36] Bergsmann O. Grundsystem, Regulation und Regulationsstörung in der Praxis der Rehabilitation. In: Pischinger A, Hrsg. Das System der Grundregulation. 11. Aufl. Stuttgart: Haug; 2009:92–132

[37] Bergsmann O, Bergsmann R. Projektionssymptome. 4. Aufl. Wien: Facultas; 1998

[38] Beyer W. Heilanästhesie und ihre Bedeutung für Chirurgie. Zentralbl Chir. 1953; 15:609–616

[39] Bhowmick S, Singh A, Flavell RA, Clark RB, O'Rourke J, Cone RE. The sympathetic nervous system modulates CD4(+)FoxP3(+) regulatory T cells via a TGF-beta-dependent mechanism. J Leukoc Biol. 2009; 86(6):1275–1283

[40] Bielefeldt K, Lamb K, Gebhart GF. Convergence of sensory pathways in the development of somatic and visceral hypersensitivity. Am J Physiol Gastrointest Liver Physiol. 2006; 291(4):G658–G665

[41] Bleys RL, Cowen T. Innervation of cerebral blood vessels: morphology, plasticity, age-related, and Alzheimer's disease-related neurodegeneration. Microsc Res Tech. 2001; 53(2):106–118

[42] Bogduk N. Klinische Anatomie von Lendenwirbelsäule und Sakrum (Rehabilitation und Prävention). Heidelberg: Springer; 2000

[43] Boissé L, Chisholm SP, Lukewich MK, Lomax AE. Clinical and experimental evidence of sympathetic neural dysfunction during inflammatory bowel disease. Clin Exp Pharmacol Physiol. 2009; 36(10):1026–1033

[44] Bonica JJ. The Management of Pain. 2nd ed. Philadelphia, PA: Lea & Febiger; 1953

[45] Bonica JJ. Clinical Application of Diagnostic and Therapeutic Nerv Blocks. Oxford: Blackwell; 1958

[46] Bouquot JE, Roberts AM, Person P, Christian J. Neuralgia-inducing cavitational osteonecrosis (NICO). Osteomyelitis in 224 jawbone samples from patients with facial neuralgia. Oral Surg Oral Med Oral Pathol. 1992; 73(3):307–319, discussion 319–320

[47] Braemer C. Neuraltherapeutische Erfahrungen bei Mensch und Tier. Erfahrungsheilkunde. 1971; 20(3):73–76, 393

[48] Braeucker W. Die Heilerfolge der gezielten neuroregulatorischen Sympathikustherapie. Ulm: Haug; 1958

[49] Brand H. Neural therapy in tinnitus [in German] Wien Med Wochenschr. 1983; 133(21):545–547

[50] Brandenburg K. Behandlung des frischen Schlaganfalls mit Novokaininfiltration des Ganglion stellatum. Med Klin. 1938; 4:29

[51] Braus H, Elze C. Anatomie des Menschen. Band 3: Periphere Leitungsbahnen II. Zentrales Nervensystem, Sinnesorgane. 2. Aufl. Berlin: Springer; 1960

[52] Breebaart AC, Bijlsma JW, van Eden W. 16-year remission of rheumatoid arthritis after unusually vigorous treatment of closed dental foci. Clin Exp Rheumatol. 2002; 20(4):555–557

[53] Brices FA. Die Behandlung chronischer Magengeschwüre mit Injektionen des Langzeitpräparats Cellnovocain durch Fibrogastroskop in die Submucosa des Magens. ZTherap Arch (Moskau). 1957; 47:97–103

[54] Briggs J, Peat FD. Die Entdeckung des Chaos. 9. Aufl. München: DTV; 2006

[55] Broggi G, Messina G, Franzini A. Cluster headache and TACs: rationale for central and peripheral neuromodulation. Neurol Sci. 2009; 30 (Suppl 1):S75–S79

[56] Brügger A. Die Erkrankungen des Bewegungsapparats und seines Nervensystems. 2. Aufl. Stuttgart: Urban & Fischer; 1986

[57] Bück F. Novokaininfiltration des Sympathikus als Frühbehandlung der Erfrierungen der Gliedmaßen. Chirurg. 1943; :347

[58] Busch V, Frese A, Bartsch T. Der trigeminozervikale Komplex. Integration peripherer und zentraler Mechanismen in primären Kopfschmerzsyndromen. Schmerz. 2004; 18(5):404–410

[59] Busch V, Jakob W, Juergens T, Schulte-Mattler W, Kaube H, May A. Occipital nerve blockade in chronic cluster headache patients and functional connectivity between trigeminal and occipital nerves. Cephalalgia. 2007; 27(11):1206–1214

[60] Bussone G. Cluster headache: from treatment to pathophysiology. Neurol Sci. 2008; 29(Suppl 1):S1–S6

[61] Carlile H. Ein mit Impletol behandelter Fall von Leberzirrhose und einiges weitere zur Neuraltherapie. Erfahrungsheilkunde. 1965; 14(11):529–536

[62] Carlile H. Angewandte Neuraltherapie bei Augenleiden und Trigeminusneuralgie. Erfahrungsheilkunde. 1969; 18(2):47–53

[63] Cassuto J, Sinclair R, Bonderovic M. Anti-inflammatory properties of local anesthetics and their present and potential clinical implications. Acta Anaesthesiol Scand. 2006; 50(3):265–282

[64] Cavanaugh JM, Lu Y, Chen C, Kallakuri S. Pain generation in lumbar and cervical facet joints. J Bone Joint Surg Am. 2006; 88(Suppl 2):63–67

[65] Cencetti S, Lagi A, Cipriani M, Fattorini L, Bandinelli G, Bernardi L. Autonomic control of the cerebral circulation during normal and impaired peripheral circulatory control. Heart. 1999; 82(3):365–372

[66] Cepeda MS, Carr DB, Lau J. Local anesthetic sympathetic blockade for complex regional pain syndrome. Cochrane Database Syst Rev. 2005(4):CD004598

[67] Challapalli V, Tremont-Lukats IW, Mc Nicol ED, Lau J, Carr DB. Systemic administration of local anesthetic agents to relieve neuropathic pain. Cochrane Database Syst Rev. 2005(4):CD003345

[68] Chien SQ, Li C, Li H, Xie W, Pablo CS, Zhang JM. Sympathetic fiber sprouting in chronically compressed dorsal root ganglia without peripheral axotomy. J Neuropathic Pain Symptom Palliation. 2005; 1(1):19–23

[69] Clara M. Das Nervensystem des Menschen. 2. Aufl. Leipzig: Barth; 1953

[70] Conn A, Buenaventura RM, Datta S, Abdi S, Diwan S. Systematic review of caudal epidural injections in the management of chronic low back pain. Pain Physician. 2009; 12(1):109–135

[71] Cousins MJ, Bridenbaugh PO, Carr DB, Horlocker TT, eds. Neural Blockade in Clinical Anesthesia and Pain Medicine. 4th ed. Philadelphia, PA: Lippincott; 2011

[72] Covino BG. Toxicity and systemic effects of local anesthetic agents. In: Strichartz GR, ed. Local Anesthetics (Handbook of Experimental Pharmacology). New York, NY: Springer; 1987

[73] Datta S, Lee M, Falco FJ, Bryce DA, Hayek SM. Systematic assessment of diagnostic accuracy and therapeutic utility of lumbar facet joint interventions. Pain Physician. 2009; 12(2):437–460

[74] Dauphin F, Linville DG, Hamel E. Cholinergic dilatation and constriction of feline cerebral blood vessels are mediated by stimulation of phosphoinositide metabolism via two different muscarinic receptor subtypes. J Neurochem. 1994; 63(2):544–551

[75] Dejung B. Triggerpunkt-Therapie. 3. Aufl. Bern; Huber; 2009

[76] Delis KT, Lennox AF, Nicolaides AN, Wolfe JH. Sympathetic autoregulation in peripheral vascular disease. Br J Surg. 2001; 88(4):523–528

[77] Descomps H. Die therapeutische Wirkung anästhesierender Infiltrationen an vegetativen Nerven im retrostyloidalen Bereich. In: Voss HF, Hrsg. Deshalb Neuraltherapie. Uelzen: ML-Verlag; 1968

[78] Van Zundert J, Hartrick C, Patijn J, Huygen F, Mekhail N, van Kleef M. Evidence-based interventional pain medicine according to clinical diagnoses. Pain Pract. 2011; 11(5):423–429

[79] Diener HC. Migräne und andere „vaskuläre Kopfschmerzen Internist. 1999; 40(2):153–161

[80] Diener HC, Katsarava Z, Limmroth V. Aktuelle Diagnostik und Therapie der Migräne. Schmerz. 2008; 22(Suppl 1):51–58, quiz 59–60

[81] Dinenno FA, Joyner MJ. Blunted sympathetic vasoconstriction in contracting skeletal muscle of healthy humans: is nitric oxide obligatory? J Physiol. 2003; 553(Pt 1):281–292

[82] Distler M, Distler J, Ciurea A, et al. Evidence-based therapy of Raynaud's syndrome [in German] Z Rheumatol. 2006; 65(4):285–289

[83] Dittmann EC, Zipf HF. Schmerzauslösung und Pharmakologie der Lokalanästhethika. In: Kilian H, Hrsg. Lokalanästhesie und Lokalanästhetika zu operativen, diagnostischen und therapeutischen Zwecken. 2. Aufl. Stuttgart: Thieme; 1988:76–144

[84] Dittmar F, Dobner E. Die neurotopische Diagnose und Therapie innerer Krankheiten. Ulm: Haug; 1964

[85] Dönges A, Fischer L, Marian F, Widmer M, Herren S, Busato A. Evaluation of Neural Therapy and Comparison with Conventional Medicine: Structure, Process and Outcomes. Bern: Universität Bern, Institut für evaluative Forschung in der orthopädischen Chirurgie und KIKOM, Dozentur Neuraltherapie; 2005

[86] Dosch P. Die Beseitigung von Commotio- und Contusio-cerebri-Folgen mit Impletol. Erfahrungsheilkunde. 1965; 14(3):101–108

[87] Dosch P. Die Anästhesie des Ganglion stellatum nach Fontaine und de Sèze in der Neuraltherapie. Hippokrates. 1965; 36(21):832–835

[88] Dosch P. Die gynäkologischen Organe als Störfeld für chronische Krankheiten. In: Voss HF, Hrsg. Deshalb Neuraltherapie. Uelzen: ML-Verlag; 1968

[89] Dosch M. Neurologie und Neuraltherapie. In: Dosch P, Hrsg. Neuraltherapie nach Huneke - Freudenstädter Vorträge. Band 6. Heidelberg: Haug; 1979:129–144

[90] Dosch M. Erste Ergebnisse des Einsatzes von Procain auf einer neurologischen Intensivstation. In: Dosch P, Hrsg. Neuraltherapie nach Huneke -Freudenstädter Vorträge. 1977/78. Band 5. Heidelberg: Haug; 1979

[91] Dosch P. Störfeldsuche bei Erkrankungen des Bewegungsapparats. In: Dosch P, Hrsg. Neuraltherapie nach Huneke - Freudenstädter Vorträge. Heidelberg: Haug; 1986:157–171

[92] Dosch P. Procain auch gegen Schlangengift? In: Dosch P, Hrsg. Aktuelle Beiträge zur Neuraltherapie nach Huneke. Band 15. Heidelberg: Haug; 1994

[93] Dosch P. Lehrbuch der Neuratherapie nach Huneke. 14. Aufl. Heidelberg: Haug; 1996

[94] Drost E. Erfahrungen mit Blockaden im sympathischen System bei der akuten Pankreatitis. Zentralbl Chir. 1957; 82(37):1563–1567

[95] Drummond PD. Mechanisms of autonomic disturbance in the face during and between attacks of cluster headache. Cephalalgia. 2006; 26(6):633–641

[96] Du Mesnil de Rochemont W, Hense IH. Messung der Hautdurchblutung am Menschen bei Einwirkung verschiedener Lokalanästhetika. Arch Exp Pathol Pharmakol. 1960; 239:464–474

[97] Dvoŕák J, Dvorak V. Manuelle Medizin. Diagnostik. 4. Aufl. Stuttgart: Thieme; 1991

[98] Ebersberger A. Pathophysiologie der Migräne Erklärungsmodelle zur Entstehung von Migränekopfschmerz. Anaesthesist. 2002; 51(8):661–667

[99] Eder M. Neuraltherapeutische Aspekte vertebragener Schmerzsyndrome. Erfahrungsheilkunde. 1983; 32(7):421–427

[100] Eder M. Herdgeschehen - Komplexgeschehen. 2. Aufl. Heidelberg: Haug; 1991

[101] Edvinsson L. Pathophysiology of primary headaches. Curr Pain Headache Rep. 2001; 5(1):71–78

[102] Egli S, Pfister M, Ludin SM, Busato A, Fischer L. Können Lokalanästhetika (Neuraltherapie) bei überwiesenen, therapieresistenten, chronischen Schmerzpatienten einen Circulus vitiosus durchbrechen?Neurophysiologie und klinische Daten [Dissertation]. Bern: Universität Bern; 2010

[103] Egloff N, Sabbioni ME, Salathé C, Wiest R, Juengling FD. Nondermatomal somatosensory deficits in patients with chronic pain disorder: clinical findings and hypometabolic pattern in FDG-PET. Pain. 2009; 145(1–2):252–258

[104] Eichholtz F, II. Toxikologie der lokalanästhetischen Stoffe. Klein Wochenschr. 1952; 30:97

[105] Eken C, Durmaz D, Erol B. Successful treatment of a persistent renal colic with trigger point injection. Am J Emerg Med. 2009; 27(2):252.e3–252.e4

[106] Elenkov IJ, Wilder RL, Chrousos GP, Vizi ES. The sympathetic nerve–an integrative interface between two supersystems: the brain and the immune system. Pharmacol Rev. 2000; 52(4):595–638

[107] el Fakir Y, Jiddane M, Abid A. Thrombophlebitis of the cavernous sinus of dental origin. Apropos of a case with a review of the literature [in French] Rev Stomatol Chir Maxillofac. 1993; 94(1):55–59

[108] Emich R. Neuraltherapie bei Herzkrankheiten In: Dosch P, Hrsg. Neuraltherapie nach Huneke - Freudenstädter Vorträge. Band 2. Heidelberg: Haug; 1975

[109] Ernsberger U, Rohrer H. Development of the cholinergic neurotransmitter phenotype in postganglionic sympathetic neurons. Cell Tissue Res. 1999; 297(3):339–361

[110] Esteller M. DNA methylation and cancer therapy: new developments and expectations. Curr Opin Oncol. 2005; 17(1):55–60

[111] Fabri GM, Siqueira SR, Simione C, Nasri C, Teixeira MJ, Siqueira JT. Refractory craniofacial pain: is there a role of periodontal disease as a comorbidity? Arq Neuropsiquiatr. 2009; 67(2B):474–479

[112] Falta W, Fenz E. Über den therarpeutischen Wert der Novokainfiltration in der inneren Medizin. Wien Med Wochenschr. 1938; 50:579–583

[113] Fanghänel J, Gedränge T. Neuroanatomie des Kiefergelenks und der Zahnregion. In: Weinschenk S, Hrsg. Handbuch Neuraltherapie. München: Elsevier; 2010:40–45
[114] Feigl EO. Neural control of coronary blood flow. J Vasc Res. 1998; 35(2):85–92
[115] Feneis H. Anatomisches Bildwörterbuch der internationalen Nomenklatur 10. Aufl. Stuttgart: Thieme; 1998
[116] Fenz E. Behandlung rheumatischer Erkrankungen durch Anästhesie. Dresden: Steinkopff; 1951
[117] Fernández-de-las-Peñas C, Cuadrado ML, Arendt-Nielsen L, Simons DG, Pareja JA. Myofascial trigger points and sensitization: an updated pain model for tension-type headache. Cephalalgia. 2007; 27(5):383–393
[118] Ferrero S, Haas S, Remorgida V, et al. Loss of sympathetic nerve fibers in intestinal endometriosis. Fertil Steril. 2010; 94(7):2817–2819
[119] Fischer L.. Neuraltherapie in der Notfallmedizin. Ärztez Naturheilverf. 1995; 9:676–685
[120] Fischer L. Einfache Untersuchungs- und Injektionstechnik am Ilio-sakralgelenk. Erfahrungsheilkunde. 1999; 48(3):159–166
[121] Fischer L.. Kopfschmerz und Sympathikus. Pathophysiologie und Therapie aus Sicht der Neuraltherapie nach Huneke. Ärztez Naturheilverf. 2002; 43(2):105–114
[122] Fischer L. Störfeld im Wandel der Zeit. Ganzheitsmed. 2002; 15:15–20
[123] Fischer L. Der Zweitschlag nach Speranski - Parallelen zur Klinik und zu neuen Wissenschaftstheorien. In: Dosch P, Barop H, Hahn Godeffroy JD, Hrsg. Neuraltherapie nach Huneke - Freudenstädter Vorträge. Band 16. Stuttgart: Haug; 2002
[124] Fischer L. Neuraltherapie nach Huneke. Stellenwert bei der Behandlung von Infektionskrankheiten. Schweiz Z Ganzheitsmed. 2003; 4:157
[125] Fischer L, ed. Der chronische Schmerz - eine interdisziplinäre Herausforderung. Bern: Peter Lang; 2006
[126] Fischer L. Pathophysiologie des Schmerzes - die Logik der Neuraltherapie. In: Fischer L, Hrsg. Der chronische Schmerz - eine interdisziplinäre Herausforderung. Bern: Peter Lang; 2006
[127] Fischer L. Wie Lokalanästhetika chronische Schmerzen kontrollieren können. Hausarztprax 2007; 40–43
[128] Fischer L. Antagonismus und Synergismus im autonomen Nervensystem -therapeutische Nutzbarkeit. In: Thurneysen A, Hrsg. Kontraste in der Medizin: Zur Dialektik gesundheitlicher Prozesse. Bern: Peter Lang; 2009
[129] Fischer L. Das Ganglion pterygopalatinum. In: Weinschenk S, Hrsg. Handbuch Neuraltherapie. München: Elsevier; 2010:505–509
[130] Fischer L. Das Ganglion stellatum. In: Weinschenk S, Hrsg. Handbuch Neuraltherapie. München: Elsevier; 2010:514–520
[131] Fischer L. Neuraltherapie. Schweiz Z Ganzheitsmed. 2010; 22:114–116
[132] Fischer L. Neurophysiologische Grundlagen: Reflexmechanismen, Schmerzgedächtnis und Neuraltherapie. In: Weinschenk S, Hrsg. Handbuch Neuraltherapie. München: Elsevier; 2010:66–72
[133] Fischer L. Neuraltherapie. In: Baron R, Koppert W, Strumpf M, Willweber-Strumpf A, Hrsg. Praktische Schmerztherapie. 2. Aufl. Heidelberg: Springer; 2011
[134] Fischer L. Neuraltherapie. Neurophysiologie, Injektionstechnik und Therapievorschläge. 4. Aufl. Stuttgart: Haug; 2014
[135] Fischer L. Physikalische und neurobiologische Grundlagen. In: Liem T, Hrsg. Morphodynamik in der Osteopathie. 2. Aufl. Stuttgart: Haug; 2014:64–86
[136] Fischer L, Barop H, Bergemann S. Health Technology Assessment Neuraltherapie nach Huneke. PEK des Schweizerischen Bundesamts für Gesundheit; 2005
[137] Fischer L, Papathanasiou G, Weinschenk S, Zieglgänsberger W. Neurophysiologie des Schmerzes. In: Weinschenk S, Hrsg. Handbuch Neuraltherapie. München: Elsevier; 2010
[138] Fischer L, Peuker E, eds. Lehrbuch Integrative Schmerztherapie. Stuttgart: Haug; 2011
[139] Fischer L, Pfister M. Wirksamkeit der Neuraltherapie bei überwiesenen Patienten mit therapieresistenten chronischen Schmerzen. Schweiz Z Ganzheitsmed. 2007; 19(1):30–35
[140] Fischl F, Huber J. Inwieweit kann die postoperative Rekonvaleszenz durch eine Prokain-Therapie verkürzt bzw. erleichtert werden? Osterr Arzteztg. 1982; 37:527–531
[141] Fleckenstein A. Die periphere Schmerzauslösung und Schmerzausschaltung. Frankfurt: Steinkopff; 1950
[142] Fleckenstein A. Mechanismus von Erregung und Erregungshemmung unter besonderer Berücksichtigung des Novocain. Anaesthesist. 1954; 3(1):15–19
[143] Fleckenstein A. Der Kalium-Natrium-Austausch als Energieprinzip im Muskel und Nerv. Berlin: Springer; 1955
[144] Fleischhacker H. Zur klinischen Bedeutung des Herdgeschehens. Osterr Z Stomatol. 1963; 60:401–409
[145] Fleischhacker H. Klinik der Herderkrankungen. Therapiewoche. 1965; 15:1274–1278
[146] Fontaine R. Irradiation im vegetativen Nervensystem. Hippokrates. 1965; 36:4
[147] Forssmann WG, Heym C. Grundriss der Neuroanatomie. Berlin: Springer; 1975
[148] Frank SM, El-Rahmany HK, Tran KM, Vu B, Raja SN. Comparison of lower extremity cutaneous temperature changes in patients receiving lumbar sympathetic ganglion blocks versus epidural anesthesia. J Clin Anesth. 2000; 12(7):525–530
[149] Freeman MD, Nystrom A, Centeno C. Chronic whiplash and central sensitization; an evaluation of the role of a myofascial trigger points in pain modulation. J Brachial Plex Peripher Nerve Inj. 2009; 4:2
[150] Freilinger T, Dichgans M. Genetics of migraine [in German] Nervenarzt. 2006; 77(10):1186–1188, 1188–1195
[151] Frese A, Schilgen M, Husstedt IW, Evers S. Pathophysiologie und Klinik zervikogener Kopfschmerzen. Schmerz. 2003; 17(2):125–130
[152] Frick H, Leonhard H, Starck D. Spezielle Anatomie II. Taschenlehrbuch der gesamten Anatomie. Band 2. 4. Aufl. Stuttgart: Thieme; 1992
[153] Fuchs J. Neuraltherapie am Auge. Therapiewoche. 1955; 6:1–2
[154] Fujita T, Kanno T, Kobayaski S. The Paraneuron. Berlin: Springer; 1988
[155] Funk R. Abortus imminens - Was ist von Prokain zu halten? Med Trib. 1980; 29:43–47
[156] Funk R. Prokain ersetzt herkömmliche Tokolyse. Sexualmed. 1985; 5:290–293
[157] Furness JB. The organisation of the autonomic nervous system: peripheral connections. Auton Neurosci. 2006; 130(1–2):1–5
[158] Gao Z, Xu Z, Hung MS, et al. Procaine and procainamide inhibit the Wnt canonical pathway by promoter demethylation of WIF-1 in lung cancer cells. Oncol Rep. 2009; 22(6):1479–1484
[159] García-Cosamalón J, del Valle ME, Calavia MG, et al. Intervertebral disc, sensory nerves and neurotrophins: who is who in discogenic pain? J Anat. 2010; 217(1):1–15
[160] García-Leiva JM, Hidalgo J, Rico-Villademoros F, Moreno V, Calandre EP. Effectiveness of ropivacaine trigger points inactivation in the prophylactic management of patients with severe migraine. Pain Med. 2007; 8(1):65–70
[161] Gay D, Dick G, Upton G. Multiple sclerosis associated with sinusitis: case-controlled study in general practice. Lancet. 1986; 1(8485):815–819
[162] Giri S, Nixdorf D. Sympathetically maintained pain presenting first as temporomandibular disorder, then as parotid dysfunction. J Can Dent Assoc. 2007; 73(2):163–167
[163] Glaser M, Türk R. Herdgeschehen, Diagnostik und Therapie. Heidelberg: Verlag für Medizin; 1982
[164] Glonti TI, Malashkiia IuA, Chkhikvishvili TsSh. On the role of chronic odontogenic infection in the genesis of neurologic disorders [in Russian] Klin Med (Mosk). 1968; 46(1):112–115
[165] Goadsby PJ, Cohen AS. Neues zur Pathophysiologie und Therapie der trigeminoautonomen Kopfschmerzsyndrome. Schmerz. 2008; 22(Suppl 1):7–10
[166] Goadsby PJ, Bartsch T, Dodick DW. Occipital nerve stimulation for headache: mechanisms and efficacy. Headache. 2008; 48(2):313–318
[167] Goebel J. Gefahren und Grenzen, Missverständnisse und Irrtümer der Neuraltherapie. In: Dosch P, Hrsg. Neuraltherapie nach Huneke Freudenstädter Vorträge. Band 2. Heidelberg: Haug; 1975
[168] Goebel J. Ein günstiger Weg für die Injektion zum Ganglion cervicale superius. In: Dosch P, Hrsg. Neuraltherapie nach Huneke - Freudenstädter Vorträge 1983/84. Band 9. Heidelberg: Haug; 1985
[169] Göbel H, Heinze A, Heinze-Kuhn K. Vorbeugung und Akutbehandlung der Migräne. Schmerz. 2006; 20(6):541–554, quiz 555–556
[170] Goecke H. Über Erfahrungen mit Neuraltherapie in der Gynäkologie und Geburtshilfe. In: Gross D, Hrsg. Therapie mit Lokalanästhetika Funktionsstörungen des oberen Verdauungstrakts und ihre Behandlung. Stuttgart: Hippokrates; 1964:153–156
[171] Gofeld M, Faclier G. Bilateral pain relief after unilateral thoracic percutaneous sympathectomy. Can J Anaesth. 2006; 53(3):258–262
[172] Gordh T. Blockade des N. suprascapularis. In: Eriksson E, Hrsg. Atlas der Lokalanästhesie. Berlin: Springer; 1980
[173] Gotsman I, Lotan C, Soskolne WA, et al. Periodontal destruction is associated with coronary artery disease and periodontal infection with acute coronary syndrome. J Periodontol. 2007; 78(5):849–858
[174] Gottschalk A, Gottschalk A. Kontinuierliche Wundinfusion von Lokalanästhetika: Stellenwert in der postoperativen Schmerztherapie. Anaesthesist. 2010; 59(12):1076–1082

[175] Graul G. Die Ergebnisse der Therapie des akuten lumbalen Radiku-lärsyndroms beim Bandscheibenvorfall mit Neuraltherapie in Form der indirekten Grenzstrang-Injektion nach Mink [Dissertation]. Berlin: Charite Universitätsmedizin Berlin; 2010
[176] Gray RL. Peripheral facial nerve paralysis of dental origin. Br J Oral Surg. 1978; 16(2):143–150
[177] Grebe KM. Editorial: regulation of the regulator: sympathetic nervous system control of regulatory T cells. J Leukoc Biol. 2009; 86(6):1269–1270
[178] Gross D. Der neurale Faktor im Herdgeschehen. Dtsch Med Wochenschr. 1954; 79(50):1853–1858
[179] Gross D. Therapeutische Lokalanästhesie. 2. Aufl. Stuttgart: Hippokrates; 1989
[180] Grüsser SM, Diers M, Flor H. Phantomschmerz: Aspekte der Neuroplastizität und Intervention. Anasthesiol Intensivmed Notfallmed Schmerzther. 2003; 38(12):762–766
[181] Grundy D. Signalling the state of the digestive tract. Auton Neurosci. 2006; 125(1-2):76–80
[182] Gutmann H. Schmerz und Schmerztherapie in der Augenheilkunde. Hippokrates. 1968; 39(21):811–815
[183] Haaks T, Tackmann W. Neuraltherapeutische Behandlung der schmerzhaften hemiparetischen Schulter. Biol Med (Paris). 1999; 28(3):130–132
[184] Haane DY, Koehler PJ, Te Lintelo MP, Peatfield R. Trigeminal autonomic cephalalgia sine headache. J Neurol. 2011; 258(4):586–589
[185] Häbler H, Eschenfelder S, Liu XG, Jänig W. Sympathetic-sensory coupling after L5 spinal nerve lesion in the rat and its relation to changes in dorsal root ganglion blood flow. Pain. 2000; 87(3):335–345
[186] Hänisch R. Das odontogene Störfeld in der Geriatrie. In: Dosch P, Hrsg. Neuraltherapie nach Huneke - Freudenstädter Vorträge 1988. Band 13. Heidelberg: Haug; 1989
[187] Hänisch R. Neuraltherapeutische Behandlung des Zahnstörfelds einschließlich dentogener Sanierung - Klinische Verläufe. Erfahrungsheilkunde. 1991; 40(10):678–683
[188] Härle P, Pongratz G, Albrecht J, Tarner IH, Straub RH. An early sympathetic nervous system influence exacerbates collagen-induced arthritis via CD4+CD25+ cells. Arthritis Rheum. 2008; 58(8):2347–2355
[189] Härle P, Straub RH, Wiest R, et al. Increase of sympathetic outflow measured by neuropeptide Y and decrease of the hypothalamic-pituitary-adrenal axis tone in patients with systemic lupus erythematosus and rheumatoid arthritis: another example of uncoupling of response systems. Ann Rheum Dis. 2006; 65(1):51–56
[190] Härtel H. Bildatlas der Herddiagnostik im Kieferbereich. Heidelberg: Haug; 1992
[191] Hahn-Godeffroy JD. Zum Zwischenfallrisiko von neuraltherapeutischen Injektionen im Kopf- und Halsbereich. In: Dosch P, Hrsg. Neuraltherapie nach Huneke - Freudenstädter Vorträge. Band 13. Heidelberg: Haug; 1989
[192] Hahn-Godeffroy JD. Procain in der Neuraltherapie nach Huneke. Literaturüberblick und zusammenfassende Bewertung. Allgemeinarzt. 1993; 15(14):876–883
[193] Hahn-Godeffroy JD. Procain in der Neuraltherapie nach Huneke. Zusammenfassende Bewertung. In: Barop H, Hahn-Godeffroy JD, Dosch P, Hrsg. Neuraltherapie nach Huneke - Freudenstädter Vorträge. Band 16. Heidelberg: Haug; 2002:36–49
[194] Hahn-Godeffroy JD. Wirkungen und Nebenwirkungen von Procain: Was ist gesichert? Komplement Integr Med. 2007; 2(7):32–34
[195] Hahn-Godeffroy JD. Procain-Reset: Ein Therapiekonzept zur Behandlung chronischer Erkrankungen. Schweiz Z Ganzheitsmed. 2011; 23:291–296
[196] Hahn-Godeffroy JD, Barop H. Zur Arzneimittelsicherheit von Procain. Dtsch Z Akupunktur. 2011; 54(4):28–29
[197] Hammer F. Segmentherapie bei Kreuz- und Gelenkschmerzen in der internistischen Praxis. In: Seithel R, ed. Neuraltherapie. Band 2. Stuttgart: Hippokrates; 1984
[198] Handwerker HO. Einführung in die Pathophysiologie des Schmerzes. Berlin: Springer; 1998
[199] Hansen K, Schliack H. Segmentale Innervation. Stuttgart: Thieme; 1962
[200] Harrer G. Kritisches zur Neuraltherapie aus neurologischer Sicht. Phys Diät Ther. 1965; 6(2):43–51
[201] Harrer G. Der neurale Faktor in der Neuraltherapie. In: Dosch P, Hrsg. Neuraltherapie nach Huneke - Freudenstädter Vorträge 1971/72. Band 1. Heidelberg: Haug; 1974
[202] Hassett AL, Clauw DJ. The role of stress in rheumatic diseases. Arthritis Res Ther. 2010; 12(3):123
[203] Heine H.. Weitreichende Wechselwirkungen als Grundlage der Homöostase. Funktionelle Aspekte der Neuratherapie. Ärztez Naturheilverf. 1987; 27:915–919
[204] Heine H. Lehrbuch der biologischen Medizin. 3. Aufl. Stuttgart: Hippokrates; 2007
[205] Hendrickson HS, van Dam-Mieras MC. Local anesthetic inhibition of pancreatic phospholipase A2 action on lecithin monolayers. J Lipid Res. 1976; 17(4):399–405
[206] Herbert MK, Holzer P. Die neurogene Entzündung - I. Grundlegende Mechanismen, Physiologie und Pharmakologie Anasthesiol Intensivmed Notfallmed Schmerzther. 2002; 37(6):314–325
[207] Herbert MK, Holzer P. Die neurogene Entzündung. II. Pathophysiologie und klinische Implikationen. Anasthesiol Intensivmed Notfallmed Schmerzther. 2002; 37(7):386–394
[208] Hess JC, Victor M. Relation between rheumatology and endodontics [in French] Ligament. 1978; 16(129):19–21
[209] Hiltunen PH, Airaksinen MS. Sympathetic cholinergic target innervation requires GDNF family receptor GFR alpha 2. Mol Cell Neurosci. 2004; 26(3):450–457
[210] Hirsch E. Pharmakodynamische Wirkung der Lokalanästhesie. In: Voss HF, ed. Deshalb Neuraltherapie. Uelzen: ML-Verlag; 1968:99–106
[211] Hollmann MW, Durieux ME. Local anesthetics and the inflammatory response: a new therapeutic indication? Anesthesiology. 2000; 93(3):858–875
[212] Holzhammer J, Wöber C. Alimentäre Triggerfaktoren bei Migräne und Kopfschmerz vom Spannungstyp. Schmerz. 2006; 20(2):151–159
[213] Hoff F. Klinische Probleme der vegetativen Regulation und der Neuralpathologie. Dtsch Med Wochenschr. 1952; 77(5):146–150
[214] Hoff F. Behandlung innerer Krankheiten. Stuttgart: Thieme; 1960
[215] Holtemann H. Klinische Erfahrungen mit nervaler Therapie von Dermatosen. Neuralmed. 1955; 3(2):89–106
[216] Hopfer F. Über die postischialgische Durchblutungsstörung nach Reichhauer. In: Voss HF, Hrsg. Deshalb Neuraltherapie. Uelzen: ML-Verlag; 1968
[217] Hopfer F.. Phänomene bei neuraltherapeutischer Tätigkeit. Ärztez Naturheilverf. 1991; 32:684–692
[218] Hopp H, Combes HJ. Stimulation or blocking of the periurethral region--an expansion of conservative therapeutic measures in irritable bladder and urge incontinence[in German] Zentralbl Gynakol. 1986; 108(14):851–856
[219] Houy-Schäfer S, Grotemeyer KH. Spannungskopfschmerz. Schmerz. 2004; 18(2):104–108
[220] Hubert G. Eigenbeobachtungen über die Wirkung der Impletolbehandlung. Hippokrates. 1948; 19(9):290–293
[221] Hülse M, Neuhuber W, Wolff HD, eds. Die obere Halswirbelsäule. Pathophysiologie und Klinik. Heidelberg: Springer; 2005
[222] Hugger A. Arthralgie der Kiefergelenke. In: Hugger A, Göbel H, Schilgen M, Hrsg. Gesichts- und Kopfschmerzen aus interdisziplinärer Sicht. Heidelberg: Springer; 2006:77–90
[223] Huneke F. Unbekannte Fernwirkung der Neuraltherapie. Med Welt. 1928; 27:1013–1014
[224] Huneke F. Focusproblem und Sekundenphänomen in seiner Behandlung für den Zahnarzt. Dtsch Zahnarztl Z. 1950; 23:1269–1278
[225] Huneke F.. Gynäkologie und Focusproblem. Ärztl Wochenschr. 1952; 7(41):967–996
[226] Huneke F. Das Focus-Problem in neuraltherapeutischer Schau. Hippokrates. 1952; 23(22):625–633
[227] Huneke F. Zahnarzt und Sekundenphänomen. Zahnärztl Referate. 1955; 56(13–14):256–259
[228] Huneke F. Neuraltherapie, Sekundenphänomen und Chirurgie. Allg Ther. 1956; 27(21):675–682
[229] Huneke F. Die Behandlung der verschiedenen Formen des Rheumatismus durch Impletol. Med Klin. 1957; 31(32):1127–1128
[230] Huneke F. Grundlegendes zum Problem der Neuraltherapie. Privatklinik und Sanatoriumsz. 1958; 12:289–293
[231] Huneke F. 35 Jahre Neuraltherapie. Phys Diät Therap. 1962; 3(5):75–80
[232] Huneke W. Besondere Erfahrungen in der Neuraltherapie. Hippokrates. 1962; 33(3):103–109
[233] Huneke W. Neuraltherapeutische Problematik und Behandlung bei Kopfschmerz. Arztl Prax. 1963; 2833:2849–2851
[234] Huneke W. Die Neuralmedizin - ein Uberblick am Beispiel der Gelenkerkrankungen. Hippokrates. 1965; 36(12):465–471
[235] Huneke F. Über die Häufigkeit des Sekundenphänomens in meiner Praxis. Hippokrates. 1969; 31(3):74–77
[236] Huneke F. Das Sekundärphänomen. 6. Aufl. Heidelberg: Haug; 1989
[237] Hutzel H. Uber zweijährige Behandlungsergebnisse mit der Segment- und Neuraltherapie in einer ambulanten chirurgischen Praxis. Therapiewoche. 1965; 15(16):855–858

[238] Iida M, Yamaguchi Y. Remission of rheumatoid arthritis following periodontal treatment. A case report [in Japanese] Nippon Shishubyo Gakkai Kaishi. 1985; 27(1):234–238

[239] Iskraut H. Neuraltherapie und Zahnheilkunde. Rundsch. 1952; 61(12):344–347

[240] Iskraut H. Grundlagen der Neuraltherapie. Hippokrates. 1953; 24(11):321–329

[241] Izumi H. Reflex parasympathetic vasodilatation in facial skin. Gen Pharmacol. 1995; 26(2):237–244

[242] Jänig W. Relationship between pain and autonomic phenomena in headache and other pain conditions. Cephalalgia. 2003; 23(Suppl 1):43–48

[243] Jänig W. The Integrative Action of the Autonomic Nervous System. Cambridge: Cambridge University Press; 2006

[244] Jänig W. Autonomic nervous system and pain. In: Firestein S, ed. The Senses: AComprehensive Reference. Amsterdam: Elsevier; 2008

[245] Jänig W, Baron R. Complex regional pain syndrome is a disease of the central nervous system. Clin Auton Res. 2002; 12(3):150–164

[246] Jänig W, Baron R. Complex regional pain syndrome: mystery explained? Lancet Neurol. 2003; 2(11):687–697

[247] Jänig W, Häbler HJ. Physiologie und Pathophysiologie viszeraler Schmerzen. Schmerz. 2002; 16(6):429–446

[248] Jänig W, Koltzenburg M. Possible ways of sympathetic afferent interaction. In: Jänig W, Schmidt RF, eds. Reflex Sympathetic Dystrophia. Pathophysiological Mechanisms and Clinical Implications. New York, NY: VCH; 1992

[249] Jänig W, Levine JD, Michaelis M. Interactions of sympathetic and primary afferent neurons following nerve injury and tissue trauma. In: Kumazawa T, Mizumura K, Krüger L, eds. Progress in Brain Research: The Polymodal Receptor: A Gateway to Pathological Pain. Amsterdam: Elsevier; 1996:161–184

[250] Jankovic D. Regionalblockaden in Klinik und Praxis. Lehrbuch und Atlas. 2. Aufl. Berlin: Blackwell; 2000

[251] Jankovic D. mTrP des Kopfes (Kaumuskulatur). In: Weinschenk S, Hrsg. Handbuch Neuraltherapie. München: Elsevier; 2010:436–438

[252] Jenker FL. Nervenblockade auf pharmakologischem und elektrischem Weg. 4. Aufl. Wien, New York: Springer; 1980:325

[253] Jessop DS. Brain-immune interactions in arthritis: an integrated systems approach. Arthritis Rheum. 2008; 58(10):2928–2930

[254] Jönsson A, Mattsson U, Tarnow P, Nellgård P, Cassuto J. Topical local anaesthetics (EMLA) inhibit burn-induced plasma extravasation as measured by digital image colour analysis. Burns. 1998; 24(4):313–318

[255] Joyner MJ, Dietz NM. Sympathetic vasodilation in human muscle. Acta Physiol Scand. 2003; 177(3):329–336

[256] Jung F. Neuraltherapie obstruktiver Blasenhalserkrankungen. In: Dosch P, ed. Neuraltherapie nach Huneke - Freudenstädter Vorträge 1980. Band 7. Heidelberg: Haug; 1981

[257] Junghans H. Die Wirbelsäule unter den Einflüssen des täglichen Lebens, der Freizeit, des Sportes. Stuttgart: Hippokrates; 1995

[258] Kahle W, Frotscher M. Taschenatlas Anatomie. Band 3: Nervensystem und Sinnesorgane. 11. Aufl. Stuttgart: Thieme; 2013

[259] Kaji A, Maeda T, Watanabe S. Parasympathetic innervation of cutaneous blood vessels examined by retrograde tracing in the rat lower lip. J Auton Nerv Syst. 1991; 32(2):153–158

[260] Kaji A, Shigematsu H, Fujita K, Maeda T, Watanabe S. Parasympathetic innervation of cutaneous blood vessels by vasoactive intestinal polypeptide-immunoreactive and acetylcholinesterase-positive nerves: histochemical and experimental study on rat lower lip. Neuroscience. 1988; 25(1):353–362

[261] Kakuyama M, Toda H, Osawa M, Fukuda K. The bilateral effect of stellate ganglion block on the facial skin blood flow. Reg Anesth Pain Med. 2000; 25(4):389–392

[262] Kano M, Moskowitz MA, Yokota M. Parasympathetic denervation of rat pial vessels significantly increases infarction volume following middle cerebral artery occlusion. J Cereb Blood Flow Metab. 1991; 11(4):628–637

[263] Käppis M. Die diagnostische und therapeutische Verwertung der paravertebralen Novokaineinspritzung. Ther Ggw. 1925; 66:335–338

[264] Kawano H, Okada R, Yano K. Histological study on the distribution of autonomic nerves in the human heart. Heart Vessels. 2003; 18(1):32–39

[265] Kawasaki H, Tsuru H. Pharmacology and physiology of perivascular nerves regulating vascular function. Preface. Jpn J Pharmacol. 2002; 88:7–8

[266] Kawashima T. The autonomic nervous system of the human heart with special reference to its origin, course, and peripheral distribution. Anat Embryol (Berl). 2005; 209(6):425–438

[267] Kellner G. Die Wirkung des Herdes auf die Labilität des humuralen Systems. Osterr Z Stomatol. 1963; 60:312

[268] Kellner G. Zur Histochemie der Narbe. Hippokrates. 1965; 36:770–785

[269] Kellner G. Wundbehandlung und Wundheilstörung. Erfahrungsheilkunde. 1971; 20(6):173–178

[270] Kellogg DL, Jr, Pérgola PE, Piest KL, et al. Cutaneous active vasodilation in humans is mediated by cholinergic nerve cotransmission. Circ Res. 1995; 77(6):1222–1228

[271] Kerr FW. Central relationships of trigeminal and cervical primary afferents in the spinal cord and medulla. Brain Res. 1972; 43(2):561–572

[272] Khader YS, Ta'ani Q. Periodontal diseases and the risk of preterm birth and low birth weight: a meta-analysis. J Periodontol. 2005; 76(2):161–165

[273] Kieper V. Die Neuraltherapie nach Huneke in der Gynäkologie und Geburtshilfe. In: Zum 100. Geburtstag von Ferdinand Huneke. Freudenstadt: Int. med. Gesellschaft für Neuraltherapie nach Huneke e. V.; 1991

[274] Kilian H, ed. Lokalanästhesie und Lokalanästhetika zu operativen, diagnostischen und therapeutischen Zwecken. 2. Aufl. Stuttgart: Thieme; 1988

[275] Kim J, Amar S. Periodontal disease and systemic conditions: a bidirectional relationship. Odontology. 2006; 94(1):10–21

[276] Kim JJ, Chung RK, Lee HS, Han JI. The changes of heart rate variability after unilateral stellate ganglion block. Korean J Anesthesiol. 2010; 58(1):56–60

[277] King HH, Jänig W, Patterson MM. Science and Clinical Application of Manual Therapy. Edinburgh: Elsevier Churchill Livingstone; 2011

[278] King MC, Triplett RG, Rees TD. Treatment of refractory facial pain diagnosed as atypical trigeminal neuralgia: a case report. Compend Contin Educ Dent. 2006; 27(2):113–120

[279] Kluge G, Neugebauer G. Grundlagen der Thermodynamik. Heidelberg: Spektrum; 1994

[280] Köck FX, Borisch N, Koester B, Grifka J. Das komplexe regionale Schmerzsyndrom Typ I (CRPS I). Ursachen, Diagnostik und Therapie. Orthopäde. 2003; 32(5):418–431

[281] Kolb BH. Spontane Remission starker Rückenschmerzen nach odontogener Sanierung. Chir Zahnheilkd. 1976; 4(35):36

[282] Koller C. Personal reminiscences of the first use of cocaine as local anesthetic in eye surgery. Curr Res Anest Anal. 1928; 7(1):9–11

[283] Kompis M, Neuner NT, Hemmeler W, Häusler R. Tinnitus [in German] Ther Umsch. 2004; 61(1):15–20

[284] Koppert W, Brueckl V, Weidner C, Schmelz M. Mechanically induced axon reflex and hyperalgesia in human UV-B burn are reduced by systemic lidocaine. Eur J Pain. 2004; 8(3):237–244

[285] Korevaar WC, Burney RG, Moore PA. Convulsions during stellate ganglion block: a case report. Anesth Analg. 1979; 58(4):329–330

[286] Kothbauer O. Über die Druckpunktdiagnostik und Neuraltherapie bei Tieren. Wien Tierarztl Monatsschr. 1961; 48:282–294

[287] Kothbauer O. Zur Behandlung von Gelenkschwellungen beim Rind durch Neuraltherapie. Wien Tierarztl Monatsschr. 1973; 60:379–381

[288] Kothbauer O. Neuraltherapie in der Veterinärmedizin. Ein Beitrag zur Ojektivierung. In: Dosch P, Hrsg. Neuraltherapie nach Huneke -Freudenstädter Vorträge. Band 2. Heidelberg: Haug; 1975

[289] Kramis RC, Roberts WJ, Gillette RG. Post-sympathectomy neuralgia: hypotheses on peripheral and central neuronal mechanisms. Pain. 1996; 64(1):1–9

[290] Kress B, Schindler M, Rasche D, et al. Trigeminusneuralgie: Wie häufig gibt es einen Gefäß-Nerven-Kontakt bei schmerzfreien Probanden? Fortsch Röntgenstr. 2006; 178(3):313–315

[291] Kulenkampff D. Die örtliche Betäubung als diagnostisches und Behandlungsmittel. Zentralbl Chir. 1949; 78:588–599

[292] Kulenkampff D. Über die örtliche Betäubung zu Behandlungszwecken bei der akuten Epididymitis. Munch Med Wochenschr. 1973; 84:1175

[293] Laewen A. Die Verwendung der Sakralanästhesie. Zentralbl Chir. 1910; 38:708

[294] Laewen A. Weitere Erfahrungen über paravertebrale Schmerzaufhebung zur Differenzialdiagnose von Erkrankungen der Gallenblase, des Magens, der Niere und des Wurmfortsatzes sowie der Behandlung postoperativer Lungenkomplikationen. Zentralbl Chir. 1923; 50:461

[295] Laurenz F. Der gynäkologische Raum in der klassischen Neuraltherapie. Phys Diät Ther. 1963; 4(6):97–100

[296] Lautenbach E. Nerven (Zahn, Mund, Kiefer). Hanau: Dausien; 1994

[297] Leicher H, Haas E. Hals-Nasen-Ohrenheilkunde, Heilanästhesie. In: Killian H, ed. Lokalanästhesie und Lokalanästhetika zu operativen, diagnostischen und therapeutischen Zwecken. Stuttgart: Thieme; 1973:544–554

[298] Leone M, Bussone G. Pathophysiology of trigeminal autonomic cephalalgias. Lancet Neurol. 2009; 8(8):755–764

[299] Leriche A. Literaturstelle über die Stellatumanästhesie bei Hirnembolie, bei Gefäßspasmen, nach Hirnoperationen und bei Hemiplegien. Rev Chir. 1936; 55:755

[300] Leriche A. Die peri- und intraarteriellen Novokaininjektionen in der Neuralmedizin. Neuralmed. 1955; 3:2–5

[301] Leriche A. Die Behandlung posttraumatischer vasomotorischer Störungen. Neuralmed. 1955; 3:15–17

[302] Leriche A. Die Chirurgie des Schmerzes. Leipzig: Barth; 1958

[303] Lewandowski L, Serafinowska A. Peripheral facial nerve palsy caused by focal dental infection [in Polish] Czas Stomatol. 1970; 23(12):1357–1360

[304] Levick SP, Murray DB, Janicki JS, Brower GL. Sympathetic nervous system modulation of inflammation and remodeling in the hypertensive heart. Hypertension. 2010; 55(2):270–276

[305] Levin M. Nerve blocks in the treatment of headache. Neurotherapeutics. 2010; 7(2):197–203

[306] Levine JD, Dardick SJ, Roizen MF, Helms C, Basbaum AI. Contribution of sensory afferents and sympathetic efferents to joint injury in experimental arthritis. J Neurosci. 1986; 6(12):3423–3429

[307] Lewit K. Manuelle Medizin. 8. Aufl. München: Elsevier/Urban & Fischer; 2006

[308] Liebeton K. Die Behandlung mit Impietol (= Procain und Koffein) bei den gynäkologischen Erscheinungen der vegetativen Dystonie [Dissertation]. Münster: Westfälische Wilhelms-Universität Münster; 1956

[309] Lippert H. Lehrbuch der Anatomie. 8. Aufl. München: Elsevier/Urban & Fischer; 2011

[310] Lobato EB, Kern KB, Paige GB, Brown M, Sulek CA. Differential effects of right versus left stellate ganglion block on left ventricular function in humans: an echocardiographic analysis. J Clin Anesth. 2000; 12(4):315–318

[311] Löfström B. Die Sakralanästhesie. In: Eriksson E, Döberl A, Hrsg. Atlas der Lokalanästhesie. 2. Aufl. Berlin: Springer; 1980

[312] Lomax AE, Sharkey KA, Furness JB. The participation of the sympathetic innervation of the gastrointestinal tract in disease states. Neurogastroenterol Motil. 2010; 22(1):7–18

[313] Loose KE. Grundlagen, Beobachtungen und Ergebnisse bei der Behandlung von 6 000Gefäßkranken. Dtsch Med Wochenschr. 1962; 87:2117

[314] Low PA, Vernino S, Suarez G. Autonomic dysfunction in peripheral nerve disease. Muscle Nerve . 2003; 27(6):646–661

[315] Lullies H, Trincker D. Taschenbuch der Physiologie. Band 1.2. Aufl. Stuttgart: Fischer; 1974

[316] Lundgren O. Sympathetic input into the enteric nervous System. Gut. 2000; 47(Suppl 4):iv :33–iv– 35

[317] Mackenzie J. Krankheitszeichen und ihre Auslegung. Leipzig: Kabitzsch; 1921

[318] McLachlan EM. Transmission of signals through sympathetic ganglia–modulation, integration or simply distribution? Acta Physiol Scand. 2003; 177(3):227–235

[319] Magis D, Bruno MA, Fumal A, et al. Central modulation in cluster headache patients treated with occipital nerve stimulation: an FDG-PET study. BMC Neurol. 2011; 11:25

[320] Mahns DA, Revington ML, Runcie MJ, Mc Closkey DI, Potter EK. Inhibition of sympathetic cholinergic vasodilatation by a selective NPY Y2 receptor agonist in the gracilis muscle of anaesthetised dogs. J Auton Nerv Syst. 1998; 68(1–2):14–20

[321] Maier C. Sympathische Reflexdystrophie - Morbus Sudeck. In: Diener HC, Maier C, Hrsg. Das Schmerztherapiebuch. 2. Aufl. München: Elsevier/Urban& Fischer; 2003

[322] Maier C, Gleim M. Diagnostik des sympathischunterhaltenen Schmerzes. In: Zenz M, Jurna I, Hrsg. Lehrbuch der Schmerztherapie. 2. Aufl. Stuttgart: Wissenschaftliche Verlagsgesellschaft; 2001:421–428

[323] Maihöfner C, Birklein F. Komplexregionale Schmerzsyndrome: Neues zu Pathophysiologie und Therapie. Fortschr Neurol Psychiatr. 2007; 75(6):331–342

[324] Malanga G, Wolff E. Evidence-informed management of chronic low back pain with trigger point injections. Spine J. 2008; 8(1):243–252

[325] Mandel F. Blockade und Chirurgie des Sympathikus. Berlin: Springer; 1953

[326] Mangos GJ, Walker BR, Kelly JJ, Lawson JA, Webb DJ, Whitworth JA. Cortisol inhibits cholinergic vasodilation in the human forearm. Am J Hypertens. 2000; 13(11):1155–1160

[327] Marmura MJ, Pello SJ, Young WB. Interictal pain in cluster headache. Cephalalgia. 2010; 30(12):1531–1534

[328] Marshall JM. The venous vessel within the skeletal muscle. Physiol. 1991; 6(1):11–15

[329] Martínez-Lavín M. Is fibromyalgia a generalized reflex sympathetic dystrophy? Clin Exp Rheumatol. 2001; 19(1):1–3

[330] Matharu MS, Zrinzo L. Deep brain stimulation in cluster headache. Expert Rev Neurother. 2011; 11(4):473–475

[331] Matsukawa K, Shindo T, Shirai M, Ninomiya I. Direct observations of sympathetic cholinergic vasodilatation of skeletal muscle small arteries in the cat. J Physiol. 1997; 500(Pt 1):213–225

[332] Matsukawa K, Shirai M, Murata J, et al. Sympathetic cholinergic vasodilation of skeletal muscle small arteries. Jpn J Pharmacol. 2002; 88(1):14–18

[333] Matsuoka H. Influence of stellate ganglion block on immune system [in Japanese] Masui. 1987; 36(3):389–401

[334] Mattle H, Mumenthaler M. Neurologie. 13. Aufl. Stuttgart: Thieme; 2012

[335] May A, Goadsby PJ. The trigeminovascular system in humans: pathophysiologic implications for primary headache syndromes of the neural influences on the cerebral circulation. J Cereb Blood Flow Metab. 1999; 19(2):115–127

[336] May A, Jürgens TP. Therapeutische Neuromodulation beiprimären Kopfschmerzsyndromen. Nervenarzt. 2011; 82(6):743–752

[337] Mayer A. Zum Störfeldgeschehen im Zahn-, Mund- und Kieferbereich. In: Dosch P, Hrsg. Neuraltherapie nach Huneke - Freudenstädter Vorträge 1975. Band 3. Heidelberg: Haug; 1976

[338] Medzhitov R. Origin and physiological roles of inflammation. Nature. 2008; 454(7203):428–435

[339] Melzack R, Stillwell DM, Fox EJ. Trigger points and acupuncture points for pain: correlations and implications. Pain. 1977; 3(1):3–23

[340] Melzack R, Wall PD. Pain mechanisms: a new theory. Science. 1965; 150(3699):971–979

[341] Merckelbach F. Neuraltherapie in der Orthopädie. Hippokrates. 1954; 25(11):356–359

[342] Merckelbach F. Die Bedeutung des Herdgeschehens in der Orthopädie. Herdtherapie. 1955; 1:4

[343] Mermod J, Fischer L, Staub L, Busato A. Patient satisfaction of primary care for musculoskeletal diseases: a comparison between neural therapy and conventional medicine. BMC Complement Altern Med. 2008; 8:33

[344] Miao FJ, Jänig W, Levine Jd. Role of sympathetic postganglionic neurons in synovial plasma extravasation induced by bradykinin. J Neurophysiol. 1996; 75(2):715–724

[345] Mink E. Behebung der Therapieresistenz beim habituellen Abort durch Neuraltherapie der Schilddrüse. Zentralbl Gynakol. 1959; 81:1311–1317

[346] Mink E. Prokaintherapie nach Huneke in der Gynäkologie. 3. Aufl. Heidelberg: Haug; 1986

[347] Minty R, Kelly L, Minty A. The occasional trigger point injection. Can Rural Med. 2007; 12(4):241–244

[348] Mönch A. Die Infiltrationsanästhesie im entzündeten Gewebe. Arztl Forsch. 1947; 18:18–19, 336–345

[349] Monnier N. Physiologie und Pathophysiologie des vegetativen Nervensystems. Band 1 und 2. Stuttgart: Hippokrates; 1963

[350] Morer G. L'arthrite du genou d'origine dentaire. Chir. 1977; 103:815–818

[351] Moreu G, Téllez L, González-Jaranay M. Relationship between maternal periodontal disease and low-birth-weight pre-term infants. J Clin Periodontol. 2005; 32(6):622–627

[352] Moskowitz MA, Cutrer FM. Possible importance of neurogenic inflammation within the meninges to migraine headaches. In: Fields HL, Liebeskind JC, eds. Pharmacological Approaches to the Treatment of Chronic Pain: New Concepts and Critical Issues. Seattle, WA: IASP Press; 1994:43–49

[353] Moskowitz MA, Macfarlane R. Autonomic and neurohumoral control of the cerebral circulation. In: Mathias CJ, Bannister R, eds. Autonomic Failure. ATextbook of Clinical Disorders of the Autonomic Nervous System. 5th ed. Oxford: Oxford University Press; 2013

[354] Moulaert P, Mertens F.. Neuraltherapeutische Beeinflussung des sympathischen Systems durch intra- und perivasale Infiltration. Ärztez Naturheilverf. 1990; 3(9):231–234

[355] Mousa SA, Shaqura M, Brendl U, Al-Khrasani M, Fürst S, Schäfer M. Involvement of the peripheral sensory and sympathetic nervous system in the vascular endothelial expression of ICAM-1 and the recruitment of opioid-containing immune cells to inhibit inflammatory pain. Brain Behav Immun. 2010; 24(8):1310–1323

[356] Müller H. Neuroplastizität und Schmerzchronifizierung. Anasthesiol Intensivmed Notfallmed Schmerzther. 2000; 35(5):274–284

[357] Müller M, Marziniak M. The linear behavior of the system middle cerebral artery flow velocity and blood pressure in patients with migraine: lack of autonomic control? Stroke. 2005; 36(9):1886–1890

[358] Müller OM, Gaul C, Katsarava Z, Sure U, Diener HC, Gasser T. Beidseitige Nervus-occipitalis-Stimulation zur Behandlung des therapierefraktären chronischen Cluster-Kopfschmerzes: eigene Fallserie und Initiierung einer prospektiven Studie. Fortschr Neurol Psychiatr. 2010; 78(12):709–714

[359] Mukharinskaia VS, Antadze ZI, Devidze NV, Emchenko VT, Nodiia EI. Neurological complications in chronic suppurative odontogenic infection [in Russian] Stomatologia (Mosk). 1981; 60(4):22–23
[360] Murata Y, Kato Y, Miyamoto K, Takahashi K. Clinical study of low back pain and radicular pain pathways by using l2 spinal nerve root infiltration: a randomized, controlled, clinical trial. Spine. 2009; 34(19):2008–2013
[361] Murayama RA, Stuginski-Barbosa J, Moraes NP, Speciali JG. Toothache referred from auriculotemporal neuralgia: case report. Int Endod J. 2009; 42(9):845–851
[362] Mumenthaler M, Mattle H. Neurologie. 13. Aufl. Stuttgart: Thieme; 2012
[363] Muschaweck R. Lokalanästhesie als Heilmethode in ihrer historischen Entwicklung. Hippokrates. 1965; 36(22):873–880
[364] Muschaweck R. Novokain zur Behandlung parvenöser Infiltrationen. Med Klin. 1964; 59:160–163
[365] Nance DM, Sanders VM. Autonomic innervation and regulation of the immune system (1987–2007). Brain Behav Immun. 2007; 21(6):736–745
[366] Narouze SN. Role of sphenopalatine ganglion neuroablation in the management of cluster headache. Curr Pain Headache Rep. 2010; 14(2):160–163
[367] Nau H. Clinical pharmacokinetics in pregnancy and perinatology. I. Placental transfer and fetal side effects of local anaesthetic agents. Dev Pharmacol Ther. 1985; 8(3):149–181
[368] Nellgård P, Jönsson A, Bojö L, Tarnow P, Cassuto J. Small-bowel obstruction and the effects of lidocaine, atropine and hexamethonium on inflammation and fluid losses. Acta Anaesthesiol Scand. 1996; 40(3):287–292
[369] Neuhuber W. Autonomes Nervensystem. In: Benninghoff A, Drenckhahn D, Hrsg. Anatomie. Band 2.16. Aufl. München: Elsevier/Urban & Fischer; 2004
[370] Nickel FT, Maihöfner C. Aktuelle Erkenntnisse zur Pathophysiologie des CRPS I. Handchir Mikrochir Plast Chir. 2010; 42(1):8–14
[371] Noble MD, Romac J, Wang Y, Hsu J, Humphrey JE, Liddle RA. Local disruption of the celiac ganglion inhibits substance P release and ameliorates caerulein-induced pancreatitis in rats. Am J Physiol Gastrointest Liver Physiol. 2006; 291(1):G128–G134
[372] Nolte H, Hagelsten J. Einseitige, doppelseitige Stellatumblockade in der Therapie der Lungenembolie. Anaesthesist. 1964; 13:160–163
[373] Noma N, Kamo H, Nakaya Y, et al. Stellate ganglion block as an early intervention in sympathetically maintained headache and orofacial pain caused by temporal arteritis. Pain Med. 2013; 14(3):392–397
[374] Nonnenbruch W. Die doppelseitigen Nierenerkrankungen. Stuttgart; Enke: 1949
[375] Nonnenbruch W. Die Lehre von Ricker und Speransky und ihre Anwendung auf eine Ganzheitsbetrachtung der Nierenpathologie. Neuralmed. 1955; 3:135–150
[376] Nonnenbruch W, Gross D. Neuralmedizin - Zeitschrift für Theorie und Praxis der neuraltherapeutischen Verfahren. 1.-4. Jahrgang. 4 Bände. Stuttgart: 1953–1956
[377] Ogawa M, Zhou S, Tan AY, et al. Left stellate ganglion and vagal nerve activity and cardiac arrhythmias in ambulatory dogs with pacing-induced congestive heart failure. J Am Coll Cardiol. 2007; 50(4):335–343
[378] Ohtori S, Yamashita M, Inoue G, et al. L2 spinal nerve-block effects on acute low back pain from osteoporotic vertebral fracture. J Pain. 2009; 10(8):870–875
[379] Ostertag D, Strittmatter M, Schimrigk K. Autonome Regulationsstörung bei Migräne und Spannungskopfschmerz. Pilotstudie. Schmerz. 1998; 12(1):25–29
[380] Papathanasiou G. Molekulare Mechanismen der zentralen Modulation von Schmerz. In: Weinschenk S, Hrsg. Handbuch Neuraltherapie. München: Elsevier; 2010
[381] Paraskevas KI, Michaloglou AA, Briana DD, Samara M. Treatment of complex regional pain syndrome type I of the hand with a series of intravenous regional sympathetic blocks with guanethidine and lidocaine. Clin Rheumatol. 2006; 25(5):687–693
[382] Park HM, Kim TW, Choi HG, Yoon KB, Yoon DM. The change in regional cerebral oxygen saturation after stellate ganglion block. Korean J Pain. 2010; 23(2):142–146
[383] Paunio K, Impivaara O, Tiekso J, Mäki J. Missing teeth and ischaemic heart disease in men aged 45–64 years. Eur Heart J. 1993; 14(Suppl K):54–56
[384] Pecher S, Böttiger BW, Graf B, Hollmann MW. "Alternative" effects of local anesthetic agents [in German] Anaesthesist. 2004; 53(4):316–325
[385] Peloso P, Gross A, Haines T, Trinh K, Goldsmith CH, Burnie S; Cervical Overview Group. Medicinal and injection therapies for mechanical neck disorders. Cochrane Database Syst Rev. 2007(3):CD000319
[386] Perger F. Einführung in die blutchemischen Wirkungen des Störfelds. Erfahrungsheilkunde. 1976; 25:269–274
[387] Perger F.. Möglichkeiten zur Objektivierung der Neuraltherapie nach Huneke. Unterschiedliche Entwicklungen der Schwermetallbelastungen (Blei, Cadmium, Quecksilber) und ihre Therapie. Ärztez Naturheilverf. 1987; 10:774–794
[388] Perger F. Die therapeutischen Konsequenzen aus der Grundregulationsforschung. In: Pischinger A, Hrsg. Das System der Grundregulation. 11. Aufl. Heidelberg: Haug; 2009:135–205
[389] Peroutka SJ. Sympathetic look at genetic basis of migraine. Headache. 2002; 42(5):378–381
[390] Peroutka SJ. Migraine: a chronic sympathetic nervous system disorder. Headache. 2004; 44(1):53–64
[391] Petersen-Felix S, Curatolo M. Neuroplasticity--an important factor in acute and chronic pain. Swiss Med Wkly. 2002; 132(21–22):273–278
[392] Pfister M, Fischer L. Die Behandlung des komplexen regionalen Schmerzsyndroms der oberen Extremität mit wiederholter Lokalanästhesie des Ganglion stellatum. Praxis (Bern). 2009; 98:247–257
[393] Piepkorn U. Ganglion-stellatum-Ausschaltung bei zentral bedingten Exremitätenschmerzen. Schweiz Med Wochenschr. 1959; 80:103
[394] Pierach A, Stotz K. Die Behandlung des Lungenödems mit Novocain-Blockaden des rechten Ganglion stellatum. Dtsch Med Wochenschr. 1952; 77(44):1344–1346
[395] Pierzga JM, Frymoyer A, Kenney WL. Delayed distribution of active vasodilation and altered vascular conductance in aged skin. J Appl Physiol (1985). 2003; 94(3):1045–1053
[396] Piotrowski H. Ganzheitstherapie bei Augenkrankheiten. 2. Aufl. Heidelberg: Haug; 1982
[397] Piotrowski H. Rheumatischer Formenkreis und Neuraltherapie. Erfahrungsheilkunde. 1983; 32(7):432–436
[398] Pipolo C, Bussone G, Leone M, Lozza P, Felisati G. Sphenopalatine endoscopic ganglion block in cluster headache: a reevaluation of the procedure after 5 years. Neurol Sci. 2010; 31(Suppl 1):S197–S199
[399] Pischinger A. Die vegetativen Grundlagen des Herdgeschehens. Osterr Z Stomatol. 1963; 60:294–311
[400] Pischinger A. System der Grundregulation. Neubearb. und hrsg. von H. Heine. 11. Aufl. Stuttgart: Haug; 2009
[401] Platzer W. Pernkopf Anatomie. Atlas der topografischen und angewandten Anatomie des Menschen. 3 Bände. 3. Aufl. München: Urban 8i Schwarzenberg; 1991
[402] Pluijms W, Huygen F, Cheng J, et al. Evidence-based interventional pain medicine according to clinical diagnoses. 18. Painful diabetic polyneuropathy. Pain Pract. 2011; 11(2):191–198
[403] Pohle S.. Odontogene Störfelder als Ursache für periphere Erkrankungen: eine neuraltherapeutische Studie. Ärztez Naturheilverf. 1992; 33(7):559–564
[404] Pongratz G, Straub RH. The B cell, arthritis, and the sympathetic nervous system. Brain Behav Immun. 2010; 24(2):186–192
[405] Pongratz G, Melzer M, Straub RH. The sympathetic nervous system stimulates anti-inflammatory B cells in collagen-type II-induced arthritis. Ann Rheum Dis. 2012; 71(3):432–439
[406] Possover M, Schneider T, Henle KP. Laparoscopic therapy for endometriosis and vascular entrapment of sacral plexus. Fertil Steril. 2011; 95(2):756–758
[407] Price DD, Long S, Wilsey B, Rafii A. Analysis of peak magnitude and duration of analgesia produced by local anesthetics injected into sympathetic ganglia of complex regional pain syndrome patients. Clin J Pain. 1998; 14(3):216–226
[408] Prochno T. Tinnitus aus Sicht der Zahnmedizin. Dtsch Arztebl. 1997; 94(7):377–379
[409] Przemek H, Grüger W. Klinische Beträge zur Neuraltherapie in der Chirurgie. Zentralbl Chir. 1949; 74:599–605
[410] Puylaert M, Kapural L, van Zundert J, et al. Evidence-based interventional pain medicine according to clinical diagnoses. 26. pain in chronic pancreatitis. Pain Pract. 2011; 9:1316–1321
[411] Quan N, Banks WA. Brain-immune communication pathways. Brain Behav Immun. 2007; 21(6):727–735
[412] Raison CL, Capuron L, Miller AH. Cytokines sing the blues: inflammation and the pathogenesis of depression. Trends Immunol. 2006; 27(1):24–31
[413] Ramer MS, French GD, Bisby MA. Wallerian degeneration is required for both neuropathic pain and sympathetic sprouting into the DRG. Pain. 1997; 72(1)(-)(2):71–78
[414] Ramien M, Ruocco I, Cuello AC, St-Louis M, Ribeiro-Da-Silva A. Parasympathetic nerve fibers invade the upper dermis following sensory denervation of the rat lower lip skin. J Comp Neurol. 2004; 469(1):83–95

[415] Ramirez RJ, Ajijola OA, Zhou W, et al. A new electrocardiographic marker for sympathetic nerve stimulation: modulation of repolarization by stimulation of stellate ganglia. J Electrocardiol. 2011; 44(6):694–699
[416] Ratner EJ, Person P, Kleinman DJ, Shklar G, Socransky SS. Jawbone cavities and trigeminal and atypical facial neuralgias. Oral Surg Oral Med Oral Pathol. 1979; 48(1):3–20
[417] Ratner EJ, Langer B, Evins ML. Alveolar cavitational osteopathosis. Manifestations of an infectious process and its implication in the causation of chronic pain. J Periodontol. 1986; 57(10):593–603
[418] Ratschow M. Kritisches zur Wirkungsbreite der Neuraltherapie (Heilanästhesie). Dtsch Med Wochenschr. 1951; 76(10):308–311
[419] Räuber A, Kopsch F, Leohard H, Tillmann B, Zilles K, eds. Anatomie des Menschen. Band 3. Nervensystem, Sinnesorgane. Stuttgart: Thieme; 1987
[420] Räuber A, Kopsch F, Leohard H, Tillmann B, Zilles K, eds. Anatomie des Menschen. Band 4. Topografie der Organsysteme, Systematik der peripheren Leitungsbahnen. Stuttgart: Thieme; 1988
[421] Rausch F. Der Herderkrankungskomplex. München: Edmund Banaschewski; 1969
[422] Reischauer F. Zur Technik der lokalen Novocainbehandlung bei Lumbago-Ischias. Dtsch Med Wochenschr. 1953; 78(40):1375–1376
[423] Reischauer F. Novokaintherapie in der Chirurgie. Langenbecks Arch Klein Chir. 1961; 298:391–404
[424] Riccabona A. Das Herdteam - Praxis und Ergebnisse umfassender Herdtherapie. Rhinolaryngologischer Beitrag. Therapiewoche. 1965; 15:1292–1294
[425] Ricker C. Pathologie als Naturwissenschaft - Relationspathologie. Berlin: Springer; 1924
[426] Ritter R. Therapie der fokalen Infektion unter der Theorie von Ricker und Speransky. Zahnarztl Welt. 1950; 2:29
[427] Roberts AM, Person P, Chandran NB, Hori JM. Further observations on dental parameters of trigeminal and atypical facial neuralgias. Oral Surg Oral Med Oral Pathol. 1984; 58(2):121–129
[428] Robertson D, Biaggioni I, Burnstock G, Low PA, Paton JFR. Primer on the Autonomic Nervous System. 3rd ed. Amsterdam: Elsevier; 2012
[429] Rohen JW. Funktionelle Anatomie des Nervensystems. 5. Aufl. Stuttgart: Schattauer; 1994
[430] von Roques KR. Die Stellung der Heilanästhesie in der Pathologie und Therapie. Munch Med Wochenschr. 1940; 87:34–37
[431] von Roques KR. Die Behandlung schwerer Tonsillenerkrankungen mittels der Stellatumanästhesie. Munch Med Wochenschr. 1959; 92:135
[432] Roslawski A. Role of infectious foci in ethiopathogenesis of chronic rheumatoid arthritis and ankylosing spondylitis [in Polish] Wiad Lek. 1972; 25(3):247–250
[433] Rost A. Objektivierung der Neuraltherapie nach Huneke durch die Thermografie. In: Dosch P, Hrsg. Neuraltherapie nach Huneke - Freudenstädter Vorträge 1986. Band 11. Heidelberg: Haug; 1987
[434] Roudenok V, Gutjar L, Antipova V, Rogov Y. Expression of vasoactive intestinal polypeptide and calcitonin gene-related peptide in human stellate ganglia after acute myocardial infarction. Ann Anat. 2001; 183(4):341–344
[435] Ruocco I, Cuello AC, Parent A, Ribeiro-da-Silva A. Skin blood vessels are simultaneously innervated by sensory, sympathetic, and parasympathetic fibers. J Comp Neurol. 2002; 448(4):323–336
[436] Sakaguchi M, Kuroda Y, Hirose M. The antiproliferative effect of lidocaine on human tongue cancer cells with inhibition of the activity of epidermal growth factor receptor. Anesth Analg. 2006; 102(4):1103–1107
[437] Samandari F. Funktionelle Anatomie der Hirnnerven und des vegetativen Nervensystems. 2. Aufl. Berlin: De Gruyter; 1993
[438] Sanders M, Zuurmond WW. Efficacy of sphenopalatine ganglion blockade in 66 patients suffering from cluster headache: a 12- to 70-month follow-up evaluation. J Neurosurg. 1997; 87(6):876–880
[439] Sanya EO, Brown CM, von Wilmowsky C, Neundörfer B, Hilz MJ. Impairment of parasympathetic baroreflex responses in migraine patients. Acta Neurol Scand. 2005; 111(2):102–107
[440] Sauer R. Neuraltherapie nach Huneke in der ärztlichen Praxis[Dissertation]. Düsseldorf: Universität Düsseldorf; 1988
[441] Schäfer M, . Physiology and pathophysiology of pain [in German]. Ther Umsch. 1999; 56(8):426–430
[442] Schattschneider J, Binder A, Siebrecht D, Wasner G, Baron R. Complex regional pain syndromes: the influence of cutaneous and deep somatic sympathetic innervation on pain. Clin J Pain. 2006; 22(3):240–244
[443] Schattschneider J, Wasner G, Binder A, Siebrecht D, Baron R. Das Symptom sympathisch unterhaltener Schmerz. Schmerz. 2003; 17(5):317–324
[444] Schiffter R. Neurologie des vegetativen Systems. Berlin: Springer; 1985
[445] Schimek JJ. Pseudoradikuläre Syndrome. In: Seithel R, Hrsg. Neuraltherapie 2. Stuttgart: Hippokrates; 1984
[446] Schleich CL. Schmerzlose Operationen. San Bernadino, CA: Ulan Press; 2012
[447] Schmidt RF. Grundriss der Neurophysiologie. 6. Aufl. Berlin: Springer; 1987
[448] Schmidt M, Hennke T, Knöchel M, et al. Can chronic irritations of the trigeminal nerve cause musculoskeletal disorders? Forsch Komplement Med. 2010; 17(3):149–153
[449] Schroeder HE. Orale Strukturbiologie. Stuttgart: Thieme; 2000
[450] Schuh E. Residual osteitis in the edentulous jaw as a focus possibility [in German] Therapiewoche. 1965; 15(23):1246–1249
[451] Schupp W. Gesichtsschmerz aus Sicht der Kieferorthopädie. Man Med. 2001; 39(6):327–336
[452] Schupp W. Kraniomandibulare Dysfunktionen und deren periphere Folgen. Eine Literaturübersicht. Man Med. 2005; 43(1):29–33
[453] Schwartz PJ. The rationale and the role of left stellectomy for the prevention of malignant arrhythmias. Ann N Y Acad Sci. 1984; 427:199–221
[454] Sciubba JJ. Neuralgia-inducing cavitational osteonecrosis: a status report. Oral Dis. 2009; 15(5):309–312
[455] Segal SS. Regulation of blood flow in the microcirculation. Microcirculation. 2005; 12(1):33–45
[456] Seithel R. Neuraltherapie 2. Stuttgart: Hippokrates; 1984
[457] Shen MJ, Shinohara T, Park HW, et al. Continuous low-level vagus nerve stimulation reduces stellate ganglion nerve activity and paroxysmal atrial tachyarrhythmias in ambulatory canines. Circulation. 2011; 123(20):2204–2212
[458] Shimizu K, Toyota Y, Koh T, Ishikawa M, Hirose Y. [A case of rheumatoid arthritis caused by focal infection from periodontal tissue [in Japanese; author's transl] Josai Shika Daigaku Kiyo. 1977; 6(6):421–424
[459] Siegen H. Theorie und Praxis der Neuraltherapie mit Impletol. Köln: Staufen; 1951
[460] Siegen H. Grundlagen der Neuraltherapie mit Impletol. Hippokrates. 1961; 32:348–357
[461] Siegen H. Das nervale Störfeld. In: Voss HF, Hrsg. Deshalb Neuraltherapie. Uelzen: ML-Verlag; 1968
[462] Siegen H. Die immunologische Ausgleichung von Spender- und Empfängerorganismus, eine klassisch-neuroregulative Aufgabe. In: Dosch P, Hrsg. Neuraltherapie nach Huneke - Freudenstädter Vorträge 1974. Band 2. Heidelberg: Haug; 1975
[463] Siegert H. Neuraltherapie nach Dr. Huneke in der Veterinärmedizin. Med Heute. 1963; 10:123–126
[464] Siegmund H. Zur Pathogenese und Pathologie von örtlichen Kälteschäden. Munch Med Wochenschr. 1942; 89:827
[465] Song JG, Hwang GS, Lee EH, et al. Effects of bilateral stellate ganglion block on autonomic cardiovascular regulation. Circ J. 2009; 73(10):1909–1913
[466] Soyka D. Kopfschmerz. 2. Aufl. Weinheim: Edition Medizin; 1989
[467] Speransky AD. Grundlage einer Theorie der Medizin. Berlin: Sänger; 1950
[468] Spernol R, Riss P. Urodynamic evaluation of the effect of neural therapy in motor and sensory urgency [in German] Geburtshilfe Frauenheilkd. 1982; 42(7):527–529
[469] Spiess G. Die Heilwirkung der Anästhetika. Ärztebl Inn Med. 1902; 23:22
[470] Spiess G. Die Bedeutung der Anästhesie in der Entzündungstheorie. Munch Med Wochenschr. 1906; 53:345–351, 967
[471] Spiess G. Die Bedeutung der Anästhesie in der Entzündungstherapie und ihre Nutzanwendung speziell bei der Behandlung der Kehlkopftuberkulose. Arch Laryngol. 1992; 21:120–125
[472] Squire LR, Berg D, Bloom FE, du Lac S, Ghosh A, Spitzer NC. Fundamental Neuroscience. 4th ed. Amsterdam: Academic Press; 2013
[473] Stacher A. Zur Wirkung der Herde auf den Gesamtorganismus. Osterr Z Stomatol. 1966; 63(8):294–303
[474] Stacher A. Über das Huneke-(Sekunden-)Phänomen und seine Objektivierung. In: Voss HF, Hrsg. Deshalb Neuraltherapie. Uelzen: ML-Verlag; 1968
[475] Stacher A, Bergsmann O. Grundlagen für eine integrative Ganzheitsmedizin. Wien: Facultas; 1993
[476] Stettbacher MA, Stettbacher A, Kammermann D. Ganzheitliche Zahnmedizin. Bulletin. 1997; 4:1–4
[477] Stoehr PH. Beobachtungen und Reflexionen zur pathologischen Histologie des vegetativen Nervensystems. Arztl Wochensch. 1946–1947; 1(1–2):8–13
[478] Stoehr PH. Bemerkung über die Endigungsweise des vegetativen Nervensystems. Acta Neuroveg (Wien). 1959; 1:74
[479] Straub RH. Autoimmune disease and innervation. Brain Behav Immun. 2007; 21(5):528–534
[480] Straub RH, Härle P. Stress, hormones, and neuronal signals in the pathophysiology of rheumatoid arthritis. The negative impact on chronic inflammation [in German] Med Klin (Munich). 2005; 100(12):794–803

[481] Straub RH, Stebner K, Härle P, Kees F, Falk W, Schölmerich J. Key role of the sympathetic microenvironment for the interplay of tumour necrosis factor and interleukin 6 in normal but not in inflamed mouse colon mucosa. Gut. 2005; 54(8):1098–1106

[482] Straub RH, Wiest R, Strauch UG, Härle P, Schölmerich J. The role of the sympathetic nervous system in intestinal inflammation. Gut. 2006; 55(11):1640–1649

[483] Straube A, May A, Kropp P, et al. Therapie primärer chronischer Kopfschmerzen: Chronische Migräne, chronischer Kopfschmerz vom Spannungstyp und andere chronische tägliche Kopfschmerzen. Schmerz. 2008; 22(5):531–534, 536–540, 542–543

[484] Strittmatter M, Grauer MT, Fischer C, et al. Autonomic nervous system and neuroendocrine changes in patients with idiopathic trigeminal neuralgia. Cephalalgia. 1996; 16(7):476–480

[485] Struzak-Wysokińska M. Peripheral paralysis of the facial nerve caused by peridental foci [in Polish] Czas Stomatol. 1967; 20(3):283–288

[486] Stüben J. Experimentelle Untersuchungen über die bakteriziden und bakteriostatischen Eigenschaften einiger Lokalanästhetika. Dtsch Zahnarztl Z. 1954; 9(11):617–628

[487] Sudeck P. Die sogenannte akute Knochenatrophie als Entzündungsvorgang. Chirurg. 1942; 15:449–457

[488] Sunder-Plassmann P. Das Leriche-Syndrom. Neuralmedizin. 1955; 3:10–15

[489] Suzuki N, Hardebo JE. Anatomical basis for a parasympathetic and sensory innervation of the intracranial segment of the internal carotid artery in man. Possible implication for vascular headache. J Neurol Sci. 1991; 104(1):19–31

[490] Suzuki N, Hardebo JE. The pathway of parasympathetic nerve fibers to cerebral vessels from the otic ganglion in the rat. J Auton Nerv Syst. 1991; 36(1):39–46

[491] Suzuki N, Hardebo JE. The cerebrovascular parasympathetic innervation. Cerebrovasc Brain Metab Rev. 1993; 5(1):33–46

[492] Tada M, Imazeki F, Fukai K, et al. Procaine inhibits the proliferation and DNA methylation in human hepatoma cells. Hepatol Int. 2007; 1(3):355–364

[493] Tada M, Yokosuka O, Fukai K, et al. Procaine functions as a demethylating agent and has growth-inhibitory effects on human hepatoma cell lines. Hepatol. 2004:52–54

[494] Tan Z, Dohi S, Ohguchi K, Nakashima S, Nozawa Y. Local anesthetics inhibit muscarinic receptor-mediated activation of extracellular signal-regulated kinases in rat pheochromocytoma PC12 cells. Anesthesiology. 1999; 91(4):1014–1024

[495] Tassarotti B. A case of spheno-palatine ganglionic syndrome of dental origin [in Italian] Rass Int Stomatol Prat. 1969; 20(5):307–313

[496] Teepker M, Schepelmann K. Atiologie und Diagnostik von Kopf- und Gesichtsschmerzen aus neurologischer Sicht. HNO. 2007; 55(7):524–531

[497] Thyaga Rajan S, Madden KS, Teruya B, Stevens SY, Felten DL, Bellinger DL. Age-associated alterations in sympathetic noradrenergic innervation of primary and secondary lymphoid organs in female Fischer 344 rats. J Neuroimmunol. 2011; 233(1–2):54–64

[498] Tilscher H, Eder M. Lehrbuch der Reflextherapie. 2. Aufl. Stuttgart: Hippokrates; 1989

[499] Tilscher H, Eder M. Schmerzsyndrome der Wirbelsäule. 5. Aufl. Stuttgart: Hippokrates; 1991

[500] Tilscher H, Eder M. Infiltrationstherapie - Therapeutische Lokalanästhesie. 4. Aufl. Wien: Maudrich; 2007

[501] Tran KM, Frank SM, Raja SN, El-Rahmany HK, Kim LJ, Vu B. Lumbar sympathetic block for sympathetically maintained pain: changes in cutaneous temperatures and pain perception. Anesth Analg . 2000; 90(6):1396–1401

[502] Travell JG, Simons DG. Myofascial Pain and Dysfunction. Vols. 1 and 2. 2nd ed. Baltimore, MD: Williams & Wilkins; 1998

[503] Treede RD, Magerl W. Zentrale nozizeptive Neurone und Bahnen. In: Egle UT, Hoffmann SO, Lehmann KA, Nix WA, Hrsg. Handbuch chronischer Schmerz. Grundlagen, Pathogenese und Therapie aus biopsychosozialer Sicht. Stuttgart: Schattauer; 2003:34–44

[504] Troeltzsch M, Troeltzsch M, Cronin RJ, Brodine AH, Frankenberger R, Messlinger K. Prevalence and association of headaches, temporomandibular joint disorders, and occlusal interferences. J Prosthet Dent. 2011; 105(6):410–417

[505] Tronnier V, Rasche D. Subkutane periphere Stimulation des N. occipitalis major zur Behandlung chronischer Kopfschmerzsyndrome. Schmerz. 2010; 24(5):441–448

[506] Truijen J, van Lieshout JJ. Parasympathetic control of blood flow to the activated human brain. Exp Physiol. 2010; 95(10):980–981

[507] Turton EP, Kent PJ, Kester RC. The aetiology of Raynaud's phenomenon. Cardiovasc Surg. 1998; 6(5):431–440

[508] Umbach W. Die Behandlung mit Lokalanästhetika in der Neurochirugie und Neurologie. In: Gross D, Hrsg. Therapie mit Lokalanästhetika -Funktionsstörungen des oberen Verdauungstrakts und ihre Behandlung. Stuttgart: Hippokrates; 1996:209–224

[509] Urbani G, Ferronato G, Bertele GP. Trigeminal neuralgia with chronic infection due to the presence of a large root fragment in the mandibular canal [in Italian] G Stomatol Ortognatodonzia. 1982; 1(2):17–20

[510] Usubiaga JE, La Iuppa M, Moya F, Wikinski JA, Velazco R. Passage of procaine hydrochloride and para-aminobenzoic acid across the human placenta. Am J Obstet Gynecol. 1968; 100(7):918–923

[511] V, an Boxern K, Cheng J, Patijn J, et al. 11. Lumbosacral ra dicular pain. Pain Pract. 2010; 10(4):339–358

[512] van der Laan L, Goris RJ. Sudeck-Syndrom. Hatte Sudeck recht? Unfallchirurg. 1997; 100(2):90–99

[513] van der Zypen E. Elektronenmikroskopische Befunde an der Endausbreitung des vegetativen Nervensystems und ihre Deutung. Acta Anat (Basel). 1967; 67:431–515

[514] van der Zypen E. Anatomie des sympathischen Nervensystems. Vasa. 1977; 6(2):115–123

[515] van Dongen R, Cohen SP, van Kleef M, Mekhail N, Huygen F. 22. Traumatic plexus lesion. Pain Pract. 2011; 11(4):414–420

[516] van Eerd M, Patijn J, Lataster A, et al. 5. Cervical facet pain. Pain Pract. 2010; 10(2):113–123

[517] Vanelderen P, Lataster A, Levy R, Mekhail N, van Kleef M, Van Zundert J. 8. Occipital neuralgia. Pain Pract. 2010; 10(2):137–144

[518] van Eijs F, Stanton-Hicks M, Van Zundert J, et al. Evidence-based interventional pain medicine according to clinical diagnoses. 16. Complex regional pain syndrome. Pain Pract. 2011; 11(1):70–87

[519] van Kleef M, Lataster A, Narouze S, Mekhail N, Geurts JW, van Zundert J. Evidence-based interventional pain medicine according to clinical diagnoses. 2. Cluster headache. Pain Pract. 2009; 9(6):435–442

[520] van Kleef M, Staats P, Mekhail N, et al. Evidence-based interventional pain medicine according to clinical diagnoses. 24. Chronic refractory angina pectoris. Pain Pract. 2011; 11(4):65–72

[521] van Kleef M, Stolker RJ, Lataster A, Geurts J, Benzon HT, Mekhail N. 10. Thoracic pain. Pain Pract. 2010; 10(4):327–338

[522] van Kleef M, Vanelderen P, Cohen SP, et al. 12. Pain originating from the lumbar facet joints. Pain Pract. 2010; 10(5):459–469

[523] van Kleef M, van Genderen WE, Narouze S, et al; World Institute of Medicine. 1. Trigeminal neuralgia. Pain Pract. 2009; 9(4):252–259

[524] van Suijlekom H, van Zundert J, Narouze S, et al. 6. Cervicogenic headache. Pain Pract. 2010; 10(2):124–130

[525] van Wijck AJ, Wallace M, Mekhail N, van Kleef M. Evidence-based interventional pain medicine according to clinical diagnoses. 17. Herpes zoster and post-herpetic neuralgia. Pain Pract. 2011; 11(1):88–97

[526] van Zundert J, Huntoon M, Patijn J, et al. 4. Cervical radicular pain. Pain Pract. 2010; 10(1):1–17

[527] Vaseghi M, Zhou W, Shi J, et al. Sympathetic innervation of the anterior left ventricular wall by the right and left stellate ganglia. Heart Rhythm. 2012; 9(8):1303–1309

[528] Villar-Garea A, Fraga MF, Espada J, Esteller M. Procaine is a DNA-demethylating agent with growth-inhibitory effects in human cancer cells. Cancer Res. 2003; 63(16):4984–4989

[529] Vissers KC, Besse K, Wagemans M, et al. 23. Pain in patients with cancer. Pain Pract. 2011; 5:453–475

[530] Voll R. Wechselbezeichnungen von Odontomen zu Organ- und Gewebssystemen. In: Dosch P, Hrsg. Neuraltherapie nach Huneke - Freudenstädter Vorträge 1974. Band 2. Heidelberg: Haug; 1975

[531] Voss HF. Was ist Neuraltherapie? Phys Diät Ther. 1963; 4(6):92–96

[532] Voss HF. Neuraltherapie und Schmerz. Erfahrungsheilkunde. 1966; 15(5):129–135

[533] Vosschulte K. Grundlagen der Schmerzbekämpfung durch Sympathikusausschaltung. Berlin: Urban & Schwarzenberg; 1949

[534] Wakai K, Ohtori S, Yamashita M, et al. Primary sensory neurons with dichotomizing axons projecting to the facet joint and the low back muscle in rats. J Orthop Sci. 2010; 15(3):402–406

[535] Wallace DE. Chronic periodontitis and a chronic swelling of the right index finger. J N Z Soc Periodontol. 1991; 71(71):15

[536] Wander R.. Blockierungsmuster bei Störfeldern im Nasen-Rachen-Raum. Ärztez Naturheilverf. 1991; 32:145–147

[537] Wander R, Ludin SM. Kiefergelenk und kraniomandibuläre Dysfunktion. In: Fischer L, Peuker ET, Hrsg. Lehrbuch Integrative Schmerztherapie. Stuttgart: Haug; 2011

[538] Watkins LR, Maier SF. Beyond neurons: evidence that immune and glial cells contribute to pathological pain states. Physiol Rev. 2002; 82(4):981–1011

[539] Weber M, Birklein F, Neundörfer B, Schmelz M. Facilitated neurogenic inflammation in complex regional pain syndrome. Pain. 2001; 91(3):251–257

[540] Weihe E, Schütz B, Hartschuh W, Anlauf M, Schäfer MK, Eiden LE. Coexpression of cholinergic and noradrenergic phenotypes in human and nonhuman autonomic nervous system. J Comp Neurol. 2005; 492(3):370–379

[541] Weinschenk S, ed. Handbuch Neuraltherapie. München: Elsevier/Urban & Fischer; 2010

[542] Werkmeister H. Neuraltherapie und Strahlenbehandlung Krebskranker. In: Dosch P, Hrsg. Neuraltherapie nach Huneke - Freudenstädter Vorträge 1974. Band 2. Heidelberg: Haug; 1975

[543] Werthman K. Neuraltherapie in meiner Kinderpraxis. In: Dosch P, Hrsg. Neuraltherapie nach Huneke - Freudenstädter Vorträge 1980. Band 7. Heidelberg: Haug; 1981

[544] Westrum LE, Canfield RC, Black RG. Transganglionic degeneration in the spinal trigeminal nucleus following removal of tooth pulps in adult cats. Brain Res. 1976; 101(1):137–140

[545] Wiener N. Kybernetik oder Regelung und Nachrichtenübertragung in Lebewesen und in der Maschine. Düsseldorf: Econ; 1992

[546] Wildner M. Sakrale epidurale Injektion. In: Weinschenk S, Hrsg. Handbuch Neuraltherapie. München: Elsevier. Urban & Fischer; 2010

[547] Wilson-Pauwels L, Stewart PA, Akesson EJ. Autonomic nerves. Hamilton: BCBecker Inc; 1997

[548] Windstosser K. Das dentale Herdgeschehen in biologisch-medizinischer Sicht. Hippokrates . 1959; 30(3):129–134

[549] Wischnewski A. Die Technik der Novokainblockade des Sympathikus im Lendenbereich. Arch Biol Wiss. 1933; 4:519–520

[550] Wischnewski A. Der Novocainblock als eine Methode der Einwirkung auf die Gewebetrophik. Zentralbl Chir. 1935; 62:735–746

[551] Wolff HD. Neurophysiologische Aspekte des Bewegungssystems. 3. Aufl. Berlin: Springer; 1996

[552] Woolf CJ, Salter MW. Neuronal plasticity: increasing the gain in pain. Science. 2000; 288(5472):1765–1769

[553] Xie YF, Zhang S, Chiang CY, Hu JW, Dostrovsky JO, Sessle BJ. Involvement of glia in central sensitization in trigeminal subnucleus caudalis (medullary dorsal horn). Brain Behav Immun. 2007; 21(5):634–641

[554] Young WB. Blocking the greater occipital nerve: utility in headache management. Curr Pain Headache Rep. 2010; 14(5):404–408

[555] Zhang JM, Li H, Munir MA. Decreasing sympathetic sprouting in pathologic sensory ganglia: a new mechanism for treating neuropathic pain using lidocaine. Pain. 2004; 109(1)(–)(2):143–149

[556] Zhang Y, Popovic ZB, Bibevski S, et al. Chronic vagus nerve stimulation improves autonomic control and attenuates systemic inflammation and heart failure progression in a canine high-rate pacing model. Circ Heart Fail. 2009; 2(6):692–699

[557] Zhou J, Scherlag BJ, Niu G, et al. Anatomy and physiology of the right interganglionic nerve: implications for the pathophysiology of inappropriate sinus tachycardia. J Cardiovasc Electrophysiol . 2008; 19(9):971–976

[558] Zhu BS, Blessing WW, Gibbins IL. Parasympathetic innervation of cephalic arteries in rabbits: comparison with sympathetic and sensory innervation. J Comp Neurol. 1997; 389(3):484–495

[559] Zieglgänsberger W. Central control of nociception. In: Mountcastle VB, Bloom FE, Geiger SR, eds. Handbook of Physiology. Section 1: The Nervous System IV. Baltimore, MD: Williams & Wilkins; 1986

[560] Zieglgänsberger W. Chronischer Schmerz: Physiologie, Pathophysiologie und Pharmakologie. Ganzheitsmed. 2002; 15(4):21–25

[561] Zieglgänsberger W. Neuronale Plastizität, Schmerzgedächtnis und chronischer Schmerz. In: Weinschenk S, Hrsg. Handbuch Neuraltherapie. München: Elsevier, Urban & Fischer; 2010

[562] Zimmermann M. Die Neuraltherapie im Licht neuerer Erkenntnisse der neurobiologischen Forschung. In: Seithel R. Neuraltherapie. Band 2. Stuttgart: Hippokrates; 1984

[563] Zimmermann M. Neuronale Mechanismen der Schmerzchronifizierung. Orthopäde. 2004; 33(5):515–524

[564] Zipf HF. Die Endoanästhesie, ein pharmakologischer Weg zur Ausschaltung innerer sensibler Rezeptoren. Dtsch Med Wochenschr. 1953; 78:1787–1792

[565] Zipf HF. Lokalanaesthetica im Lichte ihrer Allgemeinwirkungen. Arzneimittelforschung. 1957; 7(9):529–543

[566] Zipf HF. Lokalanästhetika und Nervensystem. In: Gross D, Hrsg. Therapie mit Lokalanästhetika - Funktionsstörungen des oberen Verdauungstrakts und ihre Behandlung. Therapie über das Nervensystem. Band 5. Stuttgart: Hippokrates; 1964

[567] Zipf HF. Die Allgemeinwirkungen der Lokalanästhetika. In: Killian H, Hrsg. Lokalanästhesie und Lokalanästhetika. Stuttgart: Thieme; 1973

[568] Zohmann A. Objektivierbarkeit der Neuraltherapie durch ihre Anwendung am Tier. Erfahrungsheilkunde. 1991; 40(3):150–153

[569] Zohmann A. Grundlagen und Anwendung der Neuraltherapie in Diagnostik und Behandlung. Schweiz Arch Tierheilkd. 1997; 139(3):117–125

[570] Zohmann A, Kasper M. Neuraltherapie in der Veterinärmedizin. Hannover: Schlütersche; 1994

Index

U

V

W

X